# DATA for BIOCHEMICAL RESEARCH

**REX M.C. DAWSON**
AFRC Institute of Animal Physiology, Babraham, Cambridge

**DAPHNE C. ELLIOTT**
Flinders University, Bedford Park, South Australia

**WILLIAM H. ELLIOTT**
University of Adelaide, South Australia

**KENNETH M. JONES**
University of Leicester

*Third Edition*

CLARENDON PRESS · OXFORD

Oxford University Press, Walton Street, Oxford OX2 6DP

Oxford New York Toronto
Delhi Bombay Calcutta Madras Karachi
Petaling Jaya Singapore Hong Kong Tokyo
Nairobi Dar es Salaam Cape Town
Melbourne Auckland

and associated companies in
Berlin Ibadan

Oxford is a trade mark of Oxford University Press

Published in the United States
by Oxford University Press, New York

First edition 1959
Second edition 1969
Third edition 1986
First published in paperback 1989
Reprinted 1990

British Library Cataloguing in Publication Data
Data for biochemical research.—3rd ed.
1. Biological chemistry—Technique
I. Dawson, R. M. C.
574.19'2'028   QP519.7
ISBN 0–19–855358–7
ISBN 0–19–855299–8 (pbk)

Library of Congress Cataloging in Publication Data
Main entry under title:
Data for biochemical research.
Includes bibliographies and index.
1. Biological chemistry—Handbooks, manuals, etc.
I. Dawson, R. M. C. (Rex Malcolm Chaplin)
QP520.D37 1985   574.19'2'021   85–4239
ISBN 0–19–855358–7
ISBN 0–19–855299–8 (pbk)

Printed in Great Britain by
Richard Clay Ltd
Bungay, Suffolk

# Preface

In this third edition, we again aim to supply information needed by biochemists in a form sufficiently concise to be kept in the laboratory. No attempt is made to be comprehensive. Material has been selected under the guiding principle that it should be of potential use to a reasonably large number of readers. We try, in fact, to occupy the central ground of possible interest to all biochemists. This excludes much material of use only to specialists in individual areas, but they will have more comprehensive sources of information in their own fields. Between the extremes of obvious material for inclusion, such as buffers, and for exclusion, such as rarely encountered metabolites, there is a large grey area in which subjective decisions have had to be made. Such decisions cannot suit everyone or every situation, but we have been encouraged by the sustained interest in, and demand for, the previous edition to believe that this policy is supplying a real need in the laboratory.

Much has been deleted from earlier editions to be replaced by new material of current importance to biochemistry and molecular biology. With the increase in commercial availability of biochemicals, references to preparations have been omitted as a routine; with the development of sophisticated separative technologies there is less need for references to estimations of many compounds. References are now included in the general remarks only where they appear to be of use. Alphabetical listing has been retained but functional groupings of compounds has been emphasized so that a reader can see what is available as well as find individual compounds.

Much of the revision has been done by the authors with help from people too numerous to mention individually. Some sections however have been largely revised by specialists and these are listed overleaf. It is emphasized that the final selection and presentation of material has always been made by the authors who must therefore bear the responsibility for omissions and deficiencies. Names no longer appear at the head of sections because with revisions and reorganizations it is difficult to associate any one name with a section. Acknowledgement must be made to contributors to earlier editions on whose work the current volume is based.

*Babraham, Adelaide, Bedford Park, and Leicester*       R.M.C.D.  W.H.E.
July 1984       D.C.E.  K.M.J.

# Acknowledgements

We gratefully acknowledge the help and assistance of the people listed below in the preparation of the sections listed:

9     Steroids: Dr R. Seamark, Queen Elizabeth Hospital, University of Adelaide.

10    Porphyrins and related compounds: Dr J. Barratt, Division of Plant Industry, CSIRO, Canberra.

16B   Reagents for protein modification: Dr N.M.C. Kaye, Amersham International plc (Cardiff Laboratories), Whitchurch, Cardiff.

17    Stability constants for metal complexes: Dr D. Perrin, John Curtin School of Medical Research, Australian National University, Canberra.

19    Gel electrophoresis: Dr R. Symons, Department of Biochemistry, University of Adelaide.

# Contents

# Notes on the use of this book

**I. Tables of biochemical compounds and comprehensive index of compounds**

1. The tables of biochemical compounds are arranged in sections according to the type of compound. In some instances ambiguity existed as to the correct section for a particular compound and here arbitrary decisions have been made. Few cross-references between sections or to synonyms have been included, but **there is a comprehensive index of all compounds and of their commonly used synonyms (p. 561). It is strongly advised that this index be used to determine whether a compound is included in the tables and to ascertain its location.**

2. *Melting-points and boiling-points*

The value given is that at a pressure of 760 mm of mercury, unless otherwise stated.

3. *Optical rotations*

The optical activity quoted is the specific rotation, generally for the sodium D line, with the temperature of the measurement indicated by a superscript. Where other wavelengths have been employed, the wavelength is given in Å as a subscript. Where given, the concentration of the substance is in g/100 ml.

4. *Solubility*

Solubilities are given as grams of solute dissolving in 100 ml of solvent. The temperatures at which solubility data were determined are given as superscripts. Where there is no temperature indicated, the data are for room temperature, that is in the range $15-25\,^{\circ}C$.

**II. References**

In general, references are intended to enable readers to find the relevant literature on methods and not necessarily to give credit to the main workers in the field. References are usually not given to methods of preparation of compounds which can be readily obtained commercially at a reasonable price. An abbreviated system of references has been used throughout the volume. Authors of individual papers have been omitted and for those journals and books which are mentioned most frequently the titles have been specially abbreviated as follows:

| | |
|---|---|
| *ABB* | *Archives of Biochemistry and Biophysics.* |
| *Ann.* | *Liebig's Annalen der Chemie.* |
| *ARB* | *Annual Review of Biochemistry.* |
| *BBA* | *Biochimica et Biophysica Acta.* |
| *BBRC* | *Biochemical and Biophysical Research Communications.* |
| *Ber.* | *Chemische Berichte* (prior to 1947 *Berichte der deutschen chemischen Gesellschaft*). |
| *Biochem. Preps.* | *Biochemical Preparations* (Wiley & Sons Inc., New York). |
| *BJ* | *Biochemical Journal.* |
| *BZ* | *Biochemische Zeitschrift.* |
| *EJB* | *European Journal of Biochemistry.* |
| *JACS* | *Journal of the American Chemical Society.* |
| *JBC* | *Journal of Biological Chemistry.* |

| | |
|---|---|
| *JCS* | *Journal of the Chemical Society.* |
| *JMB* | *Journal of Molecular Biology.* |
| *Meth. Biochem. Anal.* | *Methods of Biochemical Analysis,* ed. D. Glick (Wiley-Interscience Inc., N.Y.).* |
| *Meth. Enzymol.* | *Methods in Enzymology,* ed. S.P. Colowick and N.O. Kaplan (Academic Press).* |
| *PNARMB* | *Progress in Nucleic Acid Research and Molecular Biology.* |
| *PNAS* | *Proceedings of The National Academy of Sciences.* |
| *PSEBM* | *Proceedings of the Society for Experimental Biology and Medicine.* |
| *TIBS* | *Trends in Biochemical Sciences.* |
| *ZPC* | *Hoppe-Seyler's Zeitschrift für physiologische Chemie.* |

For other journals the conventional system of abbreviation has been adopted. In certain sections, works of reference which have been quoted extensively in that section only have been abbreviated and a note to this effect is included in the preamble to the section.

# Abbreviations

$[\alpha]_D^t$    specific optical rotation for sodium D line at temperature $t$

abs.    absolute, absorbance
acet.    acetone
alk.    alkaline
amorph.    amorphous
anhyd.    anhydrous
approx.    approximately
aq.    aqueous
benz.    benzene
B.p.    boiling-point
c    concentration (g/100 ml)
*ca.*    circa = approximately
cf.    compare
ch.    chapter
c.n.s.    central nervous system
col.    colourless
comp.    competitive(ly)
compd.    compound
conc.    concentrated, concentration
cryst.    crystals, crystalline, crystallization
d.    with decomposition (after M.p. or B.p.), density
decomp.    decomposition point, decomposes
deliq.    deliquescent
deriv.    derivative
diam.    diameter
dil.    dilute
dimorph.    dimorphic
DMF    dimethylformamide
DMSO    dimethylsulphoxide
ed.    editor, edition
efflor.    efflorescent
equiv.    equivalent
esp.    especially
EST.    estimation, estimated
eth.    diethyl ether
evap.    evaporates, evaporation
exptl.    experimental
extr.    extracted
F.p.    freezing-point
fluor.    fluorescence
A    excitation maximum
F    fluorescence maximum
g.i.t.    gastro-intestinal tract
gl. acetic    glacial acetic acid
GLC    gas-liquid chromatography

gp.    group
hex.    hexagonal, hexane
hygr.    hygroscopic
i.    insoluble
IDENT.    identification
i.m.    intramuscular
incl.    including
inorg.    inorganic
insol.    insoluble
i.p.    intraperitoneal
i.r.    infra-red
ISOL.    isolation, isolated
i.v.    intravenous
liq.    liquid
lt.    light
max.    maximum
min.    minimum, minute
misc.    miscible
monocl.    monoclinic
M.p.    melting-point
M.wt.    molecular weight
no.    number
opt.    optimum
org.    organic
orthorh.    orthorhombic
p., pp.    page, pages
path.    pathological
pet. eth.    petroleum ether
ppt.    precipitate
pptd.    precipitated
pract.    practically
prep.    prepared, preparation
PREP.    preparation
prism.    prismatic
pt.    point
PURIF.    purification
pyr.    pyridine
q.v.    quod vide = which see (in cross references)
recryst.    recrystallize
rect.    rectangular
ref.    reference
rel.    relative(ly)
resp.    respectively
rh.    rhombic
R.T.    room temperature
s.    soluble
sat., satd.    saturated
s.c.    subcutaneous
sens.    sensitivity

| s.g. | specific gravity | tr. | trace |
| sh | shoulder | tricl. | triclinic |
| sl. | slight, slightly | u.v. | ultra-violet |
| sl. s. | slightly soluble | v. | very |
| sol. | soluble, solubility | veg. | vegetable |
| soln. | solution | visc. | viscous |
| solv. | solvent(s) | vol. | volume |
| sp. | sparingly, species | v.s. | very soluble |
| sp. gr. | specific gravity | v. sl. s. | very slightly soluble |
| sp. s. | sparingly soluble | v/v | volume for volume |
| suppl. | supplement | wh. | white |
| SYN. | synthesis | w/v | weight for volume |
| temp. | temperature | w/w | weight for weight |
| TLC | thin-layer chromatography | yel. | yellow |
| tol. | toluene | $\infty$ | completely miscible |

# 1 Amino acids, amines, amides, peptides, and their derivatives

### Optically active compounds

For compounds exhibiting optical isomerism, information about the optical isomers (enantiomers) and the racemic (DL-) mixture, and, where they exist, about allo- and *meso*-isomers, has been included in a single entry. In most such cases, the properties of only one optical isomer, usually the one which is most abundant in natural sources, have been given in detail. The properties of the other isomer are the same *except* that the sign of optical rotation is reversed.

### Peptides

A few peptides possessing physiological activity are included in this section. Peptides used as substrates for peptidase assay are included in the Section on Artificial and natural substrates (p. 360).

### General references

J. P. Greenstein and M. Winitz, *Chemistry of the amino acids*, 3 volumes, Wiley (1961).

A. Meister, *Biochemistry of the amino acids*, 2 volumes, Academic Press (1965).

### Nomenclature

Rules of nomenclature for α-amino acids are given in *BJ* **149**, 1 (1975) and *Biochem.* **14**, 449 (1975).

Symbols for amino acid derivatives and peptides: *BJ* **126**, 773 (1972); *EJB* **27**, 201 (1972); *JBC* **247**, 977 (1972).

### p$K_a$ values

Most of the values quoted are from D. D. Perrin, *Dissociation constants of organic bases in aqueous solution*, Butterworth (1965) and D. D. Perrin, *Dissociation constants of organic bases in aqueous solution: Supplement 1972*, Butterworth (1972).

# 1 Amino acids, amines, amides, peptides, and their derivatives

| Name | Synonyms | Formula | M. wt. | Physical properties |
|------|----------|---------|--------|---------------------|
| Acetamide | Ethanamide | $CH_3 \cdot CO \cdot NH_2$ | 59.1 | col. deliq. cryst.; M.p. 81–3, B.p. 222 |
| Acetylcholine | ACh; 2-Acetyloxy-$N,N,N$-trimethyl-ethanaminium salt | $(CH_3)_3 \overset{+}{N} \cdot CH_2 \cdot CH_2 \cdot O \cdot CO \cdot CH_3$ $X^-$ | Free base as hydroxide, 163.2; Chloride, 181.7; Bromide, 226.1; Iodide, 273.1 | Chloride: v. hygr. needles or prisms; M.p. 149–52; faint amine-like odour, sharply saline taste. Bromide: hygr. prisms; M.p. 143. Iodide: non-hygr. cryst.; M.p. 161. |
| $N$-Acetyl-glutamic acid | | $HOOC \cdot CH_2 \cdot CH_2 \cdot CH \cdot COOH$ $\underset{NH \cdot CO \cdot CH_3}{\mid}$ | 189.2 | L-: cryst; M.p. 199 |
| $N$-Acetyl-5-methoxytrypt-amine | Melatonin; $N$-[2-(5-Methoxy-1$H$-indol-3-yl)-ethyl] acetamide | | 232.3 | pale yellow leaflets; M.p. 116–18; sublimes |
| Acetyl-$\beta$-methylcholine chloride | Methacholine chloride; Mecholyl chloride; 2-(Acetyloxy)-$N,N,N$-trimethylpropanaminium chloride | $(CH_3)_3 \overset{+}{N} \cdot CH_2 \cdot CH(CH_3) \cdot O \cdot CO \cdot CH_3$ $Cl^-$ | Chloride, 195.7; Bromide, 240.2; Iodide, 287.1 | Chloride: v. deliq. needles; M.p. 172–3. Bromide: hygr. cryst., M.p. 147–9. Iodide: non-hygr. cryst.; M.p. 138–9.5 |
| $S$-Adenosyl-homocysteine | 5'-$S$-(3-Amino-3-carboxypropyl)-5'-thio-adenosine; $S$-(5'-Deoxy-adenosine-5')homocysteine | | 384.4 | DL-: small prisms. L-: col. tufts of needles; M.p. 210 |
| $S$-Adenosyl-methionine | Active methionine; SAM; 5'-[(3-Amino-3-carboxypropyl) methylsulphonio-5'-deoxyadenosine; $S$-(5'-Deoxyadenosine-5')-methionine | | Free cation, 399.4; Chloride, 434.9; Bromide, 479.3; Iodide, 526.4; Hydrogen sulphate, 496.5 | Salts: cryst. solids. Chloride and bromide, hygr.; iodide, v. sl. hygr. L- chloride: M.p. 118–22d. |
| D-Adrenaline | 4-[1-Hydroxy-2-(methyl-amino)ethyl] -1,2-benzenediol; 1-(3,4-Dihydroxy-phenyl)-2-methylamino-ethanol; Epinephrine; Suprarenine | | 183.2 | wh. cryst. solid; M.p. 211–15d. |

| $[\alpha]_D^t$ | $pK_a$ at 25°C | Solubility | General remarks |
|---|---|---|---|
| | | $97.5^{20}$, $178^{60}$ H$_2$O; $25.0^{20}$, $257.1^{60}$ EtOH; v.s. glycerol; s. CHCl$_3$; sl. s. eth. | Odourless if pure, but frequently has a mousy odour. Solution neutral. Can be absorbed by cation exchange resins, *Naturwissenschaften* **42**, 580 (1955). |
| | | Chloride, bromide, iodide: v.s. H$_2$O, EtOH; s. CHCl$_3$; i. eth., benz. | Neurotransmitter substance at synapses and neuroeffector junctions, parasympathomimetic agent. Acts as transmitter of cholinergic nerve fibres. Action short-lived due to rapid breakdown of ACh by cholinesterases; action of ACh prolonged by cholinesterase inhibitors. 'Nicotinic' actions blocked by nicotine, hexamethonium, or *d*-tubocurarine (at autonomic ganglia), and by decamethonium or *d*-tubocurarine (skeletal muscle). 'Muscarinic' actions (on smooth and cardiac muscle, exocrine glands) blocked by atropine. Aq. soln. slightly acid (pH ~ 5). Aq. soln. most stable at pH 4; decomposed at alkaline pH or by heating at neutral pH. Reacts with hydroxylamine to form acethydroxamic acid. |
| L-, $-16.6^{25}$ (c = 2 in H$_2$O) $+3.9^{25}$ (c = 2 in M-NaOH) | | s. H$_2$O, alkalis, hot EtOH | |
| | | s. EtOH; sl. s. H$_2$O, benz.; v. sl. s. pet. eth. | Occurs in mammalian pineal gland. Lightens skin colour by reversing effect of MSH. $\lambda_{max}$ (in 95% EtOH) 223 nm $\epsilon$ 27 500 and 278 nm $\epsilon$ 6300. |
| L-, $+27.0^{22.5}$ (c = 2 iodide in 90% EtOH) | | v.s. H$_2$O, EtOH; s. CHCl$_3$; i. eth. | Parasympathomimetic agent; muscarinic actions, esp. on cardiovascular system, predominate, nicotinic actions negligible. Actions more prolonged than acetylcholine since less sensitive to cholinesterases. Biologically active compd. is L- isomer. Rapid decomp. by alkalis. Aq. soln. slightly acid (pH ~ 5), slowly decomp. on standing, should not be kept longer than 2 weeks at 0–4°C. Store solid airtight and protected from light. Iodide turns yellow in air and light. |
| L-, $37^{25}$ (c = 1.3 in 0.05M-H$_2$SO$_4$) $+44.5^{23}$ (c = 1 in 0.05 M-HCl) | | s. hot H$_2$O; sl. s. cold H$_2$O, EtOH; v. sl. s. eth. | Slowly oxidized to sulphoxide as solid and in soln., protected from oxidation by thiodiglycol. Store solid in inert atmosphere at low temp. Hydrolysed in acid soln., e.g. 0.1M-HCl, 100°C, 90 min., forming *S*-ribosylhomocysteine. Not hydrolysed in neutral or alkaline soln., e.g. stable in 0.1M-NaOH, R.T., 10 min., but oxidation more rapid in alkaline soln. Neutral solns. containing thiodiglycol stable for long periods at R.T. Spectrum, $\lambda_{max}$ 260 nm $\epsilon$ 16 000 at pH 7. PREP. and PURIF. *Anal. Biochem.* **15**, 323 (1966), **35**, 505 (1970); *Biochem. Preps.* **8**, 8 (1961); *J. Org. Chem.* **43**, 998 (1978). |
| L-, $+48.5^{24}$ (c = 1.8 chloride in 5M-HCl) $+16.8^{24}$ (c = 1 bromide in H$_2$O) | | L- chloride: v.s. MeOH at pH 2; s. H$_2$O; sl. s. MeOH at pH 6. Hydrogen sulphate: v.s. H$_2$O. | Compd. unstable under many conditions, presence of impurities should be expected unless special precautions have been taken. Solid halide salts unstable, iodide 12% decomp. in 1 week at 3°C, 30% at 24°C, stabilized by mixture with Li halides (10–20%). Stable solid forms include hydrogen sulphate (< 3% decomp. at 4°C in 6 months) and disulphate di-*p*-toluenesulphonate. Relatively stable in acid soln., v. unstable in alkali. At pH 2.8 after 1 week, 14% decomp. a 3°C, *more* stable in strong acid, e.g. 1M-HCl or 6M-H$_2$SO$_4$. Complete decomp. in 0.1M-NaOH at R.T. in 10 min. Slow decomp. at neutral pH, e.g. in 24 hr at 30°C, 10% decomp. at pH 6.6, 32% at pH 7.8, 70% at pH 8.8. Store solns. at $-20$°C or below at pH 2.5–4, do not store for longer than 1 month. Do not warm up solutions until immediately before use; do not mix with neutral solutions until last possible moment; in assays preferably initiate reactions by adding *S*-adenosylmethionine. Spectrum, $\lambda_{max}$ 260 nm $\epsilon$ 15 400 at pH 7, $\lambda_{max}$ 256 nm $\epsilon$ 15 200 at pH 1. Compd. has 4 stereoisomers; natural compd. is L- at $\alpha$-carbon, (−)- at sulphonium centre; see *JACS* **81**, 3975 (1959). PREP. and PURIF. *JBC* **244**, 682 (1969); *Meth. Enzymol.* **17B**, 393 (1971); *Anal. Biochem.* **15**, 323 (1966). |
| $-53.2^{22-25}$ (c = 1.2 in 0.5M-HCl) $-50.6^{17}$ (c = 7.5 in 0.37M-HCl) | 8.66 (NH) 9.95 (OH) | s. gl. acetic, mineral acids, alkalis; sl. s. H$_2$O, EtOH; i. eth., acet., CHCl$_3$ | Sympathomimetic agent, acting esp. on heart and on vascular and other smooth muscle. Predominant hormone of adrenal medulla, affecting esp. glucose and fatty acid metabolism. Configuration of natural adrenaline is D- by relation to D-mandelic acid, *JCS* **1958**, 2069. Unstable in aq. soln. at alkaline pH and when heated. Relatively stable at pH 5 in cold. Aq. soln. slightly alkaline. Solid slowly browns on exposure to air and light. |

# 1 Amino acids, amines, amides, peptides, and their derivatives

| Name | Synonyms | Formula | M. wt. | Physical properties |
|------|----------|---------|--------|---------------------|
| Alanine | 2-Aminopropanoic acid; Ala | $CH_3 \cdot CH(NH_2) \cdot COOH$ | 89.1 | needles or prisms; sublimes > 200 |
| β-Alanine | 3-Aminopropanoic acid | $H_2N \cdot CH_2 \cdot CH_2 \cdot COOH$ | 89.1 | col. prisms; M.p. 207d. (199d.); sublimes |
| Allantoin | 5-Ureidohydantoin; (2,5-Dioxo-4-imidazolidinyl)-urea | NH—CO   NH₂<br>\|         \|<br>CO         CO<br>\|         \|<br>NH—CH—NH | 158.1 | wh. prisms or plates; M.p. 238 |
| Amino acyl-transfer RNA | Amino acyl-tRNA | Transfer RNA (tRNA) with an aminoacyl group esterified with the 2′- or 3′-hydroxyl group of the terminal adenosine residue. The amino acyl group migrates rapidly between the 2′- and 3′-positions, each isomer having a half-life of 1 ms or less. The equilibrium mixture contains 2′- and 3′-isomers in a ratio of about 1:2. | | wh. amorph. powder; hygr. |
| 2-Amino-adipic acid | 2-Aminohexanedioic acid; α-Aminoadipic acid | $HOOC \cdot (CH_2)_3 \cdot CH(NH_2) \cdot COOH$ | 161.2 | cryst. solid; M.p. DL-, very variable, range 165–202d., L-, 206d. |
| 2-Amino-butyric acid | α-Aminobutyric acid; 2-Aminobutanoic acid; Butyrine | $CH_3 \cdot CH_2 \cdot CH(NH_2) \cdot COOH$ | 103.1 | leaflets; sublimes > 300 |
| 4-Amino-butyric acid | γ-Aminobutyric acid; Piperidic acid; 4-Amino-butanoic acid; GABA | $H_2N \cdot CH_2 \cdot CH_2 \cdot CH_2 \cdot COOH$ | 103.1 | monocl. tablets, plates or needles; M.p. 203d. |
| 5-Amino-imidazole-4-carboxamide | AICA; 5-Amino-1H-imidazole-4-carbox-amide |  | 126.1; Hydrochloride, 162.6 | wh. needles; M.p. 170–1. Hydrochloride: wh. needles; M.p. 255–6d. |

| $[\alpha]_D^t$ | $pK_a$ at 25°C | Solubility | General remarks |
|---|---|---|---|
| L-, + 14.6$^{25}$ (c = 2.0 in 5M-HCl) + 1.8$^{25}$ (c = 2.0 in H$_2$O) | 2.35 9.87 | DL-: 16.6$^{25}$, 32.2$^{75}$ H$_2$O; 0.084$^{25}$ 90% EtOH; 0.0087$^{25}$ EtOH; i. eth. L-: 16.65$^{25}$, 28.5$^{75}$ H$_2$O; v. sl. s. EtOH; i.eth., acet. | L-Hydrochloride, prisms, decomp. 204, $[\alpha]_D^{26}$ + 8.5 (c = 9.3 in H$_2$O). |
| | 3.55 10.24 | 54.5$^{25}$ H$_2$O; 0.017$^{25}$ EtOH; i. eth., acet., CHCl$_3$ | Decomposes in alkali at 37°C yielding ammonia and acrylic acid. $\beta$-Alanine monohydrochloride, M.p. 122.5, s. H$_2$O, sl. s. EtOH. |
| | 8.96 | 0.76$^{22}$, 3.3 hot H$_2$O; 0.2 EtOH; i. eth. | Hydrolysed to allantoic acid by alkali. Allantoic acid is unaffected by dil. alkali, but hydrolysed to glyoxylic acid and urea by 0.05M-HCl at 100°C in 2 min. Satd. aq. soln. pH 5.5. |
| | | s. H$_2$O, M-NaCl; i. EtOH | Amino acyl-tRNA compds. are obtained by the reaction between amino acids, ATP, and tRNA, catalysed by amino acyl-tRNA synthetases (amino-acid-activating enzymes). Methods for the preparation of mixed and single species of tRNAs, synthetases, and amino acyl-tRNAs are given in *Meth. Enzymol.* vols. 6, 12A, 12B, 20, 29, 30, 59 and 60. Amino acyl-tRNAs are rapidly hydrolysed to the amino acid and tRNA above pH 6; half-lives in 0.1M-Tris buffer pH 8.6 at 37°C, 2–65 min., depending on nature of the amino acid moiety. Rate of hydrolysis is increased by alkaline pH, Tris, increase in temp. or ionic strength, decreased by acylation of amino group of amino acid. For details, see *BBA*, **281** 228 (1971); *Biochimie* **56**, 383 (1974). Amino acyl groups are completely removed from tRNA (stripping) by 1–2M-Tris, pH 9–9.5, in 30–120 min. at 37°C. Store amino acyl-tRNAs in soln. or lyophilized at −20°C or below and pH 5. Spectrum as RNA, $A_{260}$ 22–24 for 1 mg/ml soln. |
| L-, + 3.2$^{25}$ (c = 2 in H$_2$O) + 25.0$^{25}$ (c = 2 in 5M-HCl) | 2.14 4.21 9.77 | 0.22$^{40}$ H$_2$O; sl. s. EtOH, eth. | Free acid cyclizes in boiling water to piperidonecarboxylic acid; DL-, M.p. 177–8; D-, $[\alpha]_D^{25}$ − 16.5 (c = 2 in H$_2$O) −41.5 (c = 2 in 6M-HCl). SYN. DL-, D- and L-, *Anal. Biochem.* **43**, 282 (1971); **55**, 411 (1973). |
| L-, + 20.6$^{25}$ (c = 1–2 in 5M-HCl) + 9.3$^{25}$ (c = 1–2 in H$_2$O) | 2.29 9.83 | DL-: 28 H$_2$O; 0.18$^{78}$ EtOH; i. eth. L-: s. H$_2$O, gl. acetic; sl. s. EtOH, eth. | L- Hydrochloride, needles, $[\alpha]_D^{19}$ + 12.9 (c = 3.64 in H$_2$O), s. H$_2$O. |
| | 4.03 10.56 | v.s. H$_2$O; sl. s. EtOH; i. eth., benz. | Inhibitory neurotransmitter in mammalian CNS and at crustacean neuromuscular junctions. Action blocked by picrotoxin. Monohydrochloride, M.p. 135–6, v.s. H$_2$O. |
| | | s. H$_2$O | Spectrum, $\lambda_{max}$ ($\epsilon$), 240 nm (9050) and 267 nm (11 200) at pH 1; 266 nm (12 700) at pH 7; 277 nm (12 500) at pH 13. Bratton-Marshall chromophore, $\lambda_{max}$ 540 nm $\epsilon$ 26 400. Riboside, 5-amino-1-($\beta$-D-ribofuranosyl)imidazole-4-carboxamide, wh. needles, M.p. 215–6, $[\alpha]_D^{26}$ −63.0 (c = 1 in H$_2$O), spectrum $\lambda_{max}$ 267 nm, $\epsilon$ 11 000 (pH 2), 12 200 (pH 7), 12 600 (pH 10.5). |

# 1 Amino acids, amines, amides, peptides, and their derivatives

| Name | Synonyms | Formula | M. wt. | Physical properties |
|---|---|---|---|---|
| 2-Aminoiso-butyric acid | α-Aminoisobutyric acid; α-Methylalanine; 2-Amino-2-methylpropanoic acid | $\begin{array}{c}CH_3\\CH_3\end{array}$C(NH$_2$)·COOH | 103.1 | col. plates or prisms; sublimes 280; M.p. 335 (sealed tube) |
| 3-Aminoiso-butyric acid | α-Methyl-β-alanine; β-Aminoisobutyric acid; 3-Amino-2-methyl-propanoic acid | $\begin{array}{c}H_2N\cdot CH_2\\CH_3\end{array}$CH·COOH | 103.1 | (±)-: col. prisms; M.p. 177–9. (−)-: cryst. plates; M.p. 194–6. |
| 5-Amino-laevulinic acid | 5-Amino-4-oxopentanoic acid; δ-Aminolaevulinic acid | HOOC·CH$_2$·CH$_2$·CO·CH$_2$·NH$_2$ | 131.1; Hydrochloride, 167.6 | cryst.; M.p. 118–9. Hydro-chloride: M.p. 144–51. |
| Angiotensin | Hypertensin; Angiotonin | Asp-Arg-Val-Tyr-Ile-His-Pro-Phe<br><br>Angiotensin II<br><br>Asp-Arg-Val-Tyr-Ile-His-Pro-Phe-His-Leu<br><br>Angiotensin I<br><br>The structures refer to angiotensins of man, pig, and horse; in ox, Ile[5] is replaced by Val. | II: 1046<br><br>I: 1297 | |
| Anthranilic acid | o-Aminobenzoic acid | [benzene ring]—COOH, —NH$_2$ | 137.1 | wh. to pale yellow cryst. leaflets; M.p. 146–9 |
| Arginine | 2-Amino-5-guanidino-pentanoic acid; N-5-Amidino-ornithine; Arg | $\begin{array}{c}HN\\H_2N\end{array}$C·NH·(CH$_2$)$_3$·CH(NH$_2$)·COOH | 174.2; Hydrate, 210.2 | DL-: M.p. 238d. L-: prisms + 2H$_2$O from H$_2$O; anhyd. plates from EtOH, decomp. 244 |
| L-Arginino-succinic acid | N-[[(4-Amino-4-carboxy-butyl)amino]iminomethyl]-L-aspartic acid | $\begin{array}{c}HN\\ \\ C \\ NH \\ (CH_2)_3 \\ CH\cdot NH_2 \\ COOH\end{array}\begin{array}{c}NH\\ \\ CH \\ CH_2 \\ COOH\end{array}$COOH | 290.3 | v.hygr. powder. Ba salt: amorphous powder |
| Asparagine | 2-Aminosuccinamic acid; Aspartic acid β-monoamide; Asn | H$_2$N·CO·CH$_2$·CH(NH$_2$)·COOH | 132.1; Hydrate, 150.1 | DL-: col. cryst. + 1H$_2$O. L-: col. cryst. + 1H$_2$O; M.p. 236d. |

| $[\alpha]_D^t$ | $pK_a$ at 25°C | Solubility | General remarks |
|---|---|---|---|
| | 2.36<br>10.21 | $13.72^{25}$ $H_2O$;<br>$0.483^{25}$ 80% EtOH;<br>i. eth. | Hydrochloride, platelets, decomp. 236–7, s. $H_2O$, EtOH. |
| (−)-, $-15.4^{27}$ (c = 1 in $H_2O$) | | s. $H_2O$ | Sublimes. Hydrochloride, (±)-, M.p. 128–9; (−)-, 134–8, $[\alpha]_D^{24}$ $-10.7$ (c = 1 in $H_2O$). (−)-Isomer found in urine. (+)-Isomer, but not (−)-, is utilized by yeast. Absolute configuration, see *JBC* **236**, 3283 (1961). PREP. (±)-, *Biochem. Preps.* **7**, 20 (1960); (−)-, *Anal. Biochem.* **57**, 82 (1974). |
| | 4.05<br>8.90 | s. $H_2O$, EtOH;<br>v. sl. s. Et acetate | Spectrum, $\lambda_{max}$ 266.5 nm $\epsilon$ 23.0. Forms a 2,5-disubstituted pyrazine in alkali. SYN. *Biochem. Preps.* **10**, 6 (1963). |
| | | s. $H_2O$, aq. solns.<br>pH 5–8, EtOH | Angiotensin II is the more active form; angiotensin I has much lower activity. Raises blood pressure (pressor action) by causing vasoconstriction in skeletal, mesenteric, and renal vascular beds; stimulates release of aldosterone from adrenal gland. Angiotensin I is formed by action of renin (proteolytic enzyme) on angiotensinogen (renin substrate) in the plasma, and is converted into angiotensin II by converting enzyme which removes C-terminal dipeptide. Angiotensin II is short-lived in blood and tissues due to further degradation by peptidases. Stable in neutral soln. Hydrolysed by strong acids and above pH 9.5. Adsorbs to glass from dilute solns. |
| | 2.05<br>4.95 | $0.35^{14}$ $H_2O$; s. hot<br>$H_2O$; $10.7^9$ EtOH;<br>$16.0^7$ eth. | Spectrum, $\lambda_{max}$ 310 nm at pH 7. |
| L-, $+27.6^{25}$ (c = 2.0 in 5M-HCl)<br>$+12.5^{25}$ (c = 2.0 in $H_2O$) | 1.82 (COOH)<br>8.99 (NH$_2$)<br>12.48 (guanido) | L-: $15^{21}$ $H_2O$; sl. s.<br>EtOH; i. eth. | Loss of arginine occurs during protein hydrolysis in the presence of carbohydrate. Unstable to hot alkali. Dihydrate loses $H_2O$ at 105°C. Hydrochloride, L-, decomp. 235, s. $H_2O$, sl. s. hot EtOH. |
| $+16.4^{24}$ (c = 2.9 in $H_2O$)<br>$+26.6^{24}$ (c = 2.9 in 0.5M-NaOH) | 1.62 (COOH)<br>2.70 (COOH)<br>4.26 (COOH)<br>9.58 ($\alpha$-NH$_2$)<br>> 12<br>(guanido) | v.s. $H_2O$. Ba salt, v.s.<br>$H_2O$; i. EtOH | Forms enzymically inactive anhydride (s. $H_2O$, EtOH), rapidly on heating or at acid pH; anhydride slowly hydrolysed to argininosuccinic acid under mildly alkaline conditions. Small amounts of second anhydride, which cannot be converted back to argininosuccinic acid, also formed on heating. Some decomp. occurs especially at neutral pH and high temp. See *BJ* **77**, 135 (1960); *Biochem.* **5**, 1821 (1966). Free amino acid and Ba salt stable for months as solid if kept dry and at 0°C. Neutral aq. solns. do not cyclize appreciably over several weeks at $-18°C$. SYN. *JBC* **204**, 95 (1953); *Biochem.* **5**, 1821 (1966). |
| L-, $+28.6^{25}$ (c = 2 in M-HCl)<br>$-5.6^{25}$ (c = 2 in $H_2O$) | 2.14<br>8.72 | DL- monohydrate:<br>$2.16^{25}$ $H_2O$;<br>i. EtOH, eth.<br>L- monohydrate:<br>$2.99^{25}$, $24.1^{75}$<br>$H_2O$; $0.0003^{25}$<br>EtOH; s. NH$_4$OH;<br>i. eth. | Stable at 100°C in $H_2O$. 23% hydrolysed in 5 min at 100°C in 5% $H_2SO_4$. |

# 1 Amino acids, amines, amides, peptides, and their derivatives

| Name | Synonyms | Formula | M. wt. | Physical properties |
|------|----------|---------|--------|---------------------|
| Aspartic acid | 2-Aminosuccinic acid; Asp | $HOOC \cdot CH_2 \cdot CH(NH_2) \cdot COOH$ | 133.1 | col. cryst.; DL-, M.p. 278–80; L-, M.p. 269–71 |
| Aspartic semialdehyde | 2-Amino-4-oxobutanoic acid; 2-Aminosuccinaldehydic acid; 4-Aspartal | $OHC \cdot CH_2 \cdot CH(NH_2) \cdot COOH$ | 117.1 | solid |
| Betaine | Glycine betaine; 1-Carboxy-$N,N,N$-trimethylmethanaminium hydroxide inner salt | $(CH_3)_3 \overset{+}{N} \cdot CH_2 \cdot COO^-$ | 117.2; Hydrate, 135.2 | col. cryst. + $1H_2O$; loses $H_2O$ 100, decomp. 310; sweet taste |
| Bradykinin | | Arg-Pro-Pro-Gly-Phe-Ser-Pro-Phe-Arg | 1060 | amorph. wh. powder |
| Butyrylcholine chloride | | $(CH_3)_3 \overset{+}{N} \cdot CH_2 \cdot CH_2 \cdot O \cdot CO \cdot (CH_2)_2 \cdot CH_3$ $Cl^-$ | 209.7 | wh. deliq. cryst. |
| Cadaverine | 1,5-Pentanediamine; Pentamethylenediamine | $H_2N \cdot CH_2 \cdot CH_2 \cdot CH_2 \cdot CH_2 \cdot CH_2 \cdot NH_2$ | 102.2; Hydrate, 138.2 | col., syrupy fuming liq., $d_4^{25}$ 0.873; M.p. 9, B.p. 178–80; forms oily hydrate + $2H_2O$ |
| Carbamylaspartic acid | Ureidosuccinic acid; Aminocarbonylaspartic acid | $HOOC \cdot CH_2 \cdot CH \cdot COOH$ $\quad\quad\quad\quad\; NH \cdot CO \cdot NH_2$ | 176.1 | wh. cryst.; M.p., DL-, 178–80, L-, 128–30 |
| Carbamylcholine chloride | Carbachol; Doryl; 2[(Aminocarbonyl)oxy]-$N,N,N$-trimethylethanamium chloride | $(CH_3)_3 \overset{+}{N} \cdot CH_2 \cdot CH_2 \cdot O \cdot CO \cdot NH_2$ $Cl^-$ | 182.6 | hard prism. cryst.; v. hygr.; M.p. 210–12; odourless. |
| γ-Carboxyglutamic acid | 4-Carboxyglutamic acid; 3-Amino-1,1,3-propanetricarboxylic acid; Gla | $\begin{matrix} HOOC \\ \quad\quad\; CH \cdot CH_2 \cdot CHNH_2 \cdot COOH \\ HOOC \end{matrix}$ | 191.2 | DL-: wh. powder; M.p. 90–2 L-: col. cryst.; M.p. 167–7.5 |
| Carnitine | γ-Trimethyl-β-hydroxybutyrobetaine; 3-Carboxy-2-hydroxy-$N,N,N$-trimethyl-1-propanaminium hydroxide inner salt. L-: Vitamin $B_T$ | $(CH_3)_3 \overset{+}{N} \cdot CH_2 \cdot CH(OH) \cdot CH_2 \cdot COO^-$ | 161.2 | DL-: hygr. cryst.; M.p. 195–7d. L-: v. hygr. cryst.; M.p. 197–8d. |

| $[\alpha]_D^t$ | $pK_a$ at 25°C | Solubility | General remarks |
|---|---|---|---|
| L-, +25.4[25] (c = 2 in 5M-HCl) +5.05[25] (c = 2 in $H_2O$) | 1.99 3.90 9.90 | DL-: 0.82[25], 4.79[75] $H_2O$; 0.032[25] 75% EtOH; i. eth. L-: 0.5[25], 2.87[75] $H_2O$; 0.00016[25] EtOH; i. eth. | Stable to hot mineral acids in the presence of carbohydrates. N-Acetyl-L-aspartic acid, oil slowly becoming microcryst., M.p. 142, $[\alpha]_D$ + 57 (in gl. acetic), v.s. $H_2O$. |
| | | s. $H_2O$, mineral acids | Unstable as dry solid and in neutral soln. Soln. stable at least for several days at 4°C or below in HCl (0.25M–4M) preferably in inert atmosphere. Stable at least 1 hr at 37°C and pH 8.6. Reacts with Tris. PREP. JBC **213**, 39 (1955), **249**, 6351 (1974). |
| | 1.83 | Hydrate: 157[19] $H_2O$; 8.6[18] EtOH; v. sl. s. eth. | pH of satd. soln. about 8. Isomerizes at M.p. giving methyl ester of dimethyl-aminoacetic acid. Hydrochloride, cryst., M.p. 232d., solubility 64.7[25] $H_2O$, 5 90% EtOH, i. eth. |
| −76.5[25] (c = 1.37 in M-acetic acid) | | s. $H_2O$, hot MeOH, 70% EtOH, gl. acetic; sl. s. cold MeOH, EtOH; v. sl. s. acet., $CHCl_3$, eth., n-BuOH | One of the plasma kinins, formed by the action of proteolytic enzymes (kallikrein, plasmin, trypsin, snake venom enzymes) on a precursor in plasma. V. potent vasodilator leading to fall in blood pressure, affects smooth muscles, increases capillary permeability, causes pain. Stable in 0.1M-HCl at 100°C for 1 hr, in 0.1M-NaOH at R.T. for 2 hr and over long periods as solid at 0°C or below. |
| | | v.s. $H_2O$, EtOH; s. $CHCl_3$; i. eth. | Rancid odour. Rapid hydrolysis in boiling acids. Substrate for pseudocholin-esterase, hydrolysed much more slowly by acetylcholinesterase. |
| | 10.05 10.93 | s. $H_2O$, EtOH; sl. s. eth. | Characteristic odour. Tends to darken on storage. Absorbs $CO_2$ from air. Dihydrochloride, hygr. cryst., M.p. 255, s. $H_2O$, MeOH, sl. s. EtOH. |
| L-, +18.9[20] (c = 3.38 in $H_2O$) +24.1[25] (c = 3 Ba salt in $H_2O$) | | s. $H_2O$ | K salt hygr., Ba and Ca salts non-hygr. PREP. L-, Chem. Pharm. Bull. Tokyo **15**, 1604 (1967); Biochem. **13**, 638 (1974). |
| | | v.s. $H_2O$; s. MeOH; sl. s. EtOH; i. $CHCl_3$, eth. | Aq. soln. neutral and stable even when heated. Parasympathomimetic action, activity not prolonged by eserine or neostigmine. Not attacked by cholin-esterases. |
| L-, +35.3[20] (c = 1 in 6M-HCl) | 1.7 3.2 4.75 9.9 | s. $H_2O$; i. eth. | Stable in alkali, e.g. in 2M-KOH at 110°C for 24 hr. Decarboxylates, yielding pyroglutamic acid, in acid soln., half-life about 10 min in 0.05M-HCl at 100°C, about 20 min in 6M-HCl at 110°C. In protein hydrolysis under standard conditions yields glutamic acid. SYN. L-: JACS, **101**, 4385 (1979); Helv. Chim. Acta **60**, 798 (1977). |
| L-, −23.9[30] (c = 0.83 in $H_2O$) | 3.80 | v.s. $H_2O$, EtOH; sl. s. acet., isopropanol; i. eth. Hydrochloride: v.s. $H_2O$; sl. s. EtOH; i. eth. | Hydrochloride, DL-: M.p. 196d., solubility in $H_2O$ 146.4[16], 234[56]; L-: M.p. 142d., $[\alpha]_D^{20}$ −23.7. O-Acetyl-L-carnitine, M.p. 145, $[\alpha]_D^{20}$ −19.5. PREP. L-: Biochem. Preps. 7, 26 (1960); ZPC **353**, 618 (1972); Appl. Environ. Microbiol. **39**, 327 (1980). Acylcarnitines: Biochem. Preps. **12**, 69 (1968); J. Org. Chem. **32**, 3989 (1967). |

# 1 Amino acids, amines, amides, peptides, and their derivatives

| Name | Synonyms | Formula | M. wt. | Physical properties |
|---|---|---|---|---|
| L-Carnosine | β-Alanyl-L-histidine | $H_2N \cdot CH_2 \cdot CH_2 \cdot CO \cdot NH \cdot CH \cdot CH_2$ with COOH, N—NH (imidazole) | 226.2 | col. needles; M.p. 260—2d. (variable) |
| Choline | 2-Hydroxy-$N,N,N$-trimethyl-ethanaminium hydroxide; (2-Hydroxyethyl)trimethyl-ammonium hydroxide; Bilineurine; Sincaline | $(CH_3)_3 \overset{+}{N} \cdot CH_2 \cdot CH_2 OH$ $OH^-$ | 121.2; Chloride, 139.6 | col. viscous syrup or col. cryst. Chloride: v. hygr. cryst. |
| ——, cytidine diphosphate derivative | Cytidine 5′-diphosphate choline; CDP-choline | $(CH_3)_3 \overset{+}{N} \cdot CH_2 \cdot CH_2 \cdot O—CDP$ $OH^-$ CDP = cytidine 5′-diphosphate residue | 506.3 | hygr. powder |
| Citrulline | $N^5$-(Aminocarbonyl)-ornithine; $N$-δ-carbamoyl-ornithine; 2-Amino-5-ureido-pentanoic acid | $O=C$ with $NH \cdot (CH_2)_3 \cdot CH(NH_2) \cdot COOH$ and $NH_2$ | 175.2 | wh. needles; M.p. 220d. |
| Cortico-tropin | ACTH; Adrenocorticotropin; Adrenocorticotrophic hormone; Corticotrophin | Ser-Tyr-Ser-Met-Glu[5]-His-Phe-Arg-Trp-Gly[10]-Lys-Pro-Val-Gly-Lys[15]-Lys-Arg-Arg-Pro-Val[20]-Lys-Val-Tyr-Pro-Asn[25]-Gly-Ala-Glu-Asp-Glu[30]-Ser-Ala-Glu-Ala-Phe[35]-Pro-Leu-Glu-Phe  Human corticotropin (Corticotropins of sheep and ox differ in having Gln[33]; that of pig in having Leu[31]) | 4541 | amorph. wh. powder |
| Creatine | $N$-(Aminoiminomethyl)-$N$-methylglycine; (α-Methyl-guanido)acetic acid; Methylglycocyamine | $HN=C$ with $NH_2$ and $N \cdot CH_2 \cdot COOH$ and $CH_3$ | 131.1; Hydrate, 149.2 | col. monocl. prisms + $1H_2O$ from $H_2O$; loses $H_2O$ 100; M.p. 303d. |
| Creatinine | 1-Methylglycocyamidine; 2-Imino-1-methyl-4-imidaz-olidinone; 2-Amino-1,5-dihydro-1-methyl-$4H$-imidazol-4-one | $HN=C$ with $NH—CO$, $N—CH_2$, $CH_3$ (ring) | 113.1; Hydrate, 149.2 | col. cryst. + $2H_2O$ on slow evap. of sat. aq. soln., or $H_2O$-free leaflets from hot sat. soln.; Anhyd., decomp. ~ 300. |
| Cystamine | Cystinamine; 2,2′-Dithiobis-ethanamine; 2,2′-Diamino-diethyldisulphide | $S \cdot CH_2 \cdot CH_2 \cdot NH_2$ \| $S \cdot CH_2 \cdot CH_2 \cdot NH_2$ | 152.3; Dihydro-chloride, 225.2 | viscous oil; B.p. 106—8[5]. Dihydrochloride: needles or plates; M.p. 217 |

| $[\alpha]_D^t$ | $pK_a$ at 25°C | Solubility | General remarks |
|---|---|---|---|
| $+21.9^{20}$ (c = 1 in $H_2O$) | 2.62 (COOH) 6.66 (imidazole) 9.24 ($NH_2$) | 32 $H_2O$; i. EtOH | Nitrate: col. needles, 222–3d.; $[\alpha]_D^{20}$ + 23.0 (c = 5.2 in $H_2O$); v.s. $H_2O$. Hydrochloride: cryst.; v.s. $H_2O$. L-Anserine (β-alanyl-1-methyl-L-histidine): v. hygr. col. cryst.; M.p. 240–2d.; $[\alpha]_D^{23}$ + 11.4 (c = 5 in $H_2O$); v.s. $H_2O$, v.sl. s. EtOH. |
| | 13.9 | v.s. $H_2O$; s. EtOH; sl. s. amyl alcohol; i. eth., $CHCl_3$ Chloride: v.s. $H_2O$, EtOH | Strongly alkaline; absorbs $CO_2$ from air. Chloride: aq. solns. approx. neutral. |
| | | CDP-choline: s. $H_2O$ | CDP-choline: M-$H_2SO_4$ at 100°C for 18 min. causes 50% hydrolysis to CMP and phosphorylcholine; 7.5% of total P released as $P_i$ after 40 min. Spectrum identical to CMP in range 245–300 nm; 280/260 = 2.17. |
| L-, $+4.0^{25}$ (c = 2 in $H_2O$) $+24.2^{25}$ (c = 2 in M-HCl) | L-, 2.43 9.69 | s. $H_2O$; i. MeOH, EtOH, eth. | Stable to acid; unstable to alkali forming ornithine, $NH_3$ and $CO_2$. Hydrochloride, L-: M.p. 185d.; $[\alpha]_D^{22}$ + 17.9 (c = 2 in $H_2O$). |
| $-150^{23}$ (c = 0.5 acetate in 0.1M-acetic acid) | | v.s. $H_2O$; sl. s. 70% EtOH, $n$-BuOH; i. cold acet. | Hormone of adenohypophysis (anterior pituitary). Stimulates secretion of cortisol, corticosterone, and aldosterone by adrenal cortex, chiefly by stimulating their synthesis, and induces growth of adrenal cortex. Aq. soln. slowly loses biological activity due to oxidation, but process reversed by mild reducing agents (e.g. $Na_2SO_3$). Stable to heat in aq. soln., e.g. stable at pH 7.5 and 100°C for at least 2 hr., and in 0.1M-HCl at 100°C for 1 hr. Loses activity in 0.1M-NaOH at 100°C in 30 min. Unstable to u.v. light in aq. soln. at alkaline pHs. Pure corticotropin contains 150–200 potency units per mg. |
| | 2.63 $14.3^{12}$ | $1.09^{10}$, $1.35^{18}$ $H_2O$; 0.0063 cold EtOH; i. eth. | Found in vertebrate muscle, small amounts in blood, absent from normal adult urine. Aq. solns. approx. neutral. In neutral and alkaline solns. forms equilibrium mixture with creatinine, see *BJ* **22**, 924 (1928); *JACS* **47**, 1179 (1925); in acid soln. completely converted into creatinine. |
| | 4.83 $9.2^{20}$ | $8.7^{16}$ $H_2O$; $0.98^{16}$ EtOH; i. eth. | Normal constituent of urine; also found in blood and muscle. Spectrum, $\lambda_{max}$ 217 nm $\epsilon$ 4500 below pH 3; $\lambda_{max}$ 234 nm $\epsilon$ 6900 at pH 6.5–12.3; $\lambda_{max}$ 225 nm $\epsilon$ 11 100 in M-KOH; *Acta Chem. Scand.* **7**, 445 (1953). |
| | $8.82^{30}$ $9.58^{30}$ | s. $H_2O$; sl. s. EtOH Dihydrochloride: s. $H_2O$; sl. s. eth. | Decomposes on distillation even in high vacuum. |

# 1 Amino acids, amines, amides, peptides, and their derivatives

| Name | Synonyms | Formula | M. wt. | Physical properties |
|---|---|---|---|---|
| L-Cysta-thionine | (R)-S-(2-Amino-2-carboxy-ethyl)-L-homocysteine | S⟨ $CH_2 \cdot CH_2 \cdot CH(NH_2) \cdot COOH$ / $CH_2 \cdot CH(NH_2) \cdot COOH$ | 222.3 | col. cryst.; darkens 270–4; decomp. 301–12 |
| Cysteamine | 2-Aminoethanethiol; 2-Mercaptoethylamine; Thioethanolamine | $HS \cdot CH_2 \cdot CH_2 \cdot NH_2$ | 77.1; Hydro-chloride, 113.6 | wh. solid., M.p. 99–100. Hydrochloride: hygr. wh. plates; M.p. 70 2. |
| L-Cysteic acid | 3-Sulpho-L-alanine; 2-Amino-3-sulphopropanoic acid | $HO_3S \cdot CH_2 \cdot CH(NH_2) \cdot COOH$ | 169.2; Hydrate, 187.2 | anhyd. col. cryst. from aq. EtOH, M.p. 260d.; prisms or needles + $1H_2O$ from $H_2O$, M.p. 289d. |
| Cysteine | 2-Amino-3-mercaptopro-panoic acid; Cys | $HS \cdot CH_2 \cdot CH(NH_2) \cdot COOH$ | 121.2; Hydrochloride, 157.6 | L-: cryst. powder, M.p. 240d. Hydrochloride: sl. hygr. cryst.; M.p. 178d. |
| L-Cysteine sulphinic acid | α-Amino-β-sulphino-propanoic acid; 3-Sulphino-L-alanine | $HO_2S \cdot CH_2 \cdot CH(NH_2) \cdot COOH$ | 153.2 | cryst.; decomp. 152–3 (foams) |
| Cystine | 3,3′-Dithiobis(2-amino-propanoic acid); Dicysteine | $S \cdot CH_2 \cdot CH(NH_2) \cdot COOH$ \| $S \cdot CH_2 \cdot CH(NH_2) \cdot COOH$ | 240.3 | DL- and L-: cryst.; M.p. 260d. |
| 2,4-Diamino-butyric acid | 2,4-Diaminobutanoic acid; γ-Aminobutyrine | $H_2N \cdot CH_2 \cdot CH_2 \cdot CH(NH_2) \cdot COOH$ | 118.1; Monohydro-chloride, 154.6; Dihydro-chloride, 191.1 | DL- and L-: Monohydro-chloride; cryst. from EtOH/ $H_2O$; M.p. 228–30d. Dihydrochloride; cryst. from conc. HCl/gl. acetic; M.p. DL-, 202–6d., L-, 197–8 |
| Diamino-pimelic acid | 2,6-Diaminoheptanedioic acid | $HOOC \cdot CH(NH_2) \cdot (CH_2)_3 \cdot CH(NH_2) \cdot COOH$ | 190.2; Hydrate, 208.2 | meso-: anhyd. cryst.; M.p. > 305. LL-: cryst. or powder + $1H_2O$ |
| L-3,4-Di-hydroxyphenyl-alanine | L-Dopa; Levodopa; 3-Hydroxy-L-tyrosine; 3-(3,4-Dihydroxyphenyl)-L-alanine | HO–⟨C6H3(OH)⟩–$CH_2 \cdot CH(NH_2) \cdot COOH$ | 197.2 | wh. cryst.; M.p. 276–86d. |

| $[\alpha]_D^t$ | $pK_a$ at 25°C | Solubility | General remarks |
|---|---|---|---|
| +23.7[24] (c = 1 in M-HCl) | | s. $H_2O$, mineral acids; i. EtOH | Configuration of molecule is designated according to configuration of 'cysteine' centre. In the allo isomers the two optical centres have opposite configurations. L-Allocystathionine, $[\alpha]_D^{21} -25$ (c = 1 in M-HCl). Separation and i.r. spectra of cystathionine and allocystathionine, *ZPC* **305**, 105 (1956). |
| | 8.35 10.81 | s. $H_2O$, 95% EtOH Hydrochloride: s. $H_2O$, EtOH | Confers protection against radiation damage. Free base v. unstable, oxidising in air, and should be used immediately after preparation. Hydrochloride more stable. *N*-Acetylcysteamine, hygr. oil, B.p. 138–40[7]. |
| +8.66 (c = 7.4 in $H_2O$) | 1.3 ($SO_3H$) 1.9 (COOH) 8.70 ($NH_2$) | v.s. $H_2O$; i. EtOH | Heated under pressure with water gives taurine. |
| L-, +6.5[25] (c = 2 in 5M-HCl) −16.5[25] (c = 2 in $H_2O$) | 1.92 (COOH) 8.37 10.70 | v.s. $H_2O$, EtOH; s. gl. acetic, $NH_4OH$; i. eth., acet. Hydrochloride: v.s. $H_2O$; s. EtOH, acet. | Aq. soln. oxidizes to cystine on contact with air at neutral or alkaline pH. Oxidation accelerated by traces of heavy metals, esp. copper and iron. Relatively stable in acid; store as hydrochloride. *S*-Carboxymethyl-L-cysteine, M.p. 197–203; $[\alpha]_D^{25}$ 0.0; PREP. *J. Org. Chem.* **23**, 1251 (1958). |
| +11(in $H_2O$) +24 (c = 1 in M-HCl) | *ca.* 2.1 | s. $H_2O$ | Forms cystine by reacting with cysteine in $H_2O$. |
| L-, −232[25] (c = 1 in 5M-HCl) −70[25] (c = 1 in M-NaOH) | < 1[35] 2.1[35] 8.02[35] 8.71[35] | DL-: 0.003[20], 0.01[50] $H_2O$. L-: 0.011[25], 0.052[75], 0.114[100] $H_2O$; s. mineral acids, alkalis, $NH_4OH$; i. EtOH, eth., $CHCl_3$ | Extensive losses occur during acid hydrolysis of proteins in the presence of carbohydrates. Spectrum, $\lambda_{max}$ 249 nm $\epsilon$ 340 (in 0.1M-NaOH). *meso*-Cystine: decomp. 200–18, solubility 0.0056[25] $H_2O$, ISOL. *JBC* **102**, 287 (1933). Dimethyl-L-cystine: M.p. 216–18; $[\alpha]_D^{22} + 75.7$ (c = 1 in M-HCl). |
| L-, +7.2[25] (c = 2 free base in $H_2O$) + 24.2[25] (c = 2 mono-hydrochloride in 5M-HCl) +14.6[18] (c = 3.67 dihydro-chloride in $H_2O$) | 1.85[20] (COOH) 8.24[20] ($NH_2$) 10.44[20] ($NH_2$) | s. $H_2O$, mineral acids | |
| *meso*-: 0.0 (in 2M-NaOH, 5M-HCl, and 12M-HCl) LL-, Mono-hydrate: + 8.1[25] (c = 5 in $H_2O$) +45.1[24] (c = 2.6 in 5M-HCl) | *meso*- and LL-: 1.8 (COOH) 2.2 (COOH) 8.8 ($NH_2$) 9.9 ($NH_2$) | *meso*-: 0.92[21] $H_2O$; s. dil. mineral acids, alkalis; i. EtOH LL-: v.s. $H_2O$; i. EtOH | The *meso*-compd. is less soluble in $H_2O$ than other stereoisomers and can easily be obtained from a mixture by crystallization. Separation of isomers, *Meth. Enzymol.* **6**, 624 (1963). The *meso*-isomer has the *erythro* configuration and the LL- and DD-isomers the *threo* configuration. |
| −39.5 (c = 1.3 in $H_2O$) −12.0[20] (c = 2 in M-HCl) | 2.32 (COOH) 8.72 ($NH_2$) 9.96 (OH) 11.79 (OH) | 0.5[20], 2.5[100] $H_2O$; s. acids and alkalis; i. EtOH, eth. | Used as a therapeutic agent in Parkinson's disease. Fully active only after decarboxylation to dopamine. Rapidly oxidised by $O_2$ in aq. soln. and as solid if moist. Store solid in dark. Spectrum, $\lambda_{max}$ 280 nm $\epsilon$ 2650 (pH 1–7). Hydrochloride, M.p. 209d. DL-3,4-Dihydroxyphenylalanine, M.p. 265–80d., solubility 0.36 $H_2O$. |

# 1 Amino acids, amines, amides, peptides, and their derivatives

| Name | Synonyms | Formula | M. wt. | Physical properties |
|---|---|---|---|---|
| 3,5-Diiodo-tyrosine | Iodogorgoic acid; 3,5-Diiodo-4-hydroxy-phenylalanine | HO—⟨ring with I at 3,5⟩—$CH_2 \cdot CH(NH_2) \cdot COOH$ | 433.0 | DL-: cryst.; M.p. 201d. L-: cryst.; M.p. 213d. |
| Dimethylamine | N-Methylmethanamine | $CH_3 \cdot NH \cdot CH_3$ | 45.1 | col. liq. or gas; M.p. −96.0, B.p. 7.4 |
| Dipicolinic acid | 2,6-Pyridine dicarboxylic acid; $\alpha,\alpha'$-Dipicolinic acid | $HOOC$—⟨pyridine ring N⟩—$COOH$ | 167.1; Hydrate, 194.1 | col. needles + $1\frac{1}{2}H_2O$; prisms when sublimed; M.p. 232d. |
| Dopamine | 3-Hydroxytyramine; 3,4-Dihydroxyphen-ethylamine | HO—, HO—⟨ring⟩—$CH_2 \cdot CH_2 \cdot NH_2$ | 153.2; Hydro-chloride, 189.7 | wh. cryst., rapidly darkening on exposure to air. HCl: cryst.; M.p. 241d. |
| $\beta$-Endorphin | C-fragment | Tyr-Gly-Gly-Phe-Met⁵-Thr-Ser-Glu- Lys¹⁰-Ser-Gln-Thr-Pro-Leu-Val¹⁵-Thr- Leu-Phe-Lys²⁰-Asn-Ala-Ile-Ile-Lys- Asn²⁵-Ala-Tyr-Lys-Lys-Gly³⁰-Gln  $\beta$-Endorphin (human) | 3464 | wh. amorph. powder |
| Enkephalin | | Tyr-Gly-Gly-Phe-Met [Met⁵]-Enkephalin | 574 | wh. amorph. powder |
| | | Tyr-Gly-Gly-Phe-Leu [Leu⁵]-Enkephalin | 556 | |
| L-Ergo-thioneine | Thioneine; Thiolhistidine trimethylbetaine | ⟨imidazole ring with SH, N=, NH⟩—$CH_2 \cdot CH \cdot COO^-$ with $^+N(CH_3)_3$ | 229.3; Hydrate, 265.3 | leaflets + $2H_2O$ from $H_2O$; anhyd. needles from EtOH, M.p. 256–7d. |
| Ethanolamine | 2-Aminoethanol; 2-Hydroxyethylamine; Colamine | $H_2N \cdot CH_2 \cdot CH_2 OH$ | 61.1 | visc. hygr. col. liq., $d_4^{20}$ 1.018; M.p. 10.5, B.p. 170.8 |
| ——, cytidine diphosphate derivative | CDP-ethanolamine; cytidine 5′-diphosphate ethanolamine | $H_2N \cdot CH_2 \cdot CH_2 \cdot O—CDP$  CDP = cytidine 5′-diphosphate residue | 446.3 | hygr. powder |
| N-Formimino-L-glutamic acid | N-Iminomethylglutamic acid | $HOOC \cdot CH_2 \cdot CH_2 \cdot CH \cdot COOH$ with $NH \cdot CH=NH$ | 174.2 | col. hygr. cryst.; M.p. 80–87d. |

| $[\alpha]_D^t$ | p$K_a$ at 25°C | Solubility | General remarks |
|---|---|---|---|
| L-, +2.9[20] (c = 5 in 4% HCl) | 2.12 (COOH)<br>5.32 (OH)<br>9.48 (NH$_2$) | DL-: 0.034[25] H$_2$O;<br>s. alkalis.<br>L-: 0.062[25] H$_2$O;<br>s. alkalis; i. EtOH, eth. | Unstable in light, losing iodine. De-iodination occurs during protein hydrolysis, esp. with acid. Spectrum, $\lambda_{max}$ 310 nm $\epsilon$ 5920 in 0.04M-KOH; $\lambda_{max}$ 285 nm $\epsilon$ 2730 in 0.04M-HCl. |
| | 10.92[20]<br>10.63[30]<br>10.35[40] | v.s. H$_2$O; s. EtOH, eth. | Hydrochloride, deliq., M.p. 171, v.s. H$_2$O, s. EtOH, CHCl$_3$, i. eth. |
| | 2.16<br>4.76 | sl. s. H$_2$O;<br>v. sl. s. EtOH | Can be sublimed. Spectrum, $\lambda_{max}$ 270 nm, shoulders at 262.5 nm and 277.5 nm (pH 7–13). Calcium salt, v.s. H$_2$O. |
| | 8.9 (OH gps)<br>10.6 (NH$_2$) | s. H$_2$O.<br>HCl: v.s. H$_2$O;<br>s. MeOH; i. eth. | Neurotransmitter in CNS. Spontaneously oxidizes in aq. soln. at alkaline pHs. Hydrobromide, cryst., M.p. 212. |
| | | | Naturally occurring opioid peptide possessing potent agonist activity at opiate receptor sites. Action antagonized by naloxone. $\beta$-Endorphin has same amino acid sequence as residues 61–91 of $\beta$-lipotropin. $\alpha$-Endorphin is residues 1–16 of $\beta$-endorphin, $\gamma$-endorphin is residues 1–17 and $\delta$-endorphin is residues 1–27; all have opioid activity. 'Endorphin' is used as a generic term for endogenous peptides possessing opioid activity; the endorphins listed here and the enkephalins are the best characterized members of the group. |
| | | | Naturally occurring opioid peptides possessing potent agonist activity at opiate receptor sites. Action antagonized by naloxone. [Met[5]]-Enkephalin has same amino acid sequence as residues 1–5 of the endorphins. Unstable in blood; Tyr is cleaved from N-terminus. The analogue, [D-Ala[2], Met[5]]-enkephalinamide, has greater and longer-lasting pharmacological activity because it is less readily degraded. |
| +115[27.5] (c = 1 in H$_2$O) | | 11.6[20], v.s. hot H$_2$O;<br>sl. s. hot EtOH;<br>i. cold EtOH, CHCl$_3$, benz. | Ergothioneine is a more powerful reducing substance than cysteine and glutathione. Yields trimethylamine and thiolimidazolyl-4-acrylic acid with strong alkali. Spectrum, $\lambda_{max}$ 258 nm $\epsilon$ 16 000 (pH 2–9). PREP. *Vitams Horm.* **17**, 155 (1959); *JCS* **1951**, 2215. |
| | 9.65[20]<br>9.35[30]<br>9.07[40] | $\infty$ H$_2$O, EtOH;<br>0.72 eth.; s. CHCl$_3$;<br>sl. s. benz.<br><br>CDP-ethanolamine:<br>s. H$_2$O | Absorbs CO$_2$ from air. Hydrochloride, deliq. cryst., M.p. 76. |
| −10.3[28] (c = 0.8 in M-HCl) | 2.7<br>4.4<br>11.3 | v.s. H$_2$O; s. MeOH, EtOH; i. eth., acet., CHCl$_3$ | Unstable in aq. soln. at alkaline pHs or when heated; neutral and acid solns. stable. Barium salt, $[\alpha]_D^{20}$ −9.8 (c = 2.5 in H$_2$O). Mercuric salt, i. H$_2$O, EtOH, eth. PREP. *Biochem. Preps.* **5**, 100 (1957). |

# 1 Amino acids, amines, amides, peptides, and their derivatives

| Name | Synonyms | Formula | M. wt. | Physical properties |
|------|----------|---------|--------|---------------------|
| Glutamic acid | 2-Aminoglutaric acid; Glu | $HOOC \cdot CH_2 \cdot CH_2 \cdot CH(NH_2) \cdot COOH$ | 147.1 | DL-: col. cryst.; M.p. 225—7d. L-: col. cryst.; M.p. 247—9d. |
| L-Glutamine | 2-Aminoglutaminic acid; Gln | $H_2N \cdot CO \cdot CH_2 \cdot CH_2 \cdot CH(NH_2) \cdot COOH$ | 146.2 | wh. needles; M.p. 185—6d. |
| L-Glutathione, reduced | L-γ-Glutamyl-L-cysteinylglycine; GSH | $CO \cdot NH \cdot CH \cdot CO \cdot NH \cdot CH_2 \cdot COOH$ $CH_2 \quad CH_2$ $CH_2 \quad SH$ $CH \cdot NH_2$ $COOH$ | 307.3 | cryst.; M.p. 190—2d. |
| ——, oxidized | GSSG | | 612.6 | wh. cryst. powder; M.p. 182—5 |
| Glycine | Aminoacetic acid; Glycocoll; Gly | $H_2N \cdot CH_2 \cdot COOH$ | 75.1 | wh. monocl. cryst., sweet taste; M.p. 292d.; darkens at 232—3 |
| Glycocyamine | Guanidoacetic acid; N-Amidinoglycine; N-(Aminoimino-methyl)glycine | $HN{=}C{\big\langle}^{NH_2}_{NH \cdot CH_2 \cdot COOH}$ | 117.1 | leaflets or needles from $H_2O$; decomp. > 300 |
| Hippuric acid | N-Benzoylglycine | $C_6H_5 \cdot CO \cdot NH \cdot CH_2 \cdot COOH$ | 179.2 | col. rh. cryst.; M.p. 187.5d. |
| Histamine | 1H-Imidazole-4-ethanamine; 4(5)-(2-aminoethyl)imidazole | $CH_2 \cdot CH_2 \cdot NH_2$ (imidazole) | 111.2 | wh. deliq. cryst.; M.p. 83—84, B.p. $209{-}10^{18}$ |
| Histidine | α-Amino-1H-imidazole-4-propanoic acid; His | $CH_2 \cdot CH(NH_2) \cdot COOH$ (imidazole) | 155.2 | cryst.; M.p. 287d. |

| $[\alpha]_D^t$ | $pK_a$ at 25°C | Solubility | General remarks |
|---|---|---|---|
| L-, +31.8[25] (c = 2 in 5M-HCl) +12.0[25] (c = 2 in $H_2O$) | 2.10 4.07 9.47 | DL-: 2.05[25], 11.86[75] $H_2O$; v. sl. s. EtOH, eth. L-: 0.86[25], 5.53[75] $H_2O$; 0.032[25] 75% EtOH; 0.00027[25] EtOH; 0.007[25] MeOH; i. eth. | In aq. soln. forms pyrrolidonecarboxylic acid slowly at room temp., more rapidly at 100°C. Stable to hot mineral acids in presence of carbohydrates. L-Glutamic acid has a meaty taste; the D-isomer is tasteless. Mono-Na L-glutamate, cryst. + $1H_2O$, v.s. $H_2O$, sl. s. EtOH. N-Carbamoyl-L-glutamic acid, M.p. 160. |
| +31.8[25] (c = 2 in M-HCl) +6.3[25] (c = 2 in $H_2O$) | 2.17 9.13 | 3.6[18], 4.25[25] $H_2O$; 0.00046[25] EtOH; 0.0035[27] MeOH; i. eth., $CHCl_3$, ethyl acetate, acet., gl. acetic | Rapidly converted in boiling neutral aq. soln. or in weak acid soln. to the ammonium salt of pyrrolidonecarboxylic acid. |
| −21.3[27] (c = 2 in $H_2O$) | 2.12 (COOH) 3.59 (COOH) 8.75 ($NH_2$) 9.65 (SH) See *Adv. Protein Chem.* **14**, 272 (1959) | s. $H_2O$; i. EtOH, eth. | Solid stable in air over long periods; aq. soln. readily oxidized in air to GSSG. REVIEW. Boyer, *et al.* (eds.), *The Enzymes*, vol. 2, p. 253 (1960). |
| GSSG: −93.9 (c = 1 in $H_2O$) −111.0$_{5461}^{16}$ (c = 1 in $H_2O$) | | GSSG: s. $H_2O$; i. EtOH, eth. | GSSG: Solid binds approx. 2 moles solvent ($H_2O$, EtOH, acet.) per mole GSSG; solvent removed only with some decomp. at high temp. (> 100°C) in v. high vacuum; not removed by lyophilization. |
| | 2.35 9.78 | 25[25], 54.4[75] $H_2O$; 0.043[25] 90% EtOH; 0.0029[25] EtOH; 0.61[20] pyr.; 0.032[25] MeOH; 0.00023[25] acet. | Acetylglycine, M.p. 206. |
| | 2.82 | 0.45[15] $H_2O$; v. sl. s. EtOH, eth. | Spectrum, $\lambda_{max}$ 214 nm $\epsilon$ 310 (in BuOH/EtOH/$H_2O$, 1:1:2, pH 8). |
| | 3.62 | 0.37[25] $H_2O$; sl. s. EtOH, eth.; 0.11[20] $CHCl_3$; i. benz., pet. eth. | Spectrum, $\lambda_{max}$ 230 nm $\epsilon$ 10 300. |
| | 6.04 (imidazole) 9.75 ($NH_2$) | s. $H_2O$, EtOH, hot $CHCl_3$; i. eth. | Potent vasodilator found in normal tissues and blood; causes contraction of other smooth muscles, e.g. gut and bronchi, stimulates gastric secretion, stimulates sensory nerve endings causing itching and pain. Dihydrochloride, M.p. 244–6, s. $H_2O$, MeOH, EtOH, i. eth., 0.005 hot $CHCl_3$. |
| L-, +11.8[25] (c = 2 in 5M-HCl) −38.5[25] (c = 2 in $H_2O$) | 1.80 (COOH) 6.04 (imidazole) 9.33 ($NH_2$) | DL-: s. $H_2O$; i. EtOH, eth., acet., $CHCl_3$ L-: 4.16[25] $H_2O$; v. sl. s. EtOH; i. eth., acet. | Losses occur during protein hydrolysis. Readily racemized on heating with $H_2SO_4$. L-Histidine dihydrochloride, cryst., M.p. 245–6, v.s. $H_2O$, i. EtOH, eth. |

| Name | Synonyms | Formula | M. wt. | Physical properties |
|---|---|---|---|---|
| Histidinol dihydro-chloride | β-Amino-1H-imidazole-4-propanol; 4-(2-Amino-3-hydroxypropyl)-imidazole | $CH_2 \cdot CH(NH_2) \cdot CH_2OH$ (imidazole ring) ·2HCl | 214.1; Free base, 141.2 | DL-: rh. plates; M.p. 193—5. L-: M.p. 198—9 |
| Homocysteine | 2-Amino-4-mercaptobutanoic acid | $HS \cdot CH_2 \cdot CH_2 \cdot CH(NH_2) \cdot COOH$ | 135.2 | cryst.; DL-: M.p. 263—5d. |
| Homocystine | 4,4'-Dithiobis(2-amino-butanoic acid) | $S \cdot CH_2 \cdot CH_2 \cdot CH(NH_2) \cdot COOH$ <br> $S \cdot CH_2 \cdot CH_2 \cdot CH(NH_2) \cdot COOH$ | 268.4 | cryst.; DL-, decomp. 263—5; L-, M.p. 282—3d. |
| Homoserine | 2-Amino-4-hydroxybutanoic acid; γ-Hydroxybutyrine | $HOCH_2 \cdot CH_2 \cdot CH(NH_2) \cdot COOH$ | 119.1 | cryst.; M.p. DL-, 186—7d., L-, 203d. |
| 3-Hydroxy-anthranilic acid | 2-Amino-3-hydroxy-benzoic acid | COOH, NH₂, OH | 153.1 | leaflets from $H_2O$; wh. needles after sublimation; M.p. 250—2d. (230—65) |
| 5-Hydroxy-indoleacetic acid | 5-Hydroxy-1H-indole-3-acetic acid; 5-Hydroxy-(hetero)auxin | HO— (indole) —$CH_2 \cdot COOH$ | 191.2 | solid; M.p. 160—6 |
| 3-Hydroxy-kynurenine | 3-(3-Hydroxyanthraniloyl)-alanine; α,2-Diamino-3-hydroxy-γ-oxobenzene-butanoic acid | $CO \cdot CH_2 \cdot CH(NH_2) \cdot COOH$, NH₂, OH | 224.2; Hydrate, 242.2 | DL-: M.p. 223d. L-: golden-yellow needles + 1$H_2O$; M.p. 180d. |
| 5-Hydroxy-lysine | δ-Hydroxylysine; 2,6-Diamino-5-hydroxy-hexanoic acid; Hyl | $CH_2 \cdot NH_2$ <br> $HC \cdot OH$ <br> $CH_2$ <br> $CH_2$ <br> $HC \cdot NH_2$ <br> COOH <br> 5-Hydroxy-L-lysine; erythro-5-Hydroxy-Lₛ-lysine    $CH_2 \cdot NH_2$ <br> $HO \cdot CH$ <br> $CH_2$ <br> $CH_2$ <br> $HC \cdot NH_2$ <br> COOH <br> Allo-5-hydroxy-L-lysine; threo-5-Hydroxy-Lₛ-lysine | 162.2; Hydro-chloride, 198.6 | Hydrochloride: wh. cryst.; M.p., DL-, 233—4d.; allo-DL-, 239—41d.; L-, 225d. |

| $[\alpha]_D^t$ | $pK_a$ at 25°C | Solubility | General remarks |
|---|---|---|---|
| L-, $-3.7^{18}$ (c = 10 in $H_2O$) D-, $+3.4^{18}$ (c = 10 in $H_2O$) | | s. $H_2O$; sl. s. EtOH, MeOH; i. eth. | PREP. Biochem. Preps. **4**, 46 (1955); BBA **273**, 18 (1972). |
| | 2.22 (COOH) 8.87 10.86 | s. $H_2O$; sl. s. EtOH; i. eth. | Readily oxidized to homocystine; can only be obtained pure in absence of $O_2$. Forms thiolactone.HCl (in a few minutes) in hot 20% HCl, JBC **112**, 149 (1935–6); thiolactone hydrolysed to homocysteine at pH 8.3. Thiolactone HCl, cryst., M.p. DL- 197–201, L- $[\alpha]_D^{26} + 21.5$ (c = 1 in $H_2O$). S-Benzyl deriv., cryst., M.p. 240–4, L- $[\alpha]_D^{26} + 27.2$ (c = 1–2 in 5M-HCl), sl. s. $H_2O$, s. mineral acids, i. MeOH, EtOH. PREP. Biochem. Preps. **5**, 93 (1957). |
| L-, $+78^{25}$ (c = 1–2 in 5M-HCl) $-16.0^{21}$ (c = 0.06 in $H_2O$) | 1.59 (COOH) 2.54 (COOH) 8.52 ($NH_2$) 9.44 ($NH_2$) | DL-: $0.02^{25}$ $H_2O$; s. mineral acids, alkalis | Preparations may contain meso-compound. PREP. Biochem. Preps. **5**, 93 (1957). |
| L-, $+18.3^{26}$ (c = 2 in 2M-HCl) $-8.8^{25}$ (c = 1–2 in $H_2O$) (freshly prepared solutions) | 2.71 9.62 | DL-: $125^{30}$ $H_2O$; v. sl. s. EtOH, eth. L-: $110^{30}$ $H_2O$; i. EtOH | Stable in neutral and alkaline aq. solns., but at acid pH is converted to a $\gamma$-lactone and/or a diketopiperazine, with an accompanying fall in optical rotation. L-$\gamma$-Lactone hydrochloride, cryst., $[\alpha]_D^{26} - 27.0$ (c = 5 in $H_2O$). |
| | | s. hot $H_2O$, alkalis; sl. s. cold $H_2O$, EtOH; i. eth. | Sublimes under reduced pressure. Spectrum, $\lambda_{max}$ ($\epsilon$) 298 nm (3000) and 235 nm (6400) in 0.1M-HCl, $\lambda_{max}$ 315–20 nm at pH 7, Z. Naturf. **4b**, 327 (1949). Hydrochloride, M.p. 227. |
| | | s. $H_2O$, EtOH, Et acetate; sl. s. eth. | Spectrum, $\lambda_{max}$ ($\epsilon$) 277 nm (5200) and 299 nm (7200) (in MeOH). |
| L-, $-34^{27}$ (c = 0.17 in $H_2O$) $+8.5^{27}$ (c = 0.17 in 0.0152 M-HCl) | | s. hot $H_2O$, acids; sl. s. cold $H_2O$, MeOH, EtOH | Soln. oxidizes spontaneously in air. Aq. soln. colourless at acid pH, yellow in alkali. Spectrum, $\lambda_{max}$ ($\epsilon$) 368 nm (4050), 267 nm (7630), 228 nm (19 000) at pH 7. Hydrobromide, DL-, s. $H_2O$, M.p. 233 d. Sulphate, DL-, M.p. 175. PREP. Biochem. Preps. **7**, 62 (1960); **9**, 79 (1962). |
| L-, $+17.8^{25}$ (c = 2 free base in 5M-HCl) $+9.2^{25}$ (c = 2 free base in $H_2O$) allo-L-, $+31.4^{25}$ (c = 2 free base in 5M-HCl) $+10.9^{25}$ (c = 2 free base in $H_2O$) | L-, $2.13^{38}$ $8.85^{25}$ $9.83^{25}$ | Normal and allo isomers: s. $H_2O$; i. MeOH, EtOH, acet., eth. | The normal isomer, which occurs in collagen and related proteins, is erythro-5-hydroxy-$L_s$-lysine. Allo-5-hydroxylysine is the threo-isomer. Most methods of synthesis yield initially a mixture of DL- and allo-DL- isomers; the normal and allo isomers can be separated by ion exchange, JBC **213**, 249 (1955). Normal 5-hydroxy-L-lysine isomerizes in 6M-HCl at 120°C to allo-5-hydroxy-D-lysine, 10% in 12 hr, 25% in 24 hr, so that isolated material is partially isomerized and gives values of $[\alpha]_D^{25}$ from $+ 14.9$ to $- 4.5$ for different preparations. PREP. of optical isomers: Biochem. Preps. **8**, 55, 62 (1961); Bull. Chem. Soc. Japan **35**, 2006 (1962). |

# 1 Amino acids, amines, amides, peptides, and their derivatives

| Name | Synonyms | Formula | M. wt. | Physical properties |
|---|---|---|---|---|
| 4-Hydroxyproline | 4-Hydroxy-2-pyrrolidine-carboxylic acid; Hyp | 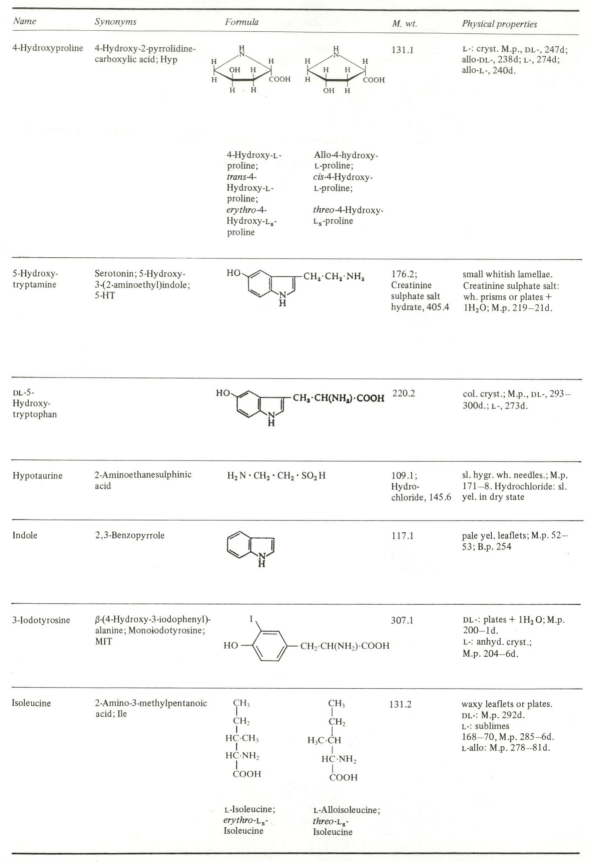 4-Hydroxy-L-proline; *trans*-4-Hydroxy-L-proline; *erythro*-4-Hydroxy-L$_s$-proline    Allo-4-hydroxy-L-proline; *cis*-4-Hydroxy-L-proline; *threo*-4-Hydroxy-L$_s$-proline | 131.1 | L-: cryst. M.p., DL-, 247d; allo-DL-, 238d; L-, 274d; allo-L-, 240d. |
| 5-Hydroxy-tryptamine | Serotonin; 5-Hydroxy-3-(2-aminoethyl)indole; 5-HT | HO—[indole]—$CH_2 \cdot CH_2 \cdot NH_2$ | 176.2; Creatinine sulphate salt hydrate, 405.4 | small whitish lamellae. Creatinine sulphate salt: wh. prisms or plates + $1H_2O$; M.p. 219—21d. |
| DL-5-Hydroxy-tryptophan | | HO—[indole]—$CH_2 \cdot CH(NH_2) \cdot COOH$ | 220.2 | col. cryst.; M.p., DL-, 293—300d.; L-, 273d. |
| Hypotaurine | 2-Aminoethanesulphinic acid | $H_2N \cdot CH_2 \cdot CH_2 \cdot SO_2H$ | 109.1; Hydro-chloride, 145.6 | sl. hygr. wh. needles.; M.p. 171—8. Hydrochloride: sl. yel. in dry state |
| Indole | 2,3-Benzopyrrole | [indole structure] | 117.1 | pale yel. leaflets; M.p. 52—53; B.p. 254 |
| 3-Iodotyrosine | β-(4-Hydroxy-3-iodophenyl)-alanine; Monoiodotyrosine; MIT | [structure] HO—[ring]—$CH_2 \cdot CH(NH_2) \cdot COOH$ | 307.1 | DL-: plates + $1H_2O$; M.p. 200—1d. L-: anhyd. cryst.; M.p. 204—6d. |
| Isoleucine | 2-Amino-3-methylpentanoic acid; Ile | $CH_3$—$CH_2$—$HC \cdot CH_3$—$HC \cdot NH_2$—$COOH$    $CH_3$—$CH_2$—$H_3C \cdot CH$—$HC \cdot NH_2$—$COOH$    L-Isoleucine; *erythro*-L$_s$-Isoleucine    L-Alloisoleucine; *threo*-L$_s$-Isoleucine | 131.2 | waxy leaflets or plates. DL-: M.p. 292d. L-: sublimes 168—70, M.p. 285—6d. L-allo: M.p. 278—81d. |

| $[\alpha]_D^t$ | $pK_a$ at 25°C | Solubility | General remarks |
|---|---|---|---|
| L-, $-50.5^{25}$ (c = 2 in 5M-HCl) $-76.0^{25}$ (c = 2 in $H_2O$) allo-L-, $-18.8^{25}$ (c = 2 in 5M-HCl) $-59.5^{25}$ (c = 2 in $H_2O$) | L-, 1.82 9.66 | DL- and allo-DL: s. $H_2O$; v. sl. s. EtOH; i. eth. L-: $36.1^{25}$, $51.7^{65}$ $H_2O$; v. sl. s. EtOH; i. eth. | Copper salt: DL-, i. $H_2O$; allo-DL-, s. $H_2O$, i. EtOH; normal and allo isomers may be separated by crystallization of the copper salt. PREP. of optical isomers, *JCS* **1945**, 429; *JBC* **195**, 383 (1952); *Biochem. Preps.* **8**, 114 (1961). |
| | 9.8 ($NH_2$) 11.1 (OH) | Creatinine sulphate salt: $2^{27}$, $10^{100}$ $H_2O$; s. gl. acetic; sl. s. MeOH, 95% EtOH; i. EtOH, acet., pyr., eth., benz., $CHCl_3$ | Pharmacologically active substance which stimulates or inhibits a variety of smooth muscles and nerves. Effects, which are chiefly on cardiovascular, respiratory and gastrointestinal systems, vary widely in different species and between individuals. Creatinine sulphate salt, soln. stable at all pHs under anaerobic conditions, oxidizes readily in air esp. at alkaline pHs; at neutral pH, soln. stable several hours at room temp. Spectrum, $\lambda_{max}$ 275 and 296 nm at pH 3.5, 275 and 322 nm at pH 11.6, $\epsilon_{275}$ 5800 at pH 7. Hydrochloride, M.p. 167–8, hygr., s. $H_2O$, unstable at room temp., photolabile. |
| L-, $-32.5^{22}$ (c = 1 in $H_2O$) $+16.0^{22}$ (c = 1 in 4M-HCl) | | $1^5$, $5.5^{100}$ $H_2O$ | Store solid under $N_2$; decomposes slowly in air. Acid soln. stable for a year or more at $-10$°C in air. At higher temps. and neutral or alkaline pH, increasingly sensitive to $O_2$. Decomp. avoided by inert atmosphere, aq. soln. may be autoclaved in absence of $O_2$. Spectrum, $\lambda_{max}$ 278 nm $\epsilon$ 5560, inflexions at 291 and 299 nm at pH 6. At pH 11, $\lambda_{max}$ 278 and 324 nm. |
| | 2.16 9.56 | v.s. $H_2O$, EtOH, acet. | Zn and Ba salts are hygr. and s. organic solvents. PREP. *Biochem. Preps.* **10**, 72 (1963). |
| | | v.s. EtOH, eth.; s. hot $H_2O$, benz., pet. eth. | Intense faecal odour unless highly purified. $\beta$-Methylene group highly reactive, coupling readily with aldehydes and phenols. |
| L-, $-4.4^{20}$ (c = 5 in M-HCl) | 2.2 (COOH) 8.7 (OH) 9.1 ($NH_2$) | sl. s. cold $H_2O$; $6.7^{100}$ $H_2O$ | Unstable in light, losing iodine. |
| L-, $+39.5^{25}$ (c = 1 in 5M-HCl) $+12.4^{25}$ (c = 1 in $H_2O$) L-allo: $+39.6^{25}$ (c = 1 in 5M-HCl) $+15.9^{25}$ (c = 1 in $H_2O$) | L-: 2.32 9.76 L-allo: 2.27 9.62 | DL-: $2.23^{25}$, $4.61^{75}$ $H_2O$; s. hot EtOH, hot gl. acetic; i. eth. L-: $4.12^{25}$, $6.08^{75}$ $H_2O$; $0.072^{20}$ EtOH; s. hot gl. acetic; i. eth. L-allo: $2.9^{20}$ $H_2O$; $0.1^{20}$ EtOH; i. eth. | Stable to hot mineral acid in the presence of carbohydrate. Commercial preparations, especially 'DL-isoleucine', may contain allo isomers. Chromatographic separation of normal and allo isomers, *JBC* **207**, 77 (1954). PREP. of optical isomers: *Biochem. Preps.* **3**, 84 (1953). |

# 1 Amino acids, amines, amides, peptides, and their derivatives

| Name | Synonyms | Formula | M. wt. | Physical properties |
|------|----------|---------|--------|---------------------|
| Kynurenic acid | 4-Hydroxy-2-quinoline-carboxylic acid; 4-Hydroxy-quinaldic acid | (structure: quinoline with OH and N–COOH) | 189.2 | yel. needles; lose $H_2O$ 140–5, decomp. 282–3 |
| Kynurenine | 3-Anthraniloylalanine; $\alpha$,2-Diamino-$\gamma$-oxobenzene-butanoic acid | (structure: benzene with $CO \cdot CH_2 \cdot CH(NH_2) \cdot COOH$ and $NH_2$) | 208.2; Hydrate, 214.2; Sulphate, 306.3; Sulphate hydrate, 324.3 | leaflets $+ \frac{1}{3}H_2O$ from $H_2O$; anhyd. needles from $H_2O$/EtOH. Sulphate, col. needles $+ 1H_2O$ from aq. solvents; M.p. DL-, 218d., Sulphate 173; L-, 191d., Sulphate 190 (178–94) |
| L-Lanthionine | Bis(2-amino-2-carboxyethyl)-sulphide; S-(2-Amino-2-carboxy-ethyl)cysteine | $S \big\langle \begin{array}{l} CH_2 \cdot CH(NH_2) \cdot COOH \\ CH_2 \cdot CH(NH_2) \cdot COOH \end{array}$ | 208.2 | hex. plates; decomp. 293–5. |
| Leucine | 2-Amino-4-methylpentanoic acid; Leu | $\begin{array}{l} CH_3 \\ CH_3 \end{array}\!\!\big\rangle CH \cdot CH_2 \cdot CH(NH_2) \cdot COOH$ | 131.2 | col. leaflets; sublimes 145–8; M.p. 293–5d. |
| Lysine | 2,6-Diaminohexanoic acid; Lys | $H_2N \cdot CH_2 \cdot (CH_2)_3 \cdot CH(NH_2) \cdot COOH$ | 146.2; Mono-HCl, 182.7; Di-HCl, 219.1 | needles or plates, M.p. L-, 224d. Mono-HCl: cryst., M.p. 263–4. Di-HCl: cryst., M.p. DL-, 187–9, L-, 192–3. |
| Methionine | 2-Amino-4-(methylthio)-butanoic acid; Met | $CH_3 \cdot S \cdot CH_2 \cdot CH_2 \cdot CH(NH_2) \cdot COOH$ | 149.2 | plates; M.p. 281d. |
| Methionine sulphone | 2-Amino-4-methyl-sulphonylbutanoic acid | $CH_3 \cdot SO_2 \cdot CH_2 \cdot CH_2 \cdot CH(NH_2) \cdot COOH$ | 181.2 | cryst.; M.p. DL-, 248–50d., L-, 257–8d. |
| Methionine sulphoxide | 2-Amino-4-methyl-sulphinylbutanoic acid | $CH_3 \cdot SO \cdot CH_2 \cdot CH_2 \cdot CH(NH_2) \cdot COOH$ | 165.2 | wh. powder; decomp. 225–31 (mixture of all four isomers) |

| $[\alpha]_D^t$ | $pK_a$ at 25°C | Solubility | General remarks |
|---|---|---|---|
| | | $0.9^{100}$ $H_2O$; s. hot EtOH, alkalis; sl. s. eth., mineral acids, 50% aq. acetic | Extremely difficult to obtain pure. Spectrum, $\lambda_{max}$ ($\epsilon$) 332 nm (9800) and 344 nm (7920) at pH 7, *BJ* **52**, 8 (1952). |
| L-, $-30.5^{25}$ (c = 1 in $H_2O$) $+10.1^{25}$ (c = 1 anhyd. sulphate in $H_2O$) | | sl. s. $H_2O$ (L > DL). Sulphate: s. $H_2O$; sl. s. EtOH. | Spectrum, $\lambda_{max}$ ($\epsilon$) 360 nm (4500) 257 nm (7500) 230 nm (18 900) at pH 7, little change in range pH 2–12. PREP. *Biochem. Preps.* **3**, 108 (1953); *JACS* **76**, 1708 (1954). $N'$-Formylkynurenine, M.p. 162, spectrum $\lambda_{max}$ ($\epsilon$) 260 nm (10 980) 321 nm (3750) at pH 7, SYN. *JCS 1952*, 137, ISOL. *BBA* **31**, 301 (1959). |
| $+8.6^{22}$ (c = 5 in 2.4M-NaOH) | | $0.15^{25}$ $H_2O$; i. EtOH, eth.; s. acids, alkalis | *meso*-Lanthionine, M.p. 306 (283–306d.), triangular plates, solubility $0.022^{25}$ $H_2O$, s. acids, alkalis, i. EtOH, eth., SYN. *JBC* **140**, 767 (1941), *Ber.* **94**, 2157 (1961), ISOL. *JBC* **144**, 87 (1942). |
| L-, $+16.0^{25}$ (c = 2.0 in 5M-HCl) $-11.0^{25}$ (c = 2.0 in $H_2O$) | 2.33 9.74 | DL-: $0.99^{25}$, $2.28^{75}$ $H_2O$; $0.13^{25}$ 90% EtOH; i. EtOH, eth. L-: $2.43^{25}$, $3.82^{75}$ $H_2O$; $0.017^{25}$ EtOH; i. eth. | Stable to hot mineral acids in the presence of carbohydrates. |
| L-, $+25.9^{25}$ (c = 2.0 in 5M-HCl) $+13.5^{25}$ (c = 2.0 in $H_2O$) | 2.16 9.06 10.54 ($\epsilon$-$NH_2$) | DL- and L-: v.s. $H_2O$; v. sl. s. EtOH; i. eth. Mono-HCl, L-: v.s. $H_2O$; s. MeOH Di-HCl, L-: v.s. $H_2O$; s. MeOH; i. EtOH | |
| L-, $+23.2^{25}$ (c = 0.5–2.0 in 5M-HCl) $-10.0^{25}$ (c = 0.5–2.0 in $H_2O$) | 2.13 9.28 | DL-: $3.38^{25}$, $10.52^{75}$ $H_2O$; s. dil. acids, alkalis. L-: s. $H_2O$; i. EtOH, eth. | Losses occur during hydrolysis of protein in presence of carbohydrate, and by oxidation. Crystals are somewhat water-repellant. |
| L-, $+13.5^{28}$ (c = 2.1 in $H_2O$) $+30.3^{28}$ (c = 2.1 in M-HCl) | | s. $H_2O$ (< sulph-oxide, > methionine); i. 95% EtOH | More stable than the sulphoxide. |
| L $l$-, $-71.6^{24-26}$ (c = 0.5–2.0 in $H_2O$) $-57.6^{24-26}$ (c = 0.5–2.0 in 5M-HCl) L $d$-, $+99.0^{24-26}$ (c = 0.5–2.0 in $H_2O$) $+127.2^{24-26}$ (c = 0.5–2.0 in 5M-HCl) | | > $66^{25}$ $H_2O$; sl. s. EtOH; i. acet., eth. | Stable in aq. soln. Four possible stereoisomers, as S atom forms asymmetric centre. These isomers are sometimes written as L $l$-, L $d$-, D $l$-, D $d$-. |

# 1 Amino acids, amines, amides, peptides, and their derivatives

| Name | Synonyms | Formula | M. wt. | Physical properties |
|------|----------|---------|--------|---------------------|
| Methylamine | Methanamine; Amino-methane | $CH_3NH_2$ | 31.1; Hydro-chloride, 67.5 | col. gas; M.p. $-93.5$, B.p. $-6.3$ |
| L-1-Methyl-histidine | N-Methylimidazole-5-alanine; $\alpha$-Amino-$\beta$-(1-methyl-5-imidazole)-propanoic acid | (ring structure) $-CH_2 \cdot CH(NH_2) \cdot COOH$ ; $N \diagdown N \cdot CH_3$ | 169.2; Hydrate, 187.2 | needles + $1H_2O$; loses $H_2O$ in vacuo and at 100; M.p. 248–9 |
| L-3-Methyl-histidine | 1-Methylimidazole-4-alanine; $\alpha$-Amino-$\beta$-(1-methyl-4-imidazole)-propanoic acid | (ring structure) $-CH_2 \cdot CH(NH_2) \cdot COOH$ ; $H_3C \cdot N \diagdown N$ | 169.2 | |
| $N^6$-Methyl-L-lysine | $\epsilon$-N-Methyl-L-lysine | $CH_3 \cdot NH \cdot (CH_2)_4 \cdot CH(NH_2) \cdot COOH$ | 160.2; Anhyd. Hydro-chloride, 196.7 | Hydrochloride: cryst.; M.p. 237–9d. |
| Methyl-methionine sulphonium bromide | Methionine methyl sulph-onium bromide; (3-Amino-3-carboxypropyl)dimethyl-sulphonium bromide | $(CH_3)_2 \cdot \overset{+}{S} \cdot CH_2 \cdot CH_2 \cdot CH(NH_2) \cdot COOH$ $Br^-$ | Free cation, 163.2; Chloride, 199.7; Bromide, 244.2 | Bromide: white needles or platelets; M.p. DL-, 139–41d., L-, 139d. |
| Noradrenaline | Arterenol; Norepinephrine; 1-(3,4-Dihydroxyphenyl)-2-aminoethanol; 4-(2-Amino-1-hydroxyethyl)-1,2-benzenediol | $HO-$(ring)$-CH(OH) \cdot CH_2 \cdot NH_2$ ; $HO-$ | 169.2; Hydro-chloride, 205.6 | col. cryst.; M.p. DL-, 188–91; D-, 215–17. |
| Norleucine | 2-Aminohexanoic acid; Glycoleucine | $CH_3 \cdot (CH_2)_3 \cdot CH(NH_2) \cdot COOH$ | 131.2 | shiny leaflets; M.p. DL-, 295d.; L-, 301d. |
| Norvaline | 2-Aminopentanoic acid | $CH_3 \cdot CH_2 \cdot CH_2 \cdot CH(NH_2) \cdot COOH$ | 117.1 | leaflets or needles; M.p. DL-, 303 (sealed tube); L-, 305d. (sealed tube) |
| Ornithine | 2,5-Diaminopentanoic acid | $H_2N \cdot CH_2 \cdot CH_2 \cdot CH_2 \cdot CH(NH_2) \cdot COOH$ | 132.2; Mono-HCl, 168.6; Di-HCl, 205.1 | syrup., cryst. only with difficulty; M.p. DL-, 195: L-, 226–7. Mono-HCl: wh. granular solid; M.p. L-, 233d. Di-HCl, L-: M.p. 190–203. |
| Oxytocin | Oxytocic hormone | CyS → Tyr → Ile → Gln → Asn → CyS— ; $H_2N$—Gly ← Leu ← Pro ← | 1007 | wh. amorph. powder |

| $[\alpha]_D^t$ | $pK_a$ at 25°C | Solubility | General remarks |
|---|---|---|---|
| | $10.79^{20}$ $10.47^{30}$ $10.16^{40}$ | $1153.9^{12.5}$ ml gas per ml $H_2O$; v. s. MeOH, EtOH; ∞ eth. | Methylamine hydrochloride, deliq. leaflets from EtOH, M.p. 227–8, B.p. $230^{15}$, v.s. $H_2O$, $23^{78}$ EtOH, i. eth., acet., $CHCl_3$. |
| $-25.8^{18}$ (c = 3.9 in $H_2O$) | 1.69 (COOH) 6.48 (imidazole) 8.85 ($NH_2$) | $20^{25}$ $H_2O$ | Appears to be some racemization during synthesis. Pauly reaction positive. PREP. *JACS* **79**, 2249 (1957). |
| $-26.5^{26}$ (c = 2.1 in $H_2O$) | 1.92 6.56 8.73 | s. $H_2O$ | Appears to be some racemization during synthesis. Pauly reaction negative. Hydrochloride, $[\alpha]_D^{27} + 13.5$ (c = 1.9 in M-HCl). PREP. *JBC* **206**, 825 (1954); *JACS* **79**, 2249 (1957). |
| $+21.9^{23}$ (c = 2 in 6M-HCl) | | Hydrochloride: s. $H_2O$, mineral acids, EtOH; v. sl. s. pyr.; i. benz. | PREP. *Biochem. Preps.* **11**, 80 (1966); *Can. J. Chem.* **42**, 2043 (1964). |
| | | s. $H_2O$; $0.439^{25}$ MeOH; $0.012^{25}$ EtOH; i. eth., acet. | Dry bromide slowly decomp. especially in light. Store cold, dry and protected from light. The free base and its salt decomp. to homoserine, methionine sulphoxide, and dimethyl sulphide in boiling aq. soln. especially in presence of alkalis. Chloride, DL-, M.p. 134–8d. Iodide, DL-, M.p. 150d. |
| D-, $-37.3^{25}$ (c = 5 in $H_2O$ + 1 equiv. HCl) | 8.64 (NH) 9.70 (OH) | s. mineral acids, alkalis; sl. s. $H_2O$, MeOH, EtOH, eth. | Sympathomimetic action. Major adrenergic effector at postganglionic effector junctions. Pressor effect, mainly due to peripheral vasoconstriction. Natural compd. has D-configuration relative to mandelic acid. Aq. solns. slowly racemize and oxidize. Stability maximal at about pH 4. Solns. may be autoclaved under anaerobic conditions at pH 3.6. Hydrochloride, DL-, M.p. 141; D-, M.p. 145–7, s. $H_2O$, $[\alpha]_D^{25} -40$ (c = 6 in $H_2O$). Bitartrate, D-, cryst. + $1H_2O$, M.p. 102–4, s. $H_2O$. |
| L-, $+24.5^{25}$ (c = 1–2 in 5M-HCl) $+4.7^{25}$ (c = 1–2 in $H_2O$) | 2.34 9.83 | DL-: $1.15^{25}$, $5.23^{100}$ $H_2O$; $0.11^{25}$ MeOH; $0.014^{25}$ EtOH; L-: $1.5^{25}$ $H_2O$; i. EtOH | Sublimes. Hydrochloride, L-: M.p. 280–5 (sublimes). |
| L-, $+24.1^{25}$ (c = 1–2 in 5M-HCl) $+7.0^{25}$ (c = 1–2 in $H_2O$) | 2.32 9.81 | DL- and L-: $10.7^{15}$ $H_2O$; sl. s. EtOH; i. acet., $CHCl_3$, eth. | Hydrochloride, L-: M.p. 223–4. |
| L-, $+28.4^{25}$ (c = 2.0 in 5M-HCl) $+12.1^{25}$ (c = 2.0 in $H_2O$) Di-HCl, L-, $+16.5^{25}$ (c = 4 in $H_2O$) | 1.71 (COOH) 8.69 ($\alpha$-$NH_2$) 10.76 ($\delta$-$NH_2$) | DL- and L-: v.s. $H_2O$, EtOH; sl. s. eth. Mono-HCl: s. $H_2O$, acids, alkalis; i. MeOH, EtOH, eth. Di-HCl: s. $H_2O$; v.s. MeOH, EtOH. | |
| $-26.2^{22}$ (c = 0.53 in $H_2O$) | Isoelectric point, 7.7 | s. $H_2O$, BuOH; sl. s. acet. | Hormone of posterior pituitary. Principal actions: causes contraction of uterine muscle, ejection of milk from lactating mammary gland and, in birds, lowering of blood pressure. Pure material contains *ca.* 500 units/mg. Stable in acid, unstable in alkali. Activity destroyed by reducing agents, e.g. thioglycollate. |

# 1 Amino acids, amines, amides, peptides, and their derivatives

| Name | Synonyms | Formula | M. wt. | Physical properties |
|---|---|---|---|---|
| Phenylalanine | 2-Amino-3-phenylpropanoic acid; Phe | $C_6H_5$—$CH_2 \cdot CH(NH_2) \cdot COOH$ | 165.2 | leaflets or needles; sublimes *in vacuo*; M.p. DL-, 271–3d.; L-, 283–4d. |
| Picolinic acid | 2-Pyridinecarboxylic acid | pyridine—COOH (2-position) | 123.1 | needles; M.p. 136 |
| L-Pipecolic acid | Pipecolinic acid; 2-Piperidinecarboxylic acid; Homoproline | piperidine ring, $CH \cdot COOH$ | 129.2 | needles or plates; sublimes *in vacuo* at 200; M.p. 270d. |
| Proline | 2-Pyrrolidinecarboxylic acid; Pro | pyrrolidine ring, $CH \cdot COOH$ | 115.1 | hygr. prisms or needles; M.p. DL-, 213d.; L-, 220–2d. |
| Propionyl-choline chloride | | $(CH_3)_3\overset{+}{N} \cdot CH_2 \cdot CH_2 \cdot O \cdot CO \cdot CH_2 \cdot CH_3$  $Cl^-$ | 195.7 | hygr. |
| Putrescine | 1,4-Butanediamine; Tetramethylenediamine | $H_2N \cdot CH_2 \cdot CH_2 \cdot CH_2 \cdot CH_2 \cdot NH_2$ | 88.2; Dihydrochloride, 161.1 | col. leaflets melting to col. liq., $d_4^{25}$ 0.877; M.p. 27–8, B.p. 158–60. |
| L-2-Pyrrolidone-5-carboxylic acid | Glutaminic acid; Pyroglutamic acid; 5-Oxo-2-pyrrolidinecarboxylic acid; 5-Oxoproline | pyrrolidinone ring, $CH \cdot COOH$ | 129.1 | col. cryst.; M.p. 162–3. |
| Quinolinic acid | Pyridine-2,3-dicarboxylic acid | pyridine—COOH, COOH (2,3-positions) | 167.1 | prisms; M.p. 190d. (rapid heating). |
| Sarcosine | *N*-Methylglycine | $CH_3 \cdot NH \cdot CH_2 \cdot COOH$ | 89.1 | deliq. col. cryst; slightly sweet taste; M.p. 212d. |
| Serine | 2-Amino-3-hydroxypropanoic acid; β-Hydroxyalanine; Ser | $D_s$–Serine: COOH / HC·NH$_2$ / CH$_2$OH  $L_s$–Serine: COOH / H$_2$N·CH / CH$_2$OH | 105.1 | prisms or plates; sweet taste; M.p. DL-, 246d.; L-, 228d. |

| $[\alpha]_D^t$ | $pK_a$ at 25°C | Solubility | General remarks |
|---|---|---|---|
| L-, $-4.47^{25}$ (c = 1–2 in 5M-HCl) $-34.5^{25}$ (c = 1–2 in $H_2O$) | 2.20 9.31 | DL-: $1.42^{25}$, $3.71^{75}$ $H_2O$; sl. s. EtOH; i. eth. L-: $2.96^{25}$, $6.62^{75}$ $H_2O$; v. sl. s. MeOH, EtOH; i. eth. | Unstable to alkali; 75% destroyed in 5 hr at 110–15°C in 5M-NaOH. Spectrum, $\lambda_{max}$ 257.5 nm, $\epsilon$ 195 in 0.1M-HCl, little change with pH; spectrum contains several minor peaks between 240 and 270 nm, see *Adv. Protein Chem.* **7**, 319 (1952). |
| | 1.07 5.25 | v.s. gl. acetic; s. $H_2O$, MeOH; $5.44^{25}$ EtOH; sl. s. benz.; i. eth., $CHCl_3$ | Sublimes. Hydrochloride, sl. s. EtOH, i. eth., M.p. 225–30d. (210–12, slow heating). |
| $-25.4^{18}$ (c = 5 in $H_2O$) $-13.3^{25}$ (c = 2 in 5M-HCl) | 2.28 10.72 | v.s. $H_2O$; s. MeOH; sl. s. EtOH; v. sl. s. acet.; i.eth. | Monohydrochloride, M.p. 258–9, v.s. $H_2O$, sl. s. EtOH, i. eth., $[\alpha]_D^{23}$ − 10.5 (c = 9.8 in $H_2O$). DL-Pipecolic acid, M.p. 264 (258–80); monohydrochloride, M.p. 257–64. PREP. DL- and L-: *Meth. Enzymol.* **17B**, 174 (1971). |
| L-, $-60.4^{25}$ (c = 1–2 in 5M-HCl) $-86.2^{25}$ (c = 1–2 in $H_2O$) | 1.95 10.64 | DL-: s. $H_2O$, EtOH; sl. s. $CHCl_3$, acet., benz.; i. eth. L-: $162.3^{25}$, $239^{65}$ $H_2O$; $67^{19}$ EtOH; i. eth. | Monohydrochloride: M.p., DL-, 159; L-, 115. |
| | | s. $H_2O$, EtOH; i. eth. | Substrate for pseudocholinesterase, hydrolysed much more slowly by acetylcholinesterase. Rapidly hydrolysed in boiling acids. Unstable in soln. Perchlorate is more stable and preferable as a standard. |
| | 1. $9.35^{20}$ $9.04^{30}$ $8.83^{40}$ 2. $10.80^{20}$ $10.50^{30}$ $10.26^{40}$ | v.s. $H_2O$, EtOH; sl. s. eth. | Dihydrochloride, col. needles or tablets, M.p. 315d., v.s. $H_2O$, hot EtOH, v. sl. s. cold EtOH, i. eth. |
| $-11.3^{20}$ (c = 2 in $H_2O$) ($-9.9$ to $-13.1$ in $H_2O$) | 3.32 | s. $H_2O$, EtOH, gl. acetic, acet.; sl. s. Et acetate; i. eth. | Hydrolysed almost completely to glutamic acid by boiling for 1–2 hr at 100°C in 2M-HCl or 0.5M-NaOH. |
| | 2.43 4.78 | $0.55^6$, s.$^{hot}$ $H_2O$; sl. s. EtOH; 0.02 eth.; i. benz. | Decomp. to nicotinic acid at 110–90°C, so mixture resolidifies and melts again at 225–36°C. Spectrum, $\lambda_{max}$ 268 nm $\epsilon$ 4000 (in acid). Copper salt, less soluble in $H_2O$ than free acid. |
| | 2.12 10.2 | 42.8 $H_2O$; sl. s. EtOH; i. eth. | Hydrochloride, col. needles from $H_2O$/EtOH, M.p. 171, v.s. $H_2O$, sl. s. EtOH, eth. |
| L-, $+15.1^{25}$ (c = 2 in 5M-HCl) $-7.5^{25}$ (c = 2 in $H_2O$) | 2.19 9.21 | DL-: $5.0^{25}$, $19.2^{75}$ $H_2O$; $0.00067^{25}$ EtOH; i. eth. L-: $25^{20}$ $H_2O$; i. EtOH, eth. | Standard compounds to which configurations of $\alpha$-amino acids are related. Serious losses occur during acid hydrolysis of protein. Destroyed by hot dil. alkali. Racemized in aq. soln. at pH 9. Store solid in desiccator. |

| Name | Synonyms | Formula | M. wt. | Physical properties |
|---|---|---|---|---|
| Somatostatin | SRIF; Somatotropin (growth hormone) release-inhibiting factor | $(H_2N)Ala \rightarrow Gly \rightarrow Cys \rightarrow Lys \rightarrow Asn \rightarrow Phe$ with disulphide bridge (S–S) from Cys to Cys, and chain Phe ↓ Phe ↓ Trp ↓ Lys ↓ Thr ↓ Phe; $(HO)Cys \leftarrow Ser \leftarrow Thr \leftarrow Phe$ | 1638 | |
| Spermidine | $N$-(3-Aminopropyl)-1,4-diaminobutane; 1,8-Diamino-4-azaoctane | $H_2N \cdot (CH_2)_3 \cdot NH \cdot (CH_2)_4 \cdot NH_2$ | 145.2; Trihydrochloride, 254.6 | cryst. Tri·HCl: cryst.; M.p. 258 |
| Spermine | $N,N'$-Bis(3-aminopropyl)-1,4-diaminobutane; 1,12-Diamino-4,9-diazadodecane | $NH \cdot (CH_2)_3 \cdot NH_2$ $(CH_2)_4$ $NH \cdot (CH_2)_3 \cdot NH_2$ | 202.3; Tetrahydrochloride, 348.2 | wh. deliq. needles; M.p. 55—60, B.p. $150^5$. Tetrahydrochloride: cryst.; M.p. 310—11d. |
| Taurine | 2-Aminoethanesulphonic acid | $H_2N \cdot CH_2 \cdot CH_2 \cdot SO_3H$ | 125.2 | needles; M.p. 320d. |
| Threonine | 2-Amino-3-hydroxybutanoic acid; Thr | L–Threonine: COOH / $H_2N \cdot CH$ / $HC \cdot OH$ / $CH_3$ ; L–Allothreonine: COOH / $H_2N \cdot CH$ / $HO \cdot CH$ / $CH_3$ | 119.1; Hydrate, 128.1 | DL- and L-: cryst. $+ \frac{1}{2}H_2O$. L-: decomp. 225—7 |
| L-Thyroxine | 3,5,3′,5′-Tetraiodothyronine; $O$-(4-Hydroxy-3,5-diiodophenyl)-3,5-diiodotyrosine; $T_4$ | $HO$—(I,I-ring)—$O$—(I,I-ring)—$CH_2 \cdot CH(NH_2) \cdot COOH$ | 776.9; Na salt, 789.9; Hydrate, 888.9 | wh. needles; M.p. 236d. Na salt: wh. cryst. $+ 5H_2O$. |
| 3,5,3′-Triiodo-L-thyronine | $T_3$; $O$-(4-Hydroxy-3-iodophenyl)-3,5-diiodo-L-tyrosine | $HO$—(I,I-ring)—$O$—(I-ring)—$CH_2 \cdot CH(NH_2) \cdot COOH$ | 651.0 | cryst.; M.p. 236—7d. |
| Trimethylamine | $N,N$-Dimethylmethanamine | $(CH_3)_3N$ | 59.1; Hydrochloride, 95.6 | col. gas; pungent fishy odour; M.p. −124, B.p. 3.5. Hydrochloride: cryst., M.p. 277—8d. |
| Trimethylamine oxide | $N,N$-Dimethylmethanamine $N$-oxide | $(CH_3)_3NO$ | 75.1; Hydrate, 111.4 | deliq. needles $+ 2H_2O$; lose $H_2O$, 96; M.p. 257 |

| $[\alpha]_D^t$ | $pK_a$ at 25°C | Solubility | General remarks |
|---|---|---|---|
| $-36^{25}$ (c = 0.5 in 1% acetic acid) | | | Inhibits release of somatotropin (growth hormone) by anterior pituitary, and of thyrotropin (but not of prolactin). Inhibits secretion of insulin, glucagon, and gastrin. Both oxidized (disulphide) and reduced (dithiol) forms have biological activity. [D-Trp[8]]-Somatostatin more active than natural, [L-Trp[8]], form. [Tyr[1]]-Somatostatin (i.e. Tyr-Gly-etc.) and Tyr-somatostatin (i.e. Tyr-Ala-Gly-etc.) used as iodinatable analogues. |
| | | s. $H_2O$ | Phosphate salt much more soluble in $H_2O$ than spermine phosphate. |
| | | s. $H_2O$, EtOH, $n$-butanol; i. eth., benz. | Strong base, absorbs $CO_2$ from air. Spermine phosphate, $C_{10}H_{26}N_4 . 2H_3PO_4 . 6H_2O$, M. wt. 506.4, col. cryst., solubility $0.037^{20}$, $1.0^{100}$ $H_2O$, s. dil. acids and alkalis, PREP. *BJ* **18**, 1263 (1924). |
| | 1.5 ($SO_3H$) 9.06 ($NH_2$) | $3.93^0$, $10.48^{25}$, $45.76^{100}$ $H_2O$; $0.0032^{17}$ EtOH; i. eth. | Stable to boiling acids. Hg salt used for isolation and identification. |
| L-, $-15.0^{25}$ (c = 1-2 in 5M-HCl) $-28.5^{25}$ (c = 1-2 in $H_2O$) L-allo, $+10.0^{25}$ (c = 1-2 in 5M-HCl) $+31.7^{25}$ (c = 1-2 in $H_2O$) | Normal isomers, 2.09 9.10 Allo isomers, 2.11 9.10 | DL-: $20^{25}$ $H_2O$; 0.07 95% EtOH; $0.0054^{25}$ EtOH; i. $CHCl_3$ L-: s. $H_2O$; i. EtOH, eth., $CHCl_3$ DL-allo: $13.9^{25}$ $H_2O$; $0.3^{25}$ 95% EtOH. L-allo: s. $H_2O$; v. sl. s. EtOH | Rapidly destroyed by hot dil. alkali and slowly destroyed by acid at high temperatures. Serious losses occur during protein hydrolysis. Store solid in desiccator. |
| $-4.5$ to $-5.7$ (in M-NaOH/EtOH, 1:2) $+15$ (c = 5 in M-HCl/95% EtOH 1:2) | 2.2 (COOH) 6.45 (OH) 10.1 ($NH_2$) | v. sl. s. $H_2O$; s. alkali; i. EtOH, eth. Na Salt: sl. s. $H_2O$ | Unstable in light, losing iodine. Slow decomp. even in cold. Deiodination occurs during protein hydrolysis, esp. with acid. Strongly adsorbed to glass from dil. solns., *BBA* **41**, 252 (1960). Forms insoluble chelates with $Mg^{2+}$, $Mn^{2+}$ and other divalent ions. Spectrum, $\lambda_{max}$ 295 nm $\epsilon$ 4160 in 0.04M-HCl, $\lambda_{max}$ ($\epsilon$) 227 nm (48 560) and 325 nm (6210) in dil. NaOH. |
| $+23.6^{24}$ (c = 5 in M-HCl/EtOH, 1:2) | 2.2 (COOH) 8.40 (OH) 10.1 ($NH_2$) | s. alkalis; v. sl. s. $H_2O$; i. EtOH | Unstable in light, losing iodine. Slow decomp. even in cold. Deiodination occurs on heating in strong acid or, less so, in alkali. Adsorbed to glass from dil. solns. Spectrum, $\lambda_{max}$ 295 nm $\epsilon$ 4090 in 0.04M-HCl, $\lambda_{max}$ ($\epsilon$) 224 nm (49 200) and 320 nm (4660) in dil. NaOH. Hydrochloride, needles, M.p. 202-3. |
| | $9.91^{20}$ $9.69^{30}$ $9.48^{40}$ | v. s. $H_2O$, EtOH; s. eth. Hydrochloride: s. $H_2O$, EtOH, $CHCl_3$; i. eth. | |
| | $4.65^{20}$ | s. $H_2O$, MeOH, EtOH, hot $CHCl_3$; i. eth. | Aq. soln. strongly alkaline. On heating decomp. to dimethylamine and formaldehyde. Hydrochloride, darkens 185, decomp. 204-26, s. $H_2O$, hot MeOH. |

# 1 Amino acids, amines, amides, peptides, and their derivatives

| Name | Synonyms | Formula | M. wt. | Physical properties |
|---|---|---|---|---|
| Tryptamine | 3-(2-Aminoethyl)indole | $CH_2 \cdot CH_2 \cdot NH_2$ (indole) | 160.2; Hydro-chloride, 196.7 | cryst.; M.p. 118 |
| Tryptophan | $\alpha$-Amino-3-indolepropanoic acid; Trp | $CH_2 \cdot CH(NH_2) \cdot COOH$ (indole) | 204.2 | col. plates; M.p. DL-, 283–5; L-, 289d. |
| Tyramine | p-(2-Aminoethyl)phenol; 4-Hydroxyphenethylamine | $HO-\langle\rangle-CH_2 \cdot CH_2 \cdot NH_2$ | 137.2; Hydro-chloride, 173.6 | needles or leaflets; M.p. 166, B.p. $205^{25}$ |
| Tyrosine | 3-(4-Hydroxyphenyl)alanine; Tyr | $HO-\langle\rangle-CH_2 \cdot CH(NH_2) \cdot COOH$ | 181.2 | needles; M.p. DL-, 316d; L-, 342–4d. |
| Urea | Carbamide | $O=C\begin{smallmatrix}NH_2\\NH_2\end{smallmatrix}$ | 60.1 | col. cryst. or needles; M.p. 132.7 |
| Urocanic acid | Urocaninic acid; 3-(1H-Imidazol-4-yl)-2-propenoic acid | $CH=CH \cdot COOH$ (imidazole) | 138.1; Hydrate, 174.1 | trans-: efflor. wh. needles or prisms + $2H_2O$; M.p. 225d. cis-: M.p. 175–9. |
| Valine | 2-Amino-3-methylbutanoic acid; Val | $\begin{smallmatrix}CH_3\\CH_3\end{smallmatrix}CH \cdot CH(NH_2) \cdot COOH$ | 117.1 | leaflets or prisms; M.p. DL-, 298d. (rapid heating, sealed tube); L-, 315d. (sealed tube), sublimes |
| Vasopressin | Pitressin; Anti-diuretic hormone | CyS → Tyr → Phe → Gln → Asn → CyS<br>$H_2N$—Gly ← Arg ← Pro<br><br>Arginine vasopressin (man, ox)<br><br>In pigs, Lys replaces Arg (lysine vasopressin) | [Arg$^8$] vaso-pressin, 1084; [Lys$^8$] vaso-pressin, 1056 | wh. amorph powder. |

| $[\alpha]_D^t$ | $pK_a$ at 25°C | Solubility | General remarks |
|---|---|---|---|
| | 10.2 | v.s. EtOH, acet.; sl. s. $H_2O$, eth. | Monohydrochloride, col. prisms from EtOH/eth., M.p. 252–3, v.s. $H_2O$, spectrum, $\lambda_{max}$ ($\epsilon$) 282 nm (6000) and 290 nm (5100) in 95% EtOH. |
| L-, +2.8[25] (c = 1–2 in M-HCl) −33.7[25] (c = 1–2 in $H_2O$) | 2.46 9.41 | DL-: 0.25[30] $H_2O$; sl. s. EtOH L-: 1.14[25], 2.8[75] $H_2O$; sl. s. EtOH; i. $CHCl_3$, eth. | Spectrum, $\lambda_{max}$ ($\epsilon$) 218 nm (33 500) 278 nm (5550) 287.5 nm (4550) in 0.1M-HCl, little change with pH. Unstable in mineral acids in the presence of carbohydrates, $CuSO_4$, $FeSO_4$, aldehydes; completely destroyed during protein hydrolysis. Stable to 5M-NaOH at 125°C provided that carbohydrate is absent. Store solid in the dark; darkens on prolonged exposure to light. |
| | 9.74 10.52 | 1.05[15] $H_2O$; 10 EtOH; s. benz.; sl. s. eth., $CHCl_3$ | Hydrochloride, cryst. from conc. HCl, M.p. 268, v.s. $H_2O$. |
| L-, −10.0[25] (c = 2 in 5M-HCl) | 2.20 (COOH) 9.21 ($NH_2$) 10.46 (OH) | DL-: 0.035[25], 0.084[50] $H_2O$; v. sl. s. EtOH; i. eth. L-: 0.045[25], 0.244[75] $H_2O$; 0.01[17] 95% EtOH; s. alkalis; i. eth., acet. | Spectrum, $\lambda_{max}$ ($\epsilon$) 223 nm (8200) and 274.5 nm (1340) in 0.1M-HCl; 240 nm (11050) and 293.5 nm (2330) in 0.1M-NaOH; spectrum affected by ionization of OH gp. in alk. soln., *Adv. Protein Chem.* **7**, 319 (1952). Pure L-tyrosine is stable in 2.5M-$H_2SO_4$ or 5M-NaOH for up to 30 hr at 100°C, but heating with acid in the presence of carbohydrate leads to destruction. There is up to 18% loss of tyrosine after hydrolysis of protein with NaOH. |
| | | 78[5], 119.3[25] $H_2O$; 15.8[20] EtOH; s. conc. HCl; v. sl. s. eth.; i. $CHCl_3$ | Nitrate, prisms, M.p. 152d., s. hot $H_2O$. Solns. of urea develop a significant concentration of reactive cyanate ions on standing, *JBC* **235**, 3177 (1960). Use fresh solns. or decompose cyanate by acidification before use. Traces of metals may be removed by treating a conc. soln. with a mixed anion-cation exchange resin. Protein denaturant. |
| | *trans-*, 3.5 5.8 *cis-*, 3.0 6.7 | 0.1[0], 0.6[37], 6.0[100] $H_2O$; s. HCl, NaOH | The *cis*-form is the less stable isomer, syntheses give mainly the *trans*-form. Slowly loses $H_2O$ at room temp., becomes anhyd. at 100°C. Spectrum, *trans-*, $\lambda_{max}$ 267 nm at pH 2, 264 nm at pH 5, 277 nm ($\epsilon$ 18 800) at pH 7.2–11, see *JBC* **201**, 775 (1953); *cis-*, $\lambda_{max}$ 269 nm at pH 2, 263 nm at pH 5, 282 nm at pH 10.7. Na salt and hydrochloride, v.s. $H_2O$. |
| L-, +28.3[25] (c = 1–2 in 5M-HCl) +5.63[25] (c = 1–2 in $H_2O$) | 2.29 9.74 | DL-: 7.04[25], 12.6[75] $H_2O$; 0.5[25] 75% EtOH; 0.015[25] EtOH; i. eth. L-: 8.85[25], 10.2[65] $H_2O$; v. sl. s. EtOH; i. eth. | |
| Lysine vasopressin, −23.8[22] (c = 0.5 in M-acetic acid) | Isoelectric point, arginine vasopressin, 10.9 | s. $H_2O$; i. acet. | Posterior pituitary hormone. Principal actions: antidiuretic, raises blood pressure. Stable in acid, unstable in alkaline solns. Activity destroyed by thioglycollate. Pure arginine vasopressin contains *ca.* 400 units/mg, lysine vasopressin *ca.* 250 units/mg. |

# 2 Carboxylic acids, alcohols, aldehydes, and ketones

Carboxylic acids and aldehydes containing seven or more carbon atoms are included in Section 8, Lipids and long-chain fatty acids.

**Optically active compounds**

For certain optically active compounds, the properties of only one optical isomer (enantiomer), usually the one which is most abundant in living organisms, have been given. The properties of the other enantiomer are the same *except* that the sign of optical rotation is reversed.

**$pK_a$ values**

Most of the values quoted are taken from G. Kortüm, W. Vogel, and K. Andrussow, *Dissociation constants of organic acids in aqueous solution*, Butterworth (1961), and E. P. Serjeant and B. Dempsey, *Ionisation constants of organic acids in aqueous solution* (IUPAC Chemical Data Series No. 23), Pergamon (1979).

**Metal chelating properties**

Metal chelating properties of carboxylic acids are included in Section 17, Stability constants for metal complexes.

## 2 Carboxylic acids, alcohols, aldehydes, and ketones

| Name | Synonyms | Formula | M. wt. | Physical properties |
|------|----------|---------|--------|---------------------|
| Acetaldehyde | Ethanal | $CH_3 \cdot CHO$ | 44.1 | col. fuming inflammable liq., s.g. $0.788_4^{16}$; M.p. $-121$, B.p. 21 |
| Acetic acid | Ethanoic acid | $CH_3 \cdot COOH$ | 60.1 | col. liq., s.g. $1.049_4^{20}$; M.p. 16.6, B.p. 118.2 |
| ——, $NH_4$ salt | | $CH_3 \cdot COO \cdot NH_4$ | 77.1 | hygr. wh. cryst. |
| ——, Na salt | | $CH_3 \cdot COO \cdot Na$ | 82.0 | hygr. whitish powder |
| ——, Na salt hydrate | | $CH_3 \cdot COO \cdot Na \cdot 3H_2O$ | 136.1 | efflorescent col. cryst. |
| ——, K salt | | $CH_3 \cdot COO \cdot K$ | 98.1 | hygr. lustrous wh. powder |
| Acetoacetic acid | 3-Oxobutanoic acid | $CH_3 \cdot CO \cdot CH_2 \cdot COOH$ | 102.1 | col. syrup or cryst.; M.p. 36–7 |
| ——, Li salt | | $CH_3 \cdot CO \cdot CH_2 \cdot COO \cdot Li$ | 108.0 | non.-hygr. cryst.; M.p. 180–90d. |
| Acetoin | 3-Hydroxy-2-butanone; Acetylmethylcarbinol | $CH_3 \cdot CO \cdot CH(OH) \cdot CH_3$ | 88.1 | $(\pm)$-: liq., s.g. $1.006_4^{20}$, pleasant odour; M.p. $-72$, B.p. 148 |
| Acetone | 2-Propanone; Dimethyl ketone | $CH_3 \cdot CO \cdot CH_3$ | 58.1 | col. inflammable liq., s.g. $0.792_4^{20}$; M.p. $-95$, B.p. 56.2 |
| Aconitic acid, cis- | 1,2,3-Propenetricarboxylic acid | $HOOC \cdot CH_2 \cdot \underset{\parallel}{C} \cdot COOH$ <br> $HC \cdot COOH$ | 174.1 | col. needles; M.p. 130 |
| ——, trans- | | $HOOC \cdot CH_2 \cdot \underset{\parallel}{C} \cdot COOH$ <br> $HOOC \cdot CH$ | 174.1 | cryst.; M.p. 190–210d. |
| Acrylic acid | 2-Propenoic acid; Vinyl-formic acid | $CH_2{=}CH \cdot COOH$ | 72.1 | col. liq., s.g. $1.062_4^{16}$, acrid odour; M.p. 13, B.p. 142, 54–6[25] |
| Adipic acid | Hexanedioic acid | $HOOC \cdot (CH_2)_4 \cdot COOH$ | 146.1 | col. cryst.; M.p. 153, B.p. 265[100] |

| $pK_a$ at 25°C | Solubility | General remarks |
|---|---|---|
| | ∞ $H_2O$, EtOH, eth., benz. | Redistilled acetaldehyde keeps indefinitely in 2M aq. soln. at −20°C. Dilute solns. keep in cold at least a week. Polymerizes readily at room temp. 2,4-Dinitrophenylhydrazone, M.p. 167, spectrum in $CHCl_3$, $\lambda_{max}$ 354 nm $\epsilon$ 22 200 (neutral), $\lambda_{max}$ 430 nm $\epsilon$ 22 500 (alkaline). |
| 4.76 | ∞ $H_2O$, EtOH, eth.; s. most organic solvents; v. sl. s. $CS_2$ | Glacial acetic acid burns skin. 1M-soln., pH 2.4, 0.1M-soln. pH 2.9. Acetic anhydride, $(CH_3 \cdot CO)_2O$, half-life in $H_2O$, 50 min at 0°C, 4.5 min at 25°C. |
| | $NH_4$ salt: 148[4] $H_2O$, decomp. hot. $H_2O$; s. EtOH; sl. s. acet. | $NH_4$ salt: Tends to lose $NH_3$. Conc. aq. soln. slightly acid. |
| | Na salt: 119[0], 170[100] $H_2O$; 2.1 EtOH | |
| | Na salt hydrate: 76.2[0], 138.5[50] $H_2O$; 2.1 EtOH; s. eth., acet. | Na salt hydrate: Loses $H_2O$ of cryst. at 120°C. Aq. soln. alkaline (0.1M soln. pH 8.9). |
| | K salt: 253[20], 492[62] $H_2O$; 33 EtOH; i. eth. | K salt: Aq. soln. alkaline (0.1M-soln. pH 9.7) |
| 3.62 | ∞ $H_2O$, EtOH; s. eth. | Unstable to heat. Cryst. stable when dry but melt on exposure to air. Salts are frequently prepared in soln. by hydrolysis of freshly distilled ethyl ester with a small excess of alkali. |
| | Li salt: s. $H_2O$, MeOH | Li salt: Stable several months in vacuo at 0–4°C. Neutral solns. stable at least 2–3 weeks at −15°C. Spectrum, $\lambda_{max}$ 273 nm $\epsilon$ 50 (in $H_2O$), $\lambda_{max}$ 267 nm $\epsilon$ 148 (in 0.1M-NaOH), $\lambda_{max}$ 247 nm $\epsilon$ 73 (in 0.1M-HCl). PREP. Biochem. Preps. 10, 1 (1963). |
| | v.s. $H_2O$, EtOH; sl. s. eth. | Reduces Fehling's soln. Forms solid dimer, M.p. 95. Dimer → monomer in aq. soln. (−)-Acetoin: $[\alpha]_D$ − 82 approx. |
| | ∞ $H_2O$, EtOH, eth., most organic solvents | 2,4-Dinitrophenylhydrazone, yel. needles, M.p. 128, spectrum in $CHCl_3$, $\lambda_{max}$ 364 nm $\epsilon$ 22 400 (neutral), $\lambda_{max}$ 431 nm $\epsilon$ 20 000 and 530 nm (alkaline). |
| 1.95[20] | s. $H_2O$; sl. s. eth. | Solid stable at least 3 months at room temp. Stable in solns. of pH 7–10 but isomerizes to trans-isomer at higher and low pHs, see J. Org. Chem. 13, 399 (1948) and BJ 38, 426 (1944). REVIEW. Adv. Carbohyd. Chem. 6, 231 (1951). |
| 2.80 4.46 | 26.4[25], 110.7[90] $H_2O$; 50[12] 88% EtOH; sl. s. eth. | Salts usually prepared by neutralization of the anhydride. |
| 4.25 | ∞ $H_2O$, EtOH, eth. | Corrosive. Polymerizes readily in the presence of $O_2$. Stabilized by addition of hydroquinone. $\lambda_{max}$ below 210 nm, $\lambda_{max}$ and $\epsilon$ vary with conc. |
| 4.44 5.44 | 1.5[15], 160[100] $H_2O$; v.s. EtOH; s. acet.; 0.6[15] eth.; i. benz. | |

## 2 Carboxylic acids, alcohols, aldehydes, and ketones

| Name | Synonyms | Formula | M. wt. | Physical properties |
|---|---|---|---|---|
| Benzoic acid | Benzenecarboxylic acid | COOH (benzene ring) | 122.1 | cryst.; M.p. 122, B.p. 249 |
| ——, Na salt | | $C_6H_5 \cdot COO \cdot Na$ | 144.1 | wh. amorph. powder |
| ——, K salt | | $C_6H_5 \cdot COO \cdot K \cdot 3H_2O$ | Hydrate, 214.3 | wh. cryst. powder |
| 2,3-Butanediol | 2,3-Butylene glycol | $CH_3$ — HCOH — HCOH — $CH_3$  *meso- (erythro-)*   $CH_3$ — HOCH — HCOH — $CH_3$  *D- (threo-)* | 90.1 | *meso-*: hygr. cryst.; M.p. 34.4, B.p. 181.7  DL-: liq., s.g. $1.003_4^{20}$; M.p. 7.6, B.p. 182.5  D-: hygr. cryst.; M.p. 34, B.p. 180–2; $[\alpha]_D^{25} - 13.2$ (pure compd.) |
| Butyraldehyde | Butanal | $CH_3 \cdot CH_2 \cdot CH_2 \cdot CHO$ | 72.1 | col. liq., s.g. $0.817_4^{20}$; M.p. —99, B.p. 75 |
| *n*-Butyric acid | Butanoic acid | $CH_3 \cdot CH_2 \cdot CH_2 \cdot COOH$ | 88.1 | col. oily liq., s.g. $0.959_4^{20}$, unpleasant, rancid odour; M.p. — 4, F.p. —19, B.p. 164 |
| ——, Na salt | | $C_4H_7O_2 \cdot Na$ | 110.1 | cryst. |
| ——, Ca salt | | $(C_4H_7O_2)_2 \cdot Ca \cdot H_2O$ | Hydrate, 232.3 | leaflets or prisms |
| Catechol | 1,2-Benzenediol; 1,2-Dihydroxybenzene; Pyrocatechol | (benzene ring)—OH —OH | 110.1 | col. leaflets; M.p. 105, B.p. 240–5 |
| Chorismic acid | | (structure) COOH, $CH_2$, O—C, H, COOH, H, OH | 226.2; Hydrate, 244.2 | cryst. + $1H_2O$; M.p. 148–9d.; $[\alpha]_D - 295$ (c = 0.2 in $H_2O$); crystals retain solvent. |
| Cinnamic acid, *trans-* | *trans*-Phenylpropenoic acid | $C_6H_5 \cdot CH{=}CH \cdot COOH$ | 148.2 | col. cryst.; M.p. 135–6, B.p. 300 |

| $pK_a$ at 25°C | Solubility | General remarks |
|---|---|---|
| 4.20 | $0.18^4$, $0.29^{20}$, $6.8^{95}$ $H_2O$; $47.1^{15}$, $66^{78}$ EtOH; $40^{15}$ eth.; 22 $CHCl_3$ | Starts to sublime at 100°C. Spectrum, $\lambda_{max}(\epsilon)$ 230 nm (11 600) and 273 nm (970) in $H_2O$; benzoate anion, 224 nm (8700) and 268 nm (560) in $H_2O$. |
| | Na salt: $66^{20}$, $74.2^{100}$ $H_2O$; $1.64^{25}$, $8.3^{78}$ EtOH | Na salt: Aq. soln. sl. alkaline (pH about 8) |
| | K salt: $52^{25}$, $112^{100}$ $H_2O$; s. anhyd. EtOH | K salt: Loses $H_2O$ at 110°C. |
| | meso-: v.s. $H_2O$; s. EtOH, eth. DL-, D- and L-: ∞ $H_2O$, EtOH; s. eth. | Three isomers, meso-(erythro-), D(−)-threo- and L(+)-threo-, are formed in fermentations by different organisms, e.g. *Aerobacter aerogenes* forms 90–95% meso- plus a small amount of L(+)-isomer, whereas *Bacillus polymyxa* forms only the D(−)-isomer. Commercial product is usually meso- or D(−)-isomer. |
| | $7.1^{25}$ $H_2O$; ∞ EtOH, eth. | 2,4-Dinitrophenylhydrazone, M.p. 123, spectrum in $CHCl_3$, $\lambda_{max}$ 358 nm $\epsilon$ 21 000 (neutral), $\lambda_{max}$ 426 nm, $\epsilon$ 20 400 (alkaline). |
| 4.82 | ∞ $H_2O$, EtOH, eth. | Volatile in steam. |
| | Na salt: s. $H_2O$; sl. s. EtOH | |
| | Anhyd. Ca salt: $18.2^{20}$, $14.9^{75}$, $15.85^{100}$ $H_2O$ | Ca salt: Solubility in $H_2O$ reaches a minimum at 75°C. |
| 9.34 ~13 | $45.1^{20}$ $H_2O$; v.s. EtOH; s. eth., benz. | Discolours in air and light. Reduces Fehling's soln and ammoniacal $AgNO_3$. Spectrum, $\lambda_{max}(\epsilon)$, 214 nm (6300) and 275.5 nm (2300) at pH 3; 236.5 nm (6800) and 292 nm (3500) at pH 11. |
| ~3 | v.s. $H_2O$, Et acetate, eth.; i. pet. eth. | Isomeric with prephenic acid. Slow decomp. in solid and solns. to give *p*-hydroxybenzoic acid plus prephenic acid; interpretation of exptl. results should allow for presence of these compds. Decomp. complete in soln. in 1 hr at 70°C and pH 10. Store solid and solns. at −15°C or below. Spectrum in $H_2O$, $\lambda_{max}$ 275 nm $\epsilon$ 2630. PREP. *Biochem. Preps.* **12**, 94 (1968). |
| 4.44 | $0.1^{20}$, $0.59^{98}$ $H_2O$; $23^{20}$ EtOH; v.s. eth.; $5.9^{15}$ $CHCl_3$ | Volatile in steam. Spectrum in EtOH, $\lambda_{max}$ 273 nm $\epsilon$ 20 000. |

## 2 Carboxylic acids, alcohols, aldehydes, and ketones

| Name | Synonyms | Formula | M. wt. | Physical properties |
|------|----------|---------|--------|---------------------|
| Citric acid | 2-Hydroxy-1,2,3-propane-tricarboxylic acid | $CH_2 \cdot COOH$<br>$\|$<br>$HO \cdot C \cdot COOH$<br>$\|$<br>$CH_2 \cdot COOH$ | 192.1<br><br>Hydrate, 210.1 | Anhyd.: monocl. cryst.; M.p. 153.<br>Monohydrate: cryst. + $1H_2O$; softens 75, melts ~100 |
| ——, $NH_4$ salt | | $C_6H_5O_7 \cdot (NH_4)_3$ | 243.2 | deliq. wh. cryst. |
| ——, Na salt | | $C_6H_5O_7 \cdot Na_3 \cdot 2H_2O$ | Hydrate, 294.1 | wh. cryst. or granules or powder |
| ——, K salt | | $C_6H_5O_7 \cdot K_3 \cdot H_2O$ | Hydrate, 324.4 | wh. cryst. or granules or powder |
| Crotonic acid, trans- | trans-2-Butenoic acid | $CH_3 \cdot CH{=}CH \cdot COOH$ | 86.1 | col. needles; M.p. 71–6, B.p. 185 |
| Diacetyl | 2,3-Butanedione; Dimethyl-glyoxal | $CH_3 \cdot CO \cdot CO \cdot CH_3$ | 86.1 | greenish-yel. liq., s.g. $0.990^{15}_{15}$; M.p. −2.4, B.p. 88. |
| Dihydroxyacetone | 1,3-Dihydroxypropanone | $HOCH_2 \cdot CO \cdot CH_2OH$ | 90.1 | cryst. as dimer, hygr.; M.p. ~80 |
| Ethanol | Ethyl alcohol | $CH_3 \cdot CH_2OH$ | 46.1 | hygr. col. liq., s.g. anhyd. $0.789^{20}_4$; M.p. −117.3, B.p. 78.5, 8.1[21] |
| Ethylene glycol | 1,2-Ethanediol; Glycol | $HOCH_2 \cdot CH_2OH$ | 62.1 | v. hygr. syrupy liq., s.g. $1.115^{20}_4$; M.p. −12, B.p. 198 |
| Formaldehyde | Methanal | $H \cdot CHO$ | 30.0 | col. gas, pungent odour; M.p. −92, B.p. −21 |
| Formic acid | Methanoic acid | $H \cdot COOH$ | 46.0 | col. liq., s.g. $1.220^{20}_4$; M.p. 8.4, B.p. 100.8 |
| ——, $NH_4$ salt | | $H \cdot COO \cdot NH_4$ | 63.1 | deliq. cryst. or granules; M.p. 116 |
| ——, Na salt | | $H \cdot COO \cdot Na$ | 68.0 | deliq. wh. cryst.; M.p. 253 |
| ——, K salt | | $H \cdot COO \cdot K$ | 84.1 | deliq. col. rhombs or granules; M.p. 167 |
| Fumaric acid | trans-Butenedioic acid | $HOOC \cdot CH$<br>$\|\|$<br>$HC \cdot COOH$ | 116.1 | col. needles or prisms; sublimes at 200 (open vessel), M.p. 300–2 (sealed tube). |
| ——, Na salt | | $C_4H_2O_4 \cdot Na_2$ | 160.0 | cryst. |

| $pK_a$ at 25°C | Solubility | General remarks |
|---|---|---|
| 3.13<br>4.76<br>6.40 | $146^{20}$, $525^{100}$ $H_2O$;<br>$62^{25}$ EtOH; $2.25^{15}$<br>eth.<br>(calculated in terms of<br>anhyd. compd.) | Below 35.8°C monohydrate is stable form.<br>Monohydrate loses $H_2O$ at 40–50°C or by standing over conc. $H_2SO_4$ in a desiccator or slowly in dry air. |
| | $NH_4$ salt: v.s. cold $H_2O$;<br>i. EtOH, eth. | $NH_4$ salt: Decomposes in hot $H_2O$. |
| | Na salt: $72^{25}$, $167^{100}$<br>$H_2O$; i. EtOH | Na salt: Loses $H_2O$ at 150°C. Aq. soln. sl. alkaline (pH ~ 8). Pentahydrate also formed. |
| | K salt: $167^{15}$, $199.7^{31}$<br>$H_2O$; v. sl. s. EtOH | K salt: Loses $H_2O$ at 180°C. Aq. soln. sl. alkaline (pH ~ 8.5). |
| 4.70 | $7.6^{20}$ $H_2O$; v.s. EtOH,<br>acet.; sl. s. ligroin | Isocrotonic acid (cis-2-butenoic acid), needles; M.p. 15.5, B.p. 169; $pK_a{}^{25}$ 4.42; s. $H_2O$; yields crotonic acid in presence of $H_2O$ and light. |
| | $25^{15}$ $H_2O$; ∞ EtOH, eth. | Forms trimers. |
| | s. $H_2O$, hot EtOH;<br>v. sl. s. cold EtOH, eth. | Reverts rapidly to monomer in aq. soln. 2,4-Dinitrophenylhydrazone, M.p. 277–8d. |
| | ∞ $H_2O$, most organic<br>solvents | Inflammable. |
| | ∞ $H_2O$, EtOH, acet.;<br>7.9 eth.; sl. s. $CHCl_3$ | General reference: Glycols, eds Curme and Johnson, A.C.S. Monograph Series No. 114, Reinhold (1952). |
| | v.s. $H_2O$, EtOH, eth. | Formalin is 37–40% (w/w) aq. soln., usually with methanol (10–15%) as stabilizer. Dilute solns. stable at 2°C for 1 week. Dimedon compound, M.p. 189. Bisulphite compd., $HOH_2C \cdot O \cdot SO_2Na$, cryst. + $1H_2O$, s. MeOH, sl. s. EtOH. 2,4-Dinitrophenylhydrazone, spectrum in $CHCl_3$, $\lambda_{max}$ 344 nm $\epsilon$ 19 000 (neutral), $\lambda_{max}$ 430 nm $\epsilon$ 15 000 (alkaline). Paraformaldehyde is a polymer of formaldehyde, cryst. powder, M.p. 121–2, solubility 0.24 cold $H_2O$, i. EtOH, eth., which forms formaldehyde on heating or on dissolving in hot $H_2O$. |
| 3.74 | ∞ $H_2O$, EtOH, eth. | |
| | $NH_4$ salt: $102^0$, $531^{80}$<br>$H_2O$; s. EtOH, eth. | |
| | Na salt: $44^0$, $97^{20}$, $160^{100}$<br>$H_2O$; sl. s. EtOH; i. eth. | Na salt: Aq. soln. neutral. |
| | K salt: $331^{18}$, $657^{90}$<br>$H_2O$; s. EtOH; i. eth. | K salt: Aq. soln. neutral. |
| 3.02<br>4.38 | $0.7^{25}$, $9.8^{100}$ $H_2O$; $5.75^{30}$,<br>$4.76^{76}$ EtOH;<br>$0.72^{25}$ eth.; v. sl. s. $CHCl_3$,<br>acet.; i. benz.<br>Na salt: $22.8^{25}$ $H_2O$ | |

## 2 Carboxylic acids, alcohols, aldehydes, and ketones

| Name | Synonyms | Formula | M. wt. | Physical properties |
|------|----------|---------|--------|---------------------|
| Glutaric acid | Pentanedioic acid | $HOOC \cdot CH_2 \cdot CH_2 \cdot CH_2 \cdot COOH$ | 132.1 | monocl. prisms or needles; M.p. 99, B.p. 304d. |
| Glyceraldehyde | 2,3-Dihydroxypropanal | *(structures: D- and L- forms, each CHO / C with H, OH / $CH_2OH$)* | 90.1 | DL-: cryst. needles as dimer, M.p. 132–45; monomer, M.p. 69–70. D-: syrup; $[\alpha]_D^{25} + 8.7$ (c = 2 in $H_2O$) + 14 (in $H_2O$) L-: syrup; $[\alpha]_D^{25} - 8.7$ (c = 2 in $H_2O$) − 14 (in $H_2O$) |
| Glyceric acid | 2,3-Dihydroxypropanoic acid | *(structure: COOH / H—C—OH / $CH_2OH$)*  D - | 106.1 | DL-: syrup D-: syrup; laevorotatory |
| ——, Ca salt | | $(C_3H_5O_4)_2 \cdot Ca \cdot 2H_2O$ | Hydrate, 286.3 | DL-: prism. cryst.; M.p. 137–8 D-: cryst.; M.p. 142–3; $[\alpha]_D^{20} + 14.5$ (c = 5 anhyd. in $H_2O$) |
| Glycerol | 1,2,3-Trihydroxypropane; 1,2,3-Propanetriol; Glycerine | *(structure: $CH_2OH$ / CHOH / $CH_2OH$)* | 92.1 | hygr. rh. cryst. or col. viscous liq., s.g. $1.261_4^{20}$; M.p. 20, F.p. ~0, B.p. 290d. |
| ——, cytidine diphosphate derivative | Cytidine 5'-diphosphate glycerol; CDP-glycerol | *(structure: $CH_2OH$ / CHOH / $CH_2O$—CDP)*  CDP = cytidine 5'-diphosphate residue | 477.2 | |
| Glycolaldehyde | Hydroxyethanal; Hydroxy-acetaldehyde | $HOCH_2 \cdot CHO$ | 60.1 | col. plates; M.p. 97 |
| Glycollic acid | Hydroxyethanoic acid; Hydroxyacetic acid | $HOCH_2 \cdot COOH$ | 76.1 | leaflets or needles, hygr.; M.p. 80 |
| Glyoxal | Ethanedial; Diformyl | $OHC \cdot CHO$ | 58.0 | yel. prisms; M.p. 15, B.p. 51 |
| Glyoxylic acid | Oxoethanoic acid | $OHC \cdot COOH$ | 74.0; Monohydrate, 92.1 | syrup or hygr. prisms |
| ——, Na salt | | $OHC \cdot COO \cdot Na \cdot H_2O$ | Hydrate, 114.0 | cryst. |
| Hexanoic acid | Caproic acid | $CH_3 \cdot (CH_2)_4 \cdot COOH$ | 116.2 | col. oily liq., s.g. $0.9272_4^{20}$; M.p. −3.4, B.p. 205 |

| $pK_a$ at 25°C | Solubility | General remarks |
|---|---|---|
| 4.35<br>5.40 | $64^{20}$ $H_2O$; v.s. EtOH, eth.; s. $CHCl_3$ | Recrystallize from benz. |
| | DL-: $3^{18}$ $H_2O$; v. sl. s. EtOH, eth.; i. benz.<br>D- and L-: s. $H_2O$ | DL-: In solid state dimer is usual. Depolymerizes in soln. M.p. depends on rate of heating. D- and L-: Polymerize rapidly. Optical rotation values up to ±14 have been reported, which fall to ±7 over a period of 1 week; fully active material can be regenerated, *JACS*, **61**, 761 (1939). Readily isomerizes to dihydroxyacetone on treatment with alkali. Dimedon deriv., M.p. 198, $[\alpha]_D^{25}$ ±210 (c = 0.6 in EtOH)(D- deriv. is dextrorotatory). PREP. *Methods Carbohyd. Chem.* **1**, 61 (1962). |
| 3.52 | ∞ $H_2O$, EtOH; v.s. acet.; i. eth. | Polymerizes and forms insoluble anhydride on long standing. Salts of D-acid are dextrorotatory and more soluble in $H_2O$ than those of D L- acid. |
| | Ca salts: DL-: $3.85^{20}$ anhyd. $H_2O$; i. EtOH, eth.<br>L-: $9.32^{20}$ anhyd. $H_2O$ | Ca salts: Lose $H_2O$ at 130°C. Optical rotation values from ±11.6 to ±15.5 (in $H_2O$) have been reported for Ca salts of D- and L-acids. D- and L-: PREP. *JACS* **61**, 2607 (1939). |
| | ∞ $H_2O$, EtOH; 0.2 eth.; i. $CHCl_3$, benz. | REVIEW. *Glycerol*, eds. Milner and Dalton, A.C.S. Monograph Series No. 117, Reinhold (1953). |
| | | CDP-glycerol: Labile in acid and alkali. Hydrolysis in 1M-HCl at 100°C for 30 min gives cytidine 5'-phosphate and a mixture of *sn*-glycerol 3-phosphate and glycerol 2-phosphate. Conc. $NH_3$ at 100°C for 1 hr gives partial hydrolysis to cytidine 5'-phosphate and *sn*-glycerol 2,3-cyclic phosphate. Glycerol phosphate moiety has *sn*-3- (or L-α-) configuration. ISOL. *BJ* **64**, 599 (1956). SYN. *JCS* **1958**, 3107; *JACS* **83**, 659 (1961). ENZYME SYN. *BJ* **110**, 565 (1968); *JBC* **239**, 3168 (1964). |
| | v.s. $H_2O$, hot EtOH; sl. s. eth. | Fresh aq. solns. contain dimeric form which becomes monomeric on standing for 24 hr. |
| 3.83 | s. $H_2O$, EtOH, eth. | |
| | v.s. $H_2O$; s. EtOH, eth. | Polymerizes rapidly on standing or in the presence of a trace of $H_2O$. Monomer obtained by distilling polyglyoxal. |
| $3.18^{30}$ | v.s. $H_2O$; sl. s. EtOH, eth. | The degree of hydration of glyoxylic acid is questionable. The common form is the monohydrate, with the hydrated oxo group, but a hemihydrate, M.p. 70–5, and an anhydrous form, M.p. 98, have also been isolated. Semicarbazone, $\lambda_{max}$ 252 nm $\epsilon$ 12 400 (in $H_2O$). |
| | Na salt: s. $H_2O$ | Na salt: Stable in neutral or sl. acid aq. soln. |
| 4.85 | $0.97^{20}$, $1.17^{60}$ $H_2O$; s. EtOH, eth. | |

## 2 Carboxylic acids, alcohols, aldehydes, and ketones

| Name | Synonyms | Formula | M. wt. | Physical properties |
|---|---|---|---|---|
| Homogentisic acid | 2,5-Dihydroxyphenylacetic acid | $CH_2 \cdot COOH$ (ring structure with OH and HO) | 168.2; Hydrate, 186.2 | anhyd. leaflets from EtOH-$CHCl_3$, M.p. 152–4; prisms $+1H_2O$ from $H_2O$ |
| p-Hydroxybenzoic acid | 4-Hydroxybenzoic acid; pOB | $COOH$ (ring with OH) | 138.1; Hydrate, 156.1 | col. monocl. cryst. $+1H_2O$; M.p. 213–14. |
| 3-Hydroxybutyric acid | 3-Hydroxybutanoic acid; $\beta$-Hydroxybutyric acid | $CH_3 \cdot CHOH \cdot CH_2 \cdot COOH$ | 104.1 | DL-: hygr. syrup D-: hygr. syrup; $[\alpha]_D^{15} - 25.3$ (c = 6.1 in $H_2O$) |
| ——, Na salt | | $C_4H_7O_3 \cdot Na$ | 126.1 | D-: hygr. wh. cryst; $[\alpha]_D^{17} - 14.2$ (c = 8.4 in $H_2O$) |
| 3-Hydroxy-3-methylglutaric acid | $\beta$-Hydroxy-$\beta$-methylglutaric acid; HMG | $HOOC \cdot CH_2 \cdot \underset{CH_3}{\overset{OH}{C}} \cdot CH_2 \cdot COOH$ | 162.2 | col. flakes; M.p. 108–9 |
| p-Hydroxyphenyl-lactic acid | | $CH_2 \cdot CH(OH) \cdot COOH$ (ring with OH) | 182.2; Hemihydrate, 191.2; Monohydrate, 200.2 | DL-: needles $+1H_2O$; M.p. anhyd. 144. L-: needles $+\frac{1}{2}H_2O$; M.p. 169–70; $[\alpha]_D - 19.6$ (c = 1.3 in $H_2O$) |
| p-Hydroxyphenyl-pyruvic acid | | $CH_2 \cdot CO \cdot COOH$ (ring with OH) | 180.2 | hex. plates; M.p. 220d. |
| Hydroxypyruvic acid | 3-Hydroxy-2-oxopropanoic acid | $HOCH_2 \cdot CO \cdot COOH$ | 104.1; Hydrate, 122.1 | wh. non-hygr. cryst. $+1H_2O$; M.p. 81–2 vigorous decomp. |
| ——, Li salt | | $HOCH_2 \cdot C(OH)_2 \cdot COO \cdot Li$ | 128.0 (hydrated diol) | col. cryst. |
| Isobutyric acid | 2-Methylpropanoic acid | $\overset{CH_3}{\underset{CH_3}{>}} CH \cdot COOH$ | 88.1 | liq., pungent odour, s.g. $0.950_4^{20}$; M.p. $-47$, B.p. 154.3 |
| ——, Na salt | | $C_4H_7O_2 \cdot Na$ | 110.1 | cryst. |
| ——, Ca salt | | $(C_4H_7O_2)_2 \cdot Ca \cdot 5H_2O$ | Hydrate, 304.4 | prisms $+5H_2O$ |

| $pK_a$ at 25°C | Solubility | General remarks |
|---|---|---|
| 4.40 | $85^{25}$ $H_2O$; s. EtOH, eth.; i. $CHCl_3$, benz. | Neutral or acid aq. soln. stable, rapidly decomposed by alkali. Spectrum, $\lambda_{max}$ 290 nm $\epsilon$ 3430 (in 0.03M-phosphate, pH 6.8). Oxidized to benzoquinone acetic acid, $\lambda_{max}$ 250 nm $\epsilon$ 10 790. Readily forms lactone (2-oxo-5-hydroxycoumaran), wh. cryst., M.p. 188—9, solubility 0.075 $H_2O$, stable in air and in acid or neutral aq. soln., decomp. by alkali, spectrum, $\lambda_{max}$ 288 nm (in $H_2O$). |
| 4.67 9.37 | $0.8^{15}$, $2.6^{75}$ $H_2O$; $39.3^{15}$ EtOH; $9.4^{17}$ eth.; $0.01^{11}$ benz.; i. $CS_2$ | No colour with $FeCl_3$. Spectrum, $\lambda_{max}(\epsilon)$ 207.5 nm (13 400) and 255 nm (13 900) in 0.1M-HCl; 245 nm (11 900), first anion at pH 8; 280 nm (16 300), second anion in M-NaOH. |
| 4.41 | DL-, D- and L-: v.s. $H_2O$, EtOH, eth. | Volatile in steam. Decomposes on dry distillation to give crotonic acid and $H_2O$. Reported that D(−)-isomer will crystallize after several months to give v. hygr. cryst., M.p. 45—8. D(−)-isomer is found in urine of diabetics and as poly-$\beta$-hydroxybutyric acid in bacteria, but intermediate in fatty acid oxidation is CoA ester of L(+)-isomer. PREP. of D- and L-isomers and salts, *Biochem. Preps.* **9**, 63 (1962). |
| | s. $H_2O$, eth. | Stable when stored dry. Anhydride, needles, M.p. 102—3, dissolves in $H_2O$ forming acid. |
| | s. $H_2O$, EtOH; sl. s. eth. | Hydrates lose $H_2O$ at 100°C, but not over conc. $H_2SO_4$. PREP. *JACS* **73**, 4972 (1951). |
| | s. EtOH, eth., Et acetate; sl. s. $H_2O$, benz. | Decomposes in hot aq. solns. in the presence of air. Rapidly oxidized in alkaline soln. forming *p*-hydroxybenzaldehyde. 2,4-Dinitrophenylhydrazone, M.p. 178. PREP. *JBC* **197**, 309 (1952); *Org. Synth.* **43**, 49 (1963). |
| | s. $H_2O$, eth., acet. | Best kept in sl. acid. soln., decomposes in alkaline soln. at pH 11.6. Free acid exists in oxo form in solid state and aq. soln. Water of crystallization cannot readily be removed. |
| | Li salt: s. $H_2O$ | Li salt: Hydrated diol in solid state, but probably oxo form in aq. soln. Solid stable for many months at 4°C. Less stable in aq. soln. particularly in presence of alkali. PREP. *Biochem. Preps.* **9**, 86 (1962). |
| 4.60 | $20^{20}$ $H_2O$; ∞ EtOH, eth. | Completely miscible with $H_2O$ above 24°C. Salts are more soluble in $H_2O$ than those of *n*-butyric acid. |
| | Na salt: s. $H_2O$; sl. s. EtOH | |
| | Anhyd. Ca salt: $20.1^{0}$, $23.1^{25}$, $28.7^{62}$, $27.0^{80}$, $26.1^{100}$ $H_2O$ | Ca salt: Solubility in $H_2O$ reaches a maximum at 62.5°C. Crystallizes + 1$H_2O$ from hot aq. soln. Transition point 62.5°C. |

## 2  Carboxylic acids, alcohols, aldehydes, and ketones

| Name | Synonyms | Formula | M. wt. | Physical properties |
|------|----------|---------|--------|---------------------|
| Isocitric acid | 1-Hydroxy-1,2,3-propane-tricarboxylic acid | COOH<br>$\mid$<br>HC·OH<br>$\mid$<br>HOOC·CH<br>$\mid$<br>CH$_2$<br>$\mid$<br>COOH<br><br>*threo*-D$_s$(+) | 192.1 | DL-: prisms; M.p. ~125<br>*threo*-D$_s$-: $[\alpha]_D$ + 30.6 (c = 1 in $H_2O$) |
| ———, KH$_2$ salt | | $C_6H_5O_7\cdot KH_2$ | 230.2 | *threo*-D$_s$-: needles or prisms; decomp. 179—86 |
| Isovaleric acid | 3-Methylbutanoic acid | CH$_3$<br>$\diagdown$CH·CH$_2$·COOH<br>CH$_3$ | 102.1 | col. liq., s.g. $0.9304_4^{20}$; M.p. −37.6, F.p. −29.3, B.p. 176.7 |
| ———, Na salt | | $C_5H_9O_2\cdot Na$ | 124.1 | hygr. col. cryst. or lumps |
| ———, Ca salt | | $(C_5H_9O_2)_2\cdot Ca\cdot 3H_2O$ | Hydrate, 296.4 | cryst. powder |
| Itaconic acid | Methylenebutanedioic acid; Methylenesuccinic acid | HOOC·C(=CH$_2$)·CH$_2$·COOH | 130.1 | hygr. wh. cryst.; M.p. 175 |
| Lactic acid | 2-Hydroxypropanoic acid; DL-, Ordinary lactic acid; L(+)-, Sarcolactic acid | COOH      COOH<br>$\mid$       $\mid$<br>HCOH   HOCH<br>$\mid$       $\mid$<br>CH$_3$    CH$_3$<br>D(−)    L(+) | 90.1 | DL-: hygr. cryst. or syrupy liq., s.g. $1.249_4^{15}$; M.p. 28—33 (18), B.p. $122^{15}$<br>D-: hygr. plates; M.p. 52—4; $[\alpha]_D^{15}$ − 2.26 (c = 1.24 in $H_2O$)<br>L-: hygr. cryst.; M.p. 53—4; $[\alpha]_D^{15}$ + 2.67 (c = 2.51 in $H_2O$) |
| ———, Li salt | | CH$_3$·CHOH·COO·Li | 96.0; Hydrate, 105.0 | DL-: anhyd. non-hygr. wh. cryst.<br>D-: plates $+\frac{1}{2}H_2O$; $[\alpha]_D^{10}$ + 13.3 (c = 0.96 anhyd. in $H_2O$) |
| ———, Na salt | | CH$_3$·CHOH·COO·Na | 112.1 | v. hygr. col. or yel. liq., s.g. $1.38_4^{20}$; M.p. 17 |
| ———, Zn salt | | DL-: (CH$_3$·CHOH·COO)$_2$ Zn·3H$_2$O<br><br>D- and L-: (CH$_3$·CHOH·COO)$_2$ Zn·2H$_2$O | Trihydrate, 297.5;<br>Dihydrate, 279.5 | DL-: deliq. wh. cryst. + 3H$_2$O<br><br>D-: needles +2H$_2$O; $[\alpha]_D^{15}$ + 8.0 (c = 2.5 anhyd. in $H_2O$)<br>L-: needles +2H$_2$O; $[\alpha]_D^{15}$ −8.0 (c = 2.5 anhyd. in $H_2O$) |
| Maleic acid | *cis*-Butenedioic acid | HC·COOH<br>$\parallel$<br>HC·COOH | 116.1 | wh. prisms; M.p. 139—40 |

| $pK_a$ at 25°C | Solubility | General remarks |
|---|---|---|
| 3.29<br>4.71<br>6.40 | | Natural compd. is *threo*-$D_s$(+)-isomer; nomenclature, see *JBC* **237**, 1739 (1962). $[\alpha]_D$ in ammonium molybdate solns., see *BJ* **45**, 578 (1949). *threo*-$D_s$(+)-acid gives laevorotatory lactone, col. needles, M.p. 156–7, $[\alpha]_D$ − 60.4 (c = 1 in $H_2O$), stable if kept dry. Lactone is used to prepare standard solns. of isocitric acid. |
| | $KH_2$ salt, *threo*-$D_s$-:<br>$3.5^0$, $50^{100}$ $H_2O$; 0.4<br>50% EtOH | $KH_2$ salt: In 2% soln., 48% converted to lactone in boiling $H_2O$, equilibrium reached after 3 hr. Solid stable at 115°C if dry at start; decomposes sharply at 179–86°C, depending on rate of heating, and isocitric lactone is the major product. PREP. *Biochem. Preps.* **3**, 44, 50, 52 (1953); **7**, 72 (1960). |
| 4.78 | $4.2^{20}$ $H_2O$; ∞ EtOH, eth., $CHCl_3$ | Salts are more soluble than those of *n*-valeric acid. |
| | Na salt: s. $H_2O$, EtOH | Na salt: Sometimes called sodium valerate. |
| | Anhyd. Ca salt: $26^0$,<br>$21.8^{20}$, $22.0^{40}$, $16.55^{100}$<br>$H_2O$ | Ca salt: Cryst. + $H_2O$ from hot aq. soln. Transition point, 45.5°C. |
| 3.63<br>5.00 | $8.3^{20}$ $H_2O$; $20^{15}$ 88%<br>EtOH; v. sl. s. eth., benz.,<br>$CHCl_3$ | |
| 3.73 | ∞ $H_2O$, EtOH, eth.;<br>i. $CHCl_3$ | Tends to polymerize esp. in conc. solns. forming cyclic dimer (lactide) and linear polymers (e.g. lactoyllactate). Polymers, esp. linear ones, hydrolyse only slowly on dilution, even on boiling. L(+)-Lactic acid is formed in animal tissues, esp. muscle, and in fermentations, e.g. by *Lactobacillus delbrueckii* and *Rhizopus oryzae*. D(−)-Lactic acid is formed by other microorganisms, e.g. *Lactobacillus leishmanii* and *Escherichia coli*. Commercial lactic acid is usually a mixture of isomers, often with the L(+)-isomer predominating. Specific rotation of lactic acid is markedly concentration dependent; its sign is reversed and it is increased in magnitude by ammonium molybdate ($[\alpha]_D$ for L-isomer, −60 to −90), see *Biochem. Preps.* **8**, 75 (1961). Salts of D(−)-acid are dextrorotatory, those of L(+)-acid laevorotatory. PREP. of D- and L- and their salts: *Biochem. Preps.* **3**, 61 (1953); **8**, 75 (1961). REVIEW. *Ann. N.Y. Acad. Sci.* **119**, 851 (1965). |
| | Li salt: s. $H_2O$; v. sl. s.<br>EtOH | Li salt: Material of choice for lactate standard. Aq. soln. about neutral. Soln. in 0.1M $H_2SO_4$ keeps indefinitely at 2–4°C. |
| | Na salt: v.s. $H_2O$, EtOH;<br>i. eth. | Na salt: Aq. soln. neutral. Commercial product is generally conc. aq. soln., proportions of isomers may vary. |
| | Zn salt, DL-: $1.67^{15}$, $16.7^{100}$<br>$H_2O$; v. sl. s. EtOH.<br>D- and L-, anhyd.: $5.0^{15}$, $9.0^{33}$<br>$H_2O$; 0.1 hot EtOH | Zn salt: Optically active forms separated from racemic salt by recrystallization at 35°C. Very readily forms supersaturated solns. $[\alpha]$ decreases markedly with increasing conc. |
| 1.97<br>6.24 | $78.8^{25}$, $392^{97.5}$ $H_2O$;<br>$69.9^{30}$ EtOH; $8^{25}$ eth.;<br>s. acet.; v. sl. s. benz. | Spectrum, $\lambda_{max}$ 210 nm $\epsilon$ 32 000 in $H_2O$. |

## 2 Carboxylic acids, alcohols, aldehydes, and ketones

| Name | Synonyms | Formula | M. wt. | Physical properties |
|---|---|---|---|---|
| Malic acid | 2-Hydroxybutanedioic acid; Hydroxysuccinic acid | $HOOC \cdot CH(OH) \cdot CH_2 \cdot COOH$ | 134.1 | DL-: col. cryst., M.p. 131. L-: col. needles, M.p. 100; $[\alpha]_D^{20} - 2.3$ (c = 9.17 in $H_2O$) $- 5.7$ (c = 3.73 in acet.) |
| Malonic acid | Propanedioic acid | $HOOC \cdot CH_2 \cdot COOH$ | 104.1 | col. cryst.; M.p. 135d. |
| Methanol | Methyl alcohol; Wood alcohol; Carbinol | $CH_3 \cdot OH$ | 32.0 | hygr. col. liq., s.g. $0.792_4^{20}$; M.p. $-93.9$, B.p. 64.7 |
| Methylglyoxal | 2-Oxopropanal; Pyruvic aldehyde | $CH_3 \cdot CO \cdot CHO$ | 72.1 | yel. liq., pungent odour, s.g. $1.046^{24}$; B.p. 72 |
| Methylmalonic acid | 2-Methylpropanedioic acid; Isosuccinic acid | $\overset{\displaystyle CH_3}{\underset{\displaystyle HOOC \cdot CH \cdot COOH}{\vert}}$ | 118.1 | col. needles; M.p. 135d. |
| Mevalonic acid | 3,5-Dihydroxy-3-methyl-pentanoic acid | $HOCH_2 \cdot CH_2 \cdot \underset{\underset{\displaystyle OH}{\vert}}{\overset{\overset{\displaystyle CH_3}{\vert}}{C}} \cdot CH_2 \cdot COOH$ | 148.2 | oil |
| cis-cis-Muconic acid | cis-cis-2,4-Hexadienedioic acid | $HOOC \cdot CH = CH \cdot CH = CH \cdot COOH$ | 142.1 | cryst.; M.p. 194—5 (rapid heating) |
| Oxalic acid | Ethanedioic acid | $HOOC \cdot COOH$ | 90.0; Hydrate, 126.1 | col. cryst. $+ 2H_2O$; sublimes 150; M.p. anhyd. 189 |
| Oxaloacetic acid | 2-Oxobutanedioic acid | $HOOC \cdot CO \cdot CH_2 \cdot COOH$ keto <br> $HOOC \cdot C(OH) = CH \cdot COOH$ enol | 132.1 | Enol: cryst.; M.p. 152—84d. |
| Oxalosuccinic acid | 1-Oxo-1,2,3-propanetri-carboxylic acid | $\underset{\underset{\displaystyle CH_2 \cdot COOH}{\vert}}{HOOC \cdot CO \cdot CH \cdot COOH}$ | 190.1 | |

| $pK_a$ at 25°C | Solubility | General remarks |
|---|---|---|
| 3.46<br>5.10 | DL-: $144^{26}$, $411^{79}$ $H_2O$;<br>$35.9^{20}$ EtOH; $0.6^{20}$ eth.;<br>i. benz.<br>L-: v.s. $H_2O$; $68.3^{20}$<br>EtOH; $1.9^{20}$ eth.; i. benz. | Optical rotation in aq. soln. depends markedly on conc. and temp. With increasing conc. the rotation decreases and solns. of L-malic acid containing more than 34 g per 100 ml of $H_2O$ at 20°C are dextrorotatory. Optical rotation is enhanced by presence of molybdate, see *BJ* **37**, 334 (1943). |
| 2.85<br>5.70 | $61.1^0$, $73.5^{20}$, $92.6^{50}$<br>$H_2O$; $57^{20}$ EtOH; $5.7^{15}$ eth. | At $10^{-2}$ M, powerful inhibitor of certain enzymes, e.g. succinate dehydrogenase, fumarate hydratase, lactate and malate dehydrogenases. |
|  | $\infty$ $H_2O$, EtOH, eth., most organic solvents. | Inflammable. Poisonous. |
|  | s. $H_2O$, EtOH, eth. | Liquid is dimeric at R.T. and rapidly polymerizes to a glassy mass. Polymer dissolves in $H_2O$ forming monomer; on heating to 50°C polymer yields either the dimeric liq. or monomeric gas. |
| 3.05<br>5.76 | $44.3^0$, $66^{20}$ $H_2O$; v.s.<br>EtOH, eth. | Crystallizes as hydrate from $H_2O$. Gives propionic acid on heating at 150°C. Does not inhibit respiration as does malonic acid. |
| 4.3 | v.s. $H_2O$; s. $CHCl_3$ | Natural isomer is (+)-, its lactone is laevorotary; (−)-isomer is biologically inactive. No distinction between acid and lactone in biological systems. $N,N'$-Dibenzylethylene-diammonium salt, cryst., M.p. 124–5. Lactone, hygr. cryst., M.p. 28, v.s. $H_2O$, most polar organic solvents, in equilibrium with acid in acid solution, rapidly hydrolysed by NaOH to give Na salt. PREP. *BJ* **69**, 146 (1958); *JACS* **79**, 2316, 3294 (1957). REVIEW. *Adv. Enzymol.* **23**, 471 (1961). |
|  | s. hot $H_2O$, hot EtOH;<br>sl. s. cold EtOH, eth. | Free acid is rapidly converted into the *cis-trans*-isomer by boiling $H_2O$, but not by boiling EtOH or MeOH, nor by alkali at R.T. or for short periods at 100°C, nor by daylight. Spectrum, $\lambda_{max}$ ($\epsilon$), 257 nm (17 300) at pH 7.0; 251 nm (23 400) 259 nm (25 600) 265 nm (23 400) in 0.1M-NaOH. PREP. of *cis-cis* and other isomers, *JCS* **1950**, 2228, 2235. |
| 1.25<br>3.67 (4.25) | $9.5^{15}$, $120^{90}$ $H_2O$; $23.7^{15}$<br>EtOH; 16.9 eth.; i. $CHCl_3$,<br>benz. | Hydrate loses $H_2O$ at 100°C. Chelates metals. Inhibits lactate dehydrogenase from heart and succinate dehydrogenase competitively. Poisonous. |
| 2.22<br>3.89<br>13.03 (enolic OH) | s. $H_2O$, EtOH; sl. s. eth.;<br>i. $CHCl_3$, benz. | Exists in keto, hydrated (*gem*-diol) and enol forms. Solid is an enol form. Compds. with M.p.s 152 and 184 have been identified as *cis*- and *trans*-enols (hydroxymaleic and hydroxyfumaric acids), but now seems probable that all solid forms are the same isomer, though doubt remains whether *cis* or *trans*, *JCS* **1961**, 5043; *ABB* **153**, 226 (1972). In soln. at pH 6–10 the dianion is 82–8% in the keto form with 7–10% enol and 5–8% hydrate; at pH 1.3 the diacid is approx. 81% hydrate, 13% keto and 6% enol, see *J. Org. Chem.* **41**, 3593 (1976). Absorbance around 260 nm is due to enol form. In ether, where oxaloacetic acid is ⩾ 90% enol, $\lambda_{max}$ 260 nm $\epsilon$ 8800. In aq. soln., $\lambda_{max}$ 255 nm, $\epsilon_{260}$ 420 (for diacid), $\epsilon_{260}$ 850 $\epsilon_{280}$ 540 (for dianion pH 6–10); effect of buffers on $\epsilon$, *JCS* **1961**, 5043. On chelation with transition metal ions $\lambda_{max}$ shifts to longer wavelengths and $\epsilon$ is increased 2–3-fold. Decarboxylates yielding pyruvate $+CO_2$, rate greatest with monoanion > dianion > diacid, max. rate at pH 3–4; decarboxylation accelerated by many di- and trivalent metal ions, with max. rate at pH 5–6.5. |
|  | s. $H_2O$ | Very unstable. Rapidly decarboxylates, esp in acid soln.; decarboxylation accelerated by metal ions. Acid keeps in neutral soln. at 0°C for a few hours. Store as Ba salt at 0°C and dry. PREP. *JBC* **174**, 115 (1948). |

## 2 Carboxylic acids, alcohols, aldehydes, and ketones

| Name | Synonyms | Formula | M. wt. | Physical properties |
|---|---|---|---|---|
| 2-Oxoadipic acid | α-Ketoadipic acid; 2-Oxo-hexanedioic acid | $HOOC \cdot CH_2 \cdot CH_2 \cdot CH_2 \cdot CO \cdot COOH$ | 160.1 | light orange cryst.; M.p. 127 |
| 3-Oxoadipic acid | β-Ketoadipic acid; 3-Oxo-hexanedioic acid | $HOOC \cdot CH_2 \cdot CH_2 \cdot CO \cdot CH_2 \cdot COOH$ | 160.1 | plates; M.p. 124—5 |
| 2-Oxobutyric acid | α-Ketobutyric acid; 2-Oxo-butanoic acid | $CH_3 \cdot CH_2 \cdot CO \cdot COOH$ | 102.1 | hygr. plates; M.p. 30—2, B.p. 85[21] |
| 2-Oxoglutaric acid | α-Ketoglutaric acid; 2-Oxo-pentanedioic acid | $HOOC \cdot CH_2 \cdot CH_2 \cdot CO \cdot COOH$ | 146.1 | cryst.; M.p. 113—16 |
| 2-Oxoisocaproic acid | 'Ketoleucine'; 4-Methyl-2-oxopentanoic acid | $\begin{array}{c} CH_3 \\ {>}CH \cdot CH_2 \cdot CO \cdot COOH \\ CH_3 \end{array}$ | 130.1 | liq.; M.p. −2, B.p. 84—5[15] |
| 2-Oxoisovaleric acid | 'Ketovaline'; 3-Methyl-2-oxobutanoic acid | $\begin{array}{c} CH_3 \\ {>}CH \cdot CO \cdot COOH \\ CH_3 \end{array}$ | 116.1 | cryst.; M.p. 31, B.p. 170 |
| 2-Oxo-3-methyl-valeric acid | 'Ketoisoleucine'; 3-Methyl-2-oxopentanoic acid | $CH_3 \cdot CH_2 \cdot CH(CH_3) \cdot CO \cdot COOH$ | 130.1 | cryst.; M.p. 38—40, B.p. 73[10] |
| Phenol | Carbolic acid | $C_6H_5 \cdot OH$ | 94.1 | col. cryst.; M.p. 43, B.p. 182 |
| Phenylacetic acid | α-Toluic acid | $C_6H_5 \cdot CH_2 \cdot COOH$ | 136.2 | col. leaflets; M.p. 76—7, B.p. 266 |
| Phenyllactic acid | α-Hydroxyhydrocinnamic acid | $C_6H_5 \cdot CH_2 \cdot CHOH \cdot COOH$ | 166.2 | L-: needles; M.p. 124; $[\alpha]_D^{24} - 21.4$ (c = 1 in $H_2O$) |
| Phenylpyruvic acid | α-Oxohydrocinnamic acid | $C_6H_5 \cdot CH_2 \cdot CO \cdot COOH$ | 164.2 | plates; M.p. 157d. |
| ———, Na salt | | $C_6H_5 \cdot CH_2 \cdot CO \cdot COO \cdot Na \cdot H_2O$ | Hydrate, 204.2 | cryst. |
| Pimelic acid | Heptanedioic acid | $HOOC \cdot (CH_2)_5 \cdot COOH$ | 160.2 | prisms; M.p. 105—6, B.p. 212[10] |
| Prephenic acid | 1-Carboxy-4-hydroxy-2,5-cyclohexadiene-1-pyruvic acid | | 226.2 | |
| ———, Ba salt | | $C_{10}H_8O_6 \cdot Ba \cdot H_2O$ | Hydrate, 379.5 | wh. cryst. |

| pK$_a$ at 25°C | Solubility | General remarks |
|---|---|---|
| | s. $H_2O$, EtOH; sl. s. eth. | PREP. *JBC* **176**, 1395 (1948); *Ber.* **88**, 316 (1955). |
| | sl. s. $H_2O$, EtOH, eth. | Violet colour with $FeCl_3$. PREP. *JCS* **1950**, 2223. |
| 2.50 | v.s. $H_2O$, EtOH; sl. s. eth. | |
| 2.47<br>4.68 | v.s. $H_2O$, EtOH; sl. s. eth. | 2,4-Dinitrophenylhydrazone, cryst., M.p. 220, spectrum, $\lambda_{max}$ 420 nm $\epsilon$ 15 400 in 1.25M-NaOH. Semicarbazone, spectrum, $\lambda_{max}$ 247–8 nm $\epsilon$ 10 000 in aq. soln. |
| | | Decomposes slowly at 0°C. Cryst. Na salt (M. wt. 152.1), stable at R.T. 2,4-Dinitrophenyl-hydrazone, M.p. 162, spectrum, $\lambda_{max}$ 435 nm $\epsilon$ 17 700 in 1.25M-NaOH. PREP. *Biochem. Preps.* **3**, 66 (1953). |
| | s. $H_2O$, EtOH, eth. | PREP. *JBC* **197**, 309 (1952); *Chem. Rev.* **41**, 585 (1947). |
| 2.3 | s. $H_2O$, EtOH, eth. | Natural compound is D-isomer. Cryst. Na salt (M.wt. 152.1), $[\alpha]_D^{26}$ + 32.6 (c = 1 in $H_2O$). PREP. *JBC* **190**, 269 (1951); *Chem. Rev.* **41**, 585 (1947). |
| 10.00 | 6.7[16], ∞[66] $H_2O$; ∞ EtOH; v.s. eth.; s. $CHCl_3$ | Colour darkens in air and light, esp. in presence of heavy metal ions. Spectrum, $\lambda_{max}(\epsilon)$ 210.5 nm (6200) and 270 nm (1450) in $H_2O$; phenate anion, 235 nm (9400) and 287 nm (2600) in $H_2O$. |
| 4.31 | 1.6[20] $H_2O$; 186 EtOH; 151 $CHCl_3$; v.s. eth. | In aq. soln. forms a complex with its Na salt. |
| | s. hot $H_2O$, EtOH, eth. | Natural compound is L-isomer. |
| | v. sl. s.[100] $H_2O$; v.s. EtOH, eth.<br>Na salt: s. $H_2O$; i. EtOH | Decomposes on storage, esp. if not kept dry. Oxidizes in air. Spectrum, $\lambda_{max}$ 320 nm $\epsilon$ 17 500 in 0.7M-NaOH.<br>Na salt: Stable in air. Water remains at 100°C. |
| 4.46<br>5.58 | 2.5[13], 5[20] $H_2O$;<br>v.s. EtOH, eth.;<br>i. cold benz. | |
| | s. $H_2O$ | Decomposed by acid to phenylpyruvic acid and $CO_2$; decomp. complete in 10 min at 37°C in 0.5M-HCl. Half-life at 0°C, 1 hr in 0.1M-HCl, 7 hr at pH 4, no detectable loss at pH 6.8. More stable to alkali, but on heating forms *p*-hydroxyphenyllactic acid. PREP. *Meth. Enzymol.* **17A**, 559 (1970). |
| | Ba salt: s. $H_2O$; i. EtOH | |

## 2 Carboxylic acids, alcohols, aldehydes, and ketones

| Name | Synonyms | Formula | M. wt. | Physical properties |
|---|---|---|---|---|
| Propionaldehyde | Propanal | $CH_3 \cdot CH_2 \cdot CHO$ | 58.1 | col. liq., s.g. $0.807_4^{20}$; M.p. $-81$, B.p. $47.5-49$ |
| Propionic acid | Propanoic acid | $CH_3 \cdot CH_2 \cdot COOH$ | 74.1 | col. liq., s.g. $0.993_4^{20}$; M.p. $-21$, B.p. 141 |
| ——, Na salt | | $CH_3 \cdot CH_2 \cdot COO \cdot Na$ | 96.1 | col. cryst. or powder |
| ——, K salt | | $CH_3 \cdot CH_2 \cdot COO \cdot K \cdot H_2O$ | Hydrate, 130.2 | hygr. wh. cryst. |
| ——, Ca salt | | $(CH_3 \cdot CH_2 \cdot COO)_2 \cdot Ca \cdot H_2O$ | Hydrate, 204.2 | col. tablets |
| Protocatechuic acid | 3,4-Dihydroxybenzoic acid | | 154.1; Hydrate, 172.1 | monocl. needles + $1H_2O$; M.p. $202-4$ |
| Pyruvic acid | 2-Oxopropanoic acid | $CH_3 \cdot CO \cdot COOH$ | 88.1 | col. liq., s.g. $1.267_4^{15}$; M.p. 13.6, B.p. 165d., $70.8^{20}$ |
| ——, Li salt | | $CH_3 \cdot C(OH)_2 \cdot COO \cdot Li$ | 112.0 | cryst. |
| ——, Na salt | | $CH_3 \cdot CO \cdot COO \cdot Na$ | 110.0 | plates |
| Quinic acid | 1,3,4,5-Tetrahydroxy-cyclohexanecarboxylic acid | | 192.2 | $(-)$-: cryst.; M.p. $173-4$; $[\alpha]_D^{20} - 44.0$ (c = 12 in $H_2O$) |
| Shikimic acid | 3,4,5-Trihydroxy-1-cyclohexenecarboxylic acid | | 174.2 | $(-)$-: cryst.; M.p. 190; $[\alpha]_D^{18} - 183.8$ (c = 4 in $H_2O$) |
| Succinic acid | Butanedioic acid | $HOOC \cdot CH_2 \cdot CH_2 \cdot COOH$ | 118.1 | col. prisms; M.p. 188 |
| ——, Na salt | | $C_4H_4O_4 \cdot Na_2 \cdot 6H_2O$ | Hydrate, 270.1 | granules or cryst. powder |
| ——, K salt | | $C_4H_4O_4 \cdot K_2 \cdot 3H_2O$ | Hydrate, 248.3 | hygr. wh. cryst. powder |

| $pK_a$ at 25°C | Solubility | General remarks |
|---|---|---|
| | $30.6^{25}$ $H_2O$; ∞ EtOH, eth. | 2,4-Dinitrophenylhydrazone, M.p. 155, spectrum in $CHCl_3$, $\lambda_{max}$ 356 nm $\epsilon$ 22 500 (neutral), $\lambda_{max}$ 438 nm $\epsilon$ 22 500 (alkaline). |
| 4.87 | ∞ $H_2O$, EtOH, eth., $CHCl_3$ | |
| | Na salt: $100^{25}$, $150^{100}$ $H_2O$; 4 EtOH | Na salt: Aq. soln. neutral or slightly alkaline. Fungicide. |
| | K salt: $207^{16}$, $360^{100}$ $H_2O$; $22^{13}$ 95% EtOH | K salt: Loses $H_2O$ at 120°C. |
| | Ca salt: $49^0$, $56^{100}$ $H_2O$; i. EtOH | Ca salt: Solubility in $H_2O$ reaches a minimum at 55°C. |
| 4.49 8.83 12.6 | $1.8^{14}$, $27^{80}$ $H_2O$; v.s. EtOH; s. eth. | Oxidizes in air. |
| 2.39 | ∞ $H_2O$, EtOH, eth. | Polymerizes and decomposes on standing unless pure and kept in air-tight container. In aq. soln., acid is 54—71% in hydrated (*gem*-diol) form, but anion is only 3—5% hydrated; no enol form present. 2,4-Dinitrophenylhydrazone, M.p. 216, spectrum, $\lambda_{max}$ 445 nm $\epsilon$ 20 400 in alkali. Semicarbazone, spectrum, $\lambda_{max}$ 246 nm $\epsilon$ 10 200 in aq. soln. |
| | Li salt: s. $H_2O$ | Li salt: Exists as *gem*-diol in solid state. |
| | Na salt: s. $H_2O$; v. sl. s. EtOH | |
| | $40^9$ $H_2O$; s. EtOH; v. sl. s. eth. | Natural isomer is laevorotatory. Forms $\gamma$-lactone (quinide) on heating to 200—50°C. |
| 4.21 | 18 $H_2O$; $2.25^{23}$ EtOH; $0.015^{28}$ eth.; i. $CHCl_3$, benz. | Natural compound is laevorotatory isomer. Spectrum, $\lambda_{max}$ 213 nm $\epsilon$ 8900 in EtOH. REVIEW. *Chem. Rev.* **65**, 435 (1965). |
| 4.21 5.72 | $6.8^{20}$, $121^{100}$ $H_2O$; $7.5^{21.5}$ EtOH; 0.3 eth.; s. MeOH, acet.; i. benz., $CHCl_3$ | Decomposition occurs at 235°C with partial conversion to succinic anhydride. |
| | Na salt: $21.5^0$, $86.6^{75}$ $H_2O$; v. sl. s. EtOH | Na salt: Hydrate stable in air, loses all $H_2O$ at 120°C. Aq. soln. neutral or slightly alkaline. |
| | K salt: v.s. $H_2O$ | K salt: Aq. soln. practically neutral. |

## 2 Carboxylic acids, alcohols, aldehydes, and ketones

| Name | Synonyms | Formula | | M. wt. | Physical properties |
|------|----------|---------|--|--------|---------------------|
| Succinic semialdehyde | 4-Oxobutanoic acid; Formyl-propionic acid | $HOOC \cdot CH_2 \cdot CH_2 \cdot CHO$ | | 102.1 | viscous col. liq.; B.p. 134–6[14] |
| Tartaric acid | 2,3-Dihydroxysuccinic acid<br>DL-: Racemic acid; Paratartaric acid<br>L(+)-: Ordinary tartaric acid; L$_g$-threo-Dihydroxybutanedioic acid<br>meso-: i-Tartaric acid; erythro-Dihydroxybutanedioic acid | COOH<br>\|<br>HC·OH<br>\|<br>HO·CH<br>\|<br>COOH<br>L(+)- | COOH<br>\|<br>HC·OH<br>\|<br>HC·OH<br>\|<br>COOH<br>meso- | 150.1;<br>Monohydrate, 168.1 | DL-: cryst. + 1H$_2$O, slightly efflor.; M.p. anhyd. 206<br>L(+)-: prisms; M.p. 171–4; $[\alpha]_D^{20}$ + 12.0 (c = 20 in H$_2$O) $[\alpha]_D$ + 0.47 (in MeOH)<br>meso-: plates +1H$_2$O; M.p. anhyd. 146–8 |
| ——, NH$_4$ salt | | $C_4H_4O_6 \cdot (NH_4)_2$ | | 184.2 | DL-: prisms or wh. granules<br>L(+)-: wh. cryst.; $[\alpha]_D^{15}$ + 34.6 (c = 1.84 in H$_2$O) |
| ——, acid Na salt | | $C_4H_4O_6 \cdot NaH \cdot H_2O$ | | Hydrate, 190.1 | DL-: wh. monocl. cryst. +1H$_2$O<br>L(+)-: wh. cryst. + 1H$_2$O; $[\alpha]_D^{19}$ + 21.8 (in H$_2$O) |
| ——, acid K salt | L-: Argol; Tartar; Cream of tartar | $C_4H_4O_6 \cdot KH$ | | 188.2 | DL-: col. cryst.<br>L-: cryst. or wh. powder; |
| ——, K salt | L-: Soluble tartar | $C_4H_4O_6 \cdot K_2 \cdot \frac{1}{2}H_2O$ | | Hydrate, 235.3 | L-: col. cryst. |
| ——, KNa salt | L-: Rochelle salt; Seignette salt | $C_4H_4O_6 \cdot KNa \cdot 4H_2O$ | | Hydrate, 282.2 | L-: cryst. or powder, slightly efflor. |
| Tartronic semi-aldehyde | 2-Hydroxy-3-oxopropanoic acid | $HOOC \cdot CHOH \cdot CHO$ | | 104.1 | |
| n-Valeric acid | Pentanoic acid | $CH_3 \cdot CH_2 \cdot CH_2 \cdot CH_2 \cdot COOH$ | | 102.1 | col. liq., s.g. $0.939_4^{20}$; M.p. −59, F.p. −33.8; B.p. 186 |

| pK$_a$ at 25°C | Solubility | General remarks |
|---|---|---|
| | s. H$_2$O | Tends to polymerize. Solns. at pH 6 or lower and 2°C stable for more than 3 months. PREP. *Meth. Enzymol.* **5**, 765 (1962). |
| DL-, D- and L-: 3.03<br>4.37<br>*meso*-: 3.17<br>4.91 | DL-: 9.23[0], 20.6[20], 185[100] H$_2$O; 3.9[25] EtOH; 1.1 eth.<br>L(+)-: 139.5[20], 343[100] H$_2$O; 20.4[15] EtOH; 0.4 eth.; s. MeOH, acet.; i. CHCl$_3$<br>*meso*-: 125[15] H$_2$O; s. EtOH; sl. s. eth. | DL-: Hydrate loses H$_2$O at 100°C. Anhyd. form is also obtained by crystallization from H$_2$O above 73°C or from EtOH.<br>L(+)-: This isomer occurs widely in fruits, wines, etc.<br>D(−)-isomer also occurs naturally, e.g. in wine, but in much smaller amounts than L-isomer. |
| | NH$_4$ salt, DL-: v.s. H$_2$O; v. sl. s. EtOH<br>L(+)-: 58.1[15], 87.2[60] H$_2$O; sl. s. EtOH | NH$_4$ salt: Crystals slowly evolve NH$_3$. Aq. soln. slightly acid, pH ∼ 6.5. |
| | NaH salt, DL-: 8.9[19] H$_2$O; i. EtOH<br>L(+)-: 6.7[18], 50[100] H$_2$O; v. sl. s. EtOH | NaH salt: Loses H$_2$O at 100°C. Decomposes without melting at 219°C (DL-) or 234°C (L(+)). Aq. soln. acid. |
| | KH salt, DL-: 0.42[25], 7.0[100] H$_2$O; i. EtOH<br>L-: 0.53[20], 6.1[100] H$_2$O; i. EtOH; s. dil. acids and alkalis | KH salt: Aq. soln. acid. |
| | K salt, L-: 150[14], 278[100] H$_2$O; v. sl. s. EtOH | K salt: Loses H$_2$O at ∼ 150°C. Aq. soln. pH 7−8. |
| | KNa salt, L-: 26[0], 66[26] H$_2$O; v. sl. s. EtOH | KNa salt: Loses 3H$_2$O at 100°C, becomes anhyd. at 130−40°C, decomp. at 220°C. Aq. soln. pH 7−8. |
| | s. H$_2$O, EtOH | Method of distinguishing between tartronic semialdehyde and its isomer, hydroxy-pyruvate, *Analyt. Biochem.* **4**, 159 (1962); *BJ* **78**, 69 (1961). PREP. *J. Biochem.* (*Tokyo*) **47**, 741 (1960); *BJ* **81**, 273 (1961). |
| 4.81 | 3.7[16] H$_2$O; s. EtOH, eth. | Salts less soluble than those of isovaleric acid. |

# 3 Phosphate esters excluding nucleotides and coenzymes

## Nomenclature

Recommendations for the nomenclature of phosphorus-containing compounds of biological importance are given in *BJ* **171**, 1 (1978); *PNAS* **74**, 2222 (1977).

In this section the term 'hydrolysis' refers to the release of phosphorus as inorganic orthophosphate, unless otherwise indicated. The proportion of phosphate released is expressed as a percentage of the *total* phosphorus in the molecule.

The abbreviation CHA signifies monocyclohexylammonium.

## Hydrates

In this section, the content of water of crystallization in the common crystalline forms of many compounds has been given. Phosphate esters and their salts are often hygroscopic and the water of crystallization in individual samples of a compound may vary widely, depending on the method of preparation and the conditions of storage. Greater reliance should therefore be placed on information supplied by the manufacturer with commercial products or, better, on analysis of the sample for its content of the compound of interest.

# 3 Phosphate esters excluding nucleotides and coenzymes

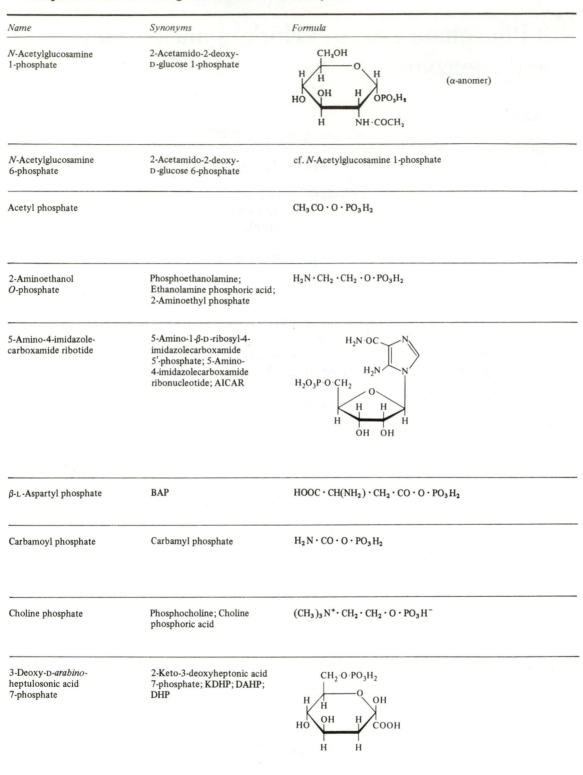

| Name | Synonyms | Formula |
|------|----------|---------|
| *N*-Acetylglucosamine 1-phosphate | 2-Acetamido-2-deoxy-D-glucose 1-phosphate | (α-anomer) |
| *N*-Acetylglucosamine 6-phosphate | 2-Acetamido-2-deoxy-D-glucose 6-phosphate | cf. *N*-Acetylglucosamine 1-phosphate |
| Acetyl phosphate | | $CH_3CO \cdot O \cdot PO_3H_2$ |
| 2-Aminoethanol *O*-phosphate | Phosphoethanolamine; Ethanolamine phosphoric acid; 2-Aminoethyl phosphate | $H_2N \cdot CH_2 \cdot CH_2 \cdot O \cdot PO_3H_2$ |
| 5-Amino-4-imidazole-carboxamide ribotide | 5-Amino-1-β-D-ribosyl-4-imidazolecarboxamide 5'-phosphate; 5-Amino-4-imidazolecarboxamide ribonucleotide; AICAR | |
| β-L-Aspartyl phosphate | BAP | $HOOC \cdot CH(NH_2) \cdot CH_2 \cdot CO \cdot O \cdot PO_3H_2$ |
| Carbamoyl phosphate | Carbamyl phosphate | $H_2N \cdot CO \cdot O \cdot PO_3H_2$ |
| Choline phosphate | Phosphocholine; Choline phosphoric acid | $(CH_3)_3N^+ \cdot CH_2 \cdot CH_2 \cdot O \cdot PO_3H^-$ |
| 3-Deoxy-D-*arabino*-heptulosonic acid 7-phosphate | 2-Keto-3-deoxyheptonic acid 7-phosphate; KDHP; DAHP; DHP | |

| M. wt. | General remarks |
|---|---|
| 301.2 | $pK_a < 1.4, 6.0$ (in $H_2O$). Both anomers completely hydrolysed in 0.1M-HCl at 100°C in 10 min. $\alpha$-Anomer 50% hydrolysed in 180 min at 37°C in 0.5M-$H_2SO_4$; $\beta$-anomer much more labile to acid. Under conditions of Fiske & Subbarow phosphate estimation (0.67M-$H_2SO_4$ at 26°C) $\beta$-anomer is completely hydrolysed in 45 min, while $\alpha$-anomer 5–6% hydrolysed in same time. $\alpha$-Anomer: $K_2$ salt + $1H_2O$, hygr. needles, $[\alpha]_D + 79$ (in $H_2O$); cryst. $Na_2$ salt. $\beta$-Anomer: anhyd. Na salt, $[\alpha]_D^{25} - 1.7$ (c = 2.9 in $H_2O$). PREP. *JACS* **78**, 5303 (1956); *JCS* **1960**, 4678; *BBA* **86**, 628 (1964). |
| 301.2 | 60% hydrolysis in 3 min at 100°C in 0.2M-alkali. $[\alpha]_D^{25} + 29.5$ (equilibrium value, c = 8 in 0.5M-Na acetate, final pH 3.0). PREP. *BJ* **84**, 185 (1962); *JBC* **230**, 497 (1958); *JACS* **78**, 1393 (1956); *Anal. Biochem.* **25**, 572 (1968). |
| 140.0 | $pK_a$ 1.2, 4.8. Rapidly hydrolysed in acid and alkaline solns. 20% hydrolysis in 30 min at pH 7 and room temp., 45% in 10 min in 0.5M-HCl. Hydrolysis in acid is accelerated by molybdate; acetyl phosphate behaves as $P_i$ in Fiske & Subbarow method. Cryst. LiK salt stable at 4°C. Solns. stable below $-30$°C. PREP. *J. Org. Chem.* **40**, 2516 (1975). |
| 141.1 | M.p. 244. $pK_a$ 5.59, 10.20. Solubility in $H_2O$, $20^{20}$ (free acid), $75^{20}$ (Na salt). Very stable to acid and alkali, 5% hydrolysis in 5 hr at 100°C in M-HCl. Free acid stable as solid at least 12 months at room temp. |
| 338.2 | Glycosidic bond more stable than that of purine nucleotides, e.g. < 5% hydrolysis in 90 min at 100°C in 0.1M-$H_2SO_4$. $pK_a$ 6.3. $\lambda_{max}$ 269 nm, $\epsilon$ 12 600 (pH 7) 9400 (pH 1). Free acid stable as solid at room temp. Soln. slowly decomposes, developing a pink colouration. PREP. *JBC* **228**, 201 (1957); *Meth. Enzymol.* **6**, 693 (1963), **51**, 189 (1978). |
| 213.1 | Somewhat less stable than acetyl phosphate. V. unstable below pH 4.5 and above pH 13. PREP. *JBC* **213**, 27 (1955). |
| 141.0 | 100% hydrolysis of $Li_2$ salt in 2 min at 100°C in water, in 10 min at room temp. in 0.1M-alkali. 50% hydrolysis in 2 hr at 30°C in $H_2O$; pH has little effect in range 1.5–9. Anhydrous salts stable several weeks over desiccant in cold but decompose slowly over long periods. Soln. of $Li_2$ salt stable frozen. $(NH_4)_2$ and $Na_2$ salts cryst. ex 32% ethanol at $-23$°C. PREP. *Biochem. Preps.* **7**, 23 (1960); *Meth. Enzymol.* **3**, 653 (1957). |
| 183.1 | Solubility in $H_2O$, $55^{20}$ (free acid) $20^{20}$ (Ca salt). Stable in acid, 15% hydrolysis in 5 hr at 100°C in M-HCl. In alkali, complete hydrolysis in 4 hr refluxing with sat. $Ba(OH)_2$. Usually obtained as Ca salt chloride, cryst. $+4H_2O$, stable at least 12 months at room temp. |
| 288.1 | $[\alpha]_D + 18$ (c = 0.5 Ca salt in $H_2O$) $+ 42$ (c = 1.47 free acid in $H_2O$). Cryst. $Ca_{1.5}$ salt, anhyd. and $Ba_{1.5}$ salt, variable hydration (2–4 $H_2O$). PREP. *JBC* **238**, 3170 (1963); *JCS Perkin I* **1975**, 600; *Meth. Enzymol.* **41**, 97 (1975). |

# 3 Phosphate esters excluding nucleotides and coenzymes

| Name | Synonyms | Formula |
|------|----------|---------|
| 2-Deoxyribose 1-phosphate | 2-Deoxy-D-*erythro*pentose 1-phosphate | 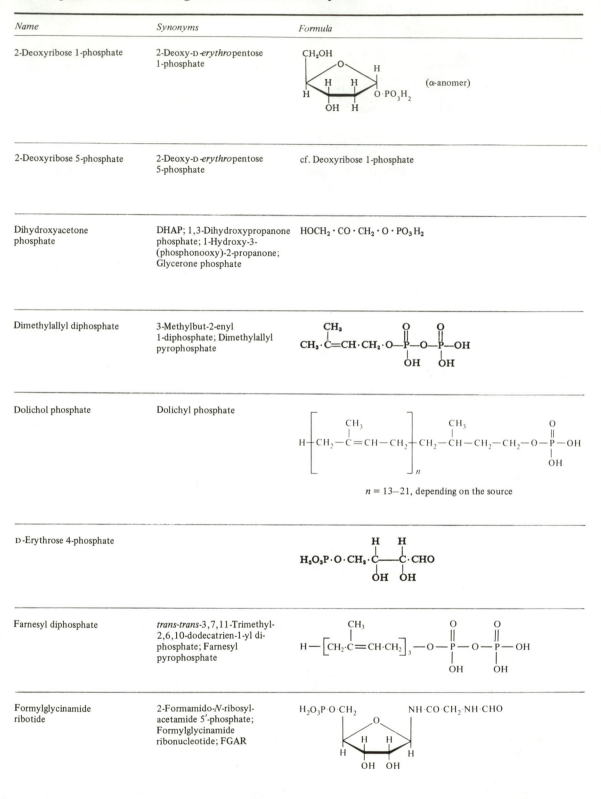 (α-anomer) |
| 2-Deoxyribose 5-phosphate | 2-Deoxy-D-*erythro*pentose 5-phosphate | cf. Deoxyribose 1-phosphate |
| Dihydroxyacetone phosphate | DHAP; 1,3-Dihydroxypropanone phosphate; 1-Hydroxy-3-(phosphonooxy)-2-propanone; Glycerone phosphate | $HOCH_2 \cdot CO \cdot CH_2 \cdot O \cdot PO_3H_2$ |
| Dimethylallyl diphosphate | 3-Methylbut-2-enyl 1-diphosphate; Dimethylallyl pyrophosphate | |
| Dolichol phosphate | Dolichyl phosphate | $n = 13-21$, depending on the source |
| D-Erythrose 4-phosphate | | |
| Farnesyl diphosphate | *trans-trans*-3,7,11-Trimethyl-2,6,10-dodecatrien-1-yl diphosphate; Farnesyl pyrophosphate | |
| Formylglycinamide ribotide | 2-Formamido-*N*-ribosyl-acetamide 5'-phosphate; Formylglycinamide ribonucleotide; FGAR | |

| M. wt. | General remarks |
|---|---|
| 214.1 | 50% hydrolysis in 10–15 min at 23°C and pH 4. $\alpha$-Anomer $[\alpha]_D$ + 38.8 (in $H_2O$), $\beta$-anomer $[\alpha]_D$ − 15.8 (in $H_2O$). Usually obtained as the $\alpha$-anomer, cryst. CHA salt. PREP. *JBC* **184**, 449 (1950); *Meth. Enzymol.* **3**, 183 (1957); *JACS* **82**, 1832 (1960), **84**, 1262 (1962). |
| 214.1 | $[\alpha]_D$ +19 (free acid in $H_2O$) + 16.5 (Ba salt in $H_2O$). In M-HCl, 45% hydrolysis in 7 min at 100°C, complete in 30 min. Cryst. $Na_2$ salt; Ba salt +$2H_2O$, v.s. $H_2O$, stable at room temp.; CHA salt of dimethyl acetal, needles, M.p. 145–50. PREP. *JBC* **215**, 389 (1955); *JACS* **81**, 3719 (1959); *Biochem. Preps.* **9**, 35 (1962); *Meth. Carbohydr. Chem.* **2**, 277 (1963); *JCS* **1964**, 5139. |
| 170.1 | $pK_a$ 1.77, 6.45. Unstable in alkali, hydrolysis complete in 20 min in M-alkali at room temp. 50% hydrolysis in 8 min at 100°C in M-HCl. Generally obtained as $(CHA)_2$ salt of dimethyl ketal, cryst. +$1H_2O$, stable at least 12 months at 4°C, converted to free compd. by treatment with Dowex 50 ($H^+$) − see *JACS* **78**, 1659 (1956); *Meth. Enzymol.* **41**, 442 (1975) − resulting soln. contains MeOH (2 moles/mole), best used at once, but stable a few days at pH 4.5 and frozen. PREP. *Biochem. Preps.* **7**, 45 (1960); *JACS* **78**, 1659 (1956); *Meth. Carbohydr. Chem.* **2**, 282 (1963). |
| 246.1 | Stability similar to farnesyl diphosphate, stable to alkali, unstable below pH 5.2. Instantaneous release of all P as pyrophosphate at pH 2. PREP. *BJ* **104**, 57 (1967); *Meth. Enzymol.* **15**, 359 (1969). |
| $n = 19$, 1462.4 | Phosphate esters of a family of polyprenols containing 14–22 isoprene units ($n = 13$–21). The principal dolichol phosphates in vertebrate tissues contain 18–20 isoprene units, in yeast 15–16 isoprene units. Stable to mild acid treatment, e.g. pH 1 at 100°C for 30 min, and to mild alkaline conditions, e.g. pH 13, 37°C for 15 min. PREP. *JBC* **249**, 6316 (1974); *Meth. Enzymol.* **50**, 122, 402 (1977). |
| 200.1 | $[\alpha]_D$ + 0.5 (c = 1 in $H_2O$). 50% hydrolysis in 20 min at 100°C in 0.5M-$H_2SO_4$. More stable at acid pH than in neutral soln. Neutral solns. should be kept cold and used at once. Ba salt of diethyl acetal, solid stable at 4°C, s. $H_2O$. Erythrose 4-phosphate tends to dimerize in soln., accelerated by Tris. PREP. *Can. J. Biochem.* **44**, 663 (1966); *Meth. Enzymol.* **9**, 35 (1966). |
| 382.3 | Labile in acid soln., rate of hydrolysis varies inversely with pH, indicating unionized compd. as labile species. At 22°C, complete hydrolysis takes about 5 days at pH 4 and less than 6 hr at pH 1. Reasonably stable in neutral and alkaline soln. At pH 8 and −20°C, 2% hydrolysis in 3 months; in 0.1M-KOH at 100°C, 15% hydrolysis in 1 hr. Cryst. Li and *S*-benzylisothiuronium salts. PREP. *Ann.* **654**, 180 (1962); *JBC* **237**, 56 (1962); *BJ* **104**, 57 (1967); *Meth. Enzymol.* **15**, 359, 445 (1969). |
| 314.2 | $pK_a$ 6.40. Formyl group hydrolysed by 0.1M-HCl at 100°C for 15 min. 25% of phosphate released in 60 min at 100°C in M-HCl, glycine and $NH_3$ released under same conditions. PREP. *JBC* **221**, 1057, 1071 (1956); *Meth. Enzymol.* **6**, 678 (1963). |

# 3 Phosphate esters excluding nucleotides and coenzymes

| Name | Synonyms | Formula |
|------|----------|---------|
| D-Fructose 1,6-bisphosphate | D-Fructose 1,6-diphosphate; Hexose diphosphate; Harden-Young ester; HDP; FDP | |
| D-Fructose 2,6-bis-phosphate | | ($\beta$-anomer) |
| D-Fructose 1-phosphate | | |
| D-Fructose 6-phosphate | Neuberg ester | cf. Fructose 1-phosphate |
| $\alpha$-D-Galactose 1-phosphate | | |
| D-Galactose 6-phosphate | | cf. Galactose 1-phosphate |
| Geranyl diphosphate | trans-3,7-Dimethyl-2,6-octadien-1-yl diphosphate; Geranyl pyrophosphate | |
| D-Gluconic acid 6-phosphate | 6-Phosphogluconic acid | |
| D-Glucosamine 6-phosphate | 2-Amino-2-deoxy-D-glucose 6-phosphate | |

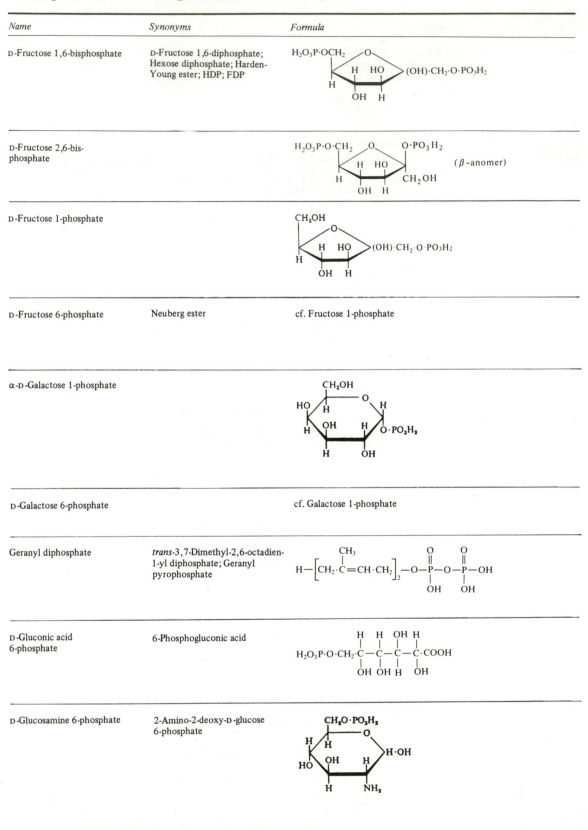

| M. wt. | General remarks |
|---|---|
| 340.1 | $[\alpha]_D^{17}$ + 4 (free acid in $H_2O$). $pK_a$ 1.48, 6.29 (each is an average value for the two phosphate groups). Half-time for hydrolysis in M-HCl at $100°C$ is 6 min for 1-phosphate and 75 min for 6-phosphate. $Na_3$ salt, cryst. + $8H_2O$, non-hygr., v.s. $H_2O$, solid stable at $4°C$, neutral soln. stable at $-15°C$. $Na_4$ salt, v. hygr. $(CHA)_4$ salt, cryst. + $10H_2O$, v.s. $H_2O$, solid stable at $4°C$. $Mg_2$ salt, solid stable, v.s. $H_2O$. $Ba_2$ and $Ca_2$ salts, solubility 0.5 $H_2O$; mono-Ba and mono-Ca salts, solubility 50 $H_2O$; Ba salts tend to decomp. on storage. Salts generally may develop a faint yellow colour on storage, but no decomp. detectable. |
| 340.1 | Natural compound is $\beta$-anomer. Unstable in acid forming fructose 6-phosphate and $P_i$; at pH 3 and $22°C$ half-life is 7 min, in 0.01 M-HCl half-life is $\sim$ 15 min at $0°C$, and less than 3 min at $20°C$. Stable in alkali, e.g. stable at $100°C$ for 30 min in 0.01 M-NaOH or for 15 min in 0.1 M-KOH. PREP. *JBC* **256**, 3171 (1981); *EJB* **117**, 319 (1981); *Meth. Enzymol.* **89**, 101 (1982). Stimulates phosphofructokinase and inhibits fructose bisphosphatase; REVIEW, *BJ* **206**, 1 (1982). |
| 260.1 | $[\alpha]_D^{20}$ $-52.5$ (free acid in $H_2O$). Complete hydrolysis in M-HCl at $100°C$ in 30 min, 50% hydrolysis in 2.8 min; at pH 4 and $37°C$, 50% hydrolysis in about 10–15 min. Cryst. Ba salt and $(CHA)_2$ salt, s. $H_2O$. $Na_2$ salt, amorph., s. $H_2O$. Salts stable at $4°C$ in dry state, sl. yellow colour may develop after storage for 6–12 months, but no decomp. detectable. Solns. should be freshly prepared. |
| 260.1 | $pK_a$ 0.97, 6.11. $[\alpha]_D^{21}$ + 2.5 (c = 3 in $H_2O$). 50% hydrolysis in 70 min in M-HCl at $100°C$. Less stable to alkali. Neutral soln. stable several weeks. $Na_2$ salt, amorph., hygr., s. $H_2O$. Ba salt, amorph., s. $H_2O$. Salts stable at room temp. if kept dry; may turn faintly yellow after long periods of storage without detectable decomp. |
| 260.1 | $pK_a$ 1.00, 6.17. $[\alpha]_D^{32}$ + 100 (c = 1.57 $K_2$ salt, $\alpha$-anomer, in $H_2O$). 50% hydrolysis in 2.1 min at $100°C$ in 0.1 M-HCl. $K_2$ salt, cryst. + 2 or $5H_2O$, s. $H_2O$. Ba salt + $3H_2O$. Salts stable at room temp. if kept dry. Neutral solns. stable for several days. $\beta$-Anomer has similar acid lability, $[\alpha]_D$ +31 (Ba salt in $H_2O$). PREP. *JACS* **72**, 4824 (1950), **79**, 5057 (1957); *Biochem. Preps.* **4**, 1(1955); *Meth. Carbohyd. Chem.* **2**, 261 (1963). |
| 260.1 | $[\alpha]_D^{20}$ +36.5 (c = 0.6 in $H_2O$), $[\alpha]_D^{25}$ +24.5 (Ba salt in $H_2O$). Ba and $Na_2$ salts, stable at room temp., s. $H_2O$. |
| 314.2 | Stability similar to farnesyl diphosphate, very labile in acid soln., reasonably stable in neutral and alkaline soln. Cryst. (ammonium)$_3$ and (*S*-benzylisothiuronium)$_2$ salts. PREP. *Ann.* **654**, 180 (1962); *BJ* **104**, 57 (1967); *Meth. Enzymol.* **15**, 359 (1969). |
| 276.1 | At $70°C$, converted to lactone for which $[\alpha]_{5461}$ +17.4. $Na_3$ salt, cryst. + $2H_2O$, solid stable at room temp., s. $H_2O$. Cryst. $(CHA)_3$ salt. Ba salt, amorph. May contain inhibitors of 6-phosphogluconate dehydrogenase. |
| 259.2 | < 1% hydrolysis in 20 min at $100°C$ in M-HCl. Decomp. 160–7. $[\alpha]_D^{25}$ + 56.0 changing to equilibrium value + 58.8 (c = 5 in $H_2O$). Readily s. $H_2O$; i. methanol, acet., eth. Unstable above pH 7. $pK_2$ 6.08, $pK_3$ 8.10. Cryst. free acid more stable than Na salt. |

## 3 Phosphate esters excluding nucleotides and coenzymes

| Name | Synonyms | Formula |
|---|---|---|

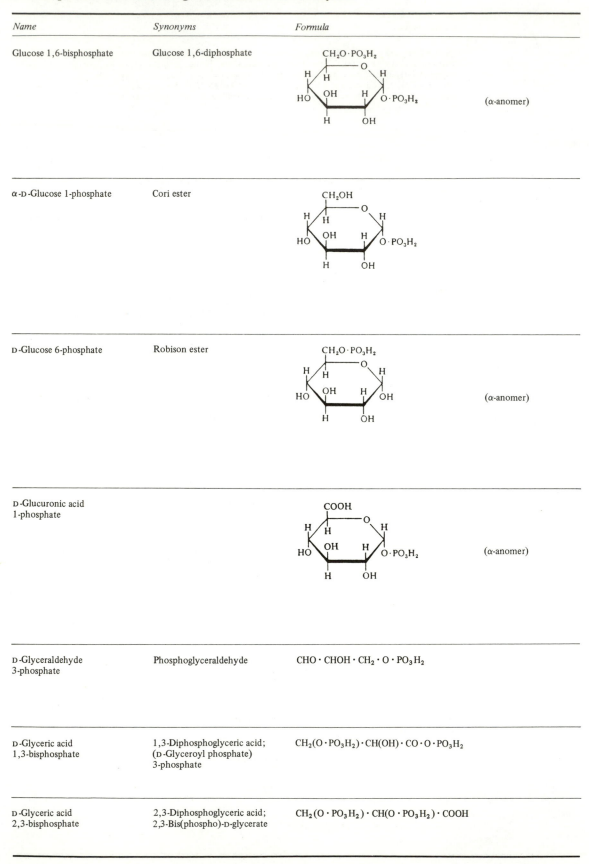

**Glucose 1,6-bisphosphate** — Glucose 1,6-diphosphate

$CH_2O \cdot PO_3H_2$ ... $O \cdot PO_3H_2$ (α-anomer)

**α-D-Glucose 1-phosphate** — Cori ester

$CH_2OH$ ... $O \cdot PO_3H_2$

**D-Glucose 6-phosphate** — Robison ester

$CH_2O \cdot PO_3H_2$ ... $OH$ (α-anomer)

**D-Glucuronic acid 1-phosphate**

$COOH$ ... $O \cdot PO_3H_2$ (α-anomer)

**D-Glyceraldehyde 3-phosphate** — Phosphoglyceraldehyde

$CHO \cdot CHOH \cdot CH_2 \cdot O \cdot PO_3H_2$

**D-Glyceric acid 1,3-bisphosphate** — 1,3-Diphosphoglyceric acid; (D-Glyceroyl phosphate) 3-phosphate

$CH_2(O \cdot PO_3H_2) \cdot CH(OH) \cdot CO \cdot O \cdot PO_3H_2$

**D-Glyceric acid 2,3-bisphosphate** — 2,3-Diphosphoglyceric acid; 2,3-Bis(phospho)-D-glycerate

$CH_2(O \cdot PO_3H_2) \cdot CH(O \cdot PO_3H_2) \cdot COOH$

| M. wt. | General remarks |
|---|---|
| 340.1 | $\alpha$-Anomer is coenzyme of phosphoglucomutase. 1-Phosphate group is slowly hydrolysed in $0.5M$-$H_2SO_4$ at $30°C$; $\alpha$-anomer, 9% of 1-phosphate in 120 min, 50% in 880 min; $\beta$-anomer, 50% of 1-phosphate in 220 min (6-phosphate is unaffected under these conditions). $\alpha$-Anomer: $[\alpha]_D^{25} + 83$ ($c = 0.6$ Na salt at pH 8); cryst. $Li_4$ salt; cryst. $(CHA)_4$ salt $+ 4H_2O$, stable indefinitely at room temp., s. $H_2O$. $\beta$-Anomer, $[\alpha]_D^{26} - 19$ ($c = 0.37$ Na salt at pH 8). PREP. *JBC* **180**, 1269 (1949); *JBC* **245**, 4031 (1970); *Meth. Enzymol.* **3**, 143 (1957), **41**, 79 (1975). |
| 260.1 | $pK_a$ 1.11, 6.13. $\alpha$-Anomer: $[\alpha]_D^{25} + 120$ ($c = 1$ free acid in $H_2O$), $+78$ ($c = 4 K_2$ salt in $H_2O$). 100% hydrolysis in $0.5M$-$H_2SO_4$ at $100°C$ in 10 min, at $33°C$ half-time for hydrolysis is 60 min. Stable at pH 8, even at $100°C$. Fairly stable in more strongly alkaline solns. Cryst. $K_2$ salt $+ 2H_2O$ and $Na_2$ salt $+ 4H_2O$, solids stable at room temp., s. $H_2O$. May contain small amounts of glucose 1,6-bisphosphate, PURIF. *JBC* **241**, 3930 (1966). $\beta$-Anomer: $[\alpha]_D^{24} + 9$ ($c = 2$ in $H_2O$). More labile to acid than $\alpha$-anomer, half-life at $33°C$ in $0.5M$-$H_2SO_4$ is 20 min. Cryst. $(CHA)_2$ salt. PREP. *Meth. Carbohyd. Chem.* **2**, 261 (1963), **6**, 389 (1972). |
| 260.1 | $pK_a$ 0.94, 6.11. $[\alpha]_D^{24} + 21.2$ ($c = 1.3 K_2$ salt in $H_2O$). More stable to acid than to alkali; 50% hydrolysis in 1400 min at $100°C$ in $M$-HCl, 60% hydrolysis in 3 min at $100°C$ in $0.2M$-NaOH. Free acid, $Na_2$, $K_2$, and Ba salts all hygr., water content very variable; stable at room temp. if kept dry. Ba salt, sp. s. $H_2O$; $Na_2$ and $K_2$ salts, v.s. $H_2O$. Mono-Na salt of $\beta$-anomer is non-hygr. and more stable to atmospheric moisture than other salts. On soln. in $H_2O$, equilibrium mixture containing 38% of $\alpha$-anomer, 62% $\beta$-anomer is immediately formed. Glucose 6-phosphate dehydrogenase is specific for $\beta$-anomer. |
| 274.1 | $\beta$-Anomer: cryst. dibrucine salt, solubility $0.4H_2O$; cryst. dibenzylamine salt, $[\alpha]_D^{20} - 14$ ($c = 2.6$ in $H_2O$). $\alpha$-Anomer: cryst. as $K_3$ salt $+ 5H_2O$, $[\alpha]_D^{20} + 51$ ($c = 2.4$ in $H_2O$), decomp. above $150°C$, sintering at $100°C$, in $0.01M$-acid at $61°C$ 50% hydrolysis occurs in 60 hr. Soln. most stable at pH 8. PREP. *JCS* **1952**, 1578, **1958**, 4128 ($\alpha$-anomer); *JBC* **197**, 863 (1952) ($\beta$-anomer). |
| 170.1 | $pK_a$ 1.42, 6.45. $[\alpha]_D + 14$ ($c = 1$ in $H_2O$). 50% hydrolysis in 8.1 min at $100°C$ in $M$-HCl. Unstable in alkaline soln. Acid solns. are stable several weeks if frozen; neutral solns. should be used as soon as possible after neutralization. Ba and $(CHA)_2$ salts of diethyl acetal, cryst., stable at $4°C$ for at least 12 months; Ba salt, sp. s. $H_2O$, $(CHA)_2$ salt $+ 1H_2O$, s. $H_2O$. Glyceraldehyde 3-phosphate regenerated from acetal by treatment with dil. HCl or Dowex 50 ($H^+$), see *Meth. Enzymol.* **41**, 443, 447 (1975); resulting solution will contain EtOH. |
| 266.0 | 50% hydrolysis in 27 min at $38°C$ and pH 7.2. Generally extremely unstable giving glyceric acid 3-phosphate. Store solns. at $-20°C$ or below. $pK_1$ 7.5, $pK_2$ 8.0. PREP. *Meth. Enzymol.* **3**, 216 (1957). |
| 266.0 | Extremely resistant to hydrolysis. Coenzyme of phosphoglyceric acid mutase. $(CHA)_5$ salt, cryst. $+ 4H_2O$, solid stable at room temp., s. $H_2O$. |

# 3 Phosphate esters excluding nucleotides and coenzymes

| Name | Synonyms | Formula |
|------|----------|---------|
| D-(+)-Glyceric acid 2-phosphate | 2-Phosphoglyceric acid | $CH_2OH \cdot CH(O \cdot PO_3H_2) \cdot COOH$ |
| D-(−)-Glyceric acid 3-phosphate | 3-Phosphoglyceric acid; Nilsson-Lohmann ester; PGA | $CH_2(O \cdot PO_3H_2) \cdot CH(OH) \cdot COOH$ |
| sn-Glycerol 3-phosphate | α-Glycerophosphoric acid; D-Glycerol 1-phosphate; L-Glycerol 3-phosphate | |
| Glycerol 2-phosphate | β-Glycerophosphoric acid | $CH_2OH \cdot CH(O \cdot PO_3H_2) \cdot CH_2OH$ |
| sn-Glycerophosphocholine | L-α-Glycerophosphorylcholine; Glycerol choline phosphate | |
| sn-Glycerophospho-ethanolamine | L-α-Glycerophosphorylethan-olamine | cf. Glycerophosphocholine<br>$X = -CH_2 \cdot CH_2NH_2$ |
| 1-(sn-Glycerophospho)-L-myo-inositol | Glycerophosphorylinositol; 1-(α-Glycerylphosphoryl)-L-myo-inositol; Glycerol inositol phosphate | cf. Glycerophosphocholine<br> |
| sn-Glycerophosphoserine | Glycerophosphorylserine | cf. Glycerophosphocholine<br>$X = -CH_2 \cdot CHNH_2 \cdot COOH$ |
| Glycollic acid phosphate | Phosphoglycollic acid | $H_2O_3P \cdot O \cdot CH_2 \cdot COOH$ |
| L-Histidinol phosphate | β-Amino-1H-imidazole-4-propanol phosphate | |

| M. wt. | General remarks |
|---|---|
| 186.1 | Slowly hydrolysed by acids. $[\alpha]_D^{22} + 3.6$ (c = 2 $Na_3$ salt in $H_2O$) + 12.9 (c = 1.8 free acid in M-HCl). Cryst. $Na_3$ salt + $6H_2O$, stable at room temp., s. $H_2O$. Cryst. $(CHA)_3$ salt. PREP. Biochem. Preps. **5**, 66 (1957); JACS **76**, 3188 (1954); BBA **141**, 445 (1967). |
| 186.1 | $[\alpha]_D^{20} - 14.5$ (in 1M-HCl) $- 745$ (in ammonium molybdate soln.). 50% hydrolysis in 35.7 hr at 100°C in M-HCl, in about 3 hr at 125°C. Cryst. acid Ba salt + $2H_2O$, sp. s. $H_2O$, s. dil. mineral acids. $Na_3$ salt, amorph., v. hygr., s. $H_2O$, stable if kept dry. $(CHA)_3$ salt, cryst. + $3H_2O$, s. $H_2O$. Solid salts stable at room temp. Solutions readily become contaminated by microorganisms unless stored frozen. May contain small amounts of glyceric acid 2,3-bisphosphate. |
| 172.1 | 2% hydrolysis in 180 min at 100°C in M-HCl. Hydrolysed by heating at 160°C in 10% $H_2SO_4$. $[\alpha]_D - 1.45$ (c = 10 Ba salt in 2M-HCl). $pK_2$ 6.66. $(CHA)_2$ salt, cryst. + $2H_2O$, s. $H_2O$, stable at 4°C. |
| 172.1 | V. slow hydrolysis at 100°C in M-HCl. $pK_1$ 1.34, $pK_2$ 6.55. Used as buffer and as substrate for assay of phosphomonoesterases, reaction followed by release of inorganic phosphate. $Na_2$ salt + $5H_2O$, s. $H_2O$. May contain small amounts of sn-glycerol 3-phosphate. |
| 275.2 | Choline completely liberated in 15 min at 100°C in M-HCl. M.p. 143, sinters 141. $[\alpha]_D^{23} - 2.85$ (c = 2.2 synthetic material in $H_2O$). V. hygr. cryst. $CdCl_2$ compound + $3H_2O$, M.p. 99. PREP. Biochem. Preps. **6**, 16 (1958), **9**, 55 (1962). |
| 215.2 | Ethanolamine completely liberated in 15 min at 100°C in M-HCl. M.p. 86–7. $[\alpha]_D^{26} - 2.9$ (c = 7.6 synthetic material in $H_2O$). Cryst. monohydrate. PREP. JACS **75**, 4510 (1953); BJ **50**, 449 (1952); Chem. Phys. Lipids **6**, 31 (1971). |
| 334.2 | Deacylation product of phosphatidylinositol. Completely decomposed in 40 min at 100°C in 0.5M-KOH giving glycerophosphate and inositol phosphate. $[\alpha]_D^{25} - 18.7$ (c = 2 free acid in water). Cryst. cyclohexyl-ammonium salt, $[\alpha]_D^{25} - 13.5$ (c = 2 in water). PREP. BJ **71**, 195 (1959); JACS **81**, 2591 (1959); JBC **236**, 1907 (1961); JCS **1959**, 3547 (DL- compound). |
| 259.2 | $[\alpha]_D^{24} + 4.5$ (c = 10 in M-HCl) $- 2.0$ (c = 10 in $H_2O$). Cryst. monohydrate. PREP. JACS **81**, 2167 (1959); BJ **71**, 195 (1959). |
| 156.0 | 7.8% hydrolysis in 2 hr at 100°C in 0.5M-$H_2SO_4$. Cryst. acid Ba salt + $1H_2O$. $(CHA)_3$ salt, cryst. + $2H_2O$, stable at room temp. |
| 221.2 | Approx. 5% hydrolysis in 4 hr at 100°C in M-NaOH or M-HCl. Approx. 20% hydrolysis at pH 4.5 and 100°C in 4 hr. Obtained as stable monohydrate. PREP. JBC **212**, 687 (1955); JBC **220**, 113 (1956). |

# 3 Phosphate esters excluding nucleotides and coenzymes

| Name | Synonyms | Formula |
|---|---|---|
| L-Homoserine phosphate | O-Phosphohomoserine | $H_2O_3P \cdot O \cdot CH_2 \cdot CH_2 \cdot CHNH_2 \cdot COOH$ |
| Hydroxypyruvic acid 3-phosphate | Phosphohydroxypyruvic acid | $H_2O_3P \cdot O \cdot CH_2 \cdot CO \cdot COOH$ |
| D-erythro-Imidazoleglycerol phosphate | IGP | |
| Indole-3-glycerol phosphate | InGP | |
| myo-Inositol hexaphosphate | Phytic acid; myo-Inositol hexakisphosphate | |
| L-myo-Inositol 1-phosphate | 1D-myo-Inositol 1-phosphate | |
| myo-Inositol 2-phosphate | | cf. Inositol hexaphosphate |
| Isopentenyl diphosphate | Isopentenyl pyrophosphate; 3-Methylbut-3-enyl 1-pyrophosphate | |
| 2-Keto-3-deoxy-6-phospho-gluconic acid | KDPG; 3-Deoxy-D-erythro-2-hexulosonic acid 6-phosphate | |

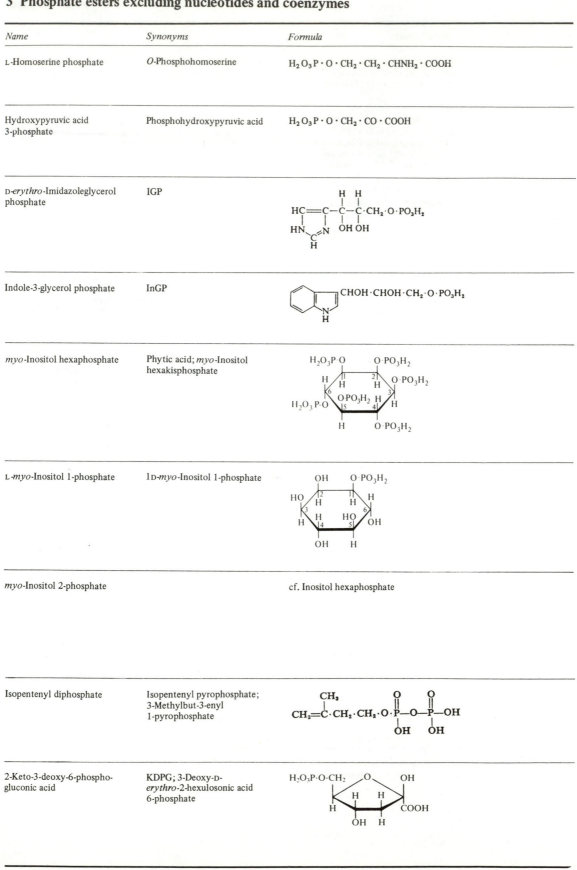

| M. wt. | General remarks |
|---|---|
| 199.1 | $[\alpha]_D^{22} + 6.2$ (c = 2.4 in $H_2O$). 12.5% hydrolysis in 1 hr at 100°C in 6m-HCl. 100% in 30 hr at 105°C in 6m-HCl. Isolated as Ba salt, probable formula $C_4H_8NO_6PBa \cdot H_2O$. PREP. *JBC* **248**, 1032 (1973); *J. Org. Chem.* **38**, 1421 (1973); *Helv. Chim. Acta* **58**, 518 (1975). |
| 184.0 | 50% hydrolysis in 20 min at 90°C in m-HCl. 50% in 15 hr at room temp. in m-alkali. (CHA)$_3$ salt of dimethyl ketal, cryst. $+1H_2O$, M.p. 183−5. Free acid regenerated by treatment with Dowex 50(H$^+$) − see refs.; resulting soln. contains MeOH. PREP. *Biochem. Preps.* **7**, 66 (1960); *Meth. Carbohyd. Chem.* **2**, 286 (1963). |
| 238.1 | Hydrolysed overnight at 100°C by 6m-HCl. Stable monohydrate. $[\alpha]_D^{20} - 12.1$ (c = 2.37 in $H_2O$, pH 7). PREP. *JBC* **228**, 131 (1957); *Meth. Enzymol.* **17B**, 15 (1971). |
| 287.2 | Not hydrolysed by m-alkali at room temp. Indole released on heating with dil. alkali; labile to dilute acid at room temp. Cryst. Ba salt + 2H$_2$O and (CHA)$_2$ salt. PREP. *JBC* **223**, 171 (1956). |
| 660.0 | 9.5% hydrolysis in 6 hr at 100°C in 0.5m-$H_2SO_4$. |
| 260.1 | The L-isomer (now correctly called the 1D-isomer) is a product of phosphodiesterase hydrolysis of phosphatidyl-inositol. The D-isomer (now 1L-) is the product of the enzyme, glucose 6-phosphate−*myo*-inositol 1-phosphate cyclase. Phosphate migrates in hot dil. acid to give a mixture of 1- and 2-phosphates. (CHA)$_2$ salt of L-isomer (1D-isomer), M.p. 200−10d., $[\alpha]_D^{25} + 3.4$ (c = 3 in $H_2O$ at pH 9) −9.8 (free acid in $H_2O$, pH 2). PREP. *JACS* **81**, 915 (1959); *Biochem. Preps.* **9**, 99 (1962); *J. Gen. Chem. U.S.S.R.* **40**, 2469 (1970) (1D-isomer); *Tetrahedron* **25**, 5681 (1969) (1L-isomer). |
| 260.1 | Monophosphate product of phytase hydrolysis of hexaphosphate. M.p. 195−7 d. Optically inactive. Stable to heating with strong alkali. Phosphate migrates in hot dil. acid to give mixture of 1- and 2-phosphates. Cryst. CHA and (CHA)$_2$ + 4H$_2$O salts, M.p. 211−13 and 203−5 respectively. PREP. *Biochem. Preps.* **2**, 65 (1952). For information on the di- and tri-phosphates of inositol, see *JBC* **236**, 1902 (1961); *J. Lipid Res.* **1**, 255 (1960); *Adv. Carbohydr. Chem.* **14**, 135 (1959). For penta-phosphates, see *BJ* **89**, 172 (1963). |
| 246.1 | Labile in 1m-HCl at 100°C for 10 min, releasing P$_i$. Cryst. Li$_3$ and (CHA)$_3$ salts. PREP. *BJ* **105**, 544 (1967); *Meth. Enzymol.* **15**, 359, 450 (1969); *JBC* **234**, 2605 (1959), **235**, 326 (1960). |
| 258.1 | 62% hydrolysis in 60 min at 100°C in m-HCl. p$K_1$ < 2.5, p$K_2$ 3.12, p$K_3$ 6.4. $[\alpha]_D^{22} + 6.5$ (Li salt in $H_2O$). Li$_3$ salt, cryst. + 2H$_2$O. PREP. *Meth. Enzymol.* **9**, 51 (1966), **41**, 97 (1975). |

# 3 Phosphate esters excluding nucleotides and coenzymes

| Name | Synonyms | Formula |
|------|----------|---------|
| α-D-Mannose 1-phosphate | α-D-Mannosyl phosphate | (structure) (α-anomer) |
| Mannose 6-phosphate | | cf. Mannose 1-phosphate |
| Mevalonic acid 5-phosphate | Phosphomevalonic acid | $HOOC \cdot CH_2 \cdot C \cdot CH_2 \cdot CH_2 \cdot O \cdot PO_3H_2$ with OH and $CH_3$ |
| Mevalonic acid 5-diphosphate | Diphosphomevalonic acid; Pyrophosphomevalonic acid; Mevalonic acid 5-pyrophosphate | cf. Mevalonic acid 5-phosphate |
| D-(+)-Pantetheine 4′-phosphate | Phosphopantetheine | $H_2O_3P \cdot O \cdot CH_2 \cdot C - C \cdot CO \cdot NH \cdot CH_2 \cdot CH_2 \cdot CO \cdot NH \cdot CH_2 \cdot CH_2 \cdot SH$ with $CH_3$, OH, $CH_3$, H |
| Pantothenic acid 4-phosphate | | $H_2O_3P \cdot O \cdot CH_2 \cdot C - C \cdot CO \cdot NH \cdot CH_2 \cdot CH_2 \cdot COOH$ with $CH_3$, OH, $CH_3$, H |
| Phosphoarginine | L-Arginine phosphate | $HN{=}C$ with $NH \cdot PO_3H_2$ and $NH \cdot (CH_2)_3 \cdot CH(NH_2) \cdot COOH$ |
| Phosphocreatine | Creatine phosphate | $HN{=}C$ with $NH \cdot PO_3H_2$ and $N \cdot CH_2 \cdot COOH$, $CH_3$ |
| Phosphoenolpyruvic acid | Phosphopyruvic acid; PEP | $CH_2{=}C(O \cdot PO_3H_2) \cdot COOH$ |
| Phosphoribosyl diphosphate | Phosphoribosyl pyrophosphate; α-D-Ribofuranose 1-pyrophosphate 5-phosphate; PRPP | (structure) |
| D-Ribitol 5-phosphate | L-Ribitol 1-phosphate | $H_2O_3P \cdot O \cdot CH_2 \cdot C - C - C \cdot CH_2OH$ with H, OH across |

| M. wt. | General remarks |
|---|---|
| 260.1 | 50% hydrolysed in 360 min in 0.95M-acid at 30 °C. $K_2$ salt, cryst. $+ 4H_2O$, s. $H_2O$, stable at room temp. for at least 1 year. $(CHA)_2$ salt, cryst. $+ 2H_2O$, $[\alpha]_D + 28.7$ (c = 2 in $H_2O$). Ba salt, cryst. $+ 2H_2O$, $[\alpha]_D^{20} + 34$ (c = 2.2 in $H_2O$), stable. PREP. *Biochem.* **12**, 5031 (1971); *Helv. Chim. Acta* **36**, 1614 (1953). |
| 260.1 | $[\alpha]_D^{22} + 13.3$ (c = 1.66 free acid in 0.1M-HCl). 50% hydrolysis in 1000 min in M-HCl at 100 °C. Cryst Ba salt $+ 3H_2O$, stable 12 months at room temp. |
| 228.1 | Natural compound laevorotatory. Stable for 7 min at 100 °C in M-HCl or M-KOH; 9% hydrolysis in 60 min in M-HCl. $pK_1$ 1.7, $pK_2$ 4.6, $pK_3$ 6.9. Cryst. $(CHA)_2$ and $(CHA)_3$ salts, M.p. 145–7 and 152–4 respectively. PREP. *Meth. Enzymol.* **6**, 506 (1963), **15**, 410 (1969). |
| 308.1 | Hydrolysis to mevalonic acid 5-phosphate and $P_i$ complete in 10 min in M-HCl at 100 °C. Acid solns. are unstable even at pH 6 and frozen; 50% hydrolysis to mevalonic acid 5-phosphate and $P_i$ may occur in 3 months. Alkaline solns. deteriorate more slowly, 3–5% in 6 months. Stable for 10 min at 100 °C in M-KOH. Store as dry Ba salt. PREP. *Meth Enzymol.* **6**, 505 (1963), **15**, 417 (1969). |
| 358.3 | Obtained as Ba salt, $[\alpha]_D^{18} + 10.8$ (c = 4.2 in water), or Li salt. PREP. *Meth. Enzymol.* **62**, 236 (1979). |
| 299.2 | 56% hydrolysis in 160 min at 100 °C in 2M-HCl. Stable for 2 hr at 100 °C in 0.05M-KOH. Ba salt, s. $H_2O$. Li salt, PREP. *Meth. Enzymol.* **62**, 236 (1979). |
| 254.2 | $pK_a$ 2.0, 4.5, 9.4, 11.2. M.p. 175–80 (free acid), 180 ($Li_2$ salt). 100% hydrolysis in 1 min at 100 °C in 0.1M-HCl. Obtained as the stable Ba salt, Ba content somewhat variable, also contains $HCO_3^-$. PREP. *BJ* **62**, 358 (1956), **92**, 429 (1964). |
| 211.1 | $pK_a$ 2.7, 4.58. Very unstable in acid; complete hydrolysis in 1 min at 100 °C in M-HCl, 50% hydrolysis in 4 min at 25 °C in 0.5M-HCl. Hydrolysis accelerated by molybdate and creatine phosphate behaves as $P_i$ in the Fiske & Subbarow phosphate estimation. Hydrolysis slow at pH 7.8, slightly alkaline solns. stable for several days in the cold, but immediate hydrolysis occurs if the soln. becomes slightly acid. Cryst. $Na_2$ and $(Tris)_2$ salts, stable in the cold, s. $H_2O$. $Na_2$ salt hydrate $+ 4H_2O$, hygr. forming hexahydrate, but stable *in vacuo* over desiccant. |
| 168.0 | 50% hydrolysis in 8.3 min at 100 °C in M-HCl. Readily hydrolysed by alkali. Sensitive to heavy metal ions. Acid salts: mono-K salt and mono-Na salt $+ 1H_2O$, non-hygr., solids stable at 4 °C, s. $H_2O$ giving acid soln. which must be neutralized at once. Neutral salts: $Na_3$ salt, anhyd. or $+ 2H_2O$; $(CHA)_3$ salt, solid stable at 4 °C for at least 1 year, s. $H_2O$ giving neutral soln. Solns. should be kept neutral and prepared fresh weekly. |
| 390.1 | $pK_a$ 5.9, 6.7. Complete loss of pyrophosphate group as inorg. pyrophosphate in 20 min at 65 °C and pH 3.0, 50% at pH 6.7. Soln. stable at pH 8 in the cold, keeps several months at pH 8 and $-20$ °C or below. $Na_4$ salt, solid stable for several months if stored dry and protected from light. PREP. *Biochem. Preps.* **8**, 110 (1961). |
| 232.1 | PREP. *JCS* **1956**, 4583; *JBC* **233**, 1049 (1958). |

# 3 Phosphate esters excluding nucleotides and coenzymes

| Name | Synonyms | Formula |
|------|----------|---------|
| Ribose 1,5-bisphosphate | α-D-Ribofuranose 1,5-diphosphate | |
| α-D-Ribose 1-phosphate | α-D-Ribofuranose 1-phosphate; α-D-Ribosyl phosphate | cf. Ribose 1,5-bisphosphate |
| D-Ribose 5-phosphate | | cf. Ribose 1,5-bisphosphate |
| D-Ribulose 1,5-bisphosphate | Ribulose 1,5-diphosphate | |
| D-Ribulose 5-phosphate | D-erythro-Pentulose 5-phosphate | cf. Ribulose 1,5-bisphosphate |
| D-Sedoheptulose 1,7-bisphosphate | | |
| D-Sedoheptulose 7-phosphate | | cf. Sedoheptulose 1,7-bisphosphate |
| Serine phosphate | O-Phosphoserine | $H_2O_3P \cdot O \cdot CH_2 \cdot CH(NH_2) \cdot COOH$ |
| Shikimic acid 5-phosphate | | |
| Sucrose 6'-phosphate | | |

| M. wt. | General remarks |
|---|---|

**310.1** 50% hydrolysis in 5 min under conditions of Fiske and Subbarow estimation. Coenzyme of phosphoribomutase. Cryst. (CHA)$_4$ salt, M.p. 171–2 d., $[\alpha]_D^{22}$ +20.8 (c = 0.43 in H$_2$O). PREP. *JBC* **245**, 4031 (1970).

**230.1** α-Anomer: Rapid hydrolysis in strong acid, 50% in 3.5 hr at 20°C in 0.01M-HCl and in 2.5 min in 0.5M-acid at 25°C. Behaves as P$_i$ in the Fiske & Subbarow phosphate estimation, where hydrolysis is complete in 2.5 min. (CHA)$_2$ salt, cryst. +1H$_2$O, solid stable at room temp., s. H$_2$O, $[\alpha]_D^{20}$ +40.3 (c = 2.37 in H$_2$O). β-Anomer: More stable to acid than α, 50% hydrolysis takes 240 min in 0.1M-acid at 26°C, $[\alpha]_D$ −13.6 (CHA salt in H$_2$O). PREP. *JBC* **167**, 477 (1947), **193**, 497 (1951); *JACS* **79**, 441 (1957), **78**, 811 (1956).

**230.1** Relatively slowly hydrolysed by acid; 59% hydrolysis in 2 hr at 100°C in M-HCl, half-time for hydrolysis at 100°C is ~17 hr in 0.01M-acid and 10 hr in 0.25M-acid. $[\alpha]_D^{20}$ +22.8 (in 0.02M-HCl) +16.5 (c = 3.35 Ba salt in 0.23M-HCl). Ba salt, cryst. +6H$_2$O, stable at room temp., s. H$_2$O. Na salt, amorph., hygr., stable at 4°C if stored dry.

**310.1** 1-Phosphate group completely hydrolysed in 20 min at 100°C in 0.5M-H$_2$SO$_4$, 50% in 12 min at 100°C in 0.1M-acid. Neutral soln. stable for weeks if frozen. Na$_4$ salt, hygr., s. H$_2$O. Ba$_2$ salt, 20–50% loss per annum when stored dry at 4°C. PREP. *Biochem. Preps.* **6**, 83 (1958); *BJ* **175**, 909 (1978). PURIF. *BJ* **159**, 563 (1976).

**230.1** 50% hydrolysis in 40 min at 100°C in 0.5M-H$_2$SO$_4$. $[\alpha]_D^{20}$ −40. Ba salt obtained about 90% pure. PREP. *Meth. Enzymol.* **9**, 41, 46 (1966); *JBC* **237**, 643 (1962).

**370.1** 50% hydrolysis in 30 min at 100°C in 0.5M-H$_2$SO$_4$, 70% in 3 hr. Na salt, cryst. PREP. *JBC* **218**, 745 (1956); *Meth. Enzymol.* **41**, 77 (1975).

**290.2** 10–15% hydrolysis in 1 hr at 100°C in 0.5M-H$_2$SO$_4$. Ba salt, cryst., $[\alpha]_D$ +5 (in H$_2$O). PREP. *Meth. Carbohydr. Chem.* **6**, 398 (1972); *Biochem. Preps.* **12**, 1 (1968).

**185.1** 61% hydrolysis in 24 hr at 100°C in M-HCl, 51% in 0.5M-NaOH. Cryst., M.p. 165–6 d. p$K_a$ 2.65, 5.91, 9.99. Solubility at 20°C in H$_2$O, 2.8 (free acid), 25 (Na salt). Ca salt, Ba salt, sp. s. H$_2$O.

**254.1** 25–30% hydrolysis in 30 min at 120°C in 0.1M-HCl. $[\alpha]_D^{29}$ −107.6 (c = 1.02 K salt in water). PREP. *JACS* **78**, 2894 (1956); *Meth. Enzymol.* **17A**, 351 (1970). 3-Enolpyruvylshikimate 5-phosphate, PREP. *JBC* **239**, 1142 (1964).

**422.3** 25% hydrolysis in 60 min at 100°C in 0.5M-H$_2$SO$_4$. Stable in hot alkali. In 0.9M-HCl at 37°C, release of reducing power is slower than with sucrose. Isolated as Ca salt. Ba salt, $[\alpha]_D$ +35.4 (in H$_2$O). PREP. *Meth. Enzymol.* **42**, 341 (1975); *Carbohydr. Res.* **21**, 283 (1972).

# 3 Phosphate esters excluding nucleotides and coenzymes

| Name | Synonyms | Formula |
|------|----------|---------|
| Undecaprenyl diphosphate | Undecaprenol pyrophosphate; $C_{55}$ polyprenol pyrophosphate | |
| D-Xylulose 5-phosphate | D-*threo*-Pentulose 5-phosphate | |

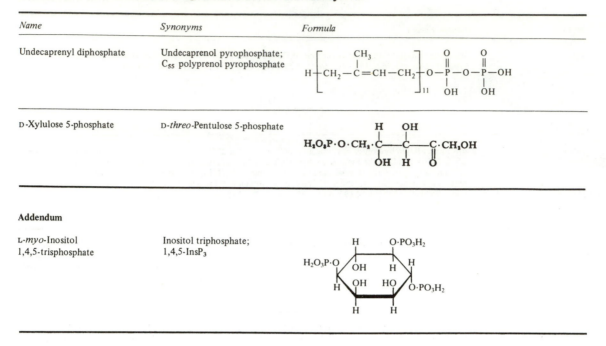

**Addendum**

| | | |
|------|----------|---------|
| L-*myo*-Inositol 1,4,5-trisphosphate | Inositol triphosphate; 1,4,5-InsP$_3$ | |

| M. wt. | General remarks |
|---|---|
| 927.3 | Mild acid conditions, e.g. pH 2 at 100°C for 1 min, cause complete hydrolysis of prenol—phosphate bond, with release of inorganic pyrophosphate. Stable in neutral and mild alkaline conditions, e.g. pH 13, 37°C for 15 min. PREP. *Meth. Enzymol.* **28**, 306 (1972). |
| 230.1 | 55% hydrolysis in 10 min at 100°C in 0.5M-$H_2SO_4$. Obtained as Na salt or Ba salt about 70% pure. PREP. *Meth. Enzymol.* **9**, 41 (1966). |
| 420.1 | $[\alpha]_D^{25} - 27.4$ (CHA salt in alkaline soln.). s. $H_2O$. Soln. of K salt at pH 7.2 stable when frozen at $-20°C$. Inositol trisphosphate is released from membrane phosphatidylinositol bisphosphate by a specific phosphodiesterase when Ca-mobilizing receptors are stimulated. It mobilizes $Ca^{2+}$ from non-mitochondrial intracellular sources. The 1,3,4-trisphosphate can also be released but this is not active in mobilizing $Ca^{2+}$ (*BJ* **223**, 237 (1984)). PREP. *BJ* **203**, 169 (1982), **222**, 269 (1984). REVIEW. *Nature (London)* **312**, 315 (1984). |

# 4 Constituents of nucleic acids and related compounds

## Nomenclature

In the literature there are two different conventions of numbering pyrimidine compounds. In the newer system uracil for example is 2,4-dihydroxypyrimidine but in the older convention uracil is 2,6-dihydroxypyrimidine. Confusion can arise because original papers may have used either system without specifying which. Thus 1-methylcytosine in *JCS* **1962**, 1348, is the same compound as 3-methylcytosine in *JACS* **85**, 4024 (1963): cytosine may be 6-amino-2-hydroxy-pyrimidine (older system) or 4-amino-2-hydroxypyrimidine (new system). A full discussion of pyrimidine nomenclature can be found in D. J. Brown, *The Pyrimidines*, Interscience, New York and London (1962). The system of numbering used here is the new one as follows:

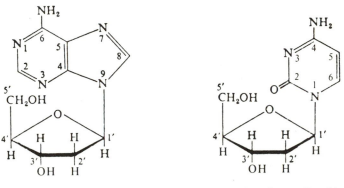

Adenine deoxyriboside    Cytosine deoxyriboside

Abbreviations and symbols for nucleic acids, polynucleotides, and their constituents are given in *BJ* **120**, 449 (1970); *JBC* **245**, 5171 (1970); *EJB* **15**, 203 (1970).

## Minor bases in Nucleic Acids

In addition to the major constituents listed in this section a large number of other purine and pyrimidine derivatives are found in small amounts; for a comprehensive review of these see *PNARMB* **12**, 49 (1972).

## $pK_a$ values

Some $pK_a$ values reported in the literature may differ from those cited here by more than ± 0.1 pH unit. For sources of $pK_a$ data see Section 5.

# 4 Constituents of nucleic acids and related compounds

| Name | Synonyms | Formula |
|------|----------|---------|
| **Adenine group** | | |
| Adenine | 6-Aminopurine | |
| Adenosine | Adenine riboside;<br>9-β-D-Ribofuranosidoadenine | |
| Adenosine 2′-phosphate | 2′-AMP; Adenylic acid a | |
| Adenosine 3′-phosphate | 3′-AMP; Yeast adenylic acid;<br>Adenylic acid b | |
| Adenosine 5′-phosphate | 5′-AMP; Muscle adenylic acid | |
| Adenosine 2′,3′-cyclic phosphate | 2′,3′-Cyclic AMP | |

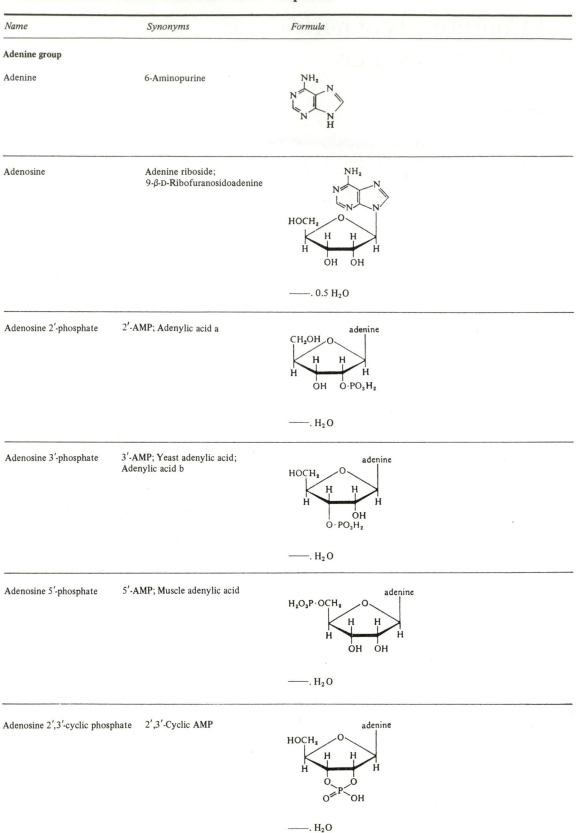

| M. wt | p$K_a$ | Solubility | General remarks |
|---|---|---|---|
| 135.1 | < 1.0<br>4.1<br>9.8 | $0.09^{25}$, $2.5^{100}$<br>$H_2O$; sl. s. EtOH;<br>i. eth., $CHCl_3$ | Released from DNA by hydrolysis with dilute acid. |
| 267.2 | 3.5<br>12.5 | s. $H_2O$; v. sl. s. EtOH | Water of cryst. lost at 100°C *in vacuo*. Readily hydrolysed in dil. mineral acids to adenine and D-ribose. Deaminated to inosine by nitrous acid. |
| 276.2 | | | |
| 347.2 | 3.8<br>6.2 | | Produced, with 3′-isomer, by the alkaline hydrolysis of RNA (0.3 M-KOH, 37°C, 16 hr). Completely hydrolysed to adenine, ribose 5-phosphate, ribose, and inorg. P by M-HCl at 100°C for 1 hr. |
| 365.2 | | | |
| 347.2 | 3.7<br>5.9 | | Produced, with 2′-isomer, by the alkaline hydrolysis of RNA (0.3M-KOH, 37°C, 16 hr). Acid hydrolysis as for adenosine 2′-phosphate. Quantitative yield of furfural when distilled from 20% HCl for 3 hr (cf. adenosine 5′-phosphate). |
| 365.2 | | | |
| 347.2 | 3.8<br>6.2–6.4 | s. hot $H_2O$ | Acid hydrolysis as for adenosine 2′-phosphate. Only traces of furfural formed when distilled from 20% HCl (cf. adenosine 3′-phosphate). |
| 365.2 | | | |
| 329.2 | | | Produced as an intermediate during hydrolysis of RNA by alkali. Readily converted to a mixture of 2′- and 3′-phosphates by dil. acid and alkali at room temp. |
| 347.2<br>346.2 | | | |

# 4 Constituents of nucleic acids and related compounds

| Name | Synonyms | Formula |
|------|----------|---------|
| Adenosine 3',5'-cyclic phosphate | 3',5'-Cyclic AMP; cAMP | |
| ——, dibutyryl deriv. | $N^6$, $O^2$-Dibutyryladenosine 3',5'-cyclic phosphate; Bu$_2$-cAMP | |
| Adenosine 5'-diphosphate | ADP | |
| Adenosine 5'-triphosphate | ATP | |
| Adenosine 3'-phosphate 5'-phosphosulphate | PAPS; 3'-Phosphoadenosine 5'-phosphosulphate; 3'-Phospho-5'-adenylyl sulphate. | |
| Adenosine 5'-phosphosulphate | APS; Adenosine 5'-sulphato-phosphate; 5'-Adenylyl sulphate | |

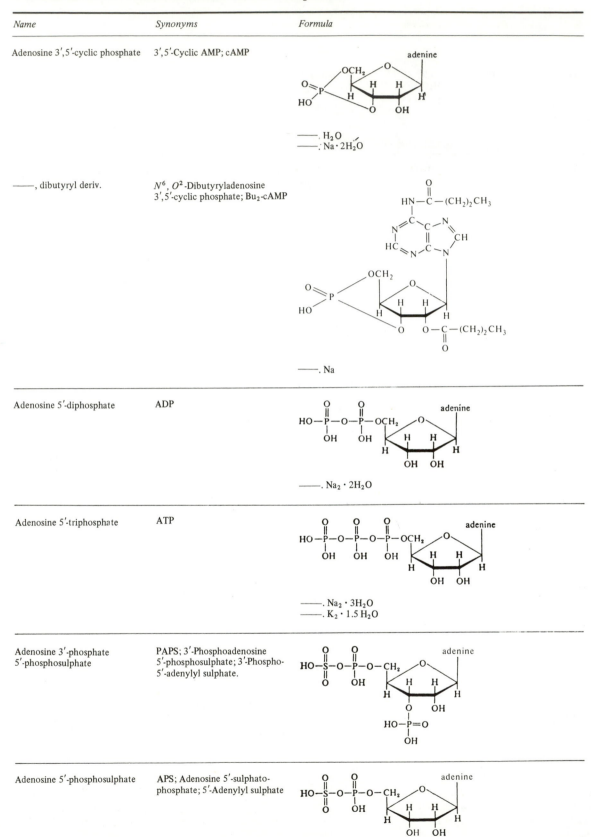

——. H$_2$O
——. Na · 2H$_2$O

——. Na

——. Na$_2$ · 2H$_2$O

——. Na$_2$ · 3H$_2$O
——. K$_2$ · 1.5 H$_2$O

| M. wt | $pK_a$ | Solubility | General remarks |
|---|---|---|---|
| 329.2 | | s. $H_2O$ | Cyclic nucleotides more acid stable than the non-cyclic monophosphates. In M-HCl at 100°C, the time for 50% liberation of adenine is 30 min for the cyclic phosphate and 2–4 min for adenosine 2'-, 3'-, or 5'-phosphate. 0.2 M-Ba(OH)$_2$ at 100°C for 30 min completely hydrolyses cyclic phosphate to give a mixture of the adenosine 3'- and 5'-phosphates in the ratio 5:1. Synthesized by adenyl cyclase in response to several hormonal stimuli; acts as 'second' messenger in cellular hormonal control via stimulation of protein kinases. $\lambda_{max}$ (pH 2) 256 ($\epsilon$ 14 500); (pH 7) 258 ($\epsilon$ 14 650). |
| 347.2 | | | |
| 387.2 | | | |
| 469.4 | | s. $H_2O$ | Dibutyryl derivative penetrates cells more effectively than cAMP and is usually employed with intact cells. $\epsilon_{273}$ (pH 7) 17 400. At pH 8.5 forms the $N^6$-mono-butyryl derivative. |
| 491.4 | | | |
| 427.2 | 3.9<br>6.1–6.7 | | In M-HCl at 100°C the terminal phosphate group is liberated in 10 min. Hydrolysis for 60 min gives adenine, ribose 5-phosphate, ribose, and inorg. P. |
| 507.2 | | | |
| 507.2 | 4.1<br>6.0–7.0 | | 66% phosphorus liberated as inorg. P in 10 min at 100°C in M-HCl. Neutral Na and K salts stable for months in soln. at −15°C, for about 1 week at 0°C, stable for several hours at 0°C in 7% trichloroacetic acid. In alkaline soln. decomposes to inorg. pyrophosphate and adenosine 5'-phosphate even at 0°C. |
| 605.2 | | | |
| 610.4 | | | |
| 507.3 | | s. $H_2O$ | Solid compd. decomposes 15–20% per day at 37°C. Store at low temp. Sulphate group is rapidly hydrolysed in acid, forming adenosine 3',5'-bisphos-phate plus sulphate; half-life 6 min in 0.1 M-HCl at 37°C. Relatively stable in alkali; no detectable hydrolysis in 0.1 M-NaOH at 37°C in 2 hr, partial hydrolysis at 100°C for 2 hr. Soln. stable at pH 8 and frozen. Reacts with $NH_4^+$ forming 5'-phosphoramidate. Spectrum similar to adenosine 5'-phosphate, $\epsilon_{260}$ 14 500. PREP. *Biochem. Preps* **10**, 3 (1963); *JBC* **239**, 2986 (1964); *BBA* **480**, 376 (1977); *Meth. Enzymol.* **6**, 766 (1963); *Molec. Pharmacol.* **2**, 56 (1966); *JBC* **249**, 2079 (1974). |
| 427.3 | | s. $H_2O$ | Solid compd. decomposes 7% per day at 37°C; store at low temp. Sulphate group rapidly hydrolysed in acid, stable in dilute alkali, as with adenosine 3'-phosphate 5'-phosphosulphate. Soln. stable at pH 8 and frozen. Spectrum similar to adenosine nucleotides, $\lambda_{max}$ 259 nm, $\epsilon$ 15 400 (pH 7). PREP. *Meth. Enzymol.* **6**, 766 (1963); *JBC* **239**, 2986 (1964); *Anal Biochem.* **42**, 207 (1971); *Z. Naturforsch. C* **34**, 346 (1979). |

# 4 Constituents of nucleic acids and related compounds

| Name | Synonyms | Formula |
|------|----------|---------|
| 2'-Deoxyadenosine | Adenine deoxyriboside; 9-β-D-2'-Deoxyribofuranosidoadenine | |
| 2'-Deoxyadenosine 3'-phosphate | Adenine deoxyribose 3'-phosphate; 3'-Deoxyadenylic acid | |
| 2'-Deoxyadenosine 5'-phosphate | Adenine deoxyribose 5'-phosphate; 5'-Deoxyadenylic acid; dAMP | |
| 2'-Deoxyadenosine 5'-triphosphate | Adenine deoxyribose 5'-triphosphate; dATP | |

**Cytosine group**

| | | |
|------|----------|---------|
| Cytosine | 4-Amino-2-hydroxypyrimidine | |
| Cytidine | Cytosine riboside; 3-β-D-Ribofuranosidocytosine | |

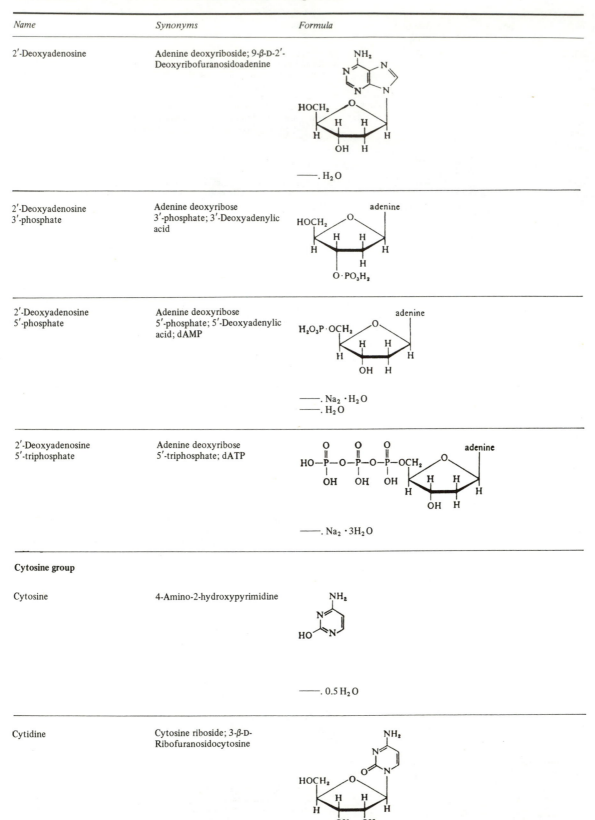

——. H$_2$O

——. Na$_2$ · H$_2$O
——. H$_2$O

——. Na$_2$ · 3H$_2$O

——. 0.5 H$_2$O

| M. wt | pK$_a$ | Solubility | General remarks |
|---|---|---|---|
| 251.2 | 3.8 | s. H$_2$O | Obtained by enzymic hydrolysis of DNA. Readily hydrolysed by dilute acids. Hydrate loses water of cryst. at 80°C *in vacuo*. |
| 269.2 | | | |
| 331.2 | 4.4<br>6.4 | | Easily hydrolysed by dilute mineral acids. Released quantitatively from DNA by use of phosphodiesterases of *Micrococcus pyogenes* and calf spleen (*JBC* **236**, 864 (1961)). |
| 331.2 | 4.4<br>6.4 | | Easily hydrolysed by dilute minerals acids. Released from heated DNA by *E. coli* diesterase (*JBC* **235**, 1479 (1960)) or by pancreatic DNA-ase followed by venom diesterase. |
| 393.2<br>349.2 | | | |
| 491.2 | 4.8<br>6.8 | | |
| 589.2 | | | |
| 111.1 | 4.4<br>12.2 | 0.77$^{25}$ H$_2$O; sl. s. EtOH; i. eth. | Water of crystallization lost at 100°C. |
| 243.2 | 4.2<br>~ 12.3 | | |

# 4 Constituents of nucleic acids and related compounds

| Name | Synonyms | Formula |
|------|----------|---------|
| Cytidine 2'-phosphate | 2'-Cytidylic acid; 2'-CMP | |
| Cytidine 3'-phosphate | 3'-Cytidylic acid; 3'-CMP | |
| Cytidine 2',3'-cyclic phosphate | 2',3'-Cyclic CMP | |
| Cytidine 5'-phosphate | 5'-Cytidylic acid; 5'-CMP | |
| Cytidine 5'-diphosphate | CDP | |
| Cytidine 5'-triphosphate | CTP | |

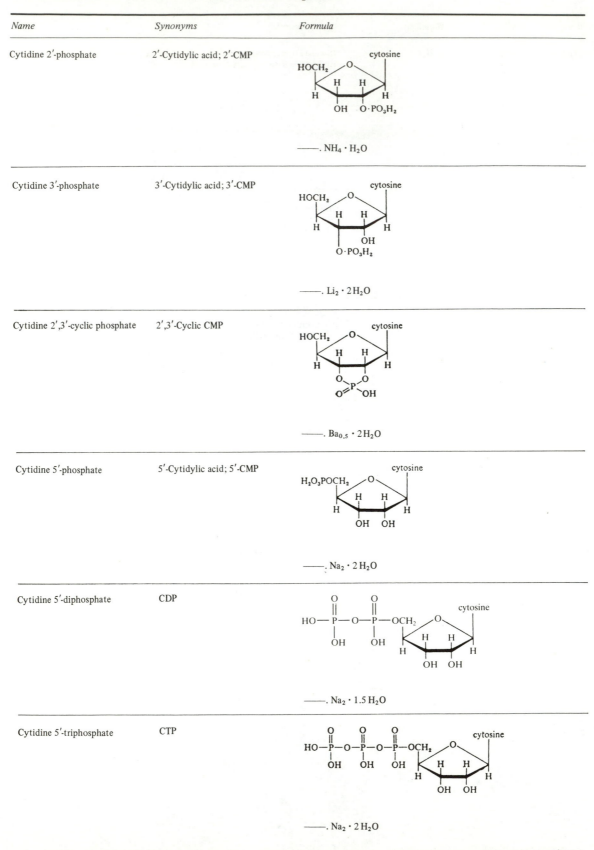

——. $NH_4 \cdot H_2O$

——. $Li_2 \cdot 2 H_2O$

——. $Ba_{0.5} \cdot 2 H_2O$

——. $Na_2 \cdot 2 H_2O$

——. $Na_2 \cdot 1.5 H_2O$

——. $Na_2 \cdot 2 H_2O$

| M. wt | p$K_a$ | Solubility | General remarks |
|---|---|---|---|
| 323.2 | 4.3<br>4.4<br>6.2 | | Only about 5% breakdown to nucleoside in M-HCl at 100°C for 1 hr. Some deamination to uridylic acid in M-NaOH at 37°C for 16 hr. |
| 358.2 | | | |
| 323.2 | 4.2<br>4.3<br>6.0 | | Only about 5% breakdown to nucleoside in M-HCl at 100°C for 1 hr, Some deamination to uridylic acid in M-NaOH at 37°C for 16 hr. |
| 371.1 | | | |
| 305.2 | | | Produced as an intermediate in the hydrolysis of RNA by pancreatic ribonuclease and by dilute alkali. Readily converted to the 3'-phosphate by pancreatic ribonuclease and to a mixture of 2'- and 3'-phosphates by dilute acid and alkali. |
| 408.9 | | | |
| 323.2 | 4.4<br>6.3 | | |
| 403.2 | | | |
| 403.2 | 4.6<br>6.4 | | 50% of total phosphorus released as inorg. P in 15 min at 100°C in 0.5M-$H_2SO_4$. |
| 474.2 | | | |
| 483.2 | 4.8<br>6.6 | | |
| 563.2 | | | |

# 4 Constituents of nucleic acids and related compounds

| Name | Synonyms | Formula |
|------|----------|---------|
| 2'-Deoxycytidine | Cytosine deoxyriboside; 3-β-D-2'-Deoxyribofuranosido-cytosine | |
| 2'-Deoxycytidine 3'-phosphate | Cytosine deoxyribose 3'-phosphate; 3'-Deoxycytidylic acid | |
| 2'-Deoxycytidine 5'-phosphate | Cytosine deoxyribose 5'-phosphate; dCMP | |
| 2'-Deoxycytidine 5'-triphosphate | Cytosine deoxyribose 5'-triphosphate; dCTP | |

**Guanine group**

| | | |
|------|----------|---------|
| Guanine | 2-Amino-6-hydroxypurine | |
| isoGuanine | 2-Hydroxy-6-aminopurine | |
| 7-Methylguanine | | |

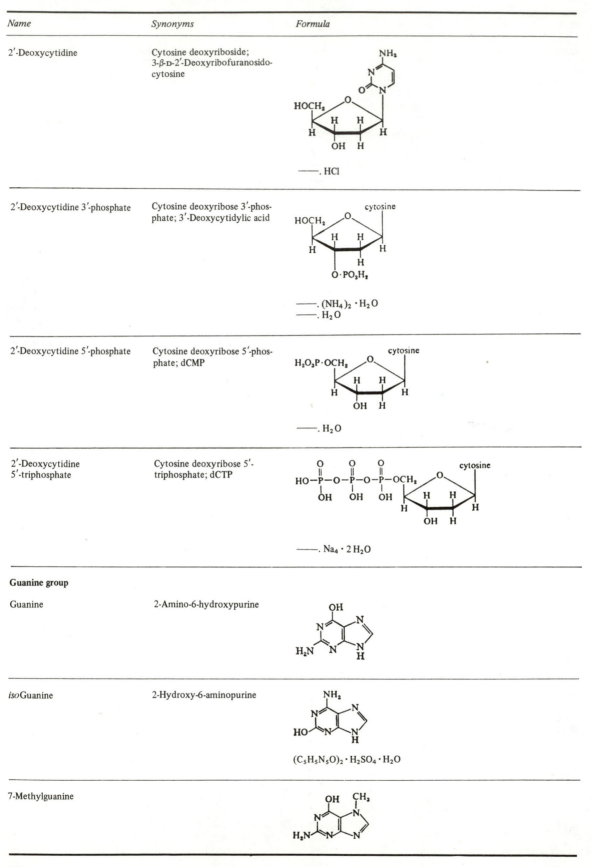

——. HCl

——. $(NH_4)_2 \cdot H_2O$
——. $H_2O$

——. $H_2O$

——. $Na_4 \cdot 2 H_2O$

$(C_5H_5N_5O)_2 \cdot H_2SO_4 \cdot H_2O$

| M. wt | pKₐ | Solubility | General remarks |
|---|---|---|---|
| 227.2 | 4.2 >13 | | |
| 263.7 | | | |
| 307.2 | | | Released quantitatively from DNA by use of phosphodiesterase of *Micrococcus pyogenes* and calf spleen (*JBC* **236**, 864 (1961)). Diesterase from *Lactobacillus acidophilus* releases 3′-phosphates from deoxyoligonucleotides (*JBC* **238**, 2789 (1963)). |
| 359.3 325.2 | | | |
| 307.2 | 4.6 6.6 13.2 | | Released from heated DNA by *E. coli* phosphodiesterase (*JBC* **235**, 1479 (1960)) or quantitatively by pancreatic DNA-ase followed by venom diesterase. |
| 325.2 | | | |
| 467.2 | | | |
| 591.2 | | | |
| 151.1 | 3.3 9.2 12.3 | s. acids and alkalis; v. sl. s. EtOH; i. $H_2O$ ($0.004^{40}$), organic acids | |
| 151.1 | 4.5 9.0 | $0.006^{25}$, $0.025^{100}$ $H_2O$ | Found as nucleoside (crotonoside) in croton bean, *JACS* **61**, 350 (1939). Water of cryst. of sulphate not lost at 130 °C *in vacuo* for 3 hr. Not deaminated by nitrous acid. Gives negligible fluorescence with u.v. light at pH 1, 7, 11, and 13 (*Anal. Biochem.* **3**, 49 (1962)). |
| 418.3 | | | |
| 165.2 | ∼0 3.5 9.9 | | Present in small amounts in urine of normal human subjects and in tRNA. Constituent of eukaryote mRNA 'cap'. |

## 4 Constituents of nucleic acids and related compounds

| Name | Synonyms | Formula |
|------|----------|---------|
| Guanosine | 9-β-D-Ribofuranosidoguanine; Vernine | |
| 7-Methylguanosine | | |
| Guanosine 2′-phosphate | 2′-Guanylic acid; 2′-GMP | |
| Guanosine 2′,3′-cyclic phosphate | 2′,3′-Cyclic GMP | |
| Guanosine 3′-phosphate | 3′-Guanylic acid; 3′-GMP | |
| Guanosine 5′-phosphate | 5′-Guanylic acid; 5′-GMP; GMP | |

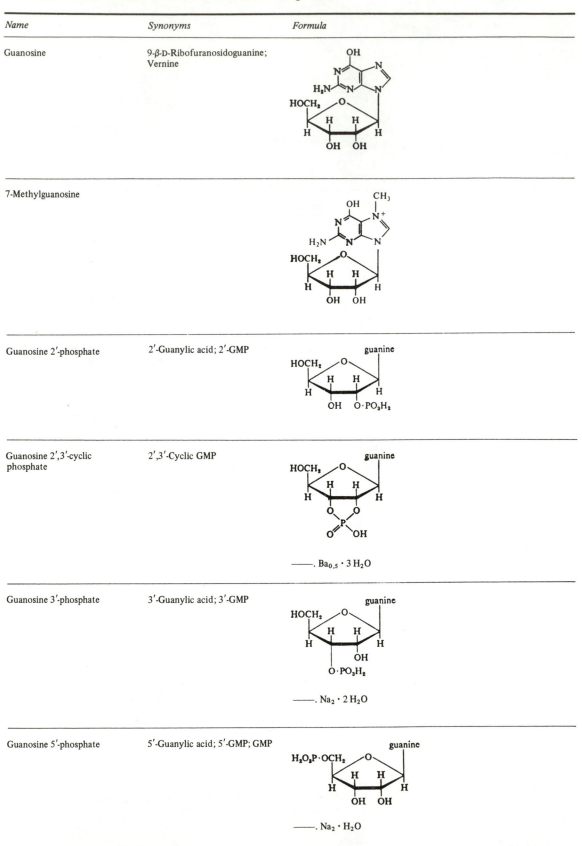

| M. wt | pK$_a$ | Solubility | General remarks |
|---|---|---|---|
| 283.2 | 1.6<br>9.2<br>12.4 | 0.08$^{18}$, 3.0$^{100}$ H$_2$O;<br>s. dil. mineral acids<br>and alkalis, hot glacial<br>acetic acid; i. eth.,<br>EtOH, CHCl$_3$, benz. | Easily hydrolysed in dil. mineral acids to guanine and D-ribose. Gives blue fluorescence at pH 1 with u.v. light but not in alkali. Deaminated to xanthosine by nitrous acid. |
| 297.3 | 7.0 | | Present in small amounts in tRNA. Hydrolysed to 7-methylguanine and D-ribose by heating at 100°C for 1 hr in water, methanol, or M-H$_2$SO$_4$. Terminus of 'capped' eukaryote mRNA (*PNAS* **72**, 1189 (1975); *Nature* **255**, 33 (1975)). |
| 363.2 | 0.7<br>2.3<br>5.9<br>9.4 | s. H$_2$O | Produced, with 3′-isomer, by the alkaline hydrolysis of RNA (0.3M-KOH, 37°C, 16 hr). Hydrolysed to guanine, ribose, and inorg. P by M-HCl at 100°C for 1 hr. pK$_a$ values are for a mixture of the 2′- and 3′- isomers. |
| 345.2 | | | Produced as an intermediate in the hydrolysis of RNA by Takadiastase T$_1$ ribonuclease and by alkali. Readily converted to the 3′-phosphate by T$_1$ and plant leaf ribonuclease and to a mixture of 2′- and 3′-phosphates by dil. acid and alkali. Not attacked by pancreatic ribonuclease. |
| 466.9 | | | |
| 363.2 | 2.3<br>5.9<br>9.7 | s. H$_2$O | As for 2′-isomer. One of the products of the action of Takadiastase T$_1$ ribonuclease on RNA. |
| 443.2 | | | |
| 363.2 | 2.4<br>6.1<br>9.4 | | Acid hydrolysis as for guanosine 2′-phosphate. |
| 425.2 | | | |

# 4 Constituents of nucleic acids and related compounds

| Name | Synonyms | Formula |
|------|----------|---------|
| Guanosine 3′,5′-cyclic phosphate | 3′,5′-Cyclic GMP; cGMP | |
| —— dibutyryl deriv. | $N^2$-2′-$O$-Dibutyrylguanosine 3′,5′-monophosphate; diBu-cGMP. | |
| Guanosine 5′-diphosphate | GDP | |
| Guanosine 5′-triphosphate | GTP | |
| Guanosine 5′-diphosphate 3′-diphosphate | ppGpp; Magic Spot I; MSI; Guanosine tetraphosphate | |
| Guanosine 5′-triphosphate 3′-diphosphate | pppGpp; Magic Spot II; MSII | c.f. ppGpp above and GTP. |

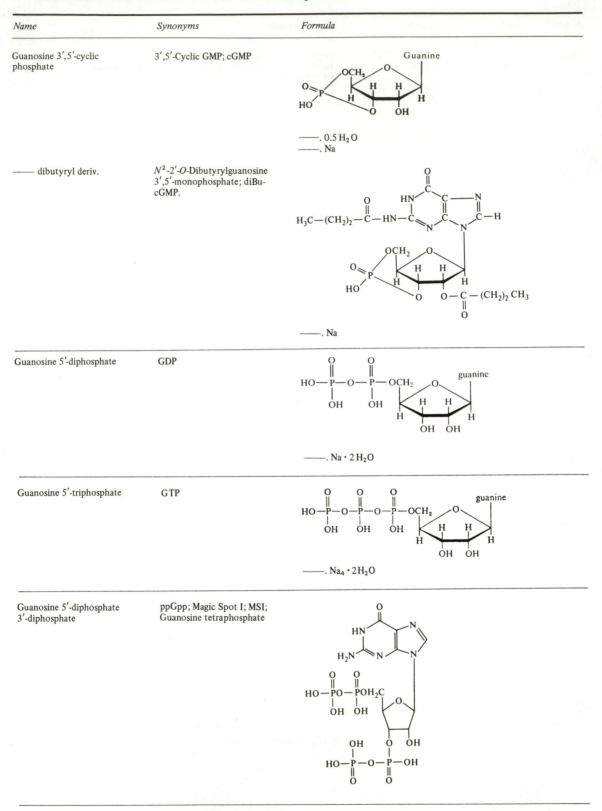

—— . 0.5 H₂O
—— . Na

—— . Na

—— . Na · 2 H₂O

—— . Na₄ · 2 H₂O

| M. wt | $pK_a$ | Solubility | General remarks |
|---|---|---|---|
| 345.2 | | | Believed to be involved in cellular control mechanisms. |
| 354.2 | | | |
| 367.2 | | | |
| 485.4 | | s. $H_2O$, MeOH | $\lambda_{max}$ (pH 7.0) 260 nm $\epsilon$ 16 700. Stable at $4\,^{\circ}$C. Penetrates cell membranes more effectively than cGMP. |
| 507.4 | | | |
| 443.2 | < 1 2.9 6.3 9.6 | | 50% of total phosphorus liberated as inorg. P in 15 min at $100\,^{\circ}$C in $0.5\text{M-}H_2SO_4$; after 1 hr converted to guanine, ribose 5-phosphate, ribose, and inorg. P. |
| 501.2 | | | |
| 523.2 | < 1 3.3 6.3 9.3 | | 66% of total phosphorus liberated as inorg. P in 15 min at $100\,^{\circ}$C in $0.5\text{M-}H_2SO_4$; after 1 hr converted into guanine, ribose 5-phosphate, ribose and inorg. P. |
| 647.2 | | | |
| 603.2 | | | Synthesized in *E. coli* by pyrophosphate transfer from ATP to GDP in response to amino acid deprivation; responsible for stringent response (inhibition of rRNA synthesis). SYNTHESIS REVIEW, *Biochem.* **14**, 981 (1975); REVIEW *PNARMB* **17**, 1 (1976). Reported to inhibit adenylosuccinate synthetase (*JBC* **254**, 2579 (1979)). 3′-Pyrophosphates more labile than 5′; store at $-70\,^{\circ}$C. ppGpp alkali labile (in 0.3 M-KOH, $t_{1/2} = 6.5$ min at $37\,^{\circ}$C). |
| 683.2 | | | As for ppGpp; synthesized from ATP and GTP. |

# 4 Constituents of nucleic acids and related compounds

| Name | Synonyms | Formula |
|------|----------|---------|

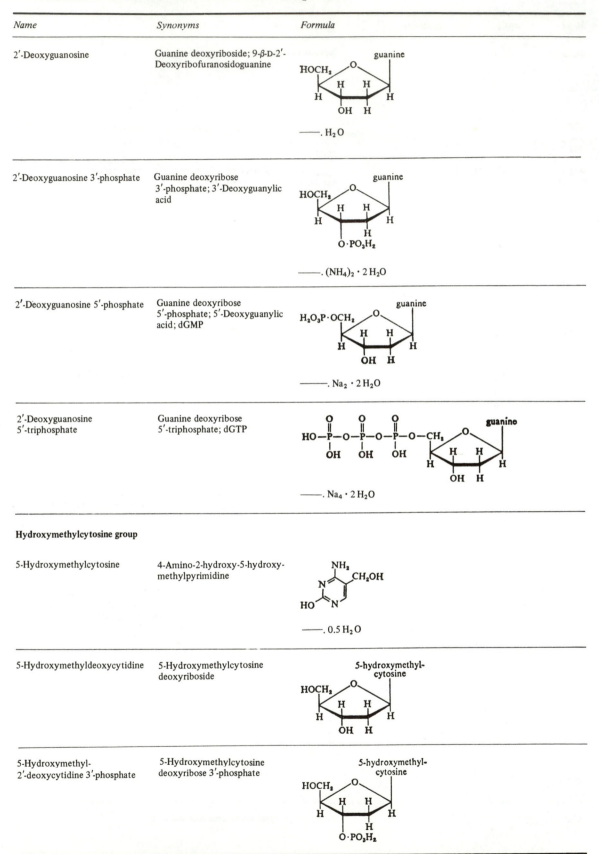

2'-Deoxyguanosine — Guanine deoxyriboside; 9-β-D-2'-Deoxyribofuranosidoguanine

——. H₂O

2'-Deoxyguanosine 3'-phosphate — Guanine deoxyribose 3'-phosphate; 3'-Deoxyguanylic acid

——. (NH₄)₂ · 2 H₂O

2'-Deoxyguanosine 5'-phosphate — Guanine deoxyribose 5'-phosphate; 5'-Deoxyguanylic acid; dGMP

——. Na₂ · 2 H₂O

2'-Deoxyguanosine 5'-triphosphate — Guanine deoxyribose 5'-triphosphate; dGTP

——. Na₄ · 2 H₂O

**Hydroxymethylcytosine group**

5-Hydroxymethylcytosine — 4-Amino-2-hydroxy-5-hydroxymethylpyrimidine

——. 0.5 H₂O

5-Hydroxymethyldeoxycytidine — 5-Hydroxymethylcytosine deoxyriboside

5-Hydroxymethyl-2'-deoxycytidine 3'-phosphate — 5-Hydroxymethylcytosine deoxyribose 3'-phosphate

| M. wt | p$K_a$ | Solubility | General remarks |
|---|---|---|---|
| 267.2 | 2.5 | s. $H_2O$ | Easily hydrolysed by dilute mineral acids. |
| 285.2 | | | |
| 347.2 | | | Readily hydrolysed by dilute mineral acids. Released quantitatively from DNA using diesterases of *Micrococcus pyogenes* and calf spleen (*JBC* **236**, 864 (1961)). Diesterase from *Lb. acidophilus* releases 3'-phosphates from deoxyoligonucleotides (*JBC* **238**, 2789 (1963)). |
| 417.3 | | | |
| 347.2 | 2.9<br>6.4<br>9.7 | | Easily hydrolysed by dilute mineral acids. Obtained by hydrolysis of heated DNA by *E. coli* phosphodiesterase (*JBC* **235**, 1479 (1960)), or by pancreatic DNA-ase followed by venom diesterase. |
| 427.2 | | | |
| 507.2 | 3.5<br>6.5<br>9.7 | | |
| 631.2 | | | |
| 141.1 | 4.3<br>~ 13 | sl. s. $H_2O$ | Isolated from acid (88% HCOOH or 6M-HCl) hydrolysates of DNA of T-even bacteriophages of *E. coli*. Destroyed if DNA heated with 72% $HClO_4$. Cryst. picrate (*JBC* **226**, 631 (1957)). |
| 150.1 | | | |
| 257.2 | 3.5 | | Isolated from acid hydrolysates (10% $HClO_4$/100°C/1 hr) of DNA of T-even bacteriophages of *E. coli*. Cryst. picrate (*JBC* **226**, 631 (1957)). |
| 337.2 | | | Isolated from T2 bacteriophage DNA degraded with diphenylamine and calf spleen diesterase. |

# 4 Constituents of nucleic acids and related compounds

| Name | Synonyms | Formula |
|---|---|---|

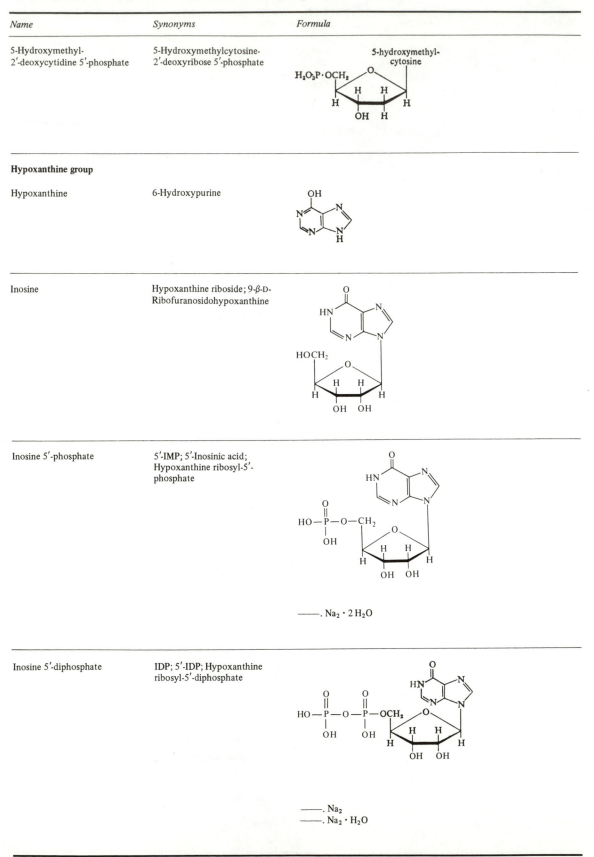

5-Hydroxymethyl-
2′-deoxycytidine 5′-phosphate

5-Hydroxymethylcytosine-
2′-deoxyribose 5′-phosphate

**Hypoxanthine group**

Hypoxanthine

6-Hydroxypurine

Inosine

Hypoxanthine riboside; 9-β-D-
Ribofuranosidohypoxanthine

Inosine 5′-phosphate

5′-IMP; 5′-Inosinic acid;
Hypoxanthine ribosyl-5′-
phosphate

——. $Na_2 \cdot 2\,H_2O$

Inosine 5′-diphosphate

IDP; 5′-IDP; Hypoxanthine
ribosyl-5′-diphosphate

——. $Na_2$
——. $Na_2 \cdot H_2O$

| M. wt | $pK_a$ | Solubility | General remarks |
|---|---|---|---|
| 337.2 | | Approx. 4.5 $\mu$mole/ml at 0°C and pH 3.0 | Distinguish from glucosylated derivative by spectra at pH 4.3 (*Science* **120**, 551 (1954)). Obtained from DNA of T2 and T6 phages by hydrolysis with *E. coli* phosphodiesterase, or non-quantitatively with pancreatic DNA-ase followed by venom diesterase. Corresponding di- and triphosphates have been synthesized (*JBC* **235**, 2688 (1960)). |
| 136.1 | 2.0 8.9 12.1 | $0.07^{19}$, $1.4^{100}$ $H_2O$; s. dil. acids and alkalis | Formed during catabolism of adenine. Less than 5% decomposition after 1 hr at 100°C in 0.5M-$H_2SO_4$ or 10M-NaOH. Formed from adenine by deamination with nitrous acid. |
| 268.2 | 1.2 8.9 12.5 | $1.6^{20}$ $H_2O$; v. sl. s. EtOH | Not a usual component of nucleic acids but may arise during isolation of components. Isolated in small amounts from yeast tRNA. Readily hydrolysed in dil. mineral acids to hypoxanthine and D-ribose. Produced by deamination of adenosine by nitrous acid. |
| 348.2 | 1.5 6.0 8.9 | s. $H_2O$, formic acid; v. sl. s. EtOH, eth. | Prepared by deamination of AMP. Hydrolysed by dil. acids to hypoxanthine, ribose 5-phosphate, D-ribose and inorg. P. |
| 428.2 | | | |
| 428.2 | | | Prepared by deamination of ADP. |
| 472.2 490.2 | | | |

# 4 Constituents of nucleic acids and related compounds

| Name | Synonyms | Formula |
|------|----------|---------|

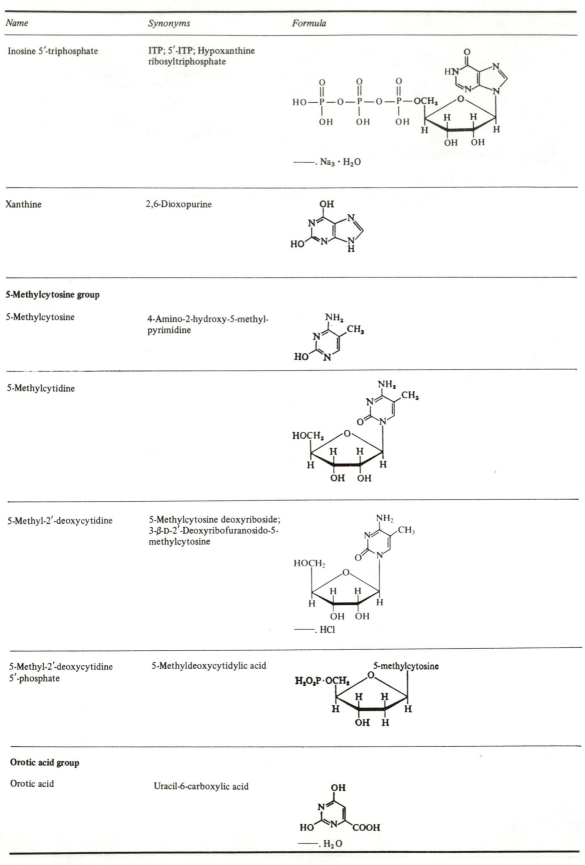

| Name | Synonyms |
|------|----------|
| Inosine 5′-triphosphate | ITP; 5′-ITP; Hypoxanthine ribosyltriphosphate |
| Xanthine | 2,6-Dioxopurine |

**5-Methylcytosine group**

| Name | Synonyms |
|------|----------|
| 5-Methylcytosine | 4-Amino-2-hydroxy-5-methyl-pyrimidine |
| 5-Methylcytidine | |
| 5-Methyl-2′-deoxycytidine | 5-Methylcytosine deoxyriboside; 3-β-D-2′-Deoxyribofuranosido-5-methylcytosine |
| 5-Methyl-2′-deoxycytidine 5′-phosphate | 5-Methyldeoxycytidylic acid |

**Orotic acid group**

| Name | Synonyms |
|------|----------|
| Orotic acid | Uracil-6-carboxylic acid |

| M. wt | $pK_a$ | Solubility | General remarks |
|---|---|---|---|
| 508.2 | 6.9 | | Prepared by deamination of ATP. 2′-Deoxyinosine 5′-triphosphate, M. wt. 492.2. |
| 592.2 | | | |
| 152.1 | ∼ 0.8<br>7.4<br>11.1 | $0.05^{20}$, $0.2^{100}$ $H_2O$;<br>sl. s. EtOH; s. alkalis;<br>i. organic solvents | Less than 10% decomposition after 1 hr at 100°C in 0.5M-$H_2SO_4$ or 10M-NaOH. Formed from guanine by deamination with nitrous acid. Riboside; ISOL. *JCS* **1933**, 662; SYN. *JCS* **1949**, 232 |
| 125.1 | 4.6<br>12.4 | $0.45^{25}$ $H_2O$ | Present up to 6% (molar) of total bases in DNA and in smaller amounts in ribosomal and tRNA from many sources. Deaminated by nitrous acid to thymine. |
| 257.2 | 4.3<br>> 13 | | Occurrence as for 5-methylcytosine. Deaminated by nitrous acid to thymine riboside |
| 241.2 | 4.4<br>> 13 | s. $H_2O$ | Isolated from wheat germ DNA. Hydrochloride loses $H_2O$ at 100°C *in vacuo* for 48 hr. |
| 277.7 | | | |
| 321.2 | 4.4 | | Obtained by hydrolysis of wheat germ DNA with pancreatic DNA-ase and venom diesterase. |
| 156.1 | 2.4<br>9.5<br>> 13.0 | $0.18^{18}$ $H_2O$ | Found in animal milk. Accumulates in large quantities during growth of mutants of *Neurospora* which require uridine, cytidine, or uracil. Ribotide is precursor in pyrimidine nucleotide biosynthesis. |
| 174.1 | | | |

# 4 Constituents of nucleic acids and related compounds

| Name | Synonyms | Formula |
|------|----------|---------|

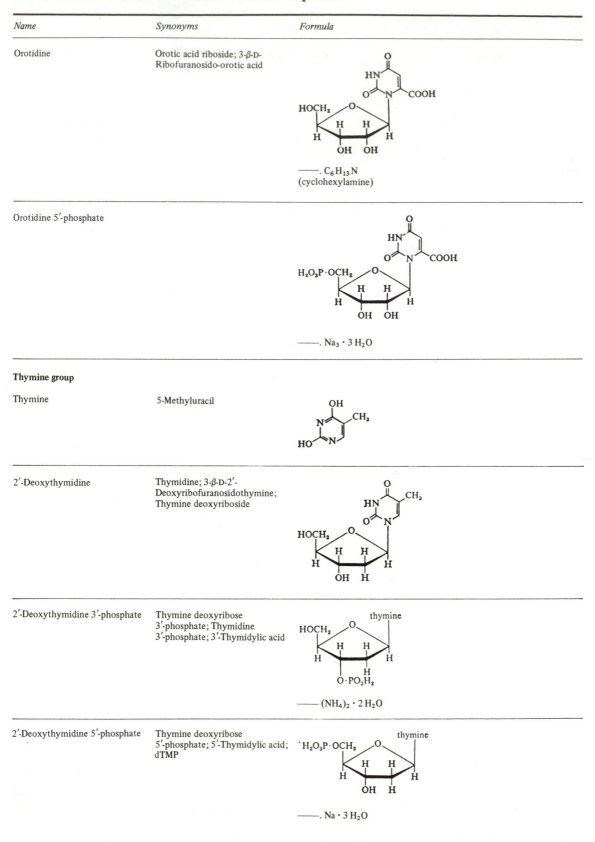

**Orotidine** — Orotic acid riboside; 3-β-D-Ribofuranosido-orotic acid

———. $C_6H_{13}N$ (cyclohexylamine)

**Orotidine 5'-phosphate**

———. $Na_3 \cdot 3 H_2O$

## Thymine group

**Thymine** — 5-Methyluracil

**2'-Deoxythymidine** — Thymidine; 3-β-D-2'-Deoxyribofuranosidothymine; Thymine deoxyriboside

**2'-Deoxythymidine 3'-phosphate** — Thymine deoxyribose 3'-phosphate; Thymidine 3'-phosphate; 3'-Thymidylic acid

——— $(NH_4)_2 \cdot 2 H_2O$

**2'-Deoxythymidine 5'-phosphate** — Thymine deoxyribose 5'-phosphate; 5'-Thymidylic acid; dTMP

———. $Na \cdot 3 H_2O$

| M. wt | $pK_a$ | Solubility | General remarks |
|---|---|---|---|
| 288.2 | | s. $H_2O$, EtOH, aq. EtOH | Hydrolyses readily in dilute mineral acids. Isolated in relatively large amounts from urine of tumour-bearing patients who have received 6-azauridine 5′-phosphate therapy. Cyclohexylamine salt M.p. 183—4. |
| 387.4 | | | |
| 368.2 | | | An intermediate in the biosynthesis of uridylic and cytidylic acids. |
| 488.2 | | | |
| 126.1 | $\sim 0$<br>9.9<br>$> 13.0$ | $0.4^{25}\,H_2O$; s. hot $H_2O$; sl. s. EtOH; v. sl. s. eth. | Not limited to DNA but found in small amounts in tRNA from many sources. Riboside also isolated (*BJ* **70**, 642 (1958)). |
| 242.2 | 9.8<br>$> 13$ | | |
| 322.2 | | | Released quantitatively from DNA by phosphodiesterases of *Micrococcus pyogenes* and calf spleen (*JBC* **236**, 864 (1961)). |
| 392.3 | | | |
| 322.2 | $\sim 1.6$<br>6.5<br>10.0 | | Obtained from heated DNA by hydrolysis with *E. coli* diesterase (*JBC* **235**, 1479 (1960)) or pancreatic DNA-ase and venom diesterase. |
| 398.2 | | | |

# 4 Constituents of nucleic acids and related compounds

| Name | Synonyms | Formula |
|------|----------|---------|

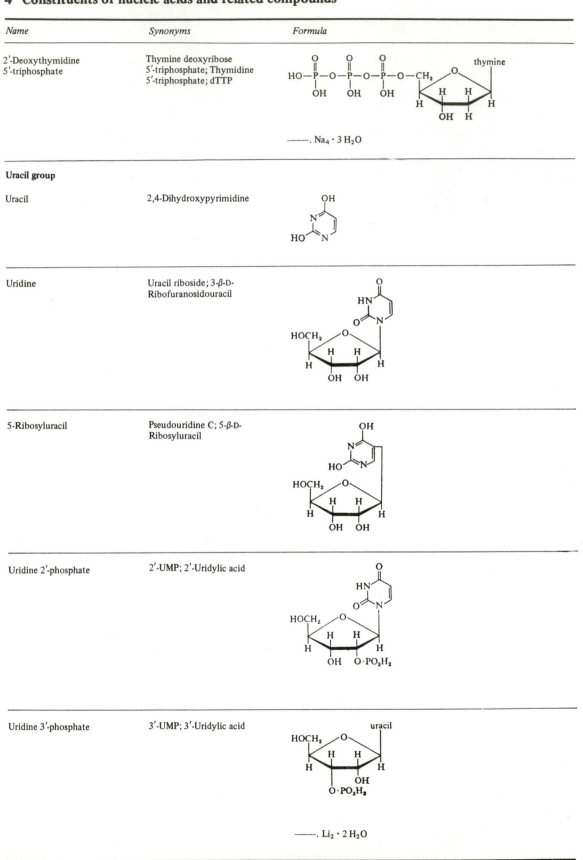

2'-Deoxythymidine 5'-triphosphate — Thymine deoxyribose 5'-triphosphate; Thymidine 5'-triphosphate; dTTP

——. Na$_4$ · 3 H$_2$O

**Uracil group**

Uracil — 2,4-Dihydroxypyrimidine

Uridine — Uracil riboside; 3-β-D-Ribofuranosidouracil

5-Ribosyluracil — Pseudouridine C; 5-β-D-Ribosyluracil

Uridine 2'-phosphate — 2'-UMP; 2'-Uridylic acid

Uridine 3'-phosphate — 3'-UMP; 3'-Uridylic acid

——. Li$_2$ · 2 H$_2$O

| M. wt | pK$_a$ | Solubility | General remarks |
|---|---|---|---|
| 482.2 | | | |
| 624.2 | | | |
| 112.1 | $\sim 0.5$<br>9.5<br>$> 13.0$ | $0.36^{25}$ H$_2$O; s. alkalis;<br>v. sl. s. EtOH; i. eth. | |
| 244.2 | 9.2<br>12.5 | s. H$_2$O;<br>sp. s. EtOH | Formed from cytidine by deamination with nitrous acid |
| 244.2 | 9.0<br>$> 13$ | | Occurs as the nucleotide in appreciable amounts in ribosomal and tRNA from many sources. Urine of patients with leukaemia, polycythaemia, or gout provides a good source of 5-ribosyluridine. See *PNARMB* **5**, 349, 399 (1966). |
| 324.2 | 1.0<br>5.9<br>9.4<br>(Equilibrium mixture of 2'- and 3'-) | v.s. H$_2$O | 40.7% of total phosphorus liberated as inorg. P in 30 hr at 100°C in 0.05M-H$_2$SO$_4$. 5% decomposition in M-HCl at 100°C for 1 hr. Slightly more alkali labile than 5'-isomer; however stable in 0.3M-KOH at 37° for 16 hr and liberated from RNA, together with 3'-isomer, under these conditions. |
| 324.2 | 1.0<br>5.9<br>9.4<br>(Equilibrium mixture of 2'- and 3'-) | s. H$_2$O | Hydrolysis in 10% H$_2$SO$_4$ gives uracil. 5% decomposition in M-HCl at 100°C for 1 hr. 81% of total phosphorus liberated as inorg. P in 30 hr at 100°C in 0.05M-H$_2$SO$_4$. Stable in 0.3M-KOH at 37°C for 16 hr and liberated, together with 2'-isomer, from RNA under these conditions. |
| 372.1 | | | |

# 4 Constituents of nucleic acids and related compounds

| Name | Synonyms | Formula |
|---|---|---|
| Uric acid | 2,6,8-Trihydroxypurine | |
| Uridine 5′-phosphate | 5′-UMP; 5′-Uridylic acid | |
| Uridine 5′-triphosphate | UTP | |

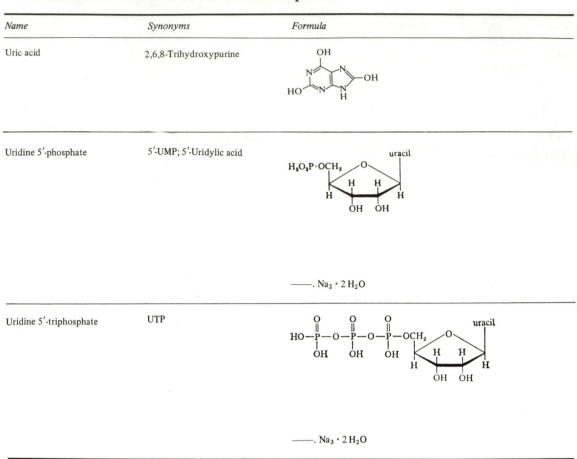

——. Na$_2$ · 2 H$_2$O

——. Na$_3$ · 2 H$_2$O

| M. wt | $pK_a$ | Solubility | General remarks |
|---|---|---|---|
| 168.1 | 5.4<br>11.3 | $0.002^{20}$, $0.05^{100}$ $H_2O$; s. alkali, glycerol; i. EtOH, eth. | Chief end-product of nitrogen metabolism of birds and reptiles. Common intermediate in purine metabolism in animals. Further metabolized in most mammals but not in man. Present in urine of all carnivorous animals. |
| 324.2 | ~1<br>6.4<br>9.4 | | |
| 404.2 | | | |
| 484.2 | ~1<br>6.6<br>9.6 | | 67% of total P liberated as inorg. P in 15 min at 100°C in 0.05 M-$H_2SO_4$. 2′-Deoxy UTP, synthesized from 2′-dUMP, M. wt. 468.2; $K_3$ salt + $5H_2O$, M. wt. 672.6. |
| 586.2 | | | |

# 5 Spectral data and p$K_a$ values for purines, pyrimidines, nucleosides, and nucleotides

**Sources of data**

All data have been compiled from the following sources:

(a) Section 7, second edition of this book;
(b) *Handbook of biochemistry and molecular biology,* third edition; Nucleic Acids, Volume 1 (ed. G. D. Fasman; CRC Press, 1975);
(c) Schwarz/Mann *Biochemical catalogue 1973/1974*;
(d) P–L Biochemicals Inc. *Catalogue, 1977.*

No references are given here but can be found in (a) and (b).

**p$K_a$ values and spectral data**

Values of 0–2 usually represent primary phosphate groups, 3–5 amino groups, and 6–7 secondary phosphate groups. Enolic hydroxyl groups titrate between pH 5 and 14 depending on the compound. p$K_a$ values are not always listed for all the titratable groups of each compound. In particular, the sugar dissociations (p$K_a$ *ca.* 13) are not always given. In the literature p$K_a$ values for some compounds may differ from those cited by more than $\pm 0.1$ pH unit, $\lambda_{max}$ and $\lambda_{min}$ values sometimes by more than $\pm 1$ nm, $\epsilon_{max}$ values by more than $\pm 5\%$ and spectral ratios by more than $\pm 10\%$. For details see reference b (above) pages 66–7.

**Numbering of purine and pyrimidine rings**

See p. 75.

**5 Spectral data and $pK_a$ values for purines, pyrimidines, nucleosides, and nucleotides**

| Name | pH | $\epsilon_{260}$ ($\times 10^{-3}$) | $\lambda_{max}$ (nm) | $\epsilon_{max}$ ($\times 10^{-3}$) | $\lambda_{min}$ (nm) | $\epsilon_{min}$ ($\times 10^{-3}$) | 250/260 | 280/260 | $pK_a$ Base | $pK_a$ Phosphate |
|---|---|---|---|---|---|---|---|---|---|---|
| **Adenine group** | | | | | | | | | | |
| Adenine | 1 | 13.0 | 262.5 | 13.2 | 229 | 2.55 | 0.76 | 0.38 | < 1 | |
| | 7 | 13.3 | 260.5 | 13.4 | 226 | 2.55 | 0.76 | 0.13 | 4.1 | |
| | 12 | 10.5 | 269 | 12.3 | 237 | 3.35 | 0.57 | 0.60 | 9.8 | |
| Adenine, $N^6$,$N^6$-dimethyl- | 1 | | 277 | 15.6 | 236 | | 0.57 | 1.36 | < 1.0 | |
| | 7 | | 275 | 17.8 | | | | | 3.9 | |
| | 13 | | 281 | 17.8 | 245 | | 0.53 | 2.61 | 10.5 | |
| Adenine, 1-methyl- | 4 | | 259 | 11.7 | 228 | | 0.80 | 0.23 | 7.2 | |
| | 9 | | 270 | 11.9 | 242 | | 0.52 | 0.87 | 11.0 | |
| | 13 | | 270 | 14.4 | 239 | | 0.55 | 0.85 | | |
| Adenine, 2-methyl- | 1 | | 266 | 12.9 | 229 | 3.3 | 0.79 | 0.56 | ~ 5.1 | |
| | 7 | | 263 | 12.7 | 226 | | 0.89 | 0.16 | | |
| | 13 | | 271 | 10.7 | 238 | 3.7 | 0.61 | 0.84 | | |
| Adenine, $N^6$-methyl- | 1 | | 267 | 15.3 | 232 | 2.7 | 0.64 | 0.70 | < 1 | |
| | 7 | | 266 | 16.2 | 231 | | 0.55 | 0.55 | 4.2 | |
| | 13 | | 273 | 15.9 | 239 | 3.6 | 0.55 | 1.19 | 10.0 | |
| Adenine, 7-methyl- | 1 | | 273 | 14.0 | 237 | | 0.60 | 1.06 | 4.2 | |
| | 12 | | 270 | 10.6 | 231 | | 0.70 | 0.80 | | |
| Adenosine | 1 | 14.3 | 257 | 14.6 | 230 | 3.5 | 0.84 | 0.22 | 3.5 | |
| | 6 | 14.9 | 260 | 14.9 | 227 | 2.3 | 0.78 | 0.14 | 12.5 | |
| | 11 | 14.9 | 259 | 15.4 | 227 | 2.3 | 0.79 | 0.15 | | |
| Adenosine, $N^6$,$N^6$-dimethyl- | 1 | | 268 | 18.4 | 234 | | 0.60 | 0.94 | 4.5 | |
| | 7 | | 275 | 18.8 | 236 | | 0.46 | 1.54 | | |
| | 13 | | 276 | 19.2 | 237 | | 0.37 | 1.68 | | |

| Compound | pH | | | | | | | | | |
|---|---|---|---|---|---|---|---|---|---|---|
| Adenosine, 1-methyl | 2 | | 258 | 13.7 | 232 | | 0.81 | 0.23 | 8.8 | |
| | 7 | | 258 | 13.9 | 232 | | 0.81 | 0.23 | | |
| | 10.5 | | 259 | 14.6 | 231 | | 0.76 | 0.35 | | |
| Adenosine, 2-methyl- | 1 | | 258 | 14.0 | 230 | | 0.84 | 0.40 | | |
| | 6 | | 264 | 14.5 | 228 | | 0.75 | 0.17 | | |
| | 13 | | 263 | 15.2 | 230 | | 0.75 | 0.17 | | |
| Adenosine, $N^6$-methyl | 1 | | 262 | 16.6 | 231 | | 0.66 | 0.41 | 4.0 | |
| | 7 | | 266 | 15.9 | 229 | | 0.57 | 0.68 | | |
| | 13 | | 266 | 15.9 | 232 | | 0.57 | 0.68 | | |
| Adenosine 2′-phosphate | 2 | 14.5 | 257 | 15.0 | 229 | 3.2 | 0.85 | 0.23 | 3.8 | 6.2 |
| | 7 | 15.3 | 259 | 15.4 | | | | 0.15 | | |
| | 12 | 15.3 | 259 | 15.4 | | | 0.80 | 0.15 | | |
| Adenosine 3′-phosphate | 1 | 14.5 | 257 | 15.1 | 230 | | 0.85 | 0.22 | 3.7 | 5.9 |
| | 7 | 15.3 | 259 | 15.4 | | | 0.80 | 0.15 | | |
| | 13 | 15.3 | 259 | 15.4 | 227 | | 0.78 | 0.22 | | |
| Adenosine 5′-phosphate | 2 | 14.5 | 257 | 15.0 | 230 | 3.5 | 0.84 | 0.22 | 3.8 | 6.2—6.4 |
| | 7 | 15.3 | 259 | 15.4 | 227 | 2.6 | 0.79 | 0.16 | | |
| | 11 | 15.3 | 259 | 15.4 | 227 | 2.6 | 0.79 | 0.15 | | |
| Adenosine 5′-diphosphate | 2 | 14.5 | 257 | 15.0 | 230 | | 0.85 | 0.21 | 3.9 | 6.1—6.7 |
| | 7 | 15.4 | 259 | 15.4 | 227 | | 0.78 | 0.16 | | |
| | 11 | 15.4 | 259 | 15.4 | 227 | | 0.78 | 0.15 | | |
| Adenosine 5′-triphosphate | 2 | 14.3 | 257 | 14.7 | 230 | 3.5 | 0.85 | 0.22 | 4.1 | 6.0—7.0 |
| | 7 | 15.4 | 259 | 15.4 | 227 | 2.5 | 0.80 | 0.15 | | |
| | 11 | 15.4 | 259 | 15.4 | 227 | 2.5 | 0.80 | 0.15 | | |
| 2′-Deoxyadenosine | 2 | | 258 | 14.5 | 228 | | 0.83 | 0.24 | 3.8 | |
| | 7 | | 260 | 15.2 | 225 | | 0.79 | 0.15 | | |
| | 13 | | 261 | 14.9 | | | | | | |
| 2′-Deoxyadenosine 3′-phosphate | 7 | | 259 | 15.0 | | | 0.79 | 0.14 | | |
| 2′-Deoxyadenosine 5′-phosphate | 2 | 14.7 | 258 | 15.0 | 228 | 3.0 | 0.81 | 0.22 | 4.4 | 6.4 |
| | 7 | 15.3 | 259 | 15.2 | 226 | 2.5 | 0.80 | 0.15 | | |

## 5 Spectral data and p$K_a$ values for purines, pyrimidines, nucleosides, and nucleotides

| Name | pH | $\epsilon_{260}$ ($\times 10^{-3}$) | $\lambda_{max}$ (nm) | $\epsilon_{max}$ ($\times 10^{-3}$) | $\lambda_{min}$ (nm) | $\epsilon_{min}$ ($\times 10^{-3}$) | 250/260 | 280/260 | p$K_a$ Base | p$K_a$ Phosphate |
|---|---|---|---|---|---|---|---|---|---|---|
| 2'-Deoxyadenosine 5'-triphosphate | 2 | 14.5 | 258 | 14.8 | 228 | 3.0 | 0.81 | 0.22 | 4.8 | 6.8 |
| | 7 | 15.3 | 259 | 15.4 | 226 | 2.5 | 0.78 | 0.15 | | |
| | 12 | 15.4 | 260 | 15.4 | 226 | 2.6 | 0.79 | 0.15 | | |
| **Cytosine group** | | | | | | | | | | |
| Cytosine | 1 | 6.0 | 276 | 10.0 | 239 | | 0.48 | 1.53 | 4.6 | |
| | 7 | 2.6 | 267 | 6.1 | 247 | | 0.78 | 0.58 | 12.2 | |
| | 14 | 2.4 | 282 | 7.9 | 251 | | 0.60 | 3.28 | | |
| Cytosine, 5-hydroxymethyl- | 1 | 4.9 | 279 | 9.7 | 241 | | 0.45 | 1.97 | 4.3 | |
| | 7 | 4.9 | 269 | 5.7 | 251 | | 0.80 | 0.80 | $\sim 13$ | |
| | 13 | 2.4 | 283 | 7.6 | 254 | | 0.83 | 2.98 | | |
| Cytosine, $N^4$-methyl- | 1 | | 277 | 10.5 | 240 | | 0.50 | 1.66 | 4.5 | |
| | 7 | | 267 | 7.2 | 248 | | 0.79 | 0.66 | 12.7 | |
| | 14 | | 286 | 8.0 | 256 | | 0.96 | 3.27 | | |
| Cytosine, 5-methyl- | 1 | 3.6 | 283 | 9.8 | 242 | | 0.40 | 2.62 | 4.6 | |
| | 7 | 4.5 | 273 | 6.2 | 252 | | 0.80 | 1.21 | 12.4 | |
| | 14 | 1.7 | 289 | 8.1 | 254 | | 0.84 | 3.64 | | |
| Cytidine | 1 | 6.4 | 280 | 13.4 | 242 | | 0.45 | 2.10 | 4.2 | |
| | 7 | 7.55 | { 229.5, 271 | { 8.3, 9.1 | { 226, 250 | | 0.86 | 0.93 | 12.5 | |
| | 13 | | 273 | 9.2 | 251 | | 0.87 | 1.02 | | |
| Cytidine, 5-methyl- | 0 | | 287 | 12.6 | 245 | | 0.33 | 3.59 | 4.3 | |
| | 7 | | 277 | 8.9 | 255 | | 1.03 | 1.45 | > 13 | |
| | 14 | | 279 | 9.0 | 256 | | 1.05 | 1.58 | | |
| Cytidine, 2-thio- | 0 | | { 229, 276 | { 17.0, 17.4 | { 213, 250 | | 0.86 | 1.30 | | |
| | 7 | | 249 | 22.3 | 220 | | 1.08 | 0.50 | | |
| | 13 | | 252 | | 229 | | 1.04 | 0.72 | | |

| Compound | pH | | λmax (nm) | | λmin (nm) | | | pK | | |
|---|---|---|---|---|---|---|---|---|---|---|
| Cytidine 2'-phosphate | 2 | 6.9 | 278 | 12.7 | 240 | 0.48 | 1.80 | 4.4 | 6.2 | |
| | 7 | 7.8 | 272 | 8.6 | 250 | 0.90 | 0.85 | | | |
| | 12 | 7.8 | 272 | 8.6 | 250 | 0.90 | 0.85 | | | |
| Cytidine 3'-phosphate | 2 | 6.6 | 279 | 13.0 | 240 | 0.45 | 2.00 | 4.3 | 6.0 | |
| | 7 | 7.6 | 270 | 9.0 | 250 | 0.86 | 0.93 | | | |
| | 12 | 7.6 | 272 | 8.9 | 250 | 0.86 | 0.93 | | | |
| Cytidine 5'-phosphate | 2 | 6.3 | 280 | 13.2 | 241 | 0.44 | 2.09 | 4.5 | 6.3 | |
| | 7 | 7.4 | 271 | 9.1 | 249 | 0.84 | 0.98 | | | |
| | 11 | 7.4 | 271 | 9.1 | 249 | 0.84 | 0.98 | | | |
| Cytidine 5'-diphosphate | 2 | 6.2 | 280 | 12.8 | 241 | 0.46 | 2.07 | 4.6 | 6.4 | |
| | 7 | 7.4 | 271 | 9.1 | 249 | 0.83 | 0.98 | | | |
| | 11 | 7.4 | 271 | 9.1 | 249 | 0.83 | 0.98 | | | |
| Cytidine 5'-triphosphate | 2 | 6.0 | 280 | 12.8 | 241 | 0.45 | 2.12 | 4.8 | 6.6 | |
| | 7 | 7.4 | 271 | 9.0 | 249 | 0.84 | 0.97 | | | |
| | 11 | 7.4 | 271 | 9.0 | 249 | 0.84 | 0.97 | | | |
| 2'-Deoxycytidine | 1 | 6.2 | 280 | 13.2 | 241 | 0.42 | 2.15 | 4.3 | | |
| | 7 | 7.4 | 271 | 9.0 | 250 | 0.83 | 0.97 | | | |
| | 11 | 7.4 | 271 | 9.0 | 250 | 0.83 | 0.97 | | | |
| 2'-Deoxycytidine, 5-hydroxylmethyl- | 1 | | 283 | 12.6 | 243 | 0.64 | 2.47 | 3.5 | | |
| | 7 | | 272 | | 247 | 0.97 | 1.17 | | | |
| | 13 | | 274 | | 252 | 0.97 | 1.17 | | | |
| 2'-Deoxycytidine, 5-methyl- | 1 | 3.2 | 287 | 12.4 | 245 | 0.42 | 2.93 | 4.4 | | |
| | 7 | 6.0 | 277 | 8.5 | 255 | 1.00 | 1.54 | >13 | | |
| | 14 | 5.3 | 279 | 8.8 | 255 | 0.98 | 1.67 | | | |
| 2'-Deoxycytidine 3'-phosphate | 2 | | 280 | 13.1 | 280 | 0.44 | 2.1 | | | |
| | 7 | | | | | 0.84 | 0.93 | | | |
| 2'-Deoxycytidine 5'-phosphate | 2 | 6.3 | 280 | 13.5 | 239 | 0.43 | 2.12 | 4.5 | 6.6 | 1.5 |
| | 7 | 7.4 | 271 | 9.3 | 249 | 0.82 | 0.99 | 13.2 | | 6.0 |
| | 12 | 7.4 | 271 | 9.0 | 250 | 0.82 | 0.99 | | | 6.1 |

## 5 Spectral data and p$K_a$ values for purines, pyrimidines, nucleosides, and nucleotides

| Name | pH | $\epsilon_{260}$ ($\times 10^{-3}$) | $\lambda_{max}$ (nm) | $\epsilon_{max}$ ($\times 10^{-3}$) | $\lambda_{min}$ (nm) | $\epsilon_{min}$ ($\times 10^{-3}$) | 250/260 | 280/260 | p$K_a$ Base | p$K_a$ Phosphate |
|---|---|---|---|---|---|---|---|---|---|---|
| 2'-Deoxycytidine | 1 | | 284 | 12.5 | 245 | | 0.44 | 2.68 | 4.4 | |
| 5'-phosphate, | 7 | 6.1 | 275 | 7.7 | 254 | | 0.90 | 1.33 | | |
| 5-hydroxymethyl- | 12 | 6.1 | 275 | 7.7 | 254 | | 0.93 | 1.31 | | |
| 2'-Deoxycytidine | 2 | | 287 | | 244 | | 0.36 | 3.14 | | |
| 5'-phosphate, 5-methyl- | 7 | | 278 | | 254 | | 0.95 | 1.52 | | |
| | 12 | | 278 | | | | | | | |
| 2'-Deoxycytidine | 2 | 6.2 | 280 | 13.1 | | | 0.44 | 2.14 | | |
| 5'-triphosphate | 7 | 7.4 | 272 | 9.1 | | | 0.82 | 0.98 | | |

### Guanine group

| Name | pH | $\epsilon_{260}$ ($\times 10^{-3}$) | $\lambda_{max}$ (nm) | $\epsilon_{max}$ ($\times 10^{-3}$) | $\lambda_{min}$ (nm) | $\epsilon_{min}$ ($\times 10^{-3}$) | 250/260 | 280/260 | p$K_a$ Base | p$K_a$ Phosphate |
|---|---|---|---|---|---|---|---|---|---|---|
| Guanine | 1 | 8.0 | {248, 276} | {11.4, 7.35} | {224, 267} | 7.15 | 1.37 | 0.84 | 3.2 | |
| | 7 | 7.2 | {246, 276} | {10.7, 8.15} | {225, 262} | 7.05 | 1.42 | 1.04 | 9.6 | |
| | 11 | 6.4 | 274 | 8.0 | 255 | 6.05 | 0.99 | 1.14 | 12.4 | |
| Guanine, $N^2$, $N^2$-dimethyl | 1 | | {256, 272} | {19.0, 17.0} | 233 | | 0.92 | 0.37 | | |
| | 7 | | {250, 283} | {17.0, 9.3} | 229 | | 1.20 | 0.62 | | |
| | 12 | | 282 | 9.2 | 265 | | 1.15 | 1.05 | | |
| Guanine, 1-methyl- | 1 | | {250, 272} | {10.2, 7.1} | {227, —} | | 1.28 | 0.81 | ~ 0 | |
| | 7 | | {248, 272} | {10.0, 7.9} | {227, 264} | | 1.24 | 0.93 | 3.1 | |
| | 13 | | 277 | 8.7 | 241 | | 0.80 | 1.19 | 10.5 | |
| Guanine, $N^2$-methyl- | 1 | | {250, 279} | {13.9, 6.2} | 228 | 6.6 | 1.34 | 0.64 | 3.3 | |
| | 7 | | {249, 277} | {14.1, 8.3} | {227, 266} | | 1.18 | 0.72 | 8.9 | |
| | 11 | | {244, 278} | {9.5, 7.2} | 263 | 6.1 | | | 12.8 | |

| Compound | pH | | λmax (nm) | ε·10⁻³ | λmin (nm) | ε·10⁻³ | ratio | ratio | pK$_a$ |
|---|---|---|---|---|---|---|---|---|---|
| Guanine, 7-methyl- | 1 | | 250, 272 | 10.6, 6.9 | 228, 268 | 4.7, 7.3 | 1.30 | 0.79 | ~0 |
| | 7 | | 248, 283 | 5.7, 7.4 | 235, 261 | 5.5, 3.9 | 1.46 | 1.87 | 3.5 |
| | 12 | | 280 | 7.4 | 257 | | 1.13 | 1.89 | 9.9 |
| Guanosine | 0.7 | | 256 | 12.3 | 228 | | 0.94 | 0.70 | 1.6 |
| | 6 | | 253 | 13.6 | 223 | | 1.15 | 0.67 | 9.2 |
| | 11.3 | | 256—66 | 11.3 | 230 | | 0.89 | 0.61 | |
| Guanosine, $N^2$, $N^2$-dimethyl- | 1 | | 265 | 17.7 | 236 | | 0.63 | 0.56 | 2.5 |
| | 7 | | 260 | 18.9 | 228 | | 0.78 | 0.57 | 9.7 |
| | 13 | | 263 | 14.3 | 242 | | 0.85 | 0.78 | |
| Guanosine, 7-methyl- | 3 | | 257 | 10.7 | 230 | | 0.88 | 0.68 | 7.0 |
| | 7 | | 258, 281 | 8.5, 7.4 | 238 | 5.5 | 0.89 | 1.04 | |
| | 9 | | 282 | 8.0 | 242 | | 0.90 | 1.46 | |
| Guanosine, $N^2$, $N^2$, 7-trimethyl- | 1 | | 266, 295 | | 240 | | 0.57 | 0.59 | |
| | 5 | | 266 | 10.3 | 239 | | 0.57 | 0.63 | |
| | 10 | | 234, 302 | | 280 | | 1.31 | 0.62 | |
| Guanosine 3'-phosphate | 1 | 11.8 | 257 | 12.2 | 228 | | 0.93 | 0.69 | 2.3 |
| | 7 | 11.4 | 252 | 13.4 | 227 | | 1.15 | 0.68 | 9.7 |
| | 10.8 | 11.2 | 257 | 11.3 | 230 | | 0.92 | 0.64 | 5.9 |
| Guanosine 5'-phosphate | 1 | 11.6 | 256 | 12.2 | 228 | | 0.96 | 0.67 | 2.4 |
| | 7 | 11.7 | 252 | 13.7 | 224 | | 1.16 | 0.66 | 9.4 |
| | 11 | 11.5 | 258 | 11.6 | 230 | | 0.90 | 0.61 | 6.1 |
| Guanosine 5'-phosphate, 7-methyl- | 2 | | 257 | 12.0 | 230 | | | | 7.1 |
| | 7.4 | | 258, 280 | 10.3 | 236 | | 0.93 | 1.43 | |
| | 8.9 | | 282 | 8.6 | 271, 242 | | | | |
| Guanosine 5'-diphosphate | 1 | 11.8 | 256 | 12.3 | 228 | | 0.95 | 0.67 | 2.9 |
| | 7 | 11.8 | 253 | 13.7 | 224 | | 1.15 | 0.66 | 9.6 |
| | 11 | 11.7 | 258 | 11.7 | 230 | | 0.91 | 0.61 | 6.3 |
| Guanosine 5'-triphosphate | 1 | 11.8 | 256 | 12.4 | 228 | | 0.96 | 0.67 | 3.3 |
| | 7 | 11.7 | 253 | 13.7 | 223 | | 1.17 | 0.66 | 9.3 |
| | 11 | 11.8 | 257 | 11.9 | 230 | | 0.92 | 0.59 | 6.5 |

## 5 Spectral data and $pK_a$ values for purines, pyrimidines, nucleosides, and nucleotides

| Name | pH | $\epsilon_{260}$ ($\times 10^{-3}$) | $\lambda_{max}$ (nm) | $\epsilon_{max}$ ($\times 10^{-3}$) | $\lambda_{min}$ (nm) | $\epsilon_{min}$ ($\times 10^{-3}$) | 250/260 | 280/260 | $pK_a$ Base | $pK_a$ Phosphate |
|---|---|---|---|---|---|---|---|---|---|---|
| Guanosine 5'-triphosphate, 7-methyl- | 2 | | 257 | 11.7 | 230 | | 0.92 | 0.66 | 7.5 | |
| | 7.4 | | 258 | 9.8 | 236 | | | | | |
| | | | 280 | 8.0 | 271 | | | | | |
| | 12 | | 281 | 8.6 | 243 | | | | | |
| 2'-Deoxyguanosine | 1 | 11.3 | 255 | 12.1 | 232 | | 1.00 | 0.69 | 2.5 | |
| | H$_2$O | 11.8 | 253 | 13.0 | 223 | 2.0 | 1.16 | 0.68 | | |
| | 12 | | 260 | 9.2 | 230 | 2.2 | 0.87 | 0.61 | | |
| 2'-Deoxyguanosine 3'-phosphate | 7 | | 253 | 13.7 | | | 1.15 | 0.67 | | |
| 2'-Deoxyguanosine 5'-phosphate | 1 | 11.5 | 255 | 11.8 | 227 | 2.7 | 1.01 | 0.71 | 2.9 | 6.4 |
| | 7 | 11.8 | 253 | 13.7 | 222 | 2.7 | 1.15 | 0.67 | 9.7 | |
| | 12 | 11.5 | 262 | 11.5 | 230 | 4.0 | 0.91 | 0.62 | | |
| 2'-Deoxyguanosine 5'-triphosphate | 1 | 11.7 | 255 | 12.3 | 227 | 2.4 | 1.01 | 0.71 | 3.5 | 6.5 |
| | 7 | 11.9 | 252 | 13.7 | 222 | 2.7 | 1.16 | 0.66 | 9.7 | |
| | 12 | 11.7 | 262 | 11.7 | 230 | 4.0 | 0.93 | 0.60 | | |
| **Hypoxanthine group** | | | | | | | | | | |
| Hypoxanthine | 0 | 7.4 | 248 | 10.8 | 215 | 1.7 | 1.45 | 0.04 | 2.0 | |
| | 6 | 7.9 | 249.5 | 10.7 | 222 | 2.6 | 1.32 | 0.09 | 8.9 | |
| | 11 | 11.0 | 259 | 11.1 | 232 | 3.8 | 0.84 | 0.12 | 12.1 | |
| Inosine | 3 | 7.1 | 248 | 12.2 | 223 | 7.1 | 1.68 | 0.25 | 1.2 | |
| | 6 | 7.1 | 248.5 | 12.3 | 223 | 3.4 | 1.68 | 0.25 | 8.8 | |
| | 11 | 11.7 | 253 | 13.1 | 224.5 | 2.6 | 1.05 | 0.18 | 12.0 | |
| Inosine 3'(2')-phosphate | 5 | | 248 | | 222 | | 1.59 | 0.29 | | |
| Inosine 5'-phosphate | 0.1 | 9.0 | 251 | 10.9 | | | 1.21 | 0.11 | 8.9 | 1.5 |
| | 6 | 7.2 | 248.5 | 12.2 | 223 | 3.4 | 1.69 | 0.25 | | 6.0 |
| | 12 | 11.5 | 253 | 12.9 | 224 | 2.7 | 1.10 | 0.24 | | |

110

| | | | | | | | | | |
|---|---|---|---|---|---|---|---|---|---|
| Inosine 5'-diphosphate | 6 | | 248.5 | 12.2 | | | 1.68 | 0.25 | |
| 2'-Deoxyinosine 5'-phosphate | 7 | | 249 | 12.2 | | | 1.68 | 0.25 | |
| 2'-Deoxyinosine 5'-triphosphate | 6 | | 269 | 12.2 | | | 1.68 | 0.25 | |
| **Orotic acid group** | | | | | | | | | |
| Orotic acid | 1 | 4.2 | 280 | 7.5 | 241 | 0.9 | 0.54 | 1.82 | 2.4 |
| | 7 | 4.5 | 279 | 7.7 | 241 | | 0.57 | 1.71 | 9.5 |
| | 12 | 3.4 | {240 / 286} | {8.9 / 6.0} | {222 / 244} | 3.4 | 0.80 | 1.71 | < 13.0 |
| Orotidine | 1 | | 267 | 9.8 | 234 | | 0.66 | 0.81 | |
| | 13 | | 266 | 7.8 | 245 | | 0.83 | 0.71 | |
| Orotidine 5'-phosphate | 7 | | 266 | | | | | 0.66 | |
| **Thymine group** | | | | | | | | | |
| Thymine | 4 | 7.4 | 264.5 | 7.9 | 233 | 1.9 | 0.67 | 0.53 | 9.9 |
| | 7 | 7.4 | 264.5 | 7.9 | 233 | 1.9 | 0.67 | 0.53 | > 13.0 |
| | 12 | 3.7 | 291 | 5.4 | 244 | 2.2 | 0.65 | 1.31 | |
| 2'-Deoxythymidine | 1 | 8.8 | 267 | 9.65 | 235 | 2.2 | 0.65 | 0.70 | 9.8 |
| | 7 | 8.8 | 267 | 9.7 | 235 | 2.2 | 0.65 | 0.70 | > 13 |
| | 12 | 6.65 | 267 | 7.4 | 241 | 4.6 | 0.74 | 0.65 | |
| 2'-Deoxythymidine 3'-phosphate | 2 | | 267 | 9.5 | 267 | | 0.65 | 0.69 | |
| | 7 | | | | | | | 0.71 | |
| 2'-Deoxythymidine 5'-phosphate | 2 | 9.3 | 267 | 9.6 | 233 | 2.3 | 0.63 | 0.71 | 10.0 |
| | 7 | 9.3 | 267 | 9.6 | 234 | 2.4 | 0.65 | 0.73 | ~ 1.6 |
| | 12 | 7.5 | 267 | 7.8 | 243 | 4.5 | 0.67 | 0.67 | 6.5 |
| 2'-Deoxythymidine 5'-triphosphate | 2 | 9.3 | 267 | 9.6 | 233 | | 0.63 | 0.71 | |
| | 7 | 9.3 | 267 | 9.6 | | | 0.65 | 0.73 | |

## 5 Spectral data and p$K_a$ values for purines, pyrimidines, nucleosides, and nucleotides

| Name | pH | $\epsilon_{260}$ ($\times 10^{-3}$) | $\lambda_{max}$ (nm) | $\epsilon_{max}$ ($\times 10^{-3}$) | $\lambda_{min}$ (nm) | $\epsilon_{min}$ ($\times 10^{-3}$) | 250/260 | 280/260 | p$K_a$ Base | Phosphate |
|---|---|---|---|---|---|---|---|---|---|---|
| **Uracil group** | | | | | | | | | | |
| Uracil | 4 | 8.2 | 259.5 | 8.2 | 227 | 1.8 | 0.84 | 0.17 | 9.5 | |
| | 7 | 8.2 | 259.5 | 8.2 | 227 | 1.8 | 0.84 | 0.17 | > 13.0 | |
| | 12 | 4.1 | 284 | 6.2 | 241 | 2.1 | 0.71 | 1.40 | | |
| Uracil, 5-hydroxy- | 2 | | 278 | 6.4 | 244 | | 0.56 | 1.63 | 8.0 | |
| | 6 | | 278 | 6.4 | 244 | | 0.54 | 1.55 | | |
| | 12 | | {239, 305} | {6.5, 5.7} | 270 | | 1.65 | 0.83 | | |
| Uracil, 5-hydroxymethyl- | 2 | | 261 | 8.0 | 231 | | 0.77 | 0.32 | 9.4 | |
| | 7 | | 261 | 8.1 | 231 | | 0.77 | 0.33 | ~ 14 | |
| | 12 | | 286 | 7.4 | 245 | | 0.67 | 1.80 | | |
| Uracil, 2-thio- | 1.5 | | 270 | 13.9 | 241 | | | | | |
| | 7.4 | | 268 | 11.8 | 240 | | | | | |
| | 11 | | {259, 307} | {10.7, 6.8} | {243, 291} | | | | | |
| Uridine | 1 | 10.0 | 262 | 10.1 | 230 | 2.0 | 0.74 | 0.35 | 9.2 | |
| | 7 | 10.0 | 262 | 10.1 | 230 | 2.0 | 0.74 | 0.35 | 12.5 | |
| | 12 | 7.4 | 262 | 7.5 | 243 | 4.5 | 0.83 | 0.29 | | |
| Uridine, 5, 6-dihydro- | H$_2$O | | 208 | 6.6 | | | | | | |
| | 13 | | 235 | 10.1 | | | | | | |
| Uridine, 5-methyl- | 1 | | 267 | 9.9 | 235 | | 0.67 | 0.74 | 9.7 | |
| | 7 | | 267 | 9.8 | 236 | | 0.67 | 0.74 | | |
| | 13 | | 268 | 7.5 | 246 | | 0.83 | 0.75 | | |
| Uridine, 2-thio- | 2 | | 279 | 16.4 | 247 | | 0.53 | 1.86 | 8.8 | |
| | 7 | | {218, 275} | {16.2, 13.6} | 247 | | 0.62 | 1.57 | | |
| | 12 | | {239, 271} | {21.0, 13.4} | | | | | | |

| Compound | pH | | λ max (nm) | | λ min (nm) | | | | pK | pK' |
|---|---|---|---|---|---|---|---|---|---|---|
| Uridine, 4-thio- | 2 | | 245, 331 | 5.2, 17.0 | 275 | | | | 8.2 | |
| | 6.5 | | { 245, 331, 316 } | { 4.0, 21.2, 19.7 } | { 225, 274, 268 } | | | | | |
| | 12 | | | | | | | | | |
| Pseudouridine (5-ribosyluracil) | 2 | 7.7 | 262 | 7.9 | 233 | 2.0 | 0.74 | 0.42 | 9.0 | |
| | 7 | 7.7 | 263 | 8.1 | 233 | 2.0 | 0.74 | 0.44 | > 13.0 | |
| | 12 | 3.4 | 286 | 7.7 | 245 | 1.7 | 0.62 | 2.06 | | |
| Uridine 3'-phosphate | 1 | 9.9 | 262 | 10.0 | 230 | 2.0 | 0.76 | 0.32 | 9.4 | 1.0 |
| | 7 | 9.9 | 262 | 10.0 | 230 | 2.0 | 0.73 | 0.35 | | 5.9 |
| | 13 | 7.3 | 261 | 7.8 | 241 | 5.4 | 0.83 | 0.28 | | |
| Uridine 2'-phosphate | 2 | | 260 | 9.9 | 230 | | 0.8 | 0.28 | | |
| | 7 | | 260 | 10.0 | 230 | | 0.78 | 0.30 | | |
| | 12 | | 261 | 7.3 | 242 | | 0.85 | 0.25 | | |
| Pseudouridine 3'-phosphate | 2 | 8.3 | 263 | 8.4 | 233 | 2.3 | 0.75 | 0.40 | 9.6 | |
| | 7 | | 263 | | 233 | | 0.74 | 0.40 | | |
| | 12 | 3.7 | 286 | 3.4 | 246 | 2.1 | 0.64 | 2.06 | | |
| Uridine 5'-phosphate | 2 | 9.9 | 262 | 10.0 | 230 | | 0.73 | 0.39 | 9.5 | 6.4 |
| | 7 | 9.9 | 262 | 10.0 | 230 | | 0.73 | 0.39 | | |
| | 11 | 7.7 | 261 | 7.8 | 241 | | 0.80 | 0.31 | | |
| Uridine 5'-diphosphate | 2 | 9.9 | 262 | 10.0 | 230 | | 0.73 | 0.39 | 9.4 | 6.5 |
| | 7 | 9.9 | 262 | 10.0 | 230 | | 0.73 | 0.39 | | |
| | 11 | 7.8 | 261 | 7.9 | 241 | | 0.80 | 0.32 | | |
| Uridine 5'-triphosphate | 2 | 9.9 | 262 | 10.0 | 230 | | 0.75 | 0.38 | 9.6 | 6.6 |
| | 7 | 9.9 | 262 | 10.0 | 230 | | 0.75 | 0.38 | | |
| | 11 | 8.0 | 261 | 8.1 | 239 | | 0.81 | 0.31 | | |
| 2'-Deoxyuridine | 1 | 10.1 | 262 | 10.2 | 231 | 2.2 | 0.74 | 0.32 | 9.3 | |
| | 7 | 10.1 | 262 | 10.2 | 231 | 2.2 | 0.74 | 0.32 | > 13 | |
| | 12 | 7.55 | 262 | 7.6 | 242 | 5.4 | 0.81 | 0.27 | | |
| 2'-Deoxyuridine, 5-hydroxymethyl- | 2 | | 264 | 9.6 | 233 | | 0.70 | 0.51 | | |
| | 7 | | 264 | 9.6 | 233 | | 0.70 | 0.51 | | |
| | 12 | | 264 | 7.0 | 243 | | 0.75 | 0.54 | | |
| 2'-Deoxyuridine 5'-phosphate | 2 | | 260 | 9.8 | 231 | | 0.72 | 0.38 | | |
| | 7 | | 260 | | 230 | | | | | |
| | 12 | 7.6 | 261 | 7.6 | 241 | | | | | |

## 5 Spectral data and p$K_a$ values for purines, pyrimidines, nucleosides, and nucleotides

| Name | pH | $\epsilon_{260}$ ($\times 10^{-3}$) | $\lambda_{max}$ (nm) | $\epsilon_{max}$ ($\times 10^{-3}$) | $\lambda_{min}$ (nm) | $\epsilon_{min}$ ($\times 10^{-3}$) | 250/260 | 280/260 | p$K_a$ Base | p$K_a$ Phosphate |
|---|---|---|---|---|---|---|---|---|---|---|
| 2'-Deoxyuridine 5'-phosphate, 5-hydroxymethyl- | 2 | | 264 | 10.2 | 234 | | 0.69 | 0.56 | | |
| | 12 | | 264 | | 244 | | 0.80 | 0.48 | | |
| 2'-Deoxyuridine 5'-triphosphate | 1 | | 262 | | | | 0.72 | 0.45 | | |
| **Xanthine group** | | | | | | | | | | |
| Xanthine | 2 | 8.9 | 267 | 10.3 | 242 | | 0.77 | 0.15 | ~ 0.8 | |
| | 6 | 8.9 | 267 | 10.3 | 239 | | 0.57 | 0.61 | 7.5 | |
| | 10 | 5.2 | 240, 277 | 8.9, 9.3 | 222, 257 | | 1.30 | 1.71 | 11.1 | |
| Xanthosine | 2 | 8.7 | 235, 263 | 8.4, 8.95 | 217, 248 | | 0.75 | 0.28 | 2.5 | |
| | 8 | 7.7 | 248, 278 | 10.2, 8.9 | 223, 264 | | 1.30 | 1.13 | 7.0 | |
| | 11 | 7.7 | 248, 278 | 10.2, 8.9 | 222, 264 | | 1.30 | 1.13 | ~ 13 | |
| Xanthosine 5'-phosphate | 10 | | 278 | 8.9 | | | 1.30 | 1.13 | | |
| Xanthosine 5'-triphosphate | 10 | | 278 | 8.9 | | | 1.30 | 1.13 | | |

# 6 Vitamins and coenzymes

## General bibliography

W. H. Sebrell and R. S. Harris (eds.), *The vitamins: chemistry, physiology, pathology, methods,* 2nd edition, vols. 1–3 and 5–7 (vol. 4 has not been published), Academic Press (1967–72).

P. D. Boyer, H. Lardy, and K. Myrbäck (eds.), *The enzymes,* 2nd edition, vols. 2 and 3, Academic Press (1960).

R. A. Morton (ed.), *Fat soluble vitamins,* Pergamon (1970).

A. F. Wagner and K. Folkers, *Vitamins and coenzymes,* Interscience (1964).

*Vitamins and Hormones,* Academic Press, a review serial published annually; vol. **1** (1943), vol. **40** (1983).

*Methods in enzymology,* Academic Press. Articles on vitamins and coenzymes appear particularly in vols. **18A** (1971), **18B** (1971), **18C** (1971), **62** (1980), **66** (1980), and **67** (1980).

## Nomenclature

Rules (or tentative rules) and recommendations for nomenclature of vitamins and coenzymes have been published in:

Trivial names: *BJ* **102**, 15 (1967); *JBC* **241**, 2987 (1966)
Folic acid compounds: *BJ* **102**, 19 (1967); *JBC* **241**, 2991 (1966)
$B_6$ compounds: *BJ* **137**, 417 (1974); *Biochem.* **13**, 1056 (1974)
Corrinoids: *BJ* **147**, 1 (1975); *Biochem.* **13**, 1555 (1974)
Tocopherols: *EJB* **123**, 473 (1982)
Cyclitols: *BJ* **153**, 23 (1976); *EJB* **57**, 1 (1975)
Vitamin D: *EJB* **124**, 223 (1982)
Retinoids: *EJB* **129**, 1 (1982)
Quinones with isoprenoid side chains: *BJ* **147**, 15 (1975); *EJB* **53**, 15 (1975)
Nicotinamide nucleotide coenzymes: *I.U.B. Enzyme Nomenclature – Recommendations (1964),* Elsevier (1965).

# 6 Vitamins and coenzymes

| Name | Synonyms | Formula | M. wt. | Physical properties |
|------|----------|---------|--------|---------------------|
| Acetyl coenzyme A | Acetyl-CoA; Acetyl-S-CoA | Cf. Coenzyme A, —SH replaced by $-S \cdot CO \cdot CH_3$ | 809.6 | wh. powder |
| Acyl coenzyme A compounds | S-Acyl coenzyme A; Acyl-CoA; Acyl-S-CoA | Cf. Coenzyme A, — SH replaced by $- S \cdot CO \cdot R$ | 749.5 + M. wt. of *acid* OR 794.5 + R | hygr. amorph. wh. solids |
| *p*-Aminobenzoic acid | pAB; pABA | | 137.1 | wh. monocl. cryst., yellows in air and light; M.p. 187; $pK_a$ 2.38, 4.89 |
| Ascorbic acid | L-Ascorbic acid; Vitamin C | | 176.1 | wh. cryst., sharp acidic taste; M.p. 192 d.; $pK_a$ 4.04, 11.34; $E_0'$ + 0.058 V (1st stage, pH 7); $[\alpha]_D^{20}$ + 23 (c = 1 in $H_2O$) |
| Biopterin | 2-Amino-4-hydroxy-6-(L-*erythro*-1,2-dihydroxy-propyl) pteridine; 6-L-*erythro*-(1,2-Dihydroxypropyl)-pterin; *Crithidia* factor | | 237.2 | yel. cryst.; decomp. 250–80; $[\alpha]_D^{25}$ − 62 (c = 0.2 in 0.1 M-HCl); $pK_a$ 2.43, 7.7 |

| Solubility | Absorption spectrum | General Remarks |
|---|---|---|
| s. $H_2O$ | $\lambda_{max}$    260 nm<br>$\epsilon$    16 400<br>$\epsilon_{232}$    8700<br>$\Delta\epsilon_{232}$ on hydrolysis 4500 | Stability, see Acyl-CoA compds. Can be heated to 100 °C for 15 min at pH 3.5 to 5 without decomp. $Li_3$ salt stable, store dry at 4 °C, no detectable decomp. in 6 months. PREP. *JACS* **75**, 2520 (1953); *Meth. Enzymol.* **3**, 931 (1957). *See also* Acyl-CoA compds. |
| s. $H_2O$, solubility decreases with increasing length of carbon chain of acyl gp. Long-chain fatty acyl-CoA pptd. from aq. soln. by acid. | In most acyl-CoAs, $\lambda_{max} \sim$ 260 nm $\epsilon$ 16 400 due to adenine, and $\sim$ 232 nm $\epsilon \sim$ 9000 due to thioester bond. Hydrolysis of thioester bond causes decrease in absorbance at 232 nm, $\Delta\epsilon_{232}$ 4500.<br>*α, β-Unsaturated acyl-CoA:*<br>Double bond shifts thioester absorbance max. to 263 nm where it is superimposed on adenine absorbance at 260 nm.<br>$\lambda_{max}$    225      260 nm<br>$\epsilon$    16 300    22 600<br>On hydrolysis of thioester bond, $\Delta\epsilon_{225}$ 8400, $\Delta\epsilon_{263}$ 6700<br>*β-Oxoacyl-CoA:* Enolate ion stabilized at pH $>$ 8 in presence of $Mg^{2+}$, giving<br>$\lambda_{max}$    260      303 nm<br>$\epsilon(C_4)$ 16 000    21 400<br>$\epsilon(C_{16})$         9900<br>*Meth. Enzymol.* **71**, 398 (1981) | *See also* Acetyl-CoA, Malonyl-CoA, Succinyl-CoA. *Stability*. Dry solids may be stored at 0 °C in a desiccator over long periods without decomp. Generally stable in neutral and moderately acid solns. even at elevated temp., hydrolysed in strong acid. (Succinyl-CoA (q.v.) is unusually labile at neutral pH.) Rapidly hydrolysed in alkaline solns.; α,β-unsaturated acyl compds. are more stable than saturated, β-hydroxyacyl somewhat more labile. Instability in alkali increases as $pK_a$ of acid decreases. React quantitatively with neutral $NH_2OH$ forming acylhydroxamic acid (β-oxoacyl compds. form isoxazolones). PREP. General methods: *JACS* **75**, 2520 (1953); *Meth. Enzymol.* **3**, 931 (1957); *Biochem. Preps.* **7**, 80 (1960); *Angew. Chem.* **65**, 186 (1953); *BZ* **335**, 540 (1962); *JBC* **236**, 2620 (1961). Certain acyl-CoAs require special methods: Acetoacetyl-CoA, *Angew. Chem.* **64**, 687 (1952); β-oxoacyl-CoA, *Anal. Biochem.* **1**, 8 (1961), *BBA* **164**, 498 (1968); Malonyl-CoA (q.v.). |
| $0.5^{25}$, v.s.$^{100}$ $H_2O$; 11 EtOH; 8 eth.; s. MeOH, $CHCl_3$, gl. acetic; sl. s. benz.; i. pet. eth. | In $H_2O$:<br>$\lambda_{max}$    266 nm<br>$\epsilon$    15 000 | Competitively counteracts sulphonamide bacteriostasis. Readily absorbed by man after oral dosage and excreted as *p*-aminohippurate, some as glucuronate. Stable as solid and in soln. |
| 33.3 $H_2O$; 2 EtOH; i. eth., $CHCl_3$, benz., pet. eth. | In $H_2O$ or neutral soln.:<br>$\lambda_{max}$    265 nm<br>$\epsilon$    7000<br>In acid:<br>$\lambda_{max}$    245 nm<br>$\epsilon$    7500<br>*JCS* **1933**, 1270 | Stable as dry solid. Aq. soln. about pH 3, acts as a monobasic acid. Powerful reducing agent, reduces Fehlings soln. in the cold; readily oxidized by many oxidizing agents. Aq. solns. stable only in absence of $O_2$. In air, aq. soln. most stable at pH 5–6, very unstable at alkaline pHs, oxidation catalyzed by Cu $>$ Fe. Used in biological systems as an H-donor in electron transport studies and to protect other readily oxidized substances e.g. tetrahydropteroylglutamate. |
| $0.07^{20}$, $0.4^{90}$ $H_2O$; v.sl.s. EtOH, eth.; s. acids, alkalis | At pH 1: $\lambda_{max}$    247      320 nm<br>     $\epsilon$    11 700    8500<br>At pH 13: $\lambda_{max}$    254      363 nm<br>     $\epsilon$    24 600    8000<br>In $H_2O$:    $\lambda_{max}$ 275 nm<br>         $A_{272}/A_{252}$ 1.9–2.1<br>*7,8-Dihydrobiopterin:*<br>$\lambda_{max}$ 258   363 nm (in 0.1M-HCl),<br>$\lambda_{max}$ 280   330 nm (pH 6.8–13),<br>$\epsilon_{330}$ 6200 (pH 6.8)<br>*5,6,7,8-Tetrahydrobiopterin:*<br>$\lambda_{max}$ 265 nm (in 0.1M-HCl);<br>        300 nm (pH 6.8) | Natural compd. is L-*erythro* isomer. Fluoresces blue in alk. soln. PREP. *Meth. Enzymol.* **18B**, 670 (1971), **66**, 508 (1980).<br>*7,8-Dihydrobiopterin*. Violet fluorescence. Soln. stable several months at −20 °C. PREP. By methods for dihydropteroylglutamic acid (q.v.), *Meth. Enzymol.* **66**, 508 (1980).<br>*5,6,7,8-Tetrahydrobiopterin*. Rapidly oxidized in soln., half-life at 24 °C and pH 6.8 $\sim$ 6 min. Store at −20 °C. PREP. By methods for tetrahydropteroylglutamate (q.v.), *JBC* **242**, 3934 (1967). |

# 6 Vitamins and coenzymes

| Name | Synonyms | Formula | M. wt. | Physical properties |
|------|----------|---------|--------|---------------------|
| Biotin | *d*-Biotin; Coenzyme R; Vitamin H | | 244.3 | wh. needles; M.p. 232–3; $[\alpha]_D^{22} + 92$ (c = 0.3 in 0.1 M-NaOH) |
| Cholecalciferol | Vitamin $D_3$; Calciol; 9,10-Secocholesta-5,7,10(19)-triene-3$\beta$-ol | | 384.7 | fine needles; M.p. 84–5; $[\alpha]_D + 51.9$ (c = 1.6 in $CHCl_3$) |
| Coenzyme A | CoA; CoA·SH | | 767.6 | wh. hygr. powder; thiol odour; $pK_a$ 4.0 (adenine $NH_2$) 6.4 ($PO_4$) 9.6 (SH) |
| ——, Li$_3$ salt | | $C_{21} H_{33} N_7 O_{16} P_3 S \cdot Li_3$ | Li$_3$ salt, 785.4 | |
| Coenzyme $B_{12}$ | 5′-Deoxyadenosylcobalamin; Adenosylcobalamin; $\alpha$-(5,6-Dimethylbenzimidazolyl)-cobamide coenzyme; $\alpha$-(5,6-Dimethylbenzimidazolyl)-5′-deoxyadenosylcobamide; DMBC coenzyme | Cf. Cyanocobalamin, –CN group replaced by | 1579.6 | flattened, diamond-shaped yel.–orange crystals, turn deep red on exposure to air; from $H_2O$ or aq. acet. contains 8–9% $H_2O$. |

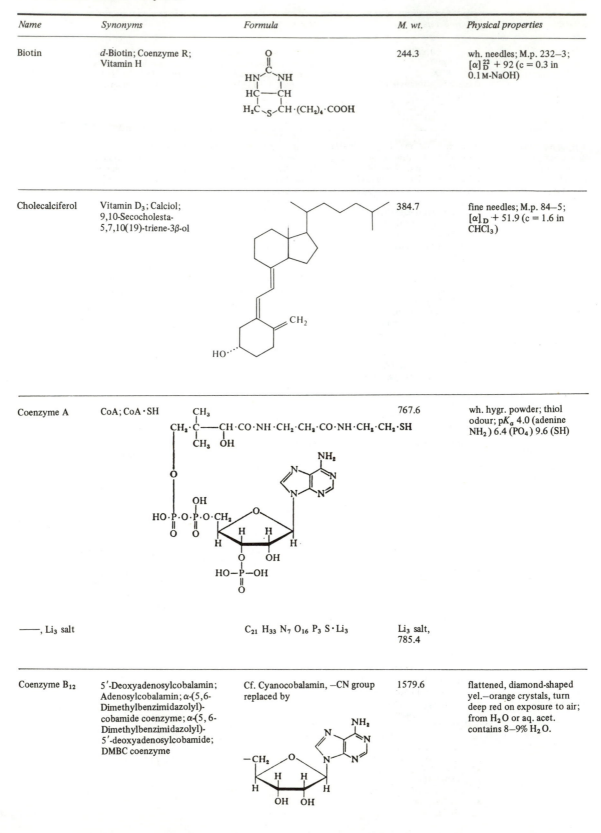

| Solubility | Absorption spectrum | General Remarks |
|---|---|---|
| $0.02^{25}$ $H_2O$; s. in hot $H_2O$ + dil. alkali; $0.08^{25}$ 95% EtOH; i. organic solvents. Na salt, v.s. $H_2O$ | | Thermostable as solid. Stable at 100 °C in moderately acid or neutral aq. soln., acidic solns. can be heat sterilized; less stable above pH 9. Inactivated by combination with avidin. *Biocytin* (ε-*N*-biotinoyl-L-lysine): cryst., s.$H_2O$, sl.s. EtOH, complete hydrolysis requires 1.5 M-$H_2SO_4$ at 120 °C for 1 hr, combines with avidin. *Avidin*; glycoprotein from egg-white, tetramer, M. wt. 66 000, v.s. $H_2O$, salt solns., stable over wide range of pH and temperature. Binds biotin (4 moles/mole; 1 per subunit); binding is effectively irreversible except by v. extreme conditions, $K$ (dissociation) $\sim 10^{-15}$ M. PREP. *BJ* 118, 67, 71 (1970); REVIEW. *Adv. Protein Chem.* 29, 85 (1975). |
| s. EtOH, acet., eth., $CHCl_3$; i. $H_2O$ | In hexane or EtOH: $\lambda_{max}$ 265 nm ε 18 200 | Sensitive to light. Oxidized in moist air within a few days. Somewhat more stable than ergocalciferol, much more stable than 7-dehydrocholesterol. Negligible decomp. of pure cryst. cholecalciferol in amber glass sealed ampoules at 0–4 °C after 1 year. Stable in soln. in propylene glycol or corn oil or as ester of 3, 5-dinitrobenzoic acid (M.p. 129). Not pptd. by digitonin. |
| s. $H_2O$; i. acet., eth., EtOH | pH 2.5– 11.0: $\lambda_{max}$ 259.5 nm ε 16 800 | Store dry at − 20 °C; free acid may decomp. $\sim$ 5% in 6 months, Li salt no detectable decomp. Purified material may contain some mixed disulphides, esp. with glutathione. Solns. unstable above pH 7, 31% of activity lost in 24 hr at pH 8 and 25 °C. Relatively stable at pH 2–6, store frozen. Readily oxidized by air to inactive disulphide; thiol may be regenerated with excess of a thiol compd. |
| $2.6^{24}$ $H_2O$; s. EtOH, phenol; i. acet., eth., dioxane | In 0.1 M-HCl: $\lambda_{max}$ 266 287 306 380 458 nm ε 41 100 23 900 22 200 8800 9400 At pH 7: $\lambda_{max}$ 262 290 318 341 376 522 nm ε 35 100 18 200 13 000 12 800 11 000 8000 | Dry cryst. stable for months at 0 °C in the dark; slowly decomp. by light at room temp. Aq. soln. rapidly decomp. by u.v. or visible light. In dark, solns. most stable at pH 6–7; dil. aq. solns. stable for months at − 10 °C. Neutral soln. red, acid soln. yellow. p$K_a$ 3.5. Heating in acid or alkaline soln. causes slow inactivation. Reacts with alkaline cyanide to give dicyanocobalamin. PREP. *Biochem. Preps.* 10, 27 (1963), 12, 124 (1968); *Meth. Enzymol.* 18C, 57 (1971). |

## 6 Vitamins and coenzymes

| Name | Synonyms | Formula | M. wt. | Physical properties |
|------|----------|---------|--------|---------------------|

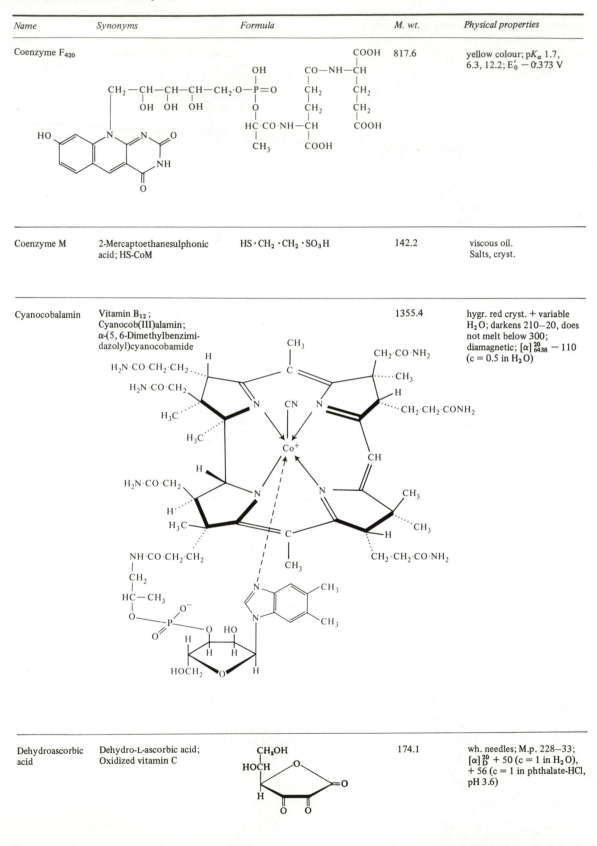

**Coenzyme F$_{420}$** — 817.6 — yellow colour; p$K_a$ 1.7, 6.3, 12.2; $E_0'$ − 0.373 V

**Coenzyme M** — 2-Mercaptoethanesulphonic acid; HS-CoM — $HS \cdot CH_2 \cdot CH_2 \cdot SO_3H$ — 142.2 — viscous oil. Salts, cryst.

**Cyanocobalamin** — Vitamin B$_{12}$; Cyanocob(III)alamin; α-(5, 6-Dimethylbenzimi-dazolyl)cyanocobamide — 1355.4 — hygr. red cryst. + variable $H_2O$; darkens 210–20, does not melt below 300; diamagnetic; $[\alpha]_{6438}^{20}$ − 110 (c = 0.5 in $H_2O$)

**Dehydroascorbic acid** — Dehydro-L-ascorbic acid; Oxidized vitamin C — 174.1 — wh. needles; M.p. 228–33; $[\alpha]_D^{20}$ + 50 (c = 1 in $H_2O$), + 56 (c = 1 in phthalate-HCl, pH 3.6)

| Solubility | Absorption spectrum | General Remarks |
|---|---|---|
| s. $H_2O$ | At pH 4.5:<br>$\lambda_{max}$ 235 250 267 395 nm<br>$\epsilon$ 41 500 24 000 25 400 27 400<br>At pH 8.9:<br>$\lambda_{max}$ 247 267 295 420 nm<br>$\epsilon$ 37 000 25 800 12 600 45 500<br>*Reduced compd.* at pH 5.7:<br>$\lambda_{max}$ 322 nm $\epsilon$ 10 500<br>At pH 8.8:<br>$\lambda_{max}$ 258 320 nm<br>$\epsilon$ 10 800 14 500 | Bright green fluorescence in oxidized form; fluorescence and visible absorbance lost on reduction, e.g. by $NaBH_4$ or dithionite at pH 7.3. Photolabile under aerobic conditions, but not in strictly anaerobic conditions, in neutral or alkaline soln. PREP. *Biochem.* **17**, 4583 (1978). |
| s. $H_2O$ | | Oxidized in air to disulphide, $\lambda_{max}$ 245 nm $\epsilon$ 380. Strong acid. PREP. *JBC* **249**, 4879 (1974); *Meth. Enzymol.* **67**, 545 (1980). |
| 1.2 $H_2O$; s. alcohols, aliphatic acids, phenols; i. eth., acet., $CHCl_3$, pyr. | In $H_2O$, pH 2–10:<br>$\lambda_{max}$ 278 305 322 361 518 550 nm<br>$\epsilon$ 16 300 9700 7900 28 100 7400 8700 | In contact with the atmosphere, usually contains 10–12% $H_2O$, removable by heating under reduced pressure. Stable as solid in the dark. Aq. solns. photolabile forming hydroxocobalamin, prolonged exposure causes irreversible destruction. Solns. most stable at pH 4–6; may be kept for years in dark at room temp. at these pHs at conc. above 0.1 $\mu$g/ml. May be autoclaved at 120°C and pH 4–6 with only sl. decomp. In strongly acid and esp. alkaline soln. slow hydrolysis of amide gps. occurs at room temp.; $B_{12}$ activity completely destroyed by heating in alk. soln., 0.1M, 100°C, 10 min. Reacts with cyanide at pH 10 to form purple dicyano-cobalamin, $\lambda_{max}$ ($\epsilon$) 367 (30 800) 550 and 580 nm (9600). Reduction with $H_2$ + Pt or electrochemically forms cob(II)alamin (Vitamin $B_{12r}$), also formed by photolysis of coenzyme $B_{12}$ and methylcobalamin. *Cob(II)alamin*, brown soln., soln. oxidized in air but solid stable, $\lambda_{max}$ ($\epsilon$) 311 (27 500) 402 (7500) 473 nm (9200). Reduction with $NaBH_4$, $CrCl_2$ at pH 9.5, Zn + HOAc gives *cob(I)alamin* (Vitamin $B_{12s}$, hydrido-cobalamin), grey–green soln., decomp. to cob(II)alamin + $H_2$ (half-time 355 min at pH 10, 87 min at pH 8), oxidized to cob(II)alamin almost instantaneously by air, $\lambda_{max}$ ($\epsilon$) 280.5 (29 100) 288 (29 400) 386 (28 000) 545 nm (2800). PREP. (of reduced compds.) *Meth. Enzymol.* **18C**, 34, 52 (1971).<br>REVIEW. Hogenkamp in *Cobalamin: Biochemistry and Pathophysiology*, ed. B. M. Babior, Wiley (1975). |
| s. hot $H_2O$, basic organic solvents; i. neutral organic solvents | No selective absorption in u.v. | Aq. solns. much less stable than ascorbic acid. pH of aq. soln. approx. neutral. PREP. *JBC* **176**, 529 (1948); *JCS* **1948**, 158; *ZPC* **351**, 52 (1970). |

## 6 Vitamins and coenzymes

| Name | Synonyms | Formula | M. wt. | Physical properties |
|------|----------|---------|--------|---------------------|
| 7-Dehydrocholesterol | Provitamin $D_3$; Cholesta-5,7-diene-3β-ol | | 384.6; Hydrate, 402.7 | plates + $1H_2O$; M.p. 150–1; $[\alpha]_D^{20} - 113.6$ (c = 1 in $CHCl_3$) |
| 3-Dehydroretinal (all-*trans*) | Retinene$_2$; Retinal$_2$; 3-Dehydroretinaldehyde; Vitamin $A_2$ aldehyde; 3,4-Didehydroretinal | | 282.4 | orange cryst.; M.p. 78–9 |
| 3-Dehydroretinol (all-*trans*) | Vitamin $A_2$; 3,4-Didehydroretinol | | 284.4 | oil; M.p. 17–19 |
| Dihydronicotinamide adenine dinucleotide | Reduced nicotinamide adenine dinucleotide; NADH; Dihydrodiphosphopyridine nucleotide; DPNH | | 665.4 | wh. amorph. powder |
| ——, Na$_2$ salt | | Na$_2$ · NADH | 709.4 | |
| Dihydro-nicotinamide adenine dinucleotide phosphate | Reduced nicotinamide adenine dinucleotide phosphate; NADPH; Dihydrotriphosphopyridine nucleotide; TPNH | Cf. Dihydronicotinamide adenine dinucleotide | 745.4 | |
| ——, Na$_4$ salt | | Na$_4$ · NADPH | 833.4 | wh. amorph. powder |
| Dihydropteroyl-glutamic acid | 7,8-Dihydropteroylglutamic acid; Dihydrofolic acid; DHFA | | 443.4; Hydrate; 488.4 | wh. needles + $2\frac{1}{2}H_2O$ when dried over $P_2O_5$ at 25 °C; turns yellow on storage. |

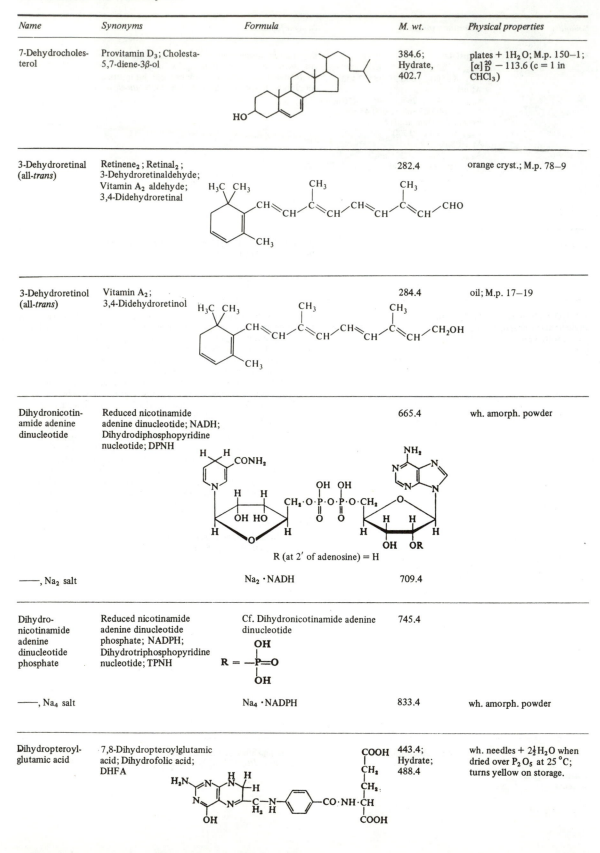

R (at 2′ of adenosine) = H

$$R = -\overset{\displaystyle OH}{\underset{\displaystyle OH}{P}}=O$$

| Solubility | Absorption spectrum | General Remarks |
|---|---|---|
| s. eth., $CHCl_3$; sl. s. MeOH; i. $H_2O$ | In EtOH:<br>$\lambda_{max}$  262  271  282<br>$\epsilon$  7700  11 250  11 900<br>$\lambda_{max}$  293.5 nm<br>$\epsilon$  6650 | Water of crystallisation tenaciously held. Oxidizes in air. Stable as paste containing 17% MeOH or when crystallized with cholesterol or as 3,5-dinitrobenzoate (M.p. 210–212). Digitonin complex insoluble. Forms cholecalciferol (Vitamin $D_3$) on u.v. irradiation. |
| s. EtOH, $CHCl_3$, eth., cyclohexane; i. $H_2O$ | In EtOH:<br>$\lambda_{max}$ 401 nm $\epsilon$ 41 450<br>$SbCl_3$ complex in $CHCl_3$:<br>$\lambda_{max}$ 740 nm falling to 705 nm.<br>$A_{1\,cm}^{1\%}$ 3720 at 705 nm | Unstable in air and acids; less stable than retinal and 3-dehydroretinol. Isomerized to cis-isomers on exposure to light. |
| s. EtOH, $CHCl_3$, eth., cyclohexane; i. $H_2O$ | In EtOH:<br>$\lambda_{max}$  276  286  350 nm<br>$\epsilon$  15 760 20 300 41 200<br>$SbCl_3$ complex in $CHCl_3$:<br>$\lambda_{max}$ 693 nm $A_{1\,cm}^{1\%}$ 4100 | More sensitive to oxygen than retinol; cryst. solid completely oxidized in air at 0 °C within 1 hr. Sensitive to light and acids. |
| s. $H_2O$ | At pH 7.5:<br>$\lambda_{max}$  259  339 nm<br>$\epsilon$  16 900  6220<br>$\lambda_{min}$  234  290 nm<br>$\epsilon$  6600  1300<br>$\epsilon_{366}$ 3300<br>$\epsilon_{339}$ falls slightly with rising temp., 6110 at 35 °C. Effect more pronounced at 366 nm | Solid stable at 0–4 °C if stored dry and protected from light. Inhibitors of lactate and other dehydrogenases readily form in solid on exposure to moist air or $CO_2$, and in solns. on freezing and thawing or on standing at 25 °C or more slowly at 4 °C. Soln. in 50 mM-Tris, pH 7.4, stable one week at 4 °C, one month at −20 °C; soln. in phosphate buffer much less stable, esp. on freezing. Stable in alkaline soln., 0.1 M-NaOH at 100 °C for 10 min has no effect. Destroyed at pH 4 or below at room temp. Stability, *Scand. J. Clin. Lab. Invest.* **33**, Suppl. 139 (1974). PURIF. *Meth. Enzymol.* **66**, 11 (1980); purified NADH has improved stability both as solid and in soln. |
| s. $H_2O$ | | |
| s. $H_2O$ | At pH 7.5:<br>$\lambda_{max}$  259  339 nm<br>$\epsilon$  16 900  6200<br>$\lambda_{min}$  236  290 nm<br>$\epsilon$  7600  1400<br>$\epsilon_{366}$ 3300 | Keep solid at 0–4 °C in the dark and in a desiccator. Stability of solns. qualitatively similar to that of NADH, i.e. stable in alk., slow decomp. at neutral pH, v. unstable in acid but NADPH is quantitatively somewhat less stable than NADH. See *JBC* **236**, 2756 (1961). |
| s. $H_2O$ | | |
| s. $H_2O$; i. $H_2O$ below pH 4 | At pH 7, $\lambda_{max}$ 282 nm $\epsilon$ 28 400 (values of 19–22 000 also reported);<br>At pH 1, $\lambda_{max}$ 282 nm $\epsilon$ 19 900;<br>At pH 13, $\lambda_{max}$ 284 nm $\epsilon$ 27 000 | Slowly oxidized by air, especially at alkaline pH. Decomp. about 50% overnight at room temp. at pH 6. Mercaptoethanol or ascorbate protects, e.g. 2.3% decomp. in 10 hr at 0 °C in Tris, pH 7.3 + 0.3M-mercaptoethanol. May be stored as solid in $O_2$-free sealed ampoules or frozen in deaerated water or as frozen suspension in dil. HCl (e.g. 0.005 M-HCl + 0.05 M-mercaptoethanol). Suspension in 0.005 M-HCl stable several days at 0–4 °C. PREP. *Nature, Lond.* **188**, 231 (1960); *Meth. Enzymol.* **6**, 801 (1963), **18B**, 726 (1971), **66**, 517 (1980). |

| Name | Synonyms | Formula | M. wt. | Physical properties |
|------|----------|---------|--------|---------------------|
| 1α, 25-Dihydroxy-cholecalciferol | 9, 10-Secocholesta-5, 7, 10(19)-triene-1α, 3β, 25-triol; 1α, 25-Dihydroxyvitamin $D_3$; Calcitriol | | 416.7 | cryst.; M.p. 84–8; $[\alpha]_D + 29$ (in eth.) |
| Dolichol | | | $n = 19$, 1382.4 | $n = 19$: col. viscous liq.; M.p. − 10 |
| Ergocalciferol | Vitamin $D_2$; Calciferol; Ercalciol | | 396.7 | col. prisms or needles; M.p. 121; $[\alpha]_D^{20} + 106$ (in EtOH) |
| Ergosterol | Provitamin $D_2$ | | 396.6; Hydrate, 414.7 | hydrated plates or needles + 1–1.5 $H_2O$; M.p. 168; $[\alpha]_D^{20} − 135$ (c = 1.6 in $CHCl_3$) |
| Flavin adenine dinucleotide | FAD | | 785.6 | orange hygr. powder; $E_0'$ −0.219V (pH 7, 30 °C) |
| ——, Na salt | | NaH·FAD | 807.6 | |

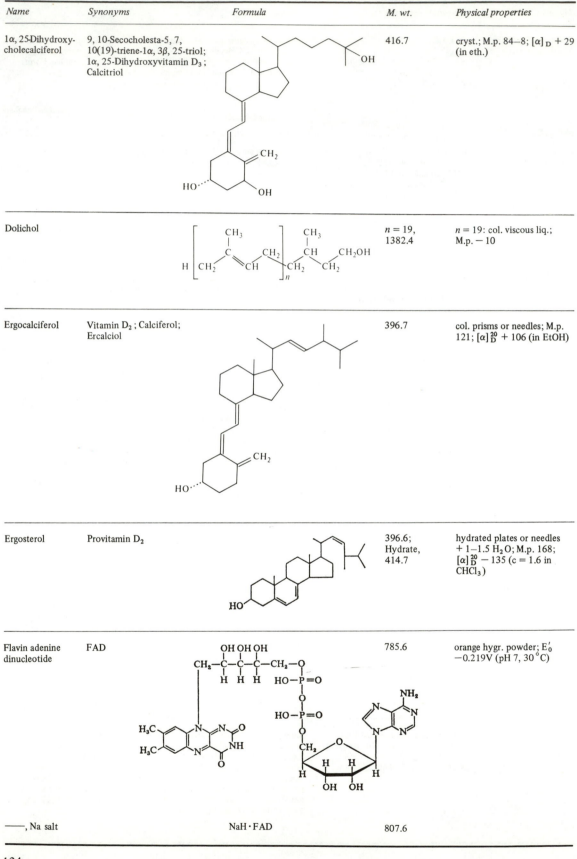

| Solubility | Absorption spectrum | General Remarks |
|---|---|---|
| i. $H_2O$; s. MeOH, EtOH, eth., $CHCl_3$ | In ether: $\lambda_{max}$ 265 nm $\epsilon$ 18 000; $\lambda_{min}$ 229 nm $\epsilon$ 10 100 | Protect from light, heat and oxygen. |
| s. eth., light pet.; sl. s. EtOH; i. $H_2O$ | p-Phenylazobenzoate: $\lambda_{max}$ 324 nm $A_{1\,cm}^{1\%}$ 171.4 p-Nitrobenzoate: $\lambda_{max}$ 256 nm $A_{1\,cm}^{1\%}$ 195 | The dolichols are a family of naturally-occurring polyprenols with the structure shown, containing 14—22 isoprene units ($n = 13$—21). The principal dolichols in vertebrates have 18—20 isoprene units and in yeast 15—16 units. |
| $28^{26}$ EtOH; $25^{26}$ acet.; s. eth., $CHCl_3$; i. $H_2O$ | In EtOH or hexane: $\lambda_{max}$ 265 nm $\epsilon$ 19 400 | Less stable than ergosterol. Sensitive to light under all conditions. Oxidized in air in a few days. Low temp. and an inert atmosphere slow down, but do not stop, decomposition. May be stored for months in sealed evacuated amber glass ampoules in the cold. Stable in soln. in propylene glycol or corn oil or as esters of various nitrobenzoic acids, e.g. 3,5-dinitrobenzoate, M.p. 146—8. Not pptd. with digitonin. |
| s. hot $CHCl_3$, benz.; sl. s. MeOH, EtOH, eth., light pet.; i. $H_2O$ | In EtOH: $\lambda_{max}$  262   271   282 $\epsilon$   7700   11 400   11 900 $\lambda_{max}$   293.5 nm $\epsilon$   6900 | Complete removal of water of crystallization is almost impossible. Oxidizes in air. Store *in vacuo*, cold and in the dark. Forms sp. s. digitonide. Forms ergocalciferol (vitamin $D_2$) on u.v. irradiation. |
| v.s. $H_2O$; s. pyr., phenol; i. EtOH, eth., acet., $CHCl_3$ | In 0.1M-$PO_4$ buffer, pH 7: $\lambda_{max}$   263   375   450 nm $\epsilon$   38 000   9300   11 300 $\epsilon_{260}$ 37 000 Fluorescence max., 525—30 nm. Fluorescence maximal at pH 2.7—3.1, much weaker (9—20%) than riboflavin or FMN. Dihydro compd., $\epsilon_{450}$ 980 | Solid and neutral aq. solns. stable indefinitely at $0\,°C$ in the dark. Cold dil. acids have no effect, but on heating (e.g. 0.1M-HCl at $100\,°C$) hydrolysis to FMN occurs. In neutral soln. at $80\,°C$ or higher and rapidly in alk. soln. hydrolysed to riboflavin 4′,5′-cyclic phosphate. In neutral soln. FAD much less photolabile than FMN or riboflavin, but v. photolabile in alk. soln. All solns. best kept dark. Reduced to colourless dihydro compound by dithionite, Na amalgam, Zn + acid or $H_2$ + catalyst; dihydro compd. v. readily autoxidizable. PREP. *Biochem. Preps.* **7**, 51 (1960); *Meth. Enzymol.* **18C**, 399 (1971). |

# 6 Vitamins and coenzymes

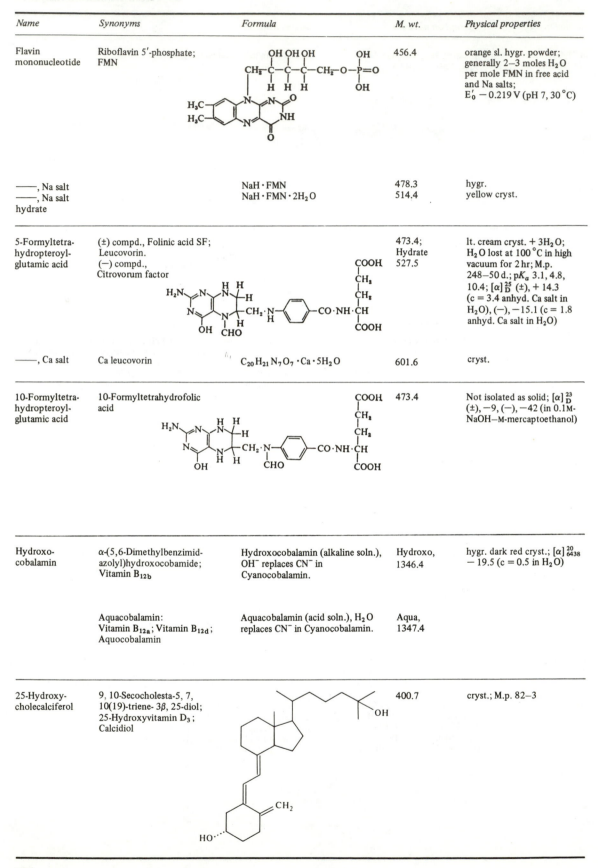

| Name | Synonyms | Formula | M. wt. | Physical properties |
|---|---|---|---|---|
| Flavin mononucleotide | Riboflavin 5'-phosphate; FMN | | 456.4 | orange sl. hygr. powder; generally 2–3 moles $H_2O$ per mole FMN in free acid and Na salts; $E_0' - 0.219\,V$ (pH 7, 30 °C) |
| ——, Na salt | | $NaH \cdot FMN$ | 478.3 | hygr. |
| ——, Na salt hydrate | | $NaH \cdot FMN \cdot 2H_2O$ | 514.4 | yellow cryst. |
| 5-Formyltetra-hydropteroyl-glutamic acid | (±) compd., Folinic acid SF; Leucovorin. (−) compd., Citrovorum factor | | 473.4; Hydrate 527.5 | lt. cream cryst. $+ 3H_2O$; $H_2O$ lost at 100 °C in high vacuum for 2 hr; M.p. 248–50 d.; $pK_a$ 3.1, 4.8, 10.4; $[\alpha]_D^{25}$ (±), + 14.3 ($c = 3.4$ anhyd. Ca salt in $H_2O$), (−), −15.1 ($c = 1.8$ anhyd. Ca salt in $H_2O$) |
| ——, Ca salt | Ca leucovorin | $C_{20}H_{21}N_7O_7 \cdot Ca \cdot 5H_2O$ | 601.6 | cryst. |
| 10-Formyltetra-hydropteroyl-glutamic acid | 10-Formyltetrahydrofolic acid | | 473.4 | Not isolated as solid; $[\alpha]_D^{23}$ (±), −9, (−), −42 (in 0.1M-NaOH–M-mercaptoethanol) |
| Hydroxo-cobalamin | α-(5,6-Dimethylbenzimid-azolyl)hydroxocobamide; Vitamin $B_{12b}$ | Hydroxocobalamin (alkaline soln.), $OH^-$ replaces $CN^-$ in Cyanocobalamin. | Hydroxo, 1346.4 | hygr. dark red cryst.; $[\alpha]_{6438}^{20}$ − 19.5 ($c = 0.5$ in $H_2O$) |
| | Aquacobalamin: Vitamin $B_{12a}$; Vitamin $B_{12d}$; Aquocobalamin | Aquacobalamin (acid soln.), $H_2O$ replaces $CN^-$ in Cyanocobalamin. | Aqua, 1347.4 | |
| 25-Hydroxy-cholecalciferol | 9, 10-Secocholesta-5, 7, 10(19)-triene- 3β, 25-diol; 25-Hydroxyvitamin $D_3$; Calcidiol | | 400.7 | cryst.; M.p. 82–3 |

| Solubility | Absorption spectrum | General Remarks |
|---|---|---|
| s. $H_2O$, gl. acetic, pyr., phenol; v. sl. s. EtOH; i. acet., eth., $CHCl_3$ | In $0.1M$-$PO_4$ buffer, pH 7:<br>$\lambda_{max}$ 266 373 445 nm<br>$\epsilon$ 31 800 10 400 12 500<br>$\lambda_{ref}$ 260 375 450 nm<br>$\epsilon$ 27 100 10 400 12 200<br>Fluorescence max., 525–30 nm<br>Dihydro compd.:<br>$\epsilon_{450}$ 870 | Most stable at about pH 6. Neutral solns. stable at $100\,°C$. In acid soln. phosphate ester bond hydrolysed, in alk. soln. ring–ribitol bond unstable. $NH_4$ salt v. unstable. Rapidly photolysed at all pHs, but esp. in alk. soln.: photolysis more rapid than riboflavin. Store in dark. Reduced to colourless dihydro compound by dithionite, Na amalgam, Zn + acid or $H_2$ + catalyst; dihydro compound v. readily autoxidizable. PURIF. Meth. Enzymol. 66, 217 (1980). |
| 11.2 (pH 6.9), 4.3 (pH 3.8) $H_2O$ | | |
| s. $H_2O$ | At pH 13:<br>$\lambda_{max}$ 282 nm<br>$\epsilon$ 32 600<br>$\lambda_{min}$ 248 nm<br>At pH 7:<br>$\lambda_{max}$ 286 nm<br>$\epsilon$ 31 800 | Solid stable indefinitely in air. In acid soln. cyclization of formyl group to 5,10-methenyltetrahydropteroylglutamic acid occurs. Stable in neutral or alk. soln.; not susceptible to oxidation by air. Naturally occurring form is $(-)$-L-compound.<br>PREP. Meth. Enzymol. 18B, 731 (1971); 66, 541, 547 (1980). |
| Ca salt: s. $H_2O$; i. EtOH | | |
| s. $H_2O$ | pH 7–9: $\lambda_{max}$ 258 nm $\epsilon$ 22 000 | Rapidly oxidized in air. Mercaptoethanol protects, soln. containing M-mercaptoethanol may be kept at $-20\,°C$ for up to 3 days. At pHs below 6, cyclizes to form 5,10-methenyltetrahydropteroylglutamic acid. On heating or prolonged standing at neutral or alkaline pHs, isomerizes to form 5-formyltetrahydropteroylglutamic acid, but strong alkali (0.1 M) removes formyl group. PREP. Readily prepared by adjusting soln. of 5,10-methenyltetrahydropteroylglutamic acid to pH 7 or above and standing for several hours. See also BJ 72, 707 (1959); Meth. Enzymol. 6, 814 (1963). Natural isomer ($(-)$-L), BBA 148, 622 (1967). 10-Formylpteroylglutamic acid, $\lambda_{max}$ 250 and 316 nm (in 98% HCOOH), $\lambda_{max}$ 256 ($\epsilon$ 46 000) and 356 nm (in 0.01 M-NaOH), PREP. BJ 72, 707 (1959); Meth. Enzymol. 66, 440 (1980). |
| s. $H_2O$, MeOH, EtOH; i. eth., acet., benz. | Hydroxocobalamin (alkaline soln.):<br>$\lambda_{max}$ 278 325 358 516 535 nm<br>$\epsilon$ 19 100 11 400 20 600 8900 9300<br>Aquacobalamin (acid soln.):<br>$\lambda_{max}$ 274 317 351 499 525 nm<br>$\epsilon$ 20 600 6100 26 500 8100 8600 | In aq. soln. hydroxo- and aquacobalamin are interconvertible by the gain/loss of a proton, $pK_a$ 7.5. Highly photolabile. Somewhat less stable than cyanocobalamin, esp. in alkaline soln. Treatment with cyanide at pH 10 yields dicyanocobalamin (see cyanocobalamin). PREP. Biochem. Preps. 12, 121 (1968). |
| i. $H_2O$; s. MeOH, EtOH, eth., $CHCl_3$ | $\lambda_{max}$ 265 nm $\epsilon$ 18 000 | Sensitive to light, heat, and $O_2$. Soln. in EtOH is stable for several weeks if protected from light, under $N_2$ and at $0\,°C$. PREP. Meth. Enzymol. 18C, 709 (1971). |

| Name | Synonyms | Formula | M. wt. | Physical properties |
|------|----------|---------|--------|---------------------|
| Hydroxyethyl-thiamin pyro-phosphate | 'Active acetaldehyde'; α-Hydroxyethyl-2-thiamin pyrophosphate; 2-Hydroxyethyl-TPP; HETPP | | 468.4 | hygr. wh. powder; $[\alpha]_D^{23} - 10$ (c = 1.5 in $H_2O$) |
| Inositol | meso-Inositol; myo-Inositol; i-Inositol | | 180.2; Hydrate 216.2 | wh. cryst. + $2H_2O$, efflor.; sweet taste; hydrate becomes anhyd. at 100°C; M.p., Hydrate 218, Anhyd. 225–7; optically inactive |
| Lipoic acid | α-(+)-Lipoic acid; Thioctic acid; 6,8-Dithiooctanoic acid; 1,2-Dithiolane-3-pentanoic acid | | 206.3 | pale yel. platelets; M.p. 47.5; $pK_a$ 4.76; $[\alpha]_D^{25} + 104$ (c = 1.88 in benz.); $E_0'$ −0.325 V (pH 7, 25 °C). DL-, M.p. 61 |
| Malonyl coenzyme A | Malonyl-CoA; Malonyl-S-CoA | Cf. Coenzyme A, −SH replaced by −S—CO·$CH_2$·COOH | 853.6 | |
| Menaquinone | n = 6: Menaquinone-6; MK-6; Vitamin $K_2(30)$ n = 7: Menaquinone-7; MK-7; Vitamin $K_2(35)$ | | MK-6, 580.9; MK-7, 649.0 | MK-6: yel. cryst., M.p. 50. MK-7: light yel. cryst. plates, M.p. 54. |
| 5,10-Methenyl-tetrahydropteroyl-glutamic acid | 'Active formate'; 5,10-Methylidynetetrahydro-pteroylglutamic acid; $N^5,N^{10}$-Anhydroformyl-tetrahydrofolic acid; Anhydroleucovorin | | Chloride, 491.9; Internal salt, 455.4 | several cryst. forms, JACS 74, 3252 (1952); chloride, M.p. 250–7d.; $[\alpha]_D^{23}$ (±), − 36, (+), + 68 (in M-HCl—M-mercaptoethanol) |

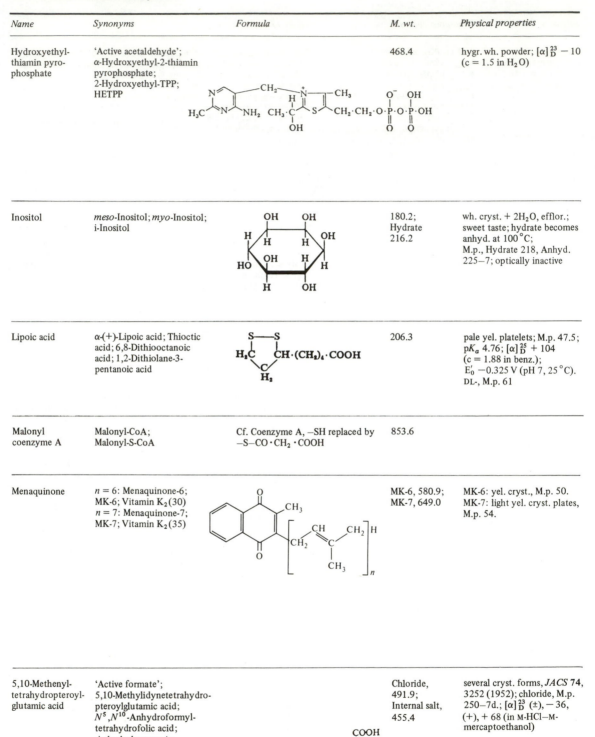

| Solubility | Absorption spectrum | General Remarks |
|---|---|---|
| s. $H_2O$ | At pH 1–3:<br>$\lambda_{max}$ 247   262 nm<br>$\epsilon$   9600<br>In $PO_4$ buffer, pH 8:<br>$\lambda_{max}$ 229   269 nm<br>$\epsilon$   9100   7500<br>$\lambda_{min}$ 248 nm<br>$\epsilon$   4450 (lower than TPP, $\epsilon_{248}$ 5900).<br>Isosbestic point (pH 2–8) 272.5 nm | Synthetic compd. is a racemic mixture of which only one isomer is enzymically active. Solid can be stored dry for several weeks at $-20\,°$C. Soln. relatively stable pH 3–8, most stable at pH 7. Decomp. in acid and esp. alk. soln.<br>PREP. *EJB* **1**, 110 (1967); *Meth. Enzymol.* **18A**, 259 (1970), **9**, 65 (1966). |
| $14^{25} H_2O$; sl. s. EtOH; i. other organic solvents | | Aq. soln. neutral. Stable to acids, alkalis and heat. Hexaacetate, M.p. 216. |
| i. $H_2O$; v.s. benz., EtOH, MeOH; sl. s. pet. eth. | In MeOH;<br>$\lambda_{max}$ 333 nm<br>$\epsilon$   150 | Reduced by borohydride to dihydrolipoic acid, $[\alpha]_D^{20}$ $-14.5$ (c = 0.6 in benz.), *Meth. Enzymol.* **3**, 944 (1957).<br>REVIEW: *Vitams Horm.* **20**, 1 (1962); *Adv. Enzymol.* **32**, 423 (1969). |
| s. $H_2O$ | *See* Acyl-CoA compds. $\Delta\epsilon_{236}$ on hydrolysis 4900 (in 0.1 M-$PO_4$ buffer, pH 7) | General methods of preparation not applicable to malonyl-CoA, *JBC* **235**, 346 (1960). PREP. *JACS* **82**, 2972 (1962); *BZ* **335**, 540 (1962). Stability, *see* Acyl-CoA compds. |
| sl.s. EtOH; s. acet., benz., eth., hexane, light petroleum; i. $H_2O$. (Slightly less soluble than phylloquinone in the same solvents) | In pet. eth.:<br>$\lambda_{max}$ 243   248   261   270   325–8 nm<br>$\epsilon$   17850 18870 17050 17150 3100<br>In EtOH:<br>$\lambda_{max}$ 242   248   260   269   325 nm<br>$\epsilon$   17930 18940 17280 17440 3080<br>*Quinol* (reduced form) (in EtOH):<br>$\lambda_{max}$ 245   325 nm<br>$\epsilon_{245}$ increases on reduction | MK-6 and MK-7 are the principal naturally occurring menaquinones with vitamin-K activity, but menaquinones with $n = 1$ to $n = 13$ are found in various organisms. Stability similar to phylloquinone (vitamin $K_1$). Extremely sensitive to light. REVIEW. *Meth. Enzymol.* **18C**, 407 (1971). |
| s. $H_2O$ | In 0.1 M-HCl;<br>$\lambda_{max}$ 286   350 nm<br>$\epsilon$   12100   24900<br>$A_{348}/A_{305} = 2.45$<br>$\lambda_{max}$ ($\epsilon$): 360 nm (25 100) (pH 3)<br>352 nm (25 000) (pH 2)<br>286 (12 400) 345 nm (26 000) (M-HCl) | Solid and acid solns. stable in air. At pH 7 and above forms 10-formyltetrahydropteroylglutamic acid; rate at pH 7 varies with buffer, maleate (half-life 40 min) < tris (9.4 min) < $PO_4$ (6 min) < pyrophosphate (4.8 min). Natural isomer is dextrorotatory. PREP. (±), *Meth. Enzymol.* **6**, 806, 814 (1963); *Anal. Biochem.* **22**, 166 (1968); **103**, 255 (1980). (+), *BBA* **148**, 622 (1967). |

| Name | Synonyms | Formula | M. wt. | Physical properties |
|------|----------|---------|--------|---------------------|
| Methylcobalamin | Methyl-B$_{12}$; α-(5,6-Dimethylbenzimid-azolyl)methylcobamide | CH$_3$ replacing CN group in Cyanocobalamin | 1344.4 | deep red needles |
| 5,10-Methylene-tetrahydropteroyl-glutamic acid | 'Active formaldehyde'; 5,10-Methylenetetrahydrofolic acid | 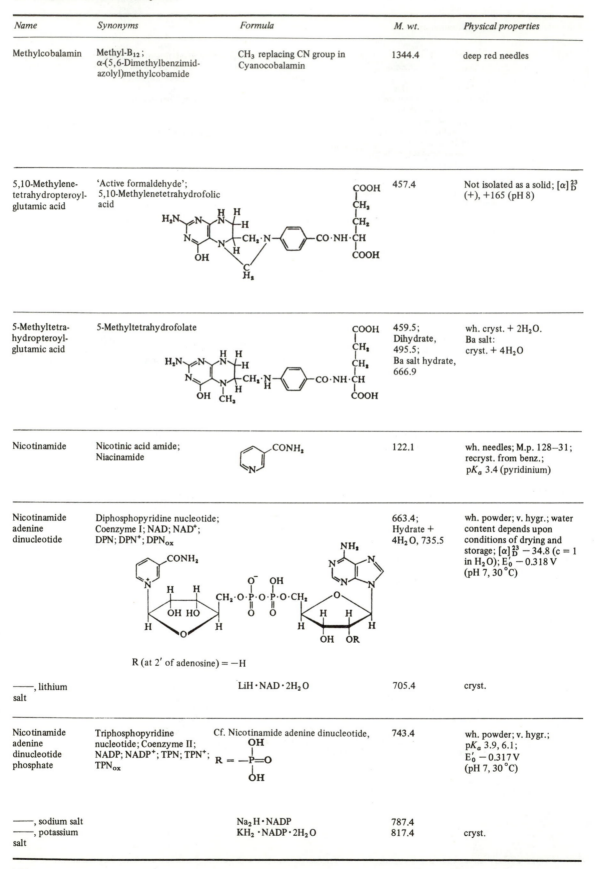 | 457.4 | Not isolated as a solid; $[\alpha]_D^{23}$ (+), +165 (pH 8) |
| 5-Methyltetra-hydropteroyl-glutamic acid | 5-Methyltetrahydrofolate | | 459.5; Dihydrate, 495.5; Ba salt hydrate, 666.9 | wh. cryst. + 2H$_2$O. Ba salt: cryst. + 4H$_2$O |
| Nicotinamide | Nicotinic acid amide; Niacinamide | | 122.1 | wh. needles; M.p. 128–31; recryst. from benz.; p$K_a$ 3.4 (pyridinium) |
| Nicotinamide adenine dinucleotide | Diphosphopyridine nucleotide; Coenzyme I; NAD; NAD$^+$; DPN; DPN$^+$; DPN$_{ox}$ | R (at 2′ of adenosine) = —H | 663.4; Hydrate + 4H$_2$O, 735.5 | wh. powder; v. hygr.; water content depends upon conditions of drying and storage; $[\alpha]_D^{23}$ −34.8 (c = 1 in H$_2$O); $E_0'$ −0.318 V (pH 7, 30 °C) |
| ——, lithium salt | | LiH·NAD·2H$_2$O | 705.4 | cryst. |
| Nicotinamide adenine dinucleotide phosphate | Triphosphopyridine nucleotide; Coenzyme II; NADP; NADP$^+$; TPN; TPN$^+$; TPN$_{ox}$ | Cf. Nicotinamide adenine dinucleotide, R = —P=O (OH)(OH) | 743.4 | wh. powder; v. hygr.; p$K_a$ 3.9, 6.1; $E_0'$ −0.317 V (pH 7, 30 °C) |
| ——, sodium salt | | Na$_2$H·NADP | 787.4 | |
| ——, potassium salt | | KH$_2$·NADP·2H$_2$O | 817.4 | cryst. |

| Solubility | Absorption spectrum | General Remarks |
|---|---|---|
| s. $H_2O$; i. acet., eth., $CHCl_3$ | In 0.1 M-HCl:<br>$\lambda_{max}$  265  284  304  380<br>458 nm<br>$\epsilon$  40 400  22 600  21 600  8000<br>9200<br>At pH 7.0:<br>$\lambda_{max}$  264  314  340  374<br>520 nm<br>$\epsilon$  18 200  12 100  12 800  10 700<br>8600 | Rapidly photolysed yielding aquacobalamin under aerobic conditions; photolysis relatively slow in absence of $O_2$, rate enhanced by thiols, EtOH. Relatively stable in acid and alkali. Does not form dicyanocobalamin with alk. cyanide. PREP. *Biochem. Preps.* **12**, 129 (1968). |
| s. $H_2O$ | At pH 7.0:<br>$\lambda_{max}$ 294 nm<br>$\epsilon$ 32 000 (also reported as 25 000)<br>$\epsilon_{340}$ 1010 | Rapidly formed by mixing excess HCHO and tetrahydropteroylglutamic acid at mildly alkaline pH (7.5–9.5). Stable in air at pH 9.5 in the cold for several days. At neutral or acid pH dissociates into HCHO and tetrahydropteroylglutamic acid; at pH 7 dissociation essentially complete in 15 min. Stable in presence of excess HCHO and mercaptoethanol or ascorbic acid. Association constant (HCHO + tetrahydropteroylglutamic acid) at 22 °C: pH 4.3, $1.3 \times 10^4$ $M^{-1}$; pH 7.2, $2.1 \times 10^4$ $M^{-1}$. Enzymically active form is (+)-L-compound. PREP. *Meth. Enzymol.* **6**, 806 (1963); **66**, 439 (1980); see also *BJ* **74**, 71 (1960); *JBC* **241**, 5851 (1966). |
| s. $H_2O$ | At pH 7.0, $\lambda_{max}$ 290 nm $\epsilon$ 31 700;<br>$A_{290}/A_{245} = 3.8$<br>In 0.1 M-HCl:<br>$\lambda_{max}$  270  294 nm<br>$\epsilon$  21 000  20 000 | Decomp. slowly in air at room temp., forming 5-methyldihydropteroylglutamic acid, $\lambda_{max}$ 249 and 290 nm. Decomp. accelerated by heavy metal ions. Solid stable under anhyd. conditions and in the dark for at least 5 yr at −80 °C and for 6 months at 4 °C. Ba salt stable indefinitely at −20 °C if anhyd. Natural isomer is (+)-L-. PREP. (±), *BJ* **105**, 633 (1967); *Anal. Biochem.* **34**, 376 (1970); *ABB* **120**, 712 (1967). (+), *Anal. Biochem.* **43**, 162 (1971), **83**, 615 (1977). |
| 100 $H_2O$;<br>66 EtOH; s. acet., $CHCl_3$; sl. s. benz., eth. | In $H_2O$:<br>$\lambda_{max}$ 261.5 nm<br>$\epsilon$ varies with pH<br>*J. Phys. Colloid Chem.* **55**, 173 (1951) | Stable as dry solid below 50 °C. In neutral aq. soln. may be autoclaved at 120 °C for 20 min but is hydrolysed to nicotinic acid in acid and alkaline solution. |
| v.s. $H_2O$; i. eth. | At pH 7:<br>$\lambda_{max}$  260 nm<br>$\epsilon$  18 000<br>$\lambda_{min}$  230 nm<br>$\epsilon$  8000<br>Cyanide adduct at pH 10:<br>$\lambda_{max}$  327 nm<br>$\epsilon$  5900 | Solid stable in desiccator at 0 °C or R.T. Neutral or sl. acid (pH between 3 and 7) soln. stable at 0 °C for at least 2 weeks. Solns. decomp. rapidly on heating. V. labile in alk. soln., decomp. accelerated by phosphate, maleate, and carbonate. Stability, see *JBC* **236**, 2756 (1961). Destroyed by u.v. light. Only β-form is enzymically active. |
| s. $H_2O$; v. sl. s. EtOH; i. eth. | At pH 7:<br>$\lambda_{max}$  260 nm<br>$\epsilon$  18 000<br>$\lambda_{min}$  231 nm<br>$\epsilon$  8100<br>Cyanide adduct at pH 10:<br>$\lambda_{max}$  327 nm<br>$\epsilon$  5900 | Solid stable over desiccant at 0 °C or R.T. Soln. of free acid stable many weeks in cold. Stability generally similar to nicotinamide adenine dinucleotide but less stable in strong acid or dil. alk. See *JBC* **236**, 2756 (1961). |

# 6 Vitamins and coenzymes

| Name | Synonyms | Formula | M. wt. | Physical properties |
|------|----------|---------|--------|---------------------|
| Nicotinamide mononucleotide | Nicotinamide ribotide; NMN | | 334.2 | $[\alpha]_D -38.3$ (c = 1 in $H_2O$) |
| Nicotinic acid | Niacin; 3-Pyridinecarboxylic acid; Pellagra — preventive factor | | 123.1 | wh. needles; melts 236—7 then sublimes; $pK_a$ 4.76 |
| Pantetheine | *Lactobacillus bulgaricus* factor; N-(Pantothenyl)-β-aminoethanethiol | | 278.4 | hygr. oil or resin; $[\alpha]_D^{20}$ +12.9 (c = 4.5 in $H_2O$) |
| Pantothenic acid | D-(+)-N-(α,γ-Dihydroxy-β,β-dimethylbutyryl)-β-alanine | | 219.2 | hygr. viscous oil; $[\alpha]_D^{25}$ +37.5 (in $H_2O$); $pK_a$ 4.4 |
| ——, Ca salt | | $(C_9H_{16}NO_5)_2 \cdot Ca$ | 476.5 | wh. cryst.; moderately hygr.; M.p. 196 d.; $[\alpha]_D^{25}$ + 28.2 (c = 5 in $H_2O$) |
| Phylloquinone | Vitamin $K_1$; 2-Methyl-3-phytyl-1,4-naphthoquinone | | 450.7 | yel. viscous oil; M.p. — 20 |
| Plastoquinone | Plastoquinone-n; PQ-n; Plastoquinone-5n. E.g. for n = 9: Plastoquinone-9; PQ-9; Plastoquinone-45; Plastoquinone A. | | PQ-9; 749.2; PQ-10, 817.3 | yellow cryst.; M.p. PQ-9, 48—9 PQ-10, 50—1 |

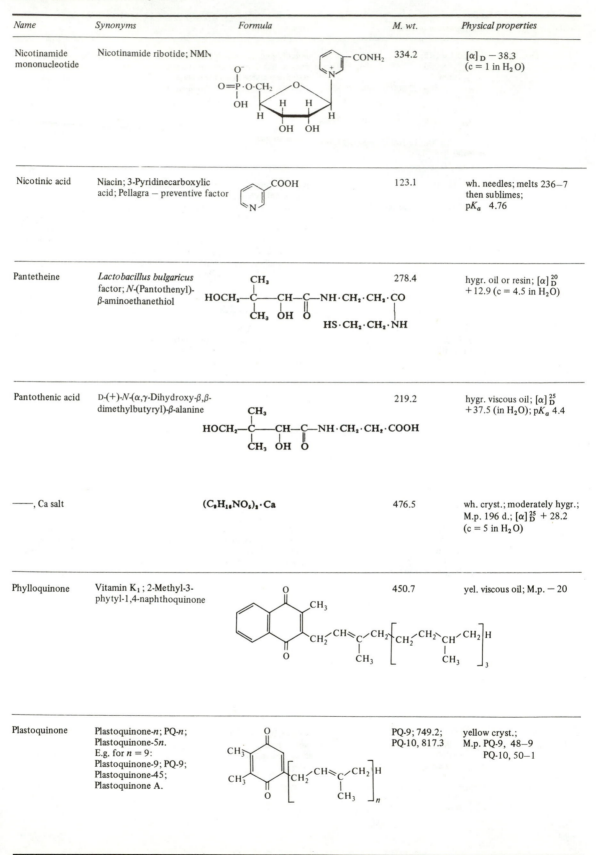

| Solubility | Absorption spectrum | General Remarks |
|---|---|---|
| s. $H_2O$; i. acet. | At pH 7.0:<br>$\lambda_{max}$ 266 nm<br>$\epsilon$ 4600<br>$\lambda_{min}$ 249 nm<br>$\epsilon$ 3600<br>Cyanide adduct:<br>$\lambda_{max}$ 325 nm<br>$\epsilon$ 6200 | Resembles NAD in reaction with cyanide. Store frozen in soln. rather than as solid. PREP. *Meth. Enzymol.* **3**, 900 (1957), **66**, 62, 71 (1980); *FEBS Lett.* **15**, 277 (1971). |
| $1.7^{20}$, $v.s.^{100}$ $H_2O$;<br>s. EtOH, alkalis;<br>sl. s. benz., eth. | In $H_2O$:<br>$\lambda_{max}$ 261.5 nm<br>$\epsilon$ varies with pH, *J. Phys. Colloid Chem.* **53**, 414 (1949) | Very stable in air. Solid nonhygroscopic. Soln. in $H_2O$ stable to autoclaving at 120 °C for 20 min. Stable in acid and alkaline solution. |
| s. $H_2O$, EtOH, eth. | | Readily oxidized to the disulphide, pantethine, $[\alpha]_D^{27}$ + 13.5 (c = 3.75 in $H_2O$); s. $H_2O$, sl. s. EtOH, i. eth., acet. Store as pantethine and regenerate pantetheine by reduction with $Na_2S$ or cysteine. S-Benzoylpantetheine, cryst., M.p. 116, $[\alpha]_D^{27}$ + 31 (in $H_2O$), s. $H_2O$, full growth promoting activity, stable in neutral aq. soln. but hydrolyses rapidly in alk. to pantetheine and benzoate. |
| v.s. $H_2O$, EtOH,<br>gl. acetic; s. eth., acet.;<br>i. benz., $CHCl_3$ | | Stable in neutral soln. Rapidly destroyed by acid, alk. or heat. |
| 14.5 $H_2O$; sl. s. EtOH,<br>acet. | | Reasonably stable in light and air. Soln. most stable at pH 5–7; not stable to autoclaving. |
| s. EtOH, acet., benz.,<br>eth., light petroleum;<br>i. $H_2O$ | In pet. eth.:<br>$\lambda_{max}$ 242 248 260 269 325 nm<br>$\epsilon$ 17850 18880 17260 17440 3065<br>Reduced form – quinol (in EtOH):<br>$\lambda_{max}$ 245 325 nm<br>$\epsilon_{245}$ increases on reduction. | Moderately stable to air, moisture and heat. Rapidly decomposed by visible and u.v. light. Unaffected by dil. acids but destroyed by alkali. Reduced to quinol by $NaBH_4$ or dithionite. |
| s. EtOH, eth., pet.<br>eth.; i. $H_2O$ | In EtOH: $\lambda_{max}$ 255 nm $\epsilon$ 15 200.<br>In pet. eth.: $\lambda_{max}$ 254 261 nm<br>$\epsilon$ 18 900<br>Quinol (in EtOH): $\lambda_{max}$ 290 nm $\epsilon$ 3450 | Plastoquinones with $n$ = 3, 4, 9, and 10 found naturally. Unstable in oxygen and light. REVIEW. *Meth. Enzymol.* **23**, 372 (1971). |

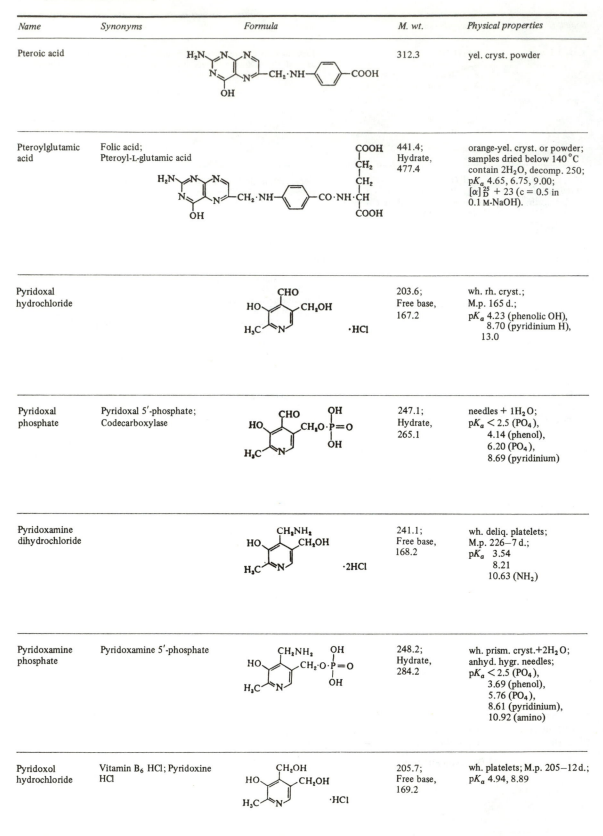

| Name | Synonyms | Formula | M. wt. | Physical properties |
|------|----------|---------|--------|---------------------|
| Pteroic acid | | | 312.3 | yel. cryst. powder |
| Pteroylglutamic acid | Folic acid; Pteroyl-L-glutamic acid | | 441.4; Hydrate, 477.4 | orange-yel. cryst. or powder; samples dried below 140 °C contain $2H_2O$, decomp. 250; $pK_a$ 4.65, 6.75, 9.00; $[\alpha]_D^{25}$ + 23 (c = 0.5 in 0.1 M-NaOH). |
| Pyridoxal hydrochloride | | | 203.6; Free base, 167.2 | wh. rh. cryst.; M.p. 165 d.; $pK_a$ 4.23 (phenolic OH), 8.70 (pyridinium H), 13.0 |
| Pyridoxal phosphate | Pyridoxal 5'-phosphate; Codecarboxylase | | 247.1; Hydrate, 265.1 | needles + $1H_2O$; $pK_a$ < 2.5 ($PO_4$), 4.14 (phenol), 6.20 ($PO_4$), 8.69 (pyridinium) |
| Pyridoxamine dihydrochloride | | | 241.1; Free base, 168.2 | wh. deliq. platelets; M.p. 226–7 d.; $pK_a$ 3.54 8.21 10.63 ($NH_2$) |
| Pyridoxamine phosphate | Pyridoxamine 5'-phosphate | | 248.2; Hydrate, 284.2 | wh. prism. cryst.+$2H_2O$; anhyd. hygr. needles; $pK_a$ < 2.5 ($PO_4$), 3.69 (phenol), 5.76 ($PO_4$), 8.61 (pyridinium), 10.92 (amino) |
| Pyridoxol hydrochloride | Vitamin $B_6$ HCl; Pyridoxine HCl | | 205.7; Free base, 169.2 | wh. platelets; M.p. 205–12 d.; $pK_a$ 4.94, 8.89 |

| Solubility | Absorption spectrum | General Remarks |
|---|---|---|
| sl. s. aq. NaOH, $Na_2CO_3$, $NaHCO_3$; i. dil. acids | At pH 7.0: $\lambda_{max}$ 280 350 nm $\epsilon$ 27 800 7180 In 0.1 M-NaOH: $\lambda_{max}$ 255 275 365 nm $\epsilon$ 26 300 23 400 8900 | Growth factor activity only for *Streptococcus faecalis* and other Enterococci. PREP. *Anal. Biochem.* **46**, 1 (1972); *J. Org. Chem.* **36**, 860 (1971). |
| Acid: $0.001^0$, $0.05^{100}$ $H_2O$; s. alkalis; i. $H_2O$ below pH 5; sl. s. gl. acetic, MeOH; v. sl. s. EtOH; i. most organic solvents. $Na_2$ salt: $1.5^0 H_2O$ | At pH 7.0: $\lambda_{max}$ 282 350 nm $\epsilon$ 27 000 7000 At pH 13: $\lambda_{max}$ 256 283 365 nm $\epsilon$ 26 900 25 100 9260 | Photolabile; inactivated by u.v. irradiation. Solid stable in dark. Alk. soln. reasonably stable in the dark. Destroyed by heat in acid or alk. soln. REVIEW. Blakley, *The biochemistry of folic acid and related pteridines*, North-Holland (1969). Naturally occurring folic acid compds. are frequently derivs. of pteroylpolyglutamates, commonly containing 2–7 γ-glutamyl residues. The polyglutamyl compds. have similar properties (e.g. solubility, spectrum) to the corresponding monoglutamyl compd. PREP. of pteroylpolyglutamates, *Meth. Enzymol.* **66**, 523 (1980); *JBC* **247**, 2266 (1972); *Vitams Horm.* **40**, 45 (1983). |
| 50 $H_2O$; 1.7 95% EtOH | At pH 7.0: $\lambda_{max}$ 252 318 nm $\epsilon$ .. 8200 In 0.1M-NaOH: $\lambda_{max}$ 300 393 nm $\epsilon$ 5800 1700 *JACS* **76**, 169 (1954) | Photolabile in soln. at neutral and particularly alk. pH. Solid and acid soln. relatively photostable. Neutral and acid solns. (up to 2.5M-$H_2SO_4$ or HCl) stable in heat, some destruction in hot strong alk. Forms Schiff bases with amines. |
| s. $H_2O$; sl. s. MeOH; v. sl. s. EtOH; i. $CHCl_3$, acet., benz. | In 0.05M-$PO_4$, pH 7.0: $\lambda_{max}$ 330 388 nm $\epsilon$ 2500 4900 In 0.1M-NaOH: $\lambda_{max}$ 305 388 nm $\epsilon$ 1100 6550 *JACS* **76**, 169 (1954) | Stable in aqueous soln. in the cold and dark, 2–3% decomposed in 3 weeks at $0°C$, only sl. greater decomp. at R.T. even in 1M-HCl or NaOH. Hydrolysed by 3 hr autoclaving at $126°C$ in 0.027M-$H_2SO_4$. Photolabile as solid and in soln. particularly at alk. pH. Forms Schiff bases with amines. Normal coenzyme form of Vitamin $B_6$. |
| 50 $H_2O$; 0.65 95% EtOH | At pH 7.0: $\lambda_{max}$ 253 325 nm $\epsilon$ 4600 7700 In 0.1M-NaOH: $\lambda_{max}$ 245 308 nm $\epsilon$ 5900 7300 *JACS* **76**, 169 (1954) | Photolabile in soln., particularly at alk. pH. Neutral, acid and alk. solns. stable to heat. |
| s. $H_2O$ | At pH 7.2: $\lambda_{max}$ 254 327 nm $\epsilon$ 5200 9400 At pH 10.0: $\lambda_{max}$ 244 312 nm $\epsilon$ 7500 8300 *JACS* **76**, 169 (1954) | Aq. solns. stable in the dark. Negligible hydrolysis in dark at room temp. or below in 3 weeks in 1M-NaOH or HCl. Complete hydrolysis by 3 hr autoclaving at $126°C$ in 0.027M-$H_2SO_4$. Photolabile in soln. particularly at alk. pH. |
| 22 $H_2O$; 1.1 EtOH; sl. s. acet.; i. eth. | At pH 6.8: $\lambda_{max}$ 254 324 nm $\epsilon$ 3700 7100 In 0.1M-NaOH: $\lambda_{max}$ 245 308 nm $\epsilon$ 6500 7000 *JACS* **76**, 169 (1954) | Cryst. stable in light, but neutral and especially alk. solns. somewhat photolabile. Sterilized by autoclaving in soln. of pH 5 or below. |

| Name | Synonyms | Formula | M. wt. | Physical properties |
|---|---|---|---|---|
| Pyrroloquinoline quinone | PQQ: Methoxatin; 2,7,9-Tricarboxy-1$H$-pyrrolo [2,3-$f$]-quinoline-4,5-dione | | 330.2 | deep red solid; $pK_a \sim 2.5$; $E_0' + 0.090$ V (pH 7.0) |
| Retinal (all-*trans*) | Retinene; Retinaldehyde; Vitamin A$_1$ aldehyde | | 284.4 | orange cryst.; M.p. 61–4 |
| Retinoic acid (all-*trans*) | Vitamin A$_1$ acid | | 300.4 | yel. needles; M.p. 179–80 |
| Retinol (all-*trans*) | Vitamin A$_1$; Axerophthol | | 286.5 | yel. prisms; M.p. 64 |
| Riboflavin | Vitamin B$_2$; Lactoflavin | | 376.4 | yel. needles; decomp. approx. 280 d.; $[\alpha]_D^{21} - 117$ (c = 0.5 in 0.1M-NaOH) strongly conc. dependent; $E_0' - 0.208$ V (pH 7, 30 °C); $pK_a$ 9.69 |
| Succinyl coenzyme A | Succinyl-CoA; Succinyl-S-CoA | Cf. Coenzyme A, —SH replaced by —S·CO·CH$_2$·CH$_2$·COOH | 867.6 | |

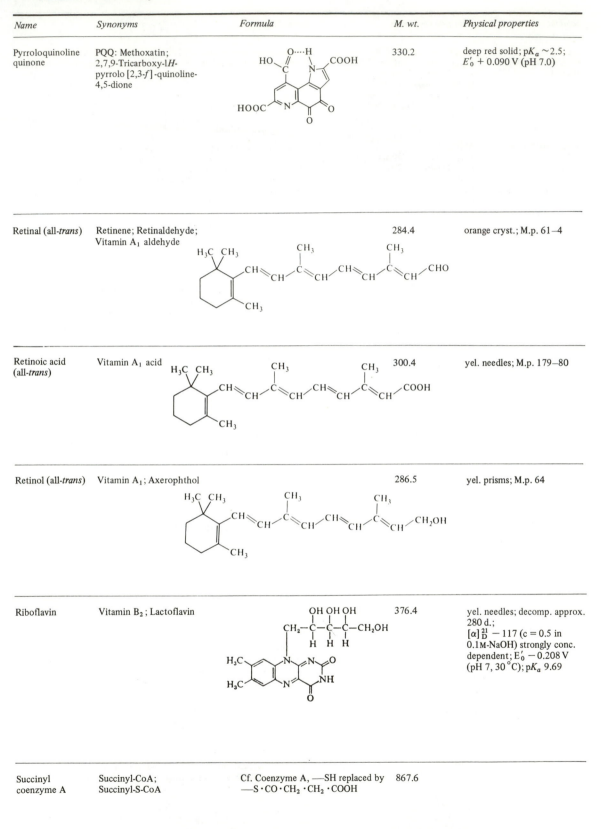

| Solubility | Absorption spectrum | General Remarks |
|---|---|---|
| s. $H_2O$; sl. s. MeOH; i. EtOH, eth., acet., $CHCl_3$ | In 0.05M-$KPO_4$, pH 7: $\lambda_{max}$ 249    275 (shoulder)    330 nm $\epsilon_{249}$ 18 400 Isosbestic points, pH 5–9: 233      259      322 nm $\epsilon$ 14 400    16 040    8960 Fluorescence at pH 7, excitation max. 225 and 365 nm, emission max. 470 nm. Intensity of absorbance and fluorescence affected by temp., EJB **125**, 69 (1982) | Prosthetic group of methanol, glucose and other dehydrogenases in bacteria. Forms fluorescent adducts at C−5 with $H_2O$ (adduct is responsible for fluorescence of PQQ), MeOH, aldehydes, $NH_3$, amines. Reduction with phenylhydrazine in 2M-HCl, $H_2$ + $PtO_2$ at pH 7 or mercaptoethanol at pH 9 forms the 4,5-quinol, $PQQH_2$; with mercapto-ethanol at pH 13 the semiquinone ($PQQH^{\cdot}$) is formed; $NaBH_4$ yields the 4,5-dihydroquinol ($PQQH_4$). PREP. Isolation, BJ **187**, 221 (1980); Synthesis, JACS **103**, 5599 (1981). EST. Anal. Biochem. **133**, 239 (1983). Semiquinone: Stable at pH 13; $\lambda_{max}$ 458 nm at pH 13. Quinol: Relatively resistant to autoxidation at low pH, rapidly oxidized at neutral or alkaline pH; $\lambda_{max}$ 302 nm $\epsilon$ 25050 at pH 7; non-fluorescent; PREP. EJB **118**, 395 (1981). REVIEW. TIBS **6**, 278 (1981). |
| s. MeOH, EtOH, $CHCl_3$, eth., cyclohexane; i. $H_2O$ | In EtOH: $\lambda_{max}$ 381 nm, $\epsilon$ 43 500 $SbCl_3$ complex in $CHCl_3$: $\lambda_{max}$ 664 nm, $A_{1cm}^{1\%}$ 3400 | Unstable in air and acid; less stable than retinol. Partially isomerized to cis-isomers by exposure to light. 11-cis-Retinal is a component of rhodopsin. PREP. BJ **42**, 516 (1948); Meth. Enzymol. **18C**, 641 (1971). |
| s. MeOH, EtOH, $CHCl_3$, eth., cyclohexane; i. $H_2O$ | In EtOH: $\lambda_{max}$ 350 nm, $\epsilon$ 45 400 $SbCl_3$ complex in $CHCl_3$: $\lambda_{max}$ 574 nm | Stability similar to retinol; unstable in air, acid and u.v. light. PREP. BJ **113**, 447 (1969). |
| s. MeOH, EtOH, $CHCl_3$, eth., cyclohexane; i. $H_2O$ | In EtOH: $\lambda_{max}$ 325 nm, $\epsilon$ 52 480 $SbCl_3$ complex in $CHCl_3$: $\lambda_{max}$ 620 nm, $A_{1cm}^{1\%}$ 4800 | Destroyed by u.v. light. Readily oxidized in air; stabilize by dissolving in oil, by addition of anti-oxidant such as α-tocopherol or hydroquinone, or by conversion to acetate or palmitate. Stable in alkali, unstable in acid. |
| $0.01^{25}$, $0.23^{100}$ $H_2O$; 0.0045 EtOH; v.s. dil. alk. with decomp., conc. HCl; s. gl. acetic, phenol; i. eth., $CHCl_3$, acet., benz. | In 0.1M-$PO_4$, pH 7: $\lambda_{max}$    266      373      445 nm $\epsilon$      32 500    10 600    12 500 $\lambda_{ref}$    260      375      450 nm $\epsilon$    27 700    10 600    12 200 Fluorescence max., 525–30 nm Maximal fluorescence in pH range 3.5–7.5 Dihydro compd., $\epsilon_{450}$  780 | Dry solid stable to diffuse light. Highly photolabile in soln. especially in alk. Neutral and acid aq. solns. stable in dark, 3% decomp. per month at 27 °C and pH 6; may be sterilized by autoclaving. Rapidly destroyed in alk. soln. Stable to mild oxidizing agents, including $O_2$. Reduced by dithionite, Na amalgam, Zn+acid or $H_2$+catalyst to colourless dihydro compd., which is v. readily autoxidizable. |
| s. $H_2O$ | See Acyl-CoA compds. $\Delta\epsilon_{232}$ on hydrolysis 4500 | Unstable at neutral pH at room temp., half-life 1–2 hr in bicarbonate buffer pH 7.5, slower decomp. in $PO_4$ buffer. Hydrolysis v. rapid if heated, complete hydrolysis in 1–2 min at 100 °C. Neutral soln. may be stored at −15 °C with negligible decomp. Stable at pH 1. PREP. Biochem. Preps. **5**, 30 (1957). See also Acyl-CoA compds. |

| Name | Synonyms | Formula | M. wt. | Physical properties |
|------|----------|---------|--------|---------------------|
| Tetrahydro-pteroylglutamic acid | 5,6,7,8-Tetrahydropteroyl-glutamic acid; Tetrahydro-folic acid; THFA; THF | | 445.4; + 2 Acetic acid, 565.4 | fluffy wh. powder, becoming darker due to degradation; when prepd. from acetic acid contains $2CH_3 \cdot COOH$; $E_0'$ $-0.19$ V (for DHFA/THFA); $pK_a$ 3.5 (COOH), 4.8 (COOH), 4.8 ($N^5$), 10.5 ($N^3$); $[\alpha]_D^{27}$ ($\pm$), $+14.9$ (in 0.1 M-NaOH), ($-$), $-16.9$ (in 0.1 M-NaOH). |
| Thiamin chloride hydrochloride | Thiamin hydrochloride; Vitamin $B_1 \cdot HCl$; Aneurin $\cdot$ HCl | | 337.3; Hydrate, 355.3 | monocl. plates; hygr., usually $+\frac{1}{2}$ or $1H_2O$; yeast-like odour; M.p. 247–8 d; $pK_a$ 4.8, 9.2 |
| Thiamin pyrophosphate | Diphosphothiamin; Cocarboxylase; TPP | | Free cation, 425.3; Chloride, 460.8; Hydrate, 478.8 | Chloride, cryst.$+ 1H_2O$ from EtOH; M.p. 240–4 d.; $pK_a$ 5.0 |
| Tocopherol | Vitamin E. α-Tocopherol: 5, 7, 8-Trimethyltocol. β-Tocopherol: 5, 8-Dimethyltocol. γ-Tocopherol: 7, 8-Dimethyltocol. δ-Tocopherol: 8-Methyltocol | | α: 430.7 β: 416.7 γ: 416.7 δ: 402.7 | pale yellow oils; M.p. α, 2.5 to 3.5 γ, $-3$ to $-2$; optical activity weakly *dextro* in EtOH, sign of rotation may depend on solvent. |
| Ubiquinone | Ubiquinone-*n*; Q-*n*; Coenzyme $Q_n$; $CoQ_n$ Ubiquinone-5*n*. E.g. for *n* = 10: Ubiquinone-10; Q-10; Coenzyme $Q_{10}$; $CoQ_{10}$; Ubiquinone-50 | | Q-6, 590.9; Q-7, 659.0; Q-8, 727.1; Q-9, 795.3; Q-10, 863.4 | orange cryst.; M.p. Q-6, 19–20, Q-7, 31–2, Q-8, 37–8, Q-9, 44–5, Q-10, 49 |

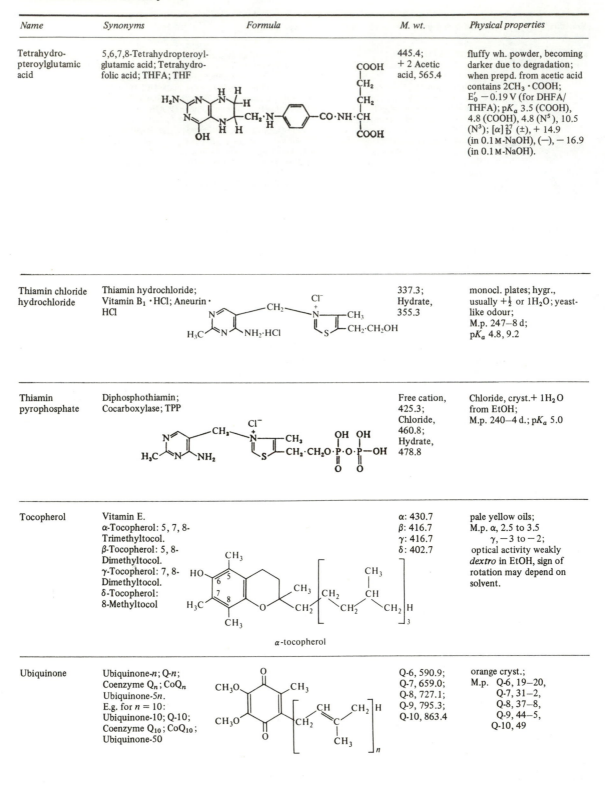

α-tocopherol

| Solubility | Absorption spectrum | General Remarks |
|---|---|---|

s. $H_2O$, gl. acetic; i. eth.

At pH 7: $\lambda_{max}$ 297 nm $\epsilon$ 29 100
pH 11: $\lambda_{max}$ 290 nm $\epsilon$ 21 600
pH 3: $\lambda_{max}$    270        290 nm
     $\epsilon$    25 400    22 800
On decomp. $\lambda_{max}$ shifts to 282 nm due to formation of dihydropteroyl-glutamic acid.

Solid slowly oxidizes in air, becoming darker in colour. Storage in vacuum or inert atmosphere, in the dark and cold under anhyd. conditions, greatly slows but does not entirely halt decomp. Rapidly oxidized in soln. to dihydropteroylglutamic acid; further decomp. occurs more slowly, causing colouration of soln. Decomp. catalysed by light, acid, base and heavy metal ions (Cu, Fe). Most stable at pH 5–6. Stability affected by buffer; most stable in veronal, tris, triethanolamine, least stable in phosphate or maleate. Solns. stabilized by ascorbate or mercaptoethanol or by bubbling with $N_2$ or Ar. Half-life without stabilizer in phosphate buffer pH 7.5, 200 min at 0 °C, 40 min at 23 °C. Solns. containing ascorbate or mercaptoethanol stable for months at −20 °C, hours at 0 °C, 1–2 hr at 23 °C, up to 15 min in tris buffer at 100 °C. Solns. can be kept for months without significant degradation in 0.2 M-mercaptoethanol at pH 7 and 4 °C under vacuum or (without mercaptoethanol) in $10^{-3}$ M-EDTA, pH 5–6, in inert atmosphere and frozen. Natural isomer is (−)-L-. PREP. (±), *BJ* **65**, 331 (1957); *Biochem. Preps.* **7**, 89 (1960); *Meth. Enzymol.* **6**, 802 (1963); **18B**, 728 (1971); **66**, 519 (1980); *Biochem.* **5**, 303 (1964); *BBRC* **4**, 180 (1961); *Anal. Biochem.* **103**, 255 (1980). (−), *Meth. Enzymol.* **6**, 805 (1963); *JBC* **249**, 4100 (1972).

---

100 $H_2O$; 0.35 EtOH; s. MeOH; i. eth., benz., $CHCl_3$

In $H_2O$:
At pH 7 and above:
$\lambda_{max}$    235        267 nm
$\epsilon$    11 300      8300
At pH 5.5 and below:
$\lambda_{max}$    247 nm
$\epsilon$    14 200

Commercial samples contain about 4% $H_2O$ removable at 100 °C. Dry solid stable in air. Soln. at pH 3.5 stable at 120 °C. Solns. above pH 5 unstable, especially to heat, above pH 7 unstable on standing at room temp. Unstable to reducing and oxidizing agents. Solutions acid.

---

s. $H_2O$

At pH 1–3:
$\lambda_{max}$ 247 nm $\epsilon$ 13 000
In $PO_4$ buffer pH 8:
$\lambda_{max}$    233        267 nm
$\epsilon$    10 800      7800
$\lambda_{min}$ 248 nm
Isosbestic point (pH 2–8), 272.5 nm

Solid stable when dry. Solns. somewhat less stable than thiamin chloride hydrochloride. REVIEW: *Ann. N.Y. Acad. Sci.* **98**, 383 et seq. (1962).

---

s. acet., EtOH, $CHCl_3$, eth., oils; i. $H_2O$.

In EtOH:
$\alpha$, $\lambda_{max}$ 292 nm $\epsilon$ 3260
$\beta$, $\lambda_{max}$ 296 nm $\epsilon$ 3720
$\gamma$, $\lambda_{max}$ 298 nm $\epsilon$ 3810
$\delta$, $\lambda_{max}$ 298 nm $\epsilon$ 3510
Strong fluorescence, excitation max. 295 nm, emission max. 340 nm.

Slowly oxidized by air, rapidly in the presence of alkali or on heating. In absence of $O_2$, stable to heat up to ~200 °C and to alkali. Not affected by acids up to 100 °C. Darken gradually on exposure to light, sensitive to u.v. Active as anti-oxidants; $\delta$-tocopherol is the most potent anti-oxidant of the group. Esters, e.g. acetate, allophanate, *p*-nitrophenyl-urethane, are much more stable to light and $O_2$ than free tocopherols. $\alpha$-*Tocopheryl acetate*; yel. cryst., M.p. 28, $\lambda_{max}$ 284 nm $\epsilon$ 2050. The corresponding tocotrienols, with $-CH_2 \cdot CH = C(CH_3) \cdot CH_2-$ units in the side chains, are also found in natural sources; spectra similar to the corresponding tocopherol.

---

s. EtOH, eth., hexane, pet. eth., cyclohexane; i. $H_2O$

All homologues:
In EtOH: $\lambda_{max}$ 275    405 nm
         $\lambda_{min}$ 236 nm
Quinol, $\lambda_{max}$ 290 nm
In pet. eth.: $\lambda_{max}$ 270 nm
In hexane: $\lambda_{max}$ 272 nm
$\epsilon$ values:

| | 270 nm (pet. eth.) | 275 nm (EtOH) | $\Delta\epsilon_{ox-red}$ (275 nm in EtOH) |
|---|---|---|---|
| Q-6 | 15 370 | 14 900 | 12 400 |
| Q-7 | 15 090 | 14 800 | 12 600 |
| Q-8 | 14 980 | 14 900 | 12 700 |
| Q-9 | 14 870 | 14 700 | 12 500 |
| Q-10 | 15 190 | 14 600 | 12 500 |

Slowly destroyed by oxygen, u.v. light or sunlight. Rapidly oxidized in alkali, but stable to alkali in presence of pyrogallol to remove oxygen. Reduced by dithionite, borohydride or Zn + acid to quinol, which is slowly reoxidized by air. REVIEWS. *Vitams Horm.* **24**, 291 et seq. (1966); *Meth. Enzymol.* **18C**, 137 (1971), **53**, 591 (1978).

# 7 Carbohydrates and related compounds

## Nomenclature

Rules of carbohydrate nomenclature are reported in *BJ* **125**, 673 (1971); *EJB* **21**, 455 (1971); *BBA* **244**, 223 (1971); *JBC* **247**, 613 (1971).

The configuration of a monosaccharide (designated by the letters D- and L-) is decided by the configuration of the highest numbered asymmetric carbon atom and is related to the configuration of glyceraldehyde, which is known. D-Glyceraldehyde has the same absolute configuration as D-serine and D-lactic acid.

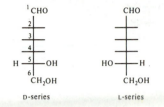

The relationship between the Fischer projection formula for the open-chain form of a sugar and the Haworth representation of the ring form is shown below for the example of D-glucose and its pyranose ring form.

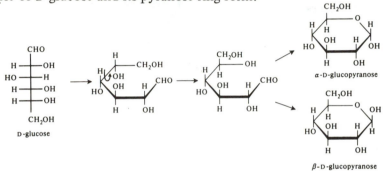

## Reference works

W. W. Pigman and D. Horton (eds.), *The carbohydrates: chemistry and biochemistry*, 2nd edition, Academic Press, vols. IA (1972), IB (1980), IIA (1970), and IIB (1970).

R. L. Whistler and others (eds.), *Methods in carbohydrate chemistry*, Academic Press, vols. 1–5 (1962–5), 6 (1972), 7 (1976) and 8 (1980).

S. Coffey (ed.), *Rodd's Chemistry of carbon compounds*, 2nd edition, Elsevier, vol. 1F (1967), Supplement 1FG (1983).

Tollens and Elsner, *Kurzes Handbuch der Kohlenhydrate*, J. A. Barth Verlag, Leipzig (1935).

F. J. Bates *et al.*, *Polarimetry, Saccharimetry, and the Sugars*, U.S. Department of Commerce, National Bureau of Standards, Washington, D.C. (1942).

*Beilstein's Handbuch der Organischen Chemie*, vol. 31, Springer, Berlin (1938).

*Advances in Carbohydrate Chemistry and Biochemistry* (until 1968, *Advances in Carbohydrate Chemistry*), Academic Press, published annually, vol. 1 (1945), 41 (1983).

## Abbreviations

The sign → is used to signify mutarotation.

*Meth. Carbohydr. Chem.* refers to R. L. Whistler and others (eds.), *Methods in Carbohydrate Chemistry*, Academic Press, vols. 1–8 (1962–80).

| Name | Synonyms | Formula | M. wt. |
|------|----------|---------|--------|

**TETROSES AND RELATED SUBSTANCES**

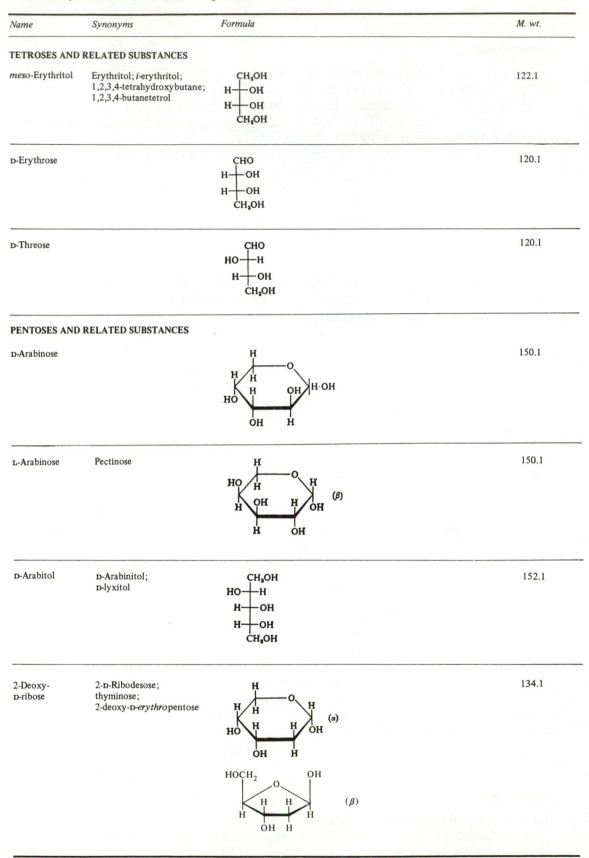

*meso*-Erythritol — Erythritol; *i*-erythritol; 1,2,3,4-tetrahydroxybutane; 1,2,3,4-butanetetrol — 122.1

D-Erythrose — — 120.1

D-Threose — — 120.1

**PENTOSES AND RELATED SUBSTANCES**

D-Arabinose — — 150.1

L-Arabinose — Pectinose — (β) 150.1

D-Arabitol — D-Arabinitol; D-lyxitol — 152.1

2-Deoxy-D-ribose — 2-D-Ribodesose; thyminose; 2-deoxy-D-*erythro*pentose — (α) (β) 134.1

| Physical properties | Solubility | General Remarks |
|---|---|---|
| wh. prisms; M.p. 126; optically inactive | v.s. $H_2O$; s. hot EtOH; sl. s. cold EtOH, pyr.; i. eth. | Non-reducing. Sweet taste (2 × sucrose). |
| col. syrup; $[\alpha]_D - 15.9 \rightarrow -23.1$ (c = 1.9 in $H_2O$) | s. $H_2O$, MeOH, EtOH | Reduces Fehling's soln. slowly in the cold. Not fermented by yeasts. PREP. *JCS* **1955**, 1212; *JACS* **81**, 2838 (1959); *Can. J. Chem.* **33**, 1216 (1955); *Meth. Carbohydr. Chem.* **1**, 64 (1962). |
| v. hygr. col. needles; M.p. 126–32; $[\alpha]_D^{27} - 12.9$ (c = 2.3 in $H_2O$) | v.s. $H_2O$; s. MeOH; sl. s. EtOH; i. eth., pet. eth. | PREP. *JCS* **1955**, 1212; *Can. J. Chem.* **34**, 541 (1956); *Meth. Carbohydr. Chem.* **1**, 68 (1962). |
| rh. cryst.; M.p. 159–60; $[\alpha]_D - 175 \rightarrow -104.5$ (c = 1 in $H_2O$) | s. $H_2O$; v. sl. s. EtOH; i. eth. | Not fermented by yeasts. |
| obtained as β-form; rh. cryst., M.p. 160; $[\alpha]_D + 190.6 \rightarrow + 104.5$ (c = 4.3 in $H_2O$) | s. $H_2O$; v. sl. s. EtOH; i. eth. | Not fermented by yeasts. |
| prisms; M.p. 103; $[\alpha]_D^{20} + 7.82$ (in saturated borax soln.) | v.s. $H_2O$; s. 90% EtOH | Sweet taste. |
| slightly hygr. cryst. (α) M.p. 78–82; $[\alpha]_D^{25} - 56$ (final c = 1 in $H_2O$). (β) M.p. 96–8; $[\alpha]_D - 91 \rightarrow - 58$ (c = 1 in $H_2O$) | s. $H_2O$; sl. s. EtOH; v. sl. s. isopropanol | Free sugar exists in pyranose ring form, but in combination in nucleosides adopts the furanose ring structure. Gives Molisch test. Gives Dische test for deoxy sugars. Negative anthrone reaction. Best stored as the anilide, M.p. 175–7; deoxyribose regenerated by the action of benzaldehyde. |

# 7 Carbohydrates and related compounds

| Name | Synonyms | Formula | M. wt. |
|---|---|---|---|
| Ribitol | Adonitol | | 152.1 |
| D-Ribonic acid | | | 166.1 |
| D-Ribose | | | 150.1 |
| D-Ribulose | Adonose;<br>D-riboketose;<br>D-arabulose;<br>D-araboketose;<br>D-*erythro*pentulose | | 150.1 |
| Xylitol | | | 152.1 |
| D-Xylose | Wood sugar | | 150.1 |
| D-Xylulose | D-Xyloketose,<br>D-lyxoketose,<br>D-*threo*pentulose | | 150.1 |

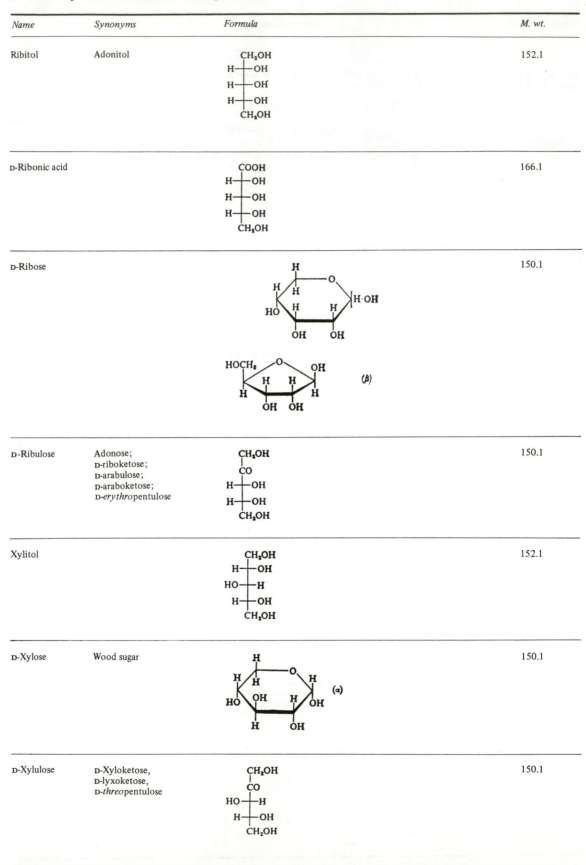

| Physical properties | Solubility | General Remarks |
|---|---|---|
| cryst.; M.p. 102; optically inactive | s. $H_2O$, EtOH; i. eth. | Non-reducing. |
| M.p. 112–13;<br>$[\alpha]_D^{25} - 17.3$ (c = 4 in MeOH) | s. $H_2O$, MeOH, EtOH | Unstable at room temp. 1,4-Lactone, M.p. 72–8, $[\alpha]_D +18.4$ (in $H_2O$). |
| v. hygr. cryst.; M.p. 86–7;<br>$[\alpha]_D^1 - 23.1 \rightarrow - 23.7$<br>(c = 4 in $H_2O$) (mutarotation complex) | s. $H_2O$; v. sl. s. EtOH | Occurs in combination as the furanose form. Solutions contain a mixture of pyranose and furanose forms. Normal cryst. form is $\beta$-D-ribopyranose. Not fermented by common yeasts. |
| syrup;<br>$[\alpha]_D^{21} - 16.3$ (in $H_2O$) | s. $H_2O$ | Gives Seliwanoff test. Reduces Fehling's soln. in the cold.<br>PREP. *Meth. Enzymol.* **9**, 39 (1966); **41**, 103 (1975). |
| cryst.; M.p. 93–4.5 (stable form), 61–1.5 (unstable form); optically inactive. | s. $H_2O$, hot EtOH, MeOH | Sweetest polyol known. |
| obtained as $\alpha$-form;<br>wh. needles; M.p. 145;<br>$[\alpha]_D^{20} + 93.6 \rightarrow + 18.8$<br>(c = 4 in $H_2O$) | 125 $H_2O$; s. EtOH, pyr., gl. acetic; i. eth. | Not fermented by yeasts. Very sweet taste. |
| syrup;<br>$[\alpha]_D^{18} - 33.2$ (c = 2.5 in $H_2O$) | s. $H_2O$ | Reduces Fehling's soln. in the cold. Gives Seliwanoff's test. Prepared and stored as *O*-isopropylidene deriv., M.p. 70–1; $[\alpha]_D^{25} + 1.7$ (in acet.).<br>PREP. *Meth. Carbohydr. Chem.* **1**, 94, 98 (1962); *Meth. Enzymol.* **9**, 39 (1966). |

| Name | Synonyms | Formula | M. wt. |
|---|---|---|---|
| L-Xylulose | L-Xyloketose, L-lyxoketose, L-*threo*pentulose.. Formerly known as *d*-xylulose | | 150.1 |

**DEOXYHEXOSES**

| | | | |
|---|---|---|---|
| 2-Deoxy-D-glucose | D-2-Glucodesose, 2-deoxy-D-*arabino*hexose | | 164.2 |
| 6-Deoxy-D-glucose | D-Glucomethylose, D-*iso*rhamnose, D-*epi*rhamnose, *iso*rhodeose, chinovose, quinovose | | 164.2 |
| D-Fucose | D-Rhodeose, D-galactomethylose, 6-deoxy-D-galactose | | 164.2 |
| L-Fucose | L-Rhodeose, L-galactomethylose, 6-deoxy-L-galactose | | 164.2 |
| L-Rhamnose | L-Mannomethylose, 6-deoxy-L-mannose | | 164.2; Hydrate, 182.2 |

**HEXOSES AND RELATED SUBSTANCES**

| | | | |
|---|---|---|---|
| *N*-Acetyl-D-galactos-amine | *N*-Acetylchondrosamine; 2-acetamido-2-deoxy-D-galactose | | 221.2 |

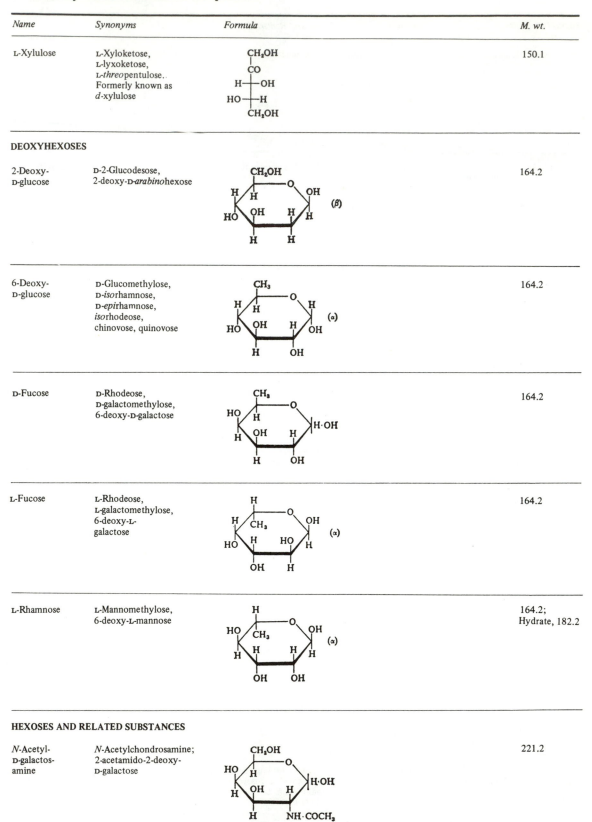

| Physical properties | Solubility | General Remarks |
|---|---|---|
| syrup; $[\alpha]_D^{20} + 33.1$ (c = 2 in $H_2O$) | s. $H_2O$ | Reduces Fehling's soln. in the cold. Gives Seliwanoff's test. PREP. *Meth. Carbohydr. Chem.* **1**, 98 (1962); *J. Org. Chem.* **30**, 458 (1965); *Meth. Enzymol.* **9**, 39 (1966). |
| obtained as β-form; cryst., M.p. 148; $[\alpha]_D^{17} + 38.5 \rightarrow + 45.9$ (c = 0.5 in $H_2O$) | s. $H_2O$, EtOH | α-Form has been prepared. |
| obtained as α-form; cryst., M.p. 146; $[\alpha]_D^{20} + 73.3 \rightarrow + 29.7$ (c = 8 in $H_2O$) | s. $H_2O$, EtOH; i. eth., acet. | PREP. *Meth. Carbohydr. Chem.* **1**, 198 (1962); **6**, 177 (1972); *Carbohydr. Res.* **36**, 392 (1974). |
| (α) needles; M.p. 145; $[\alpha]_D^{20} + 153 \rightarrow + 76$ (c = 4 in $H_2O$) | s. $H_2O$; sl. s. EtOH; i. eth. | Not fermented by yeasts. Sweet taste. |
| obtained as α-form; needles, M.p. 145; $[\alpha]_D^{20} - 152.6 \rightarrow - 75.9$ (c = 4 in $H_2O$) | s. $H_2O$; sl. s. EtOH | Not fermented by yeasts. |
| (α) col. cryst. + $1H_2O$ from $H_2O$; M.p. 94; $[\alpha]_D^{20} - 8.6 \rightarrow + 8.2$ (c = 4 hydrate in $H_2O$) (β) anhyd. needles from acet., hygr., M.p. 123–6; $[\alpha]_D^{20} + 38.4 \rightarrow + 8.9$ (c = 4 in $H_2O$) | $57^{18}$, $109^{40}$ $H_2O$; s. EtOH, MeOH; i. eth., benz. | Not fermented by yeasts. Very sweet taste. Hydrate of α-anomer loses $H_2O$ and is converted to β-form on heating. β-Anomer is converted to α- in moist air. |
| (α) cryst.; M.p. 172–3; $[\alpha]_D + 115 \rightarrow + 86$ (in $H_2O$) | s. $H_2O$ | Lower M.p.s have been recorded. Form with M.p. 120–2 may be monohydrate. Gives positive Morgan–Elson reaction. PREP. *JACS* **76**, 301 (1954), **79**, 4737 (1957); *Meth. Carbohydr. Chem.* **7**, 32 (1976). |

# 7 Carbohydrates and related compounds

| Name | Synonyms | Formula | M. wt. |
|------|----------|---------|--------|
| *N*-Acetyl-D-glucosamine | 2-Acetamido-2-deoxy-D-glucose | 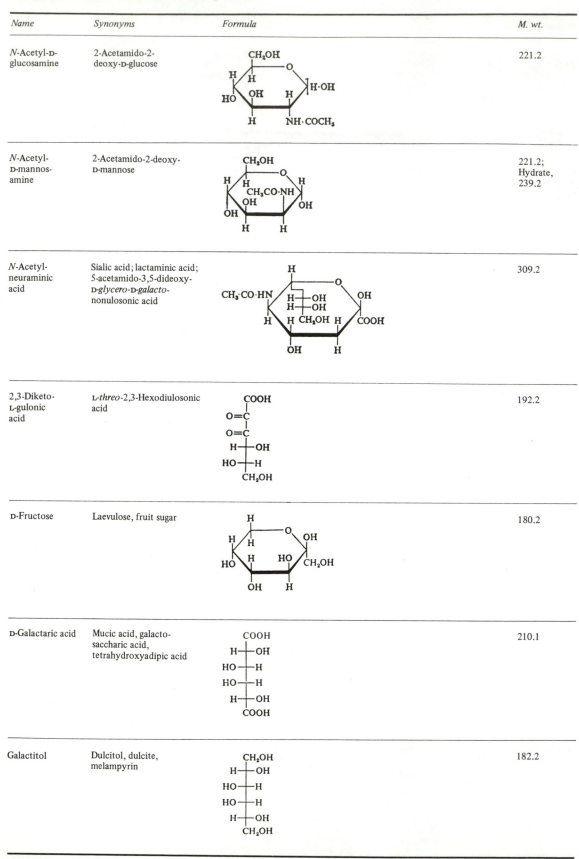 | 221.2 |
| *N*-Acetyl-D-mannosamine | 2-Acetamido-2-deoxy-D-mannose | | 221.2; Hydrate, 239.2 |
| *N*-Acetyl-neuraminic acid | Sialic acid; lactaminic acid; 5-acetamido-3,5-dideoxy-D-*glycero*-D-*galacto*-nonulosonic acid | | 309.2 |
| 2,3-Diketo-L-gulonic acid | L-*threo*-2,3-Hexodiulosonic acid | | 192.2 |
| D-Fructose | Laevulose, fruit sugar | | 180.2 |
| D-Galactaric acid | Mucic acid, galacto-saccharic acid, tetrahydroxyadipic acid | | 210.1 |
| Galactitol | Dulcitol, dulcite, melampyrin | | 182.2 |

| Physical properties | Solubility | General Remarks |
|---|---|---|
| ($\alpha$) col. needles; M.p. 205; $[\alpha]_D^{21} + 75 \rightarrow + 41$ (c = 2 in $H_2O$) ($\beta$) cryst; M.p. 182–3.5; $[\alpha]_D - 22 \rightarrow + 41.3$ (in $H_2O$) | s. $H_2O$ | Gives positive Morgan–Elson reaction. PREP. *Biochem. Preps.* **11**, 1 (1966). |
| large prisms + 1$H_2O$; M.p. 128–9; $[\alpha]_D^{20} - 9.4 \rightarrow + 9.7$ (c = 10 in $H_2O$) | s. $H_2O$ | Gives positive Morgan–Elson reaction. |
| cryst.; M.p. 185–7d.; $[\alpha]_D^{22} - 32$ (c = 2 in $H_2O$); $pK_a$ 2.60 | s. $H_2O$, MeOH; sl. s. EtOH; i. eth., acet., $CHCl_3$ | The sialic acids are acylated derivatives of neuraminic acid. Naturally occurring sialic acids all contain an *N*-acetyl or *N*-glycolyl substituent; some also contain one or two *O*-acetyl groups on *O*-9, *O*-7 or *O*-4. *O*-Acetyl groups are very labile, most stable at pH 3.5–4.5. *N*-Acetyl groups are more stable, greatest stability at pH 4.5, moderately stable in mild alkali, e.g. pH 11 at 25 °C. *N*-Glycolylneuraminic acid: M.p. 189–91d.; $[\alpha]_D - 33.6$ (in $H_2O$); $pK_a$ 2.75. PREP. *Biochem. Preps.* **7**, 1 (1960); *Meth. Enzymol.* **6**, 453 (1963), **8**, 131 (1966), **50**, 64 (1978); *BBA* **338**, 369 (1974); *Ann.* **659**, 156 (1962). |
| Ba, Ca salts amorphous; $[\alpha]_D^{22} - 6.8$ (Ba salt in 0.1m-HCl), $- 8.3$ (Ca salt in 0.1m-HCl) | s. $H_2O$ | Free acid known only in solution. $\gamma$-Lactone is dehydroascorbic acid. PREP. *BJ* **39**, 1 (1945); *JBC* **216**, 539 (1955). |
| obtained as $\beta$-form; v. hygr. col. prisms or needles; M.p. 103–5d.; $[\alpha]_D^{20} - 132.2 \rightarrow - 92.4$ (c = 4 in $H_2O$) | $375^{20}$, $740^{55}$ $H_2O$; s. MeOH, EtOH, pyr., acet., gl. acetic | Anhyd. form stable above 21.4 °C. Tends to hydrate forming hemihydrate (and dihydrate) below 20 °C. Recrystallize from MeOH. Gives Seliwanoff's test. Cryst. sugar is $\beta$-D-pyranose, but in soln. at least 15% of furanose form and appreciable amounts of the open chain form are present. In combination only the furanose form is found. Sweet taste. |
| col. cryst. or wh. powder; M.p. 255 (225); optically inactive; $pK_a$ 3.08, 3.63 | $0.33^{14}$ $H_2O$; s. alkalis; sp. s. eth., EtOH | Recrystallize from $H_2O$. M.p. depends markedly on rate of heating. Reduces ammoniacal $AgNO_3$ but not Fehling's soln. |
| col. monocl. prisms; M.p. 188–9; optically inactive | $3.0^{14}$ $H_2O$; sp. s. EtOH, eth. | Slightly sweet taste. |

| Name | Synonyms | Formula | M. wt. |
|---|---|---|---|
| D-Galactonic acid | D-Lactonic acid | 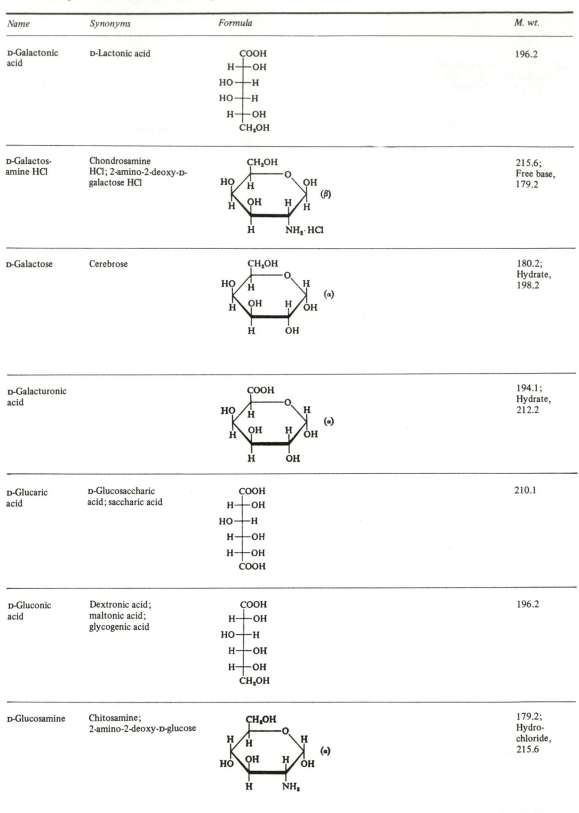 | 196.2 |
| D-Galactos-amine HCl | Chondrosamine HCl; 2-amino-2-deoxy-D-galactose HCl | | 215.6; Free base, 179.2 |
| D-Galactose | Cerebrose | | 180.2; Hydrate, 198.2 |
| D-Galacturonic acid | | | 194.1; Hydrate, 212.2 |
| D-Glucaric acid | D-Glucosaccharic acid; saccharic acid | | 210.1 |
| D-Gluconic acid | Dextronic acid; maltonic acid; glycogenic acid | | 196.2 |
| D-Glucosamine | Chitosamine; 2-amino-2-deoxy-D-glucose | | 179.2; Hydrochloride, 215.6 |

| Physical properties | Solubility | General Remarks |
|---|---|---|
| anhyd. needles from EtOH, M.p. 148; + $\frac{1}{2}H_2O$ from aq. EtOH, M.p. 140–2; + $2H_2O$ from $H_2O$, M.p. 118–20; $[\alpha]_D^{20} - 13 \to - 46$ (in $H_2O$) | s. $H_2O$ | Dihydrate readily loses $H_2O$ by air drying. Salts usually prepared by neutralization of $\gamma$-lactone. K salt, cryst. + $1H_2O$, s. $H_2O$. Ca salt, cryst. + $5H_2O$, s. $H_2O$, loses part of $H_2O$ at $100\,^{\circ}C$. $\gamma$-Lactone (1,4-lactone), needles + $1H_2O$, M.p. 66 (hydrate) 133–5 (anhyd.), $[\alpha]_D^{20} - 77.4 \to - 63.7$ (anhyd. in $H_2O$). |
| ($\alpha$) needles; M.p. 185; $[\alpha]_D^{20} + 121 \to + 95$ (in $H_2O$) ($\beta$) cryst.; M.p. 187; $[\alpha]_D^{20} + 44.5 \to + 95$ (in $H_2O$) p$K_a$ 7.70 | s. $H_2O$ | Usually obtained as $\beta$-form. Reducing sugar. Gives ninhydrin reaction. Negative Molisch test. |
| ($\alpha$) prisms or needles + $1H_2O$ from $H_2O$, M.p. 118–20; anhyd. plates from EtOH, M.p. 168; $[\alpha]_D^{20} + 150.7 \to + 80.2$ (c = 5 in $H_2O$) ($\beta$) cryst.; M.p. 167; $[\alpha]_D^{20} + 52.8 \to + 80.2$ (c = 4 in $H_2O$) | $10^0$, $68^{25}$ $H_2O$; v. sl. s. MeOH; $5.45^{25}$ pyr. | Generally obtained as $\alpha$-form. |
| ($\alpha$) needles + $1H_2O$, sinters 110–11, M.p. 159–60d.; $[\alpha]_D^{20} + 107.0 \to + 51.9$ (c = 4 hydrate in $H_2O$) ($\beta$) anhyd., M.p. 160d.; $[\alpha]_D^{20} + 31.1 \to + 56.7$ (c = 4 anhyd. in $H_2O$) | ($\alpha$) s. $H_2O$, hot EtOH; sp. s. cold EtOH; i. eth. | Generally obtained as $\alpha$-form or as mixture of $\alpha$- and $\beta$-forms. Na salt, obtained as $\beta$-form, cryst., $[\alpha]_D^{20} + 11.5 \to + 36.0$ (c = 4 in $H_2O$), s. $H_2O$, i. EtOH. Ca salt, obtained as $\alpha$-form, cryst. + $1H_2O$, $[\alpha]_D^{20} + 75.0 \to + 36.8$ (c = 1.4 anhyd. in $H_2O$), solubility $4.9^{20}$, $10^{100}$ $H_2O$, i. EtOH. |
| deliq. needles; M.p. 125–6d.; $[\alpha]_D + 6.86 \to + 20.6$ (c = 2.8 in $H_2O$); p$K_a$ 3.01, 3.94 | v.s. $H_2O$, EtOH; v. sl. s. eth. | Crystals lactonize spontaneously to a mixture of lactones. Reduces ammoniacal $AgNO_3$ but not Fehling's soln. Dilactone and methyl esters of monolactones reduce Fehling's soln. 1,4-Lactone, M.p. 98. 3,6-Lactone, M.p. 144, $[\alpha]_D + 37.9 \to + 22.5$ (in $H_2O$). 1,4-3,6-Dilactone, M.p. 134. KH salt, cryst., $[\alpha]_D^{20} + 5.1$ (c = 0.8 in $H_2O$). |
| cryst.; M.p. 132; $[\alpha]_D^{20} - 6.7 \to + 12$ (in $H_2O$); p$K_a$ 3.76 | s. $H_2O$; sl. s. EtOH; i. eth. | Mildly acid taste. In aq. soln. acid is partly transformed into a mixture of lactones. Lactones partially hydrolysed to acid on soln. in $H_2O$. $\gamma$-Lactone (1,4-lactone), M.p. 133–5, $[\alpha]_D^{20} + 68 \to + 17.7$ (c = 5 in $H_2O$). $\delta$-Lactone (1,5-lactone), M.p. 153, $[\alpha]_D^{25} + 66.7 \to + 8.5$ (c = 5 in $H_2O$), s. $H_2O$, sl. s. EtOH, sweet taste. Na salt, cryst., s. $H_2O$. Ca salt, cryst. + $2H_2O$, sl. s. $H_2O$, i. EtOH. |
| p$K_a$ 7.75 ($\alpha$) wh. cryst. powder, M.p. 88; $[\alpha]_D^{20} + 100 \to + 47.5$ (c = 1 in $H_2O$) Hydrochloride: cryst., decomp. 190–210; $[\alpha]_D + 100 \to + 72.5$ (c = 1 in $H_2O$) ($\beta$) needles, M.p. 120; $[\alpha]_D^{20} + 14 \to + 47.5$ (c = 1 in $H_2O$) Hydrochloride: $[\alpha]_D + 25 \to + 72.5$ (c = 1 in $H_2O$) | v.s. $H_2O$; s. hot MeOH; sl. s. EtOH; i. eth., $CHCl_3$ HCl, sl. s. $H_2O$ | Generally obtained as $\alpha$-form. Reducing sugar. Gives ninhydrin reaction. Negative Molisch test. |

| Name | Synonyms | Formula | M. wt. |
|---|---|---|---|
| D-Glucose | Dextrose; grape sugar | | 180.2;<br>Hydrate,<br>198.2 |
| D-Glucuronic acid | | | 194.1 |
| L-Iduronic acid | | | 194.1 |
| 2-Keto-D-gluconic acid | 2-Oxo-D-gluconic acid;<br>D-glucosonic acid;<br>fructuronic acid;<br>D-*arabino*hexulosonic acid | | 194.1 |
| 5-Keto-D-gluconic acid | 5-Oxo-D-gluconic acid;<br>L-sorburonic acid;<br>D-*xylo*hexulosonic acid. | | 194.1 |
| 2-Keto-L-gulonic acid | 2-Oxo-L-gulonic acid;<br>L-*xylo*-2-hexulosonic acid | | 194.1 |
| D-Mannitol | D-Mannite | | 182.2 |

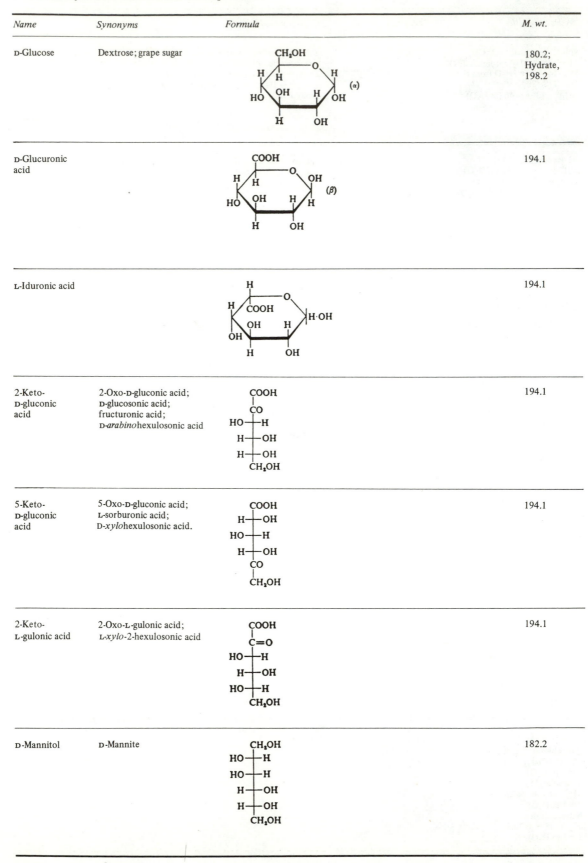

| Physical properties | Solubility | General Remarks |
|---|---|---|
| (α) plates + $1H_2O$ from $H_2O$, M.p. 83; anhyd. cryst. from MeOH, M.p. 146; $[\alpha]_D^{20} + 112.2 \rightarrow + 52.7$ (c = 3.9 anhyd. in $H_2O$) (β) cryst.; M.p. 148−50; $[\alpha]_D^{20} + 18.7 \rightarrow + 52.7$ (c = 3.9 in $H_2O$) | (α) Hydrate, $32.3^0$, $82.0^{25}$ $H_2O$; sl. s. EtOH, MeOH; i. eth., acet. (β) $154^{15}$ $H_2O$; sl. s. EtOH; i. eth. | Glucose of commerce is generally largely α-glucose · $H_2O$. α-Glucose crystallizes as hydrate below 50°C, in anhyd. form above 50°C. |
| obtained as β-form; needles, M.p. 165d.; $[\alpha]_D + 11.7 \rightarrow + 36.3$ (in $H_2O$); $pK_a$ 3.18 | s. $H_2O$, EtOH | Crystallization usually gives a mixture of acid and lactone. In aq. soln. acid and lactone are interconverted. Equilibrium is reached slowly (2 months) at room temp., but rapidly at high temp. (2 hr at 100°C). At equilibrium mixture contains 20% lactone at room temp., 60% lactone at 100°C. Reduces Fehling's soln. Na salt, cryst. + $1H_2O$, s. $H_2O$, $H_2O$ remains *in vacuo* over $CaCl_2$. K salt, cryst. + $2H_2O$, s. $H_2O$, loses $1H_2O$ *in vacuo* over $CaCl_2$. 6 → 3-Lactone (D-glucurone), plates, M.p. 176−8, $[\alpha]_D^{20} + 19.2$ (in $H_2O$), solubility 26.9 $H_2O$, 2.8 MeOH, 0.7 EtOH, exists in furanose form. |
| cryst., M.p. 131−2; $[\alpha]_D^{25} + 37 \rightarrow + 33$ (c = 3 in $H_2O$) | s. $H_2O$, MeOH | PREP. *Meth. Carbohydr. Chem.,* **2**, 32 (1962); **8**, 177 (1980). 6 → 3-Lactone, syrup, $[\alpha]_D^{18} + 30$ (in $H_2O$). |
| syrup or hygr. cryst.; $[\alpha]_D$ −99.6 (K salt in HCl) | s. $H_2O$ | Ca salt, cryst. + $3H_2O$, M.p. 153d., $[\alpha]_D^{20} − 70.8$ (c = 2 in $H_2O$), s. $H_2O$. |
| unstable; turns black and evolves gas; $[\alpha]_D^{20}$ −14.4 (in $H_2O$) | s. $H_2O$ | Reduces Fehling's solution. Ca salt, cryst. + $3H_2O$, $[\alpha]_D − 11.7$ (in dil. HCl), solubility 0.2 $H_2O$ |
| cryst. + $1H_2O$; M.p. 171; $[\alpha]_D − 48$ (c = 1 in $H_2O$) | s. $H_2O$ | In soln. mainly 2,6-lactol ring compd. plus a very little free acid. Solid either free acid or 1,4-lactone, both + $1H_2O$. Rapidly reduces boiling Fehling's soln. 1,4-Lactone is keto-tautomer of ascorbic acid. |
| needles; M.p. 166−8; $[\alpha]_D + 28.6$ (in borax soln.) | $15.6^{18}$ $H_2O$; s. hot EtOH; sl. s. pyr.; i. eth. | Sweetish taste. |

| Name | Synonyms | Formula | M. wt. |
|---|---|---|---|
| D-Mannosamine HCl | | | 215.6; Free base, 179.2 |
| D-Mannose | Seminose, carubinose | | 180.2 |
| D-Mannuronic acid | Mannurone | | 194.1 |
| α-Methyl D-galacto-pyranoside | α-Methyl galactoside | | 194.2; Hydrate, 212.2 |
| β-Methyl D-galacto-pyranoside | β-Methyl galactoside | | 194.2 |
| α-Methyl D-gluco-pyranoside | α-Methyl glucoside | | 194.2 |
| β-Methyl D-gluco-pyranoside | β-Methyl glucoside | | 194.2 |

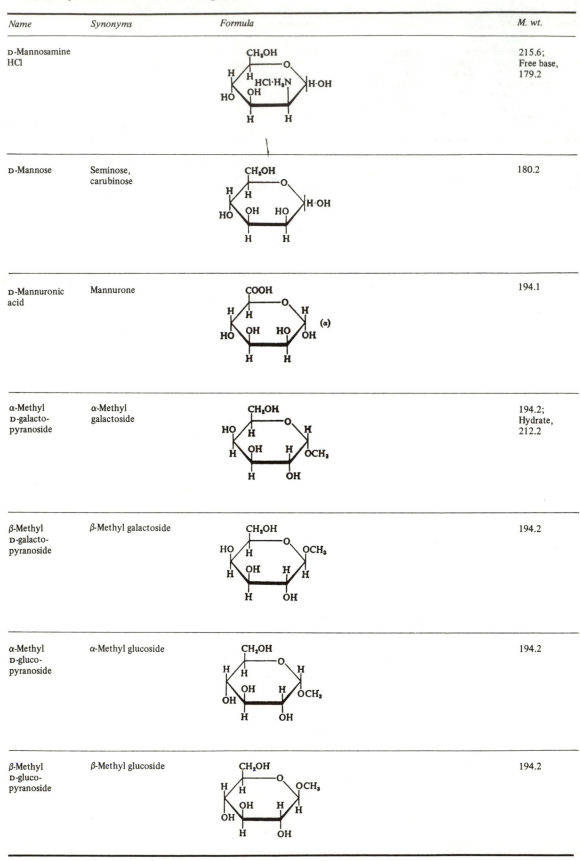

| Physical properties | Solubility | General Remarks |
|---|---|---|
| cryst.; M.p. 178–80; $[\alpha]_D^{20} - 4.6$ (c = 10 in 5% HCl); $pK_a$ 7.28 | s. $H_2O$, MeOH | Reducing. |
| obtained as α- or β-form (α) cryst. mass; M.p. 133; $[\alpha]_D^{20} + 29.3 \rightarrow + 14.2$ (c = 4 in $H_2O$) (β) needles; M.p. 132; $[\alpha]_D^{20} - 17.0 \rightarrow + 14.2$ (c = 4 in $H_2O$) | $248^{17}$ $H_2O$; sp. s. EtOH, MeOH; i. eth. | |
| (α) v. hygr. microneedles + 1$H_2O$; sinters 110, darkens 120–30; $[\alpha]_D^{25} + 16.01 \rightarrow - 6.05$ (in $H_2O$) (β) microcryst.; M.p. 165–7; $[\alpha]_D^{25} - 47.9 \rightarrow - 23.94$ (in $H_2O$) | (α) s. $H_2O$ (β) s. $H_2O$ | Readily forms 6 → 3-lactone. PREP. *Meth. Carbohydr. Chem.,* **2**, 35 (1963); *JCS* **1944**, 587. 6 → 3-Lactone (D-mannurone), cryst., M.p. 197–9, $[\alpha]_D^{21} + 71 \rightarrow + 92$ (c = 1 in $H_2O$). Na salt, cryst. powder, s. $H_2O$. K salt, cryst. + 1$H_2O$, s. $H_2O$. |
| needles + 1$H_2O$; M.p. 111–12 (anhyd.); $[\alpha]_D + 196$ (in $H_2O$, anhyd. form) | s. $H_2O$, MeOH | Non-reducing. |
| cryst., M.p. 178–80; $[\alpha]_D + 0.61$ (in $H_2O$) | s. $H_2O$, MeOH | Non-reducing. |
| cryst. mass, M.p. 168; $[\alpha]_D^{20} + 158$ (c = 10 in $H_2O$) | s. $H_2O$, MeOH, hot EtOH | Non-reducing. |
| cryst. + ½$H_2O$, M.p. 110 (anhyd.); $[\alpha]_D - 31$ (c = 8 in $H_2O$, anhyd. form) | s. $H_2O$, MeOH | Non-reducing |

# 7  Carbohydrates and related compounds

| Name | Synonyms | Formula | M. wt. |
|------|----------|---------|--------|
| Muramic acid | 2-Amino-3-O-(1-carboxyethyl)-2-deoxy-D-glucose | | 251.2; Hydrate, 269.2 |
| D-Sorbitol | Sorbitol; D-glucitol | | 182.2; Hydrate, 200.2 |
| L-Sorbose | L-Sorbinose, 2-oxo-L-xylohexose | | 180.2 |

**HEPTOSES AND RELATED SUBSTANCES**

| | | | |
|------|----------|---------|--------|
| D-manno-Heptulose | D-mannoKeto-heptose | | 210.2 |
| Sedoheptulose | D-altroHeptulose | | 210.2 |

**OLIGOSACCHARIDES**

| | | | |
|------|----------|---------|--------|
| Allolactose | 6-O-β-D-Galactopyran-osyl-D-glucopyranose | | 342.3 |

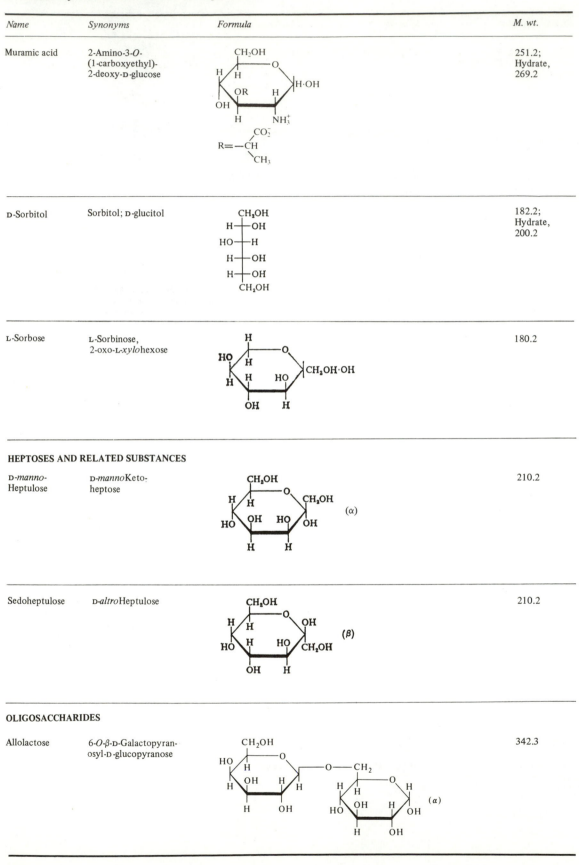

| Physical properties | Solubility | General Remarks |
|---|---|---|
| cryst. + 1$H_2O$ from aq. EtOH; M.p. 152–4d.; $[\alpha]_D^{20}$ + 155 → + 110 (in $H_2O$) | s. $H_2O$, MeOH; v. sl. s. EtOH | Natural isomer is $\alpha$-form. Reducing sugar. Positive Morgan—Elson reaction. PREP. *Biochem. Preps.* **10**, 106, 109 (1963); *Meth. Carbohydr. Chem.* **1**, 250 (1962); *JCS* **1965**, 2975; *J. Org. Chem.* **30**, 448 (1965). *N*-Acetyl deriv., M.p. 119–20; $[\alpha]_D^{20}$ + 60 → + 40 (c = 1.2 in $H_2O$). |
| needles + 1$H_2O$, sl. hygr.; M.p. 75 (hydrate), 97 (anhyd.); $[\alpha]_D$ − 2.0 (in $H_2O$) + 6.5 (in borax) + 30.9 (in $NH_4$ molybdate) | v.s. $H_2O$; s. hot EtOH; v. sl. s. cold EtOH; i. eth. | Sweet taste (60% of sucrose). |
| rh. cryst., M.p. 165; $[\alpha]_D^{20}$ − 43.7 → − 43.4 (c = 12 in $H_2O$) (mutarotation complex) | $55^{17}$ $H_2O$; sp. s. hot EtOH, MeOH | Not fermented by yeasts. Gives Seliwanoff's test. Sweetness similar to sucrose. |
| prisms; M.p. 152; $[\alpha]_D$ + 29.2 (in $H_2O$) | s. $H_2O$; sp. s. EtOH | Not fermented by yeasts. PREP. *Meth. Carbohydr. Chem.* **1**, 173, 175 (1962). |
| syrup; $[\alpha]_D$ + 8.2 (in $H_2O$) | s. $H_2O$; sp. s. EtOH | Sugar forms anhydro compd. (sedoheptulosan) in soln., esp. in acid. Not fermented by yeasts. Sedoheptulosan (2,7-anhydro-D-*altro*heptulose): prisms + 1$H_2O$, M.p. 101–2; anhyd. prisms from MeOH, M.p. 155–6; $[\alpha]_D^{20}$ − 146 (c = 2 anhyd. in $H_2O$); s. $H_2O$. Non-reducing. Anhyd. form stable in desiccator, hydrate stable in air. In soln., stable to alkali; in acid partially hydrolysed to sedoheptulose (9% sedoheptulose at 20°C). PREP. *Meth. Carbohydr. Chem.* **1**, 167 (1962). |
| needles; M.p. 174–6d.; $[\alpha]_D^{18}$ + 54.2 → + 30.7 (in $H_2O$) | s. $H_2O$ | PREP. *Ber.* **66**, 806 (1933); *Meth. Carbohydr. Chem.* **1**, 303 (1962). |

# 7 Carbohydrates and related compounds

| Name | Synonyms | Formula | M. wt. |
|---|---|---|---|
| Cellobiose | Cellose; 4-*O*-β-D-glucopyranosyl-D-glucopyranose | | 342.3 |
| Chondrosine | 2-Amino-2-deoxy-3-*O*-(β-D-glucopyranosyluronic acid)-D-galactopyranose | | 355.3 |
| *N,N′*-Diacetyl-chitobiose | Chitobiose; 2-acetamido-2-deoxy-4-*O*-(2-acetamido-2-deoxy-β-D-glucopyranosyl)-D-glucopyranose | | 424.4 |
| Gentiobiose | Amygdalose; 6-*O*-β-D-glucopyranosyl-D-glucopyranose | | 342.3 |
| Hyalobiuronic acid | 2-Amino-2-deoxy-3-*O*-(β-D-glucopyranosyluronic acid)-D-glucopyranose | | 355.3; Hydrate, 373.3 |
| Isomaltose | Brachyose; 6-*O*-α-D-glucopyranosyl-D-glucose | | 342.3 |

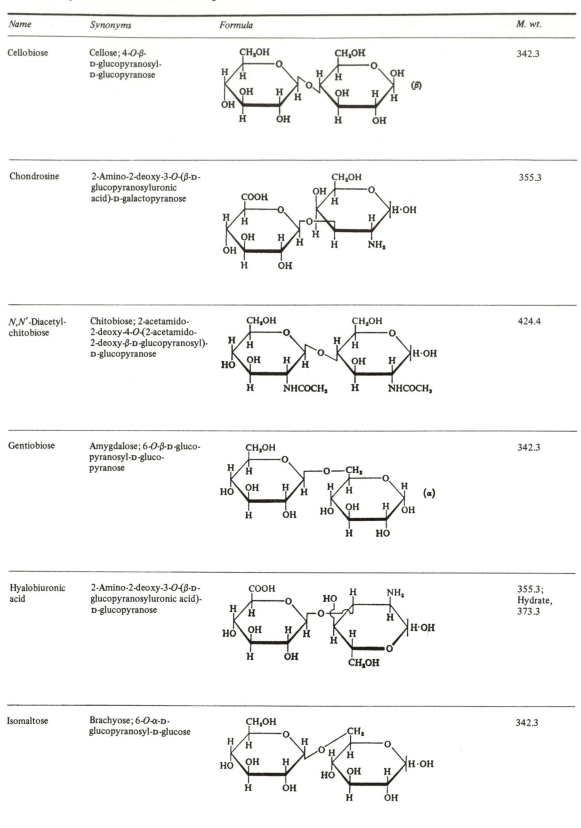

158

| Physical properties | Solubility | General Remarks |
|---|---|---|
| obtained as $\beta$-form; col. needles, darkens 180, decomp. 225; $[\alpha]_D^{20} + 14.2 \rightarrow + 34.6$ (c = 8 in $H_2O$) | s. $H_2O$; i. EtOH, eth. | Reducing sugar. Not fermented by yeasts. |
| fine needles, $[\alpha]_D^{24} + 42$ (c = 2 in $H_2O$) + 40 (c = 1 in 0.05M-HCl) | s. dil. acid | Reducing sugar. PREP. *JACS* **74**, 1491 (1952), **76**, 5686 (1954), **84**, 3029 (1962). *N*-Acetylchondrosine, $[\alpha]_D^{25} + 32.5$ (in $H_2O$), PREP. *JBC* **240**, 992 (1965). |
| cryst.; M.p. 245–7 and 260–4; $[\alpha]_D^{27} + 32.3 \rightarrow + 16.0$ (c = 0.74 in $H_2O$) | s. $H_2O$ | Reducing sugar; acetyl-free sugar isol. but not characterized. PREP. *Biochem. Preps.* **13**, 14 (1971); *BBA* **83**, 245 (1964); *Meth. Carbohydr. Chem.* **1**, 305 (1962). |
| ($\alpha$) cryst. + 2MeOH, M.p. 86; $[\alpha]_D^{20} + 21.4 \rightarrow + 8.7$ (c = 5 alcoholate in $H_2O$) ($\beta$) cryst., M.p. 190–5; $[\alpha]_D^{20} - 11 \rightarrow + 9.6$ (in $H_2O$) | s. $H_2O$, hot EtOH, hot MeOH | Generally obtained as $\beta$-form. Reducing sugar. Not fermented by top yeasts. |
| crystalline + $1H_2O$, lost over $P_2O_5$ at 80°C, M.p. 190d.; $[\alpha]_D + 22.5^{23}$ (c = 1 in 1.0M-HCl) + 34 $\rightarrow$ + 30$^{24}$ (c = 1 in 0.1M-HCl) | s. dil. acid | Reducing sugar. PREP. *JBC* **205**, 205 (1953); *JACS* **84**, 3029, 3030 (1962). *N*-Acetyl, $[\alpha]_D + 31$ to + 32 (in $H_2O$). |
| amorphous, M.p. 120; $[\alpha]_D^{25} + 119 \rightarrow + 122$ (in $H_2O$) | s. $H_2O$, MeOH | Reducing sugar: not fermented by yeasts. PREP. *Biochem. Preps.* **10**, 86 (1963); *Meth. Carbohydr. Chem.* **1**, 316, 319 (1962). |

# 7 Carbohydrates and related compounds

| Name | Synonyms | Formula | M. wt. |
|---|---|---|---|
| Lactose | Milk sugar; lactobiose; 4-*O*-β-D-galactopyranosyl-D-glucopyranose | | 342.3; Hydrate, 360.3 |
| Maltose | Malt sugar; maltobiose; 4-*O*-α-D-glucopyranosyl-D-glucopyranose | | 342.3; Hydrate, 360.3 |
| Melibiose | 6-*O*-α-D-Galactopyranosyl-D-glucopyranose | | 342.3; Dihydrate, 378.3 |
| Raffinose | 6$^G$-α-Galactosylsucrose | α-D-Galactosyl*p*-(1 → 6)-α-D-glucosyl*p*-(1 → 2)-β-D-fructoside*f* | 504.4; Hydrate, 594.5 |
| Stachyose | Lupeose; 6$^{Gal}$-α-Galactosyl-raffinose | α-D-Galactosyl*p*-(1 → 6)-α-D-galactosyl*p*-(1 → 6)-α-D-glucosyl*p*-(1 → 2)-β-D-fructoside*f* | 666.6; Hydrate, 738.7 |
| Sucrose | Cane sugar; saccharose; 1-*O*-α-D-glucopyranosyl-β-D-fructofuranoside | | 342.3 |
| α,α-Trehalose | Mycose, 1-*O*-α-D-gluco-pyranosyl-α-D-gluco-pyranoside | | 342.3; Hydrate 378.3 |
| Xylobiose | 4-*O*-β-D-Xylopyranosyl-β-D-xylose | | 282.3 |

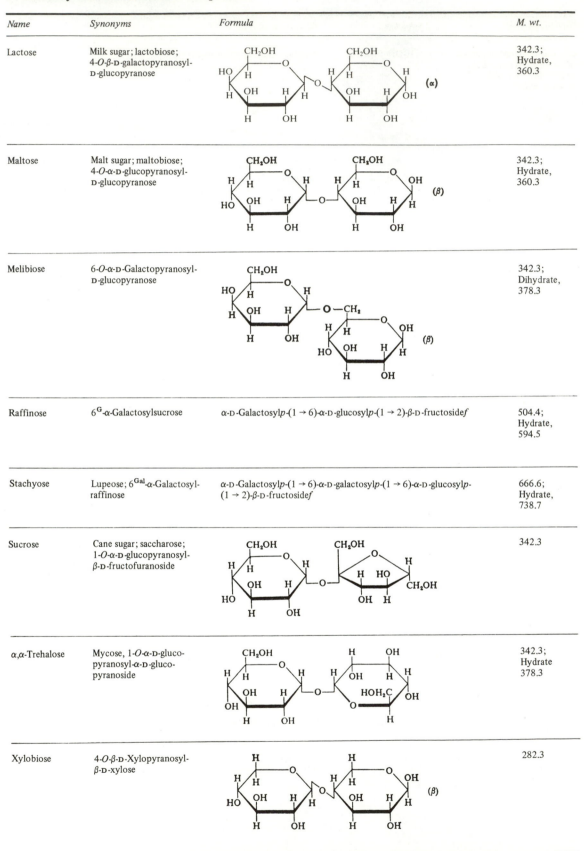

| Physical properties | Solubility | General Remarks |
|---|---|---|
| ($\alpha$) cryst. + 1$H_2O$; M.p. 202 (hydrate) 223 (anhyd.); $[\alpha]_D^{20}$ + 85.0 → + 52.6 (c = 7.6 hydrate in $H_2O$) [+ 89.4 → + 55.4 on anhyd. basis] ($\beta$) anhyd.; M.p. 252; $[\alpha]_D^{20}$ + 34.9 → + 55.4 (c = 4 in $H_2O$) | 21.6[25], 139[89] $H_2O$; sl. s. gl. acetic; i. MeOH, EtOH, eth. | Generally obtained as $\alpha$-lactose · $H_2O$ which loses $H_2O$ at 130°C and at 70°C *in vacuo*. Anhyd. forms of $\alpha$- and $\beta$- are hygr. Reducing sugar. Fermented by lactose yeasts and lactose-adapted yeasts. |
| obtained as $\beta$-form; fine needles + 1$H_2O$, M.p. 102–3 (hydrate), 160–5 (anhyd.); $[\alpha]_D^{20}$ + 111.7 → + 130.4 (c = 4 hydrate in $H_2O$) | 108[20] $H_2O$; v. sl. s. EtOH; i. eth. | Reducing sugar. Fermented by yeasts in presence of glucose. |
| ($\alpha$) cryst. + 1$H_2O$; M.p. 179–81; $[\alpha]_D^{23}$ + 157 → + 137 (c = 1 hydrate in $H_2O$) ($\beta$) cryst. + 2$H_2O$; M.p. 82–5d.; $[\alpha]_D^{20}$ + 111.7 → + 129.5 (c = 4 hydrate in $H_2O$) | s. $H_2O$; v. sl. s. EtOH | Originally obtained as $\beta$-anomer, but commercial samples may be $\alpha$-form. Reducing sugar. Fermented by bottom yeasts but not by most top yeasts. |
| wh. prisms + 5$H_2O$; M.p. 78 (hydrate) 118–20 (anhyd.); $[\alpha]_D^{20}$ + 104.8 (hydrate in $H_2O$) | 14.3[20] $H_2O$; 9.8 MeOH; v.s. pyr.; i. EtOH | Non-reducing. Fermented by bottom yeasts. |
| fine cryst. + 4$H_2O$; M.p. 101–5 (hydrate); $[\alpha]_D^{25}$ + 132 (c = 9 in $H_2O$) | s. $H_2O$ | Non-reducing. PREP. *Meth. Carbohydr. Chem.* **1**, 368 (1962). |
| exists in A and B forms (A) cryst. from EtOH and most solvents, M.p. 188 (B) cryst. from MeOH, M.p. 169–70 $[\alpha]_D^{20}$ + 66.53 (c = 26 in $H_2O$) | 180[0], 197[15], 487[100] $H_2O$; sl. s. EtOH, MeOH; i. eth., benz., acet., $CHCl_3$ | A form is the stable cryst. form. Non-reducing. Fermented by yeasts. An alkaline soln. of diazouracil turns blue-green only in the presence of sucrose or other oligosaccharides having sucrose as a component, e.g. raffinose (Raybin test). |
| cryst. + 2$H_2O$, M.p. 97; anhyd., M.p. 203; $[\alpha]_D$ + 178.3 (c = 7 in $H_2O$) | s. $H_2O$, hot EtOH; i. eth. | Non-reducing. Fermented by most yeasts. |
| cryst., M.p. 186–7; $[\alpha]_D^{25}$ − 32 → − 25 (c = 1 in $H_2O$) | s. $H_2O$ | Reducing sugar. Not fermented by yeasts. PREP. *JACS* **74**, 3059, 3609 (1952); *JCS* **1961**, 3674; *J. Org. Chem.* **26**, 4609 (1961). |

# 7 Carbohydrates and related compounds

## NUCLEOSIDE DIPHOSPHOSUGARS

The nucleoside diphosphate derivatives of most common sugars have the same basic structure and have very similar chemical and physical properties. These common features and representative examples of nucleoside diphosphosugars possessing them are included in the first entry 'Common properties'. Related nucleotide

| Name | Structure | M. wt. |
|---|---|---|

**Common properties**

Nucleoside diphosphosugar
[NDP-sugar;
Nucleoside 5'-diphosphosugar;
Nucleoside diphosphate sugar;
Nucleoside 5'-(sugar pyrophosphate)]

Structure illustrated by uridine 5'-diphospho-α-D-glucopyranose (UDP-glucose)

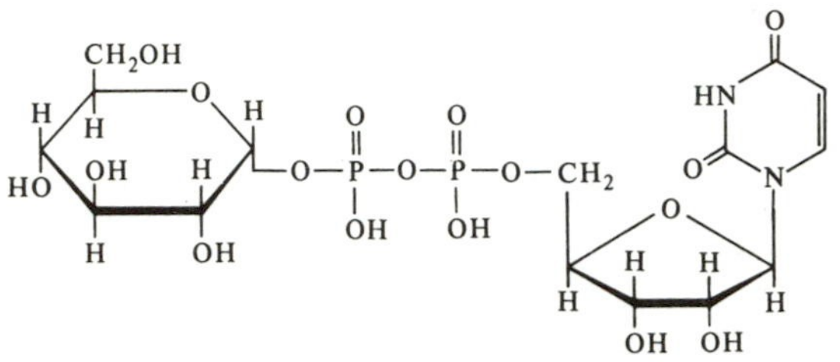

**Properties of representative individual compounds**

| Name | Structure | M. wt. |
|---|---|---|
| ADP-glucose | Adenosine 5'-diphospho-α-D-glucopyranose | 589.3 |
| GDP-fucose | Guanosine 5'-diphospho-β-L-fucose | 589.3 |
| GDP-glucose | Guanosine 5'-diphospho-α-D-glucopyranose | 605.3 |
| GDP-mannose | Guanosine 5'-diphospho-α-D-mannopyranose | 605.3 |
| (d)TDP-glucose | Thymidine 5'-diphospho-α-D-glucopyranose | 564.4 |
| (d)TDP-rhamnose | Thymidine 5'-diphospho-β-L-rhamnose | 548.4 |
| UDP-N-acetylgalactosamine | Uridine 5'-diphospho-2-acetamido-2-deoxy-α-D-galactopyranose | 607.4 |
| UDP-N-acetylglucosamine | Uridine 5'-diphospho-2-acetamido-2-deoxy-α-D-glucopyranose | 607.4 |
| UDP-galactose | Uridine 5'-diphospho-α-D-galactopyranose | 566.4 |
| UDP-galacturonic acid | Uridine 5'-diphospho-α-D-galacturonic acid | 580.3 |

derivatives of carbohydrate compounds having different structures and/or properties are dealt with in separate entries.

REVIEW. *Adv. Carbohydr. Chem. Biochem.* **28**, 307 (1973); **26**, 352 (1971).

---

*General Remarks*

---

*Structure*: The nucleoside moiety in naturally occurring compounds may be adenosine, guanosine, cytidine, uridine, or (deoxy)thymidine. The sugar is linked to phosphate through its anomeric carbon atom, i.e. C-1 in aldoses and their derivatives. In the naturally occurring compounds the glycosidic link usually has the α-configuration with D-sugars and the β-configuration with L-sugars. The sugar ring is usually pyranose.

*Solubility*: s. $H_2O$; i. MeOH, EtOH, eth., acet.

*Spectrum*: The spectrum is the same as that of the nucleoside diphosphate moiety of the molecule.

*Stability*: The sugar-phosphate in nucleoside diphosphosugar compounds is more labile to acid than in the corresponding sugar 1-phosphate. Completely hydrolysed by 0.01M-HCl in 10–15 min at 100°C to give nucleoside 5'-diphosphate plus sugar. Longer time or stronger acid, e.g. M-HCl at 100°C for 15 min, gives nucleoside 5'-phosphate, $P_i$ and sugar. Alkaline hydrolysis, e.g. 2 min at 100°C at pH 8.5 or 30 min at 0°C in conc. $NH_3$, of UDP-α-D-glucose forms uridine 5'-phosphate and glucose 1,2-cyclic phosphate. Compounds which can form a 1,2-cyclic phosphate are labile to alkali, but those which cannot, either because of the absence of a 2-hydroxyl group or because of an unfavourable steric relationship of substituents on C-1 and C-2, e.g. NDP-α-D-mannose, are stable to alkali. Solid salts (Na, K, Li, Ba, etc.) are hygr., but stable if stored dry at 4°C or below.

*Preparation*: Methods described in the following references are chemical syntheses applicable to most nucleoside diphosphosugars. *JACS* **83**, 659 (1961); *Meth. Enzymol.* **8**, 136, 142 (1966); *BBA* **91**, 1 (1964); *Analyt. Biochem.* **13**, 405 (1965). Methods applicable to individual compounds, e.g. isolation procedures and enzymic methods, are noted in the individual entries below.

---

Labile in alkali forming AMP and glucose 1,2-cyclic phosphate. Synthesised enzymically from ATP and α-D-glucose 1-phosphate. Functions in the synthesis of starch. PREP. *ABB* **106**, 371 (1964); *Meth. Enzymol.* **28**, 279 (1972).

---

Formed by NADPH – dependent reduction of GDP-mannose. PREP. *JBC* **243**, 1110 (1968), **246**, 5154 (1971); *Meth. Enzymol.* **8**, 293 (1966), **28**, 285 (1972).

---

PREP. *JBC* **237**, 1260 (1960).

---

Stable to mild alkali treatment. Formed enzymically from GTP and α-D-mannose 1-phosphate. PREP. *Meth. Enzymol.* **6**, 777 (1963), **8**, 145 (1966), **28**, 281 (1972); *Anal. Biochem.* **18**, 464 (1967); *ABB* **122**, 17 (1967).

---

Formed from TTP and glucose 1-phosphate. PREP. *JBC* **236**, 1791 (1961), **237**, 3014 (1962); *Meth. Enzymol.* **28**, 287 (1972).

---

Labile in alkali forming (d)TMP and L-rhamnose 1,2-cyclic phosphate. Formed enzymically from TDP-glucose. PREP. *BBA* **44**, 478 (1960); *BJ* **81**, 114 (1961); *JBC* **236**, 1795 (1961).

---

$[\alpha]_D^{25} + 81.7$ (c = 0.8 Li salt in $H_2O$). Stable to mild alkaline conditions. PREP. *Biochem.* **3**, 402 (1964); *Meth. Enzymol.* **8**, 147 (1966), **28**, 271, 274 (1972); *Anal. Biochem.* **91**, 490 (1978).

---

$[\alpha]_D^{25} + 54.6$ (c = 1.0 anhyd. Li salt in $H_2O$). Stable to alkaline hydrolysis. PREP. *Meth. Enzymol.* **6**, 777 (1963), **28**, 271 (1972); *Meth. Biochem. Anal.* **10**, 107 (1962); *Anal. Biochem.* **91**, 490 (1978).

---

Labile to alkali. Formed enzymically by epimerization of UDP-glucose or from UTP and α-D-galactose 1-phosphate. PREP. *JACS* **81**, 6514 (1959); *Anal. Biochem.* **8**, 362 (1964); *J. Biochem., Tokyo* **56**, 145 (1964).

---

Formed enzymically by epimerization of UDP-glucuronic acid. PREP. *ABB* **78**, 401 (1958); *PNAS* **54**, 1626 (1965); *JBC* **235**, 910 (1960).

# 7 Carbohydrates and related compounds

| Name | Structure | M. wt. |
|------|-----------|--------|
| UDP-glucose | Uridine 5′-diphospho-α-D-glucopyranose | 566.4 |
| UDP-glucuronic acid | Uridine 5′-diphospho-α-D-glucuronic acid | 580.3 |
| UDP-xylose | Uridine 5′-diphospho-α-D-xylopyranose | 536.3 |

**Other related nucleotides**

Cytidine 5′-diphosphoribitol
   [CDP-ribitol; Cytidine
   5′-(L-ribitol 1-diphosphate)]
      537.3

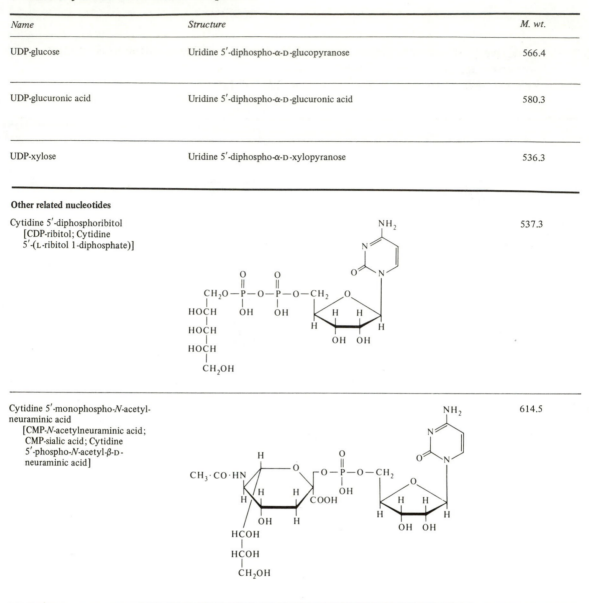

Cytidine 5′-monophospho-N-acetyl-
neuraminic acid
   [CMP-N-acetylneuraminic acid;
   CMP-sialic acid; Cytidine
   5′-phospho-N-acetyl-β-D-
   neuraminic acid]
      614.5

*General Remarks*

Formed enzymically from UTP and α-D-glucose 1-phosphate. PREP. *BBA* **26**, 146 (1957), **104**, 594 (1965); *Meth. Enzymol.* **6**, 777 (1963); *Biochem. Preps.* **8**, 125 (1961).

$[\alpha]_D^{25}$ + 54.5 (c = 1 anhyd. Li salt in $H_2O$), $pK_a$ (COOH) 4.4. Solid decomposes slowly at room temp. Hydrolysis with 0.01M-HCl at 100°C for 15 min gives mainly UDP + glucuronic acid but also small amounts of UMP and glucuronic acid 1-phosphate. PREP. *ABB* **78**, 401 (1958); *JBC* **235**, 910 (1960); *Biochem.* **1**, 1171 (1961).

Formed enzymically from UTP and α-D-xylose 1-phosphate or (together with UDP-L-arabinose) by decarboxylation of UDP-glucuronic acid. PREP. *JBC* **223**, 977 (1956); *Meth. Enzymol.* **6**, 782 (1963).

Functions in the synthesis of teichoic acids in Gram-positive bacteria. Very labile in both acid and alkali. 19% hydrolysis at pH 2 and 20°C after 18 hr. Complete hydrolysis to cytidine 5'-phosphate and ribitol 1,2-cyclic phosphate in 8M-$NH_4OH$ at 100°C in 30 min. Ribitol 1-phosphate moiety has L-configuration (equivalent to D-ribitol 5-phosphate). PREP. *JBC* **241**, 639 (1966); **239**, 3178 (1964); *BJ* **82**, 297 (1962); *JACS* **83**, 653 (1961); *Meth. Enzymol.* **8**, 423 (1966).

Wh. amorph. powder; s. $H_2O$; i. MeOH, acet., eth. In dry state, decomp. at −20°C, 5–10% per day to CMP and *N*-acetylneuraminic acid. Extremely labile to acid; completely hydrolysed within 1 hr at 37°C at pH 4 and below, in 0.01M-HCl at 23°C, 83% hydrolysis in 5 min. More stable at neutral and mildly alkaline pH, but completely decomp. in a few min at neutral pH and 100°C and slowly destroyed at high pH and room temp. PREP. *JBC* **237**, 3527 (1962), **241**, 5637 (1966); *Meth. Enzymol.* **8**, 208 (1966); *Exptl. Cell Res.* **69**, 384 (1971); *ZPC* **353**, 883 (1972); *BJ* **177**, 1 (1979).

# 8 Lipids and long-chain fatty acids

Please note: fat-soluble vitamins, carotenoids, steroid hormones, and fatty acids with less than 8 carbon atoms are dealt with in other sections.

## General bibliography

G. B. Ansell, J. N. Hawthorne, and R. M. C. Dawson, *Form and functions of phospholipids,* 2nd edition, Elsevier (1973).

M. Kates, *Techniques of lipidology: isolation, analysis, and identification of lipids,* North-Holland (1972).

M. I. Gurr and A. T. James, *Lipid biochemistry,* 2nd edition, Chapman Hall (1975).

F. D. Gunstone, *An introduction to the chemistry and biochemistry of fatty acids and their glycerides,* 2nd edition, Chapman Hall (1967).

W. W. Christie, *Lipid analysis,* Pergamon (1973).

C. Hitchcock and B. W. Nichols, *Plant lipid biochemistry,* Academic Press (1971).

A. R. Johnson and J. B. Davenport (eds.), *Biochemistry and methodology of lipids,* Wiley Interscience (1971).

G. V. Marinetti (ed.) *Lipid chromatographic analysis,* 2nd edition Vols. 1, 2, 3, Marcel Dekker (1976).

## Nomenclature

Rules for the nomenclature of lipids are given in *EJB* **2**, 127 (1967); *BJ* **105**, 897 (1967); *BJ* **171**, 21 (1978).

# 8 Lipids and long-chain fatty acids

| Name | Synonyms | Formula | M. wt. |
|------|----------|---------|--------|
| Arachidic acid | *n*-Eicosanoic; eicosoic, eicosanic acids | $CH_3 \cdot (CH_2)_{18} \cdot COOH$ | 312.5 |
| Arachidonic acid | 5:6, 8:9, 11:12, 14:15-Eicosa-tetraenoic acid | $CH_3 \cdot (CH_2)_4 \cdot (CH{=}CH \cdot CH_2)_3 \cdot CH$ $\overset{\parallel}{CH}$ $\mid$ $(CH_2)_3$ $\mid$ $COOH$ | 304.5 |
| Azelaic acid | Nonanedioic, heptamethylene-1,7-dicarboxylic, lepargylic acids | $HOOC \cdot (CH_2)_7 \cdot COOH$ | 188.2 |
| Behenic acid | *n*-Docosanoic acid | $CH_3 \cdot (CH_2)_{20} \cdot COOH$ | 340.6 |
| Capric acid | *n*-Decanoic, decoic acids | $CH_3 \cdot (CH_2)_8 \cdot COOH$ | 172.3 |
| Caprylic acid | *n*-Octanoic, octoic acids | $CH_3 \cdot (CH_2)_6 \cdot COOH$ | 144.2 |
| Cardiolipin | CL; Dipnosphatidyl-glycerol; bis-(1, 2-diacyl-*sn*-glycero-3-phospho)-1′, 3′-*sn*-glycerol; | $R_1 R_2 R_3 R_4 =$ fatty acid residues | 508.3 $+ R_1 + R_2$ $+ R_3 + R_4$ |

| M.p | $[\alpha]_D^t$ | Solubility | General Remarks |
|---|---|---|---|
| 75.4 | | $0.45^{20}$ EtOH; s. $CHCl_3$, benz., eth. | Cryst. plates from EtOH. Found in vegetable and fish oils and milk. |
| −49.5 | | i. $H_2O$; s. eth. | Occurs only in animal fats. 'Essential' fatty acid produced *in vivo* from linoleic acid. Precursor of prostaglandins. |
| 107 B.p. $225.5^{10}$, $286.5^{100}$ | | $0.1^0$, $0.212^{22}$, $1.648^{55}$ $H_2O$; s. eth.; v.s. EtOH | Col. needles or leaflets. Product of oxidative cleavage of oleic acid. |
| 81 | | sp. s. $H_2O$, EtOH; sl. s. eth.; s. $CHCl_3$ | Col. needles. Occurs in peanut, rape seed, and mustard oils. |
| 31.6 B.p. 268–70 | | At 20°C: 0.015 $H_2O$, 398 benz., 326 $CHCl_3$, 210 $CCl_4$, 510 MeOH, 407 acet., 567 gl. acetic, 289 Et acetate | Col. needles, rancid odour. Found in butter, coconut oil, and head of sperm whale. |
| 16.7 B.p. 237.5 | | At 20°C: 0.068 $H_2O$; ∞ benz., $CHCl_3$, $CCl_4$, MeOH, acet., Et acetate | Col. leaflets or liq. with rancid odour. $pK_a$ 4.85. Pb salt, i. $H_2O$. Cu and Zn salts, sp. s. $H_2O$. |
| | $+5.8^{25}$ (in EtOH) | i. $H_2O$; s. acet., $CHCl_3$, eth., EtOH | Free acid unstable. Na salt stored 18 months shows no loss of serological activity. Found in mitochondria and some bacteria. |

## 8 Lipids and long-chain fatty acids

| Name | Synonyms | Formula | M. wt. |
|------|----------|---------|--------|
| Cerebrosides | Glyco-sphingosides | $CH_3 \cdot (CH_2)_{12} \cdot CH{=}CH \cdot CH(OH)$<br>$R \cdot CO \cdot NH \cdot CH$ 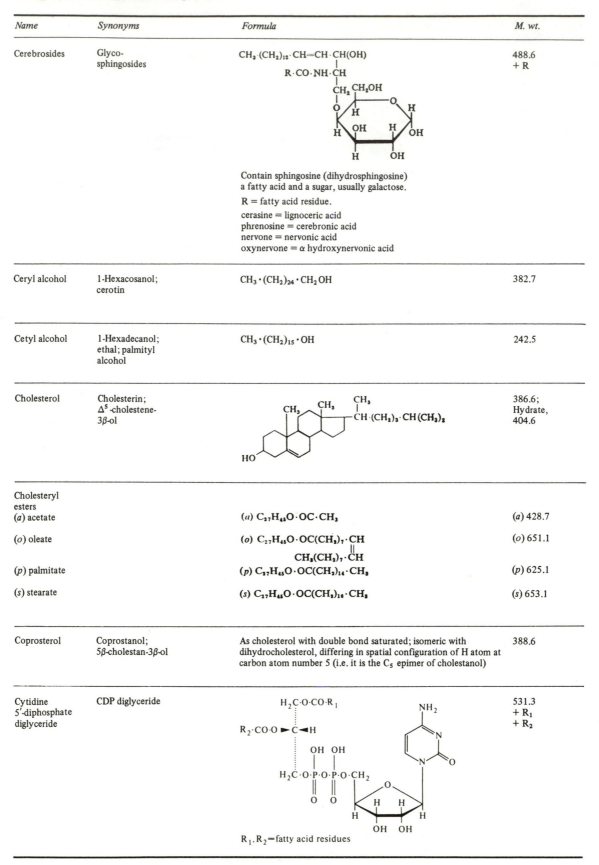<br>Contain sphingosine (dihydrosphingosine) a fatty acid and a sugar, usually galactose.<br>R = fatty acid residue.<br>cerasine = lignoceric acid<br>phrenosine = cerebronic acid<br>nervone = nervonic acid<br>oxynervone = α hydroxynervonic acid | 488.6 + R |
| Ceryl alcohol | 1-Hexacosanol; cerotin | $CH_3 \cdot (CH_2)_{24} \cdot CH_2 OH$ | 382.7 |
| Cetyl alcohol | 1-Hexadecanol; ethal; palmityl alcohol | $CH_3 \cdot (CH_2)_{15} \cdot OH$ | 242.5 |
| Cholesterol | Cholesterin; $\Delta^5$-cholestene-3β-ol | | 386.6; Hydrate, 404.6 |
| Cholesteryl esters<br>(a) acetate | | (a) $C_{27}H_{45}O \cdot OC \cdot CH_3$ | (a) 428.7 |
| (o) oleate | | (o) $C_{27}H_{45}O \cdot OC(CH_2)_7 \cdot CH$<br>$\quad\quad CH_3(CH_2)_7 \cdot CH$ | (o) 651.1 |
| (p) palmitate | | (p) $C_{27}H_{45}O \cdot OC(CH_2)_{14} \cdot CH_3$ | (p) 625.1 |
| (s) stearate | | (s) $C_{27}H_{45}O \cdot OC(CH_2)_{16} \cdot CH_3$ | (s) 653.1 |
| Coprosterol | Coprostanol; 5β-cholestan-3β-ol | As cholesterol with double bond saturated; isomeric with dihydrocholesterol, differing in spatial configuration of H atom at carbon atom number 5 (i.e. it is the $C_5$ epimer of cholestanol) | 388.6 |
| Cytidine 5'-diphosphate diglyceride | CDP diglyceride | $R_1, R_2$ = fatty acid residues | 531.3 + $R_1$ + $R_2$ |

| M.p | $[\alpha]_D^t$ | Solubility | General Remarks |
|---|---|---|---|
| Phrenosine melts finally 212–15; Cerasine melts finally 185–7; Nervone melts finally 180 | Diverse values reported which probably depend on purity. *See* H. Deuel, *The Lipids*, vol. 1, p. 485 Interscience, New York (1951) | i. $H_2O$, eth., pet. eth.; sl. s. EtOH; s. pyr., acet., gl. acetic, $CHCl_3$ | Wax-like white powders. Resistant to hydrolysis with boiling sat. $Ba(OH)_2$. |
| 79–80 | | i. $H_2O$; s. EtOH, eth. | Crystalline form, rh. plates. Widely distributed in various waxes of plant and animal origin, usually esterified with fatty acids. |
| 49.3 B.p. $190^{15}$ | | i. $H_2O$; s. EtOH, MeOH, eth., benz. | Leaflets from EtOH. Found in various marine oils, often esterified to fatty acids. |
| 148.5 (anhyd.) | $-31.1^{15}$ (in eth.) | sp. s. $H_2O$, EtOH; s. eth., $CHCl_3$, benz., pet. eth., pyr., Et acetate, hot EtOH | Monocl. leaflets $+ 1H_2O$ from 95% EtOH; needles from anhyd. solvents. Slowly oxidizes in air causing yellowing and changes in solubility and M.p. Shows birefringence. Dibromide, needles, M.p. 109–11, or 123–4. |
| (a) 115  (o) cis, 44.5  (p) 90.5  (s) 82.5 | (a) $-47.4^{20}$  (o) $-23.4^{20}$  (p) $-25.1^{20}$  (s) $-24.3^{20}$ | sp. s. EtOH; sl. s. acet.; s. hot EtOH, hot acet., eth., $CHCl_3$ | (a) Plates or needles from EtOH–eth.  (o) thin needles  (s) wh. plates  Exhibit mesomorphism on heating and change to turbid liq. state before melting. |
| 101 | $+ 28^{25}$ (in $CHCl_3$) | s. eth., $CHCl_3$, benz.; sl. s. MeOH; i. $H_2O$ | Found in faeces; produced by action of intestinal micro-organisms on cholesterol. Acetate, M.p. 89. Benzoate, M.p. 125. |
| Dipalmitoyl (di-$NH_4$ salt) 171–2 | | Free acid s. $CHCl_3$, K salt clear dispersion in $H_2O$ | K salt stable at low temperatures $< 0°C$ as dry solid or in aqueous dispersion. Free acid unstable in $CHCl_3$ solution at room temperature. On alkaline methanolysis gives initially cytidine monophosphate and cyclic glycerophosphate. |

## 8 Lipids and long-chain fatty acids

| Name | Synonyms | Formula | M. wt. |
|---|---|---|---|
| Diglyceride | Diacyl glycerol | 1,2 ($\alpha\beta$) $CH_2OCOR_1$ / $CHOCOR_2$ / $CH_2OH$  1,3 ($\alpha\alpha'$) $CH_2OCOR_1$ / $CHOH$ / $CH_2OCOR_2$  $R_1, R_2$ = fatty acid residues | $146.1 + R_1 + R_2$ Dimyristin 512.8 Dipalmitin 568.9 Distearin 625.0 Diolein 621.0 |
| Dihydro-cholesterol | Cholestanol; 5$\alpha$-cholestan-3$\beta$-ol | As cholesterol with saturated double bond; isomeric with coprosterol, differing in spatial configuration at carbon atom number 5 | 388.6 Hydrate, 406.6 |
| Dihydro-sphingosine | Sphinganine; *erythro*-1,3-dihydroxy-2-aminooctadecene | As sphingosine with saturated double bond | 301.5 |
| Diphospho-inositide | DPI; 1-phosphatidyl-(inositol-4-phosphate); 1,2-diacyl-*sn*-glycero-3-phosphoryl-L-1-*myo*-inositol-4-phosphate | $R_1, R_2$ = fatty acid residues | 468.2 $+ R_1 + R_2$ |
| Elaeostearic acid ($\alpha$ or *cis*, and $\beta$ or *trans*) | 9:10, 11:12, 13:14-Octadecatrienoic acid | $CH_3 \cdot (CH_2)_3 \cdot (CH=CH)_3 \cdot (CH_2)_7 \cdot COOH$ | 278.4 |
| Erucic acid (*cis* and *trans*) | 13-Docosenoic acid; *trans*-isomer, brassidic acid; *iso*erucic acid | $CH_3 \cdot (CH_2)_7 \cdot CH=CH \cdot (CH_2)_{11} \cdot COOH$ | 338.6 |

| M.p | $[\alpha]_D^t$ | Solubility | General Remarks |
|---|---|---|---|
| 1,2-dimyristin 58.9 1,2-dipalmitin 68.9 1,3-dipalmitin 69.5 1,2-distearin 76.7 1,3-distearin 79 | −3.3 (in CHCl₃) −2.9 (in CHCl₃) −2.8 (in CHCl₃) | i. H₂O; sl. s. EtOH, gl. acetic; s. eth., CHCl₃, CCl₄, pet. eth. If residues (R₁, R₂) contain unsaturation generally more soluble in organic solvents | Diglyceride in tissues or formed from phospholipids is generally 1,2 diacyl-*sn*-glycerol although 1,3 isomer can be present. Acyl migration can occur on storage especially under acid conditions. |
| 142–3 | + 27.4²⁰ (in CHCl₃) | s. CHCl₃, eth. | Hex. plates from EtOH; +1H₂O from 95% EtOH. Forms insol. digitonin complex but does not give colour reactions of cholesterol which depend on double bond. Acetate, M.p. 111. Benzoate, M.p. 135. |
| 85–7 | | s. EtOH, eth. | Col. cryst from pet. eth. and Et acetate. Occurs in cerebrosides of brain, spinal cord, and wheat flour. Tribenzoyl deriv., M.p. 142–4. Triacetyl deriv., M.p. 102–3. *N*-acetyl deriv., M.p. 122–4. |
| | | Free lipid, s. MeOH, EtOH, CHCl₃. Na salt, s. H₂O, wet CHCl₃; i. MeOH, acet., eth. | Present in mammalian nervous system. PREP. *JBC* 239, 1369 (1964). |
| *cis* α, 48–9 *trans* β, 71.5–71.8 | | *cis*, i. H₂O; s. EtOH, eth., CS₂, hot gl. acetic. *trans*, i. H₂O; sl. s. EtOH; s. hot gl. acetic, eth., CS₂ | *cis* Leaflets or needles from EtOH; *trans* plates or needles from EtOH. *cis*-Form is naturally occurring acid and is easily converted to *trans*-isomer by light, heat, catalysts such as I or S. α-Tetrabromide, M.p. 115. |
| *cis*, 33.5 *trans*, 60 | | *cis*, s. EtOH, eth. *trans*, sl. s. H₂O, EtOH; s. eth. | *cis*-Form isomerized by treatment with aq. sulphurous acid, 24 hr at 200°C. *cis*, Col. needles from EtOH. |

# 8 Lipids and long-chain fatty acids

| Name | Synonyms | Formula | M. wt. |
|------|----------|---------|--------|

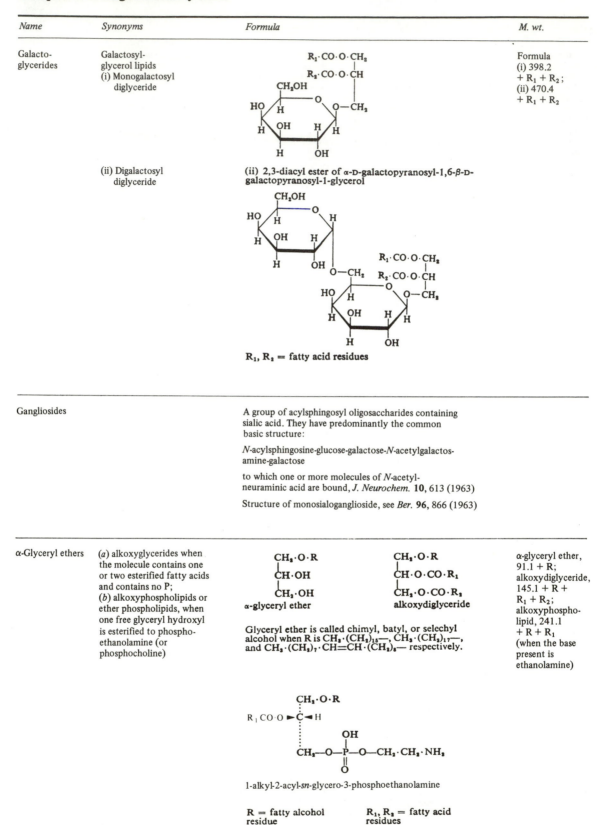

Galacto-glycerides — Galactosyl-glycerol lipids (i) Monogalactosyl diglyceride

$R_1 \cdot CO \cdot O \cdot CH_2$
$R_2 \cdot CO \cdot O \cdot CH$

Formula (i) 398.2 + $R_1$ + $R_2$; (ii) 470.4 + $R_1$ + $R_2$

(ii) Digalactosyl diglyceride

(ii) 2,3-diacyl ester of α-D-galactopyranosyl-1,6-β-D-galactopyranosyl-1-glycerol

$R_1 \cdot CO \cdot O \cdot CH_2$
$R_2 \cdot CO \cdot O \cdot CH$

$R_1, R_2$ = fatty acid residues

---

**Gangliosides**

A group of acylsphingosyl oligosaccharides containing sialic acid. They have predominantly the common basic structure:

N-acylsphingosine-glucose-galactose-N-acetylgalactos-amine-galactose

to which one or more molecules of N-acetyl-neuraminic acid are bound, *J. Neurochem.* **10**, 613 (1963)

Structure of monosialoganglioside, see *Ber.* **96**, 866 (1963)

---

**α-Glyceryl ethers** — (a) alkoxyglycerides when the molecule contains one or two esterified fatty acids and contains no P; (b) alkoxyphospholipids or ether phospholipids, when one free glyceryl hydroxyl is esterified to phospho-ethanolamine (or phosphocholine)

$CH_2 \cdot O \cdot R$
$CH \cdot OH$
$CH_2 \cdot OH$
α-glyceryl ether

$CH_2 \cdot O \cdot R$
$CH \cdot O \cdot CO \cdot R_1$
$CH_2 \cdot O \cdot CO \cdot R_2$
alkoxydiglyceride

Glyceryl ether is called chimyl, batyl, or selechyl alcohol when R is $CH_3 \cdot (CH_2)_{15}—$, $CH_3 \cdot (CH_2)_{17}—$, and $CH_3 \cdot (CH_2)_7 \cdot CH{=}CH \cdot (CH_2)_8—$ respectively.

α-glyceryl ether, 91.1 + R; alkoxydiglyceride, 145.1 + R + $R_1$ + $R_2$; alkoxyphospho-lipid, 241.1 + R + $R_1$ (when the base present is ethanolamine)

$CH_2 \cdot O \cdot R$
$R_1 CO \cdot O \blacktriangleright C \blacktriangleleft H$
$CH_2—O—\overset{OH}{\underset{O}{P}}—O—CH_2 \cdot CH_2 \cdot NH_2$

1-alkyl-2-acyl-sn-glycero-3-phosphoethanolamine

R = fatty alcohol residue          $R_1, R_2$ = fatty acid residues

| M.p | $[\alpha]_D^t$ | Solubility | General Remarks |
|---|---|---|---|
| Mono-galactosyl-glycerol, 139—40 Digalactosyl-glycerol, 182—4 | Mono-galactosyl-glycerol + 3.77[27] Digalactosyl-glycerol, + 86.4[27] | (i) s. MeOH (ii) s. $H_2O$ | Crystalline from alcohol—water mixtures. Found in lipids of green leaves, peas, wheat flour, algae. (i) Occurs in nervous tissue. In bacteria galactose can occur in furanose form; *Bacteriol. Rev.* **34**, 365 (1970). Fatty acids present include a high content of linoleic acid (wheat flour) and of linolenic acid (leaves). |
| | | Form micellar aggregates in aqueous solution | Complex lipids present in brain, spleen, and erythrocytes. |
| Chimyl alcohol, 60.5—61.5; Batyl alcohol, 70—71. (Selechyl alcohol is liquid) | | (*a*) s. in fat solvents | Glyceryl ethers and alkoxydiglycerides found in liver oils of Elasmobranch fishes, bone marrow, spleen, milk and neonatal depot fat of calves. Alkoxyphospholipids found in brain, erythrocytes, egg yolk, and slugs. |

| Name | Synonyms | Formula | M. wt. |
|------|----------|---------|--------|
| Heptadecanoic acid | Margaric; daturic; heptadecylic; heptadecoic acids | $CH_3 \cdot (CH_2)_{15} \cdot COOH$ | 270.4 |
| 2-Hydroxy-stearic acid | α-Hydroxystearic; 2-hydroxy-octadecanoic acids | $\overset{\displaystyle OH}{\underset{\displaystyle |}{}}$ $CH_3 \cdot (CH_2)_{15} \cdot CH \cdot COOH$ | 300.4 |
| 10-Hydroxy-stearic acid | Rosilic; 10-hydroxyocta-decanoic acids | $\overset{\displaystyle OH}{\underset{\displaystyle |}{}}$ $CH_3 \cdot (CH_2)_7 \cdot CH \cdot (CH_2)_8 \cdot COOH$ | 300.4 |
| Lanosterol | Lanosta-8, 24-dien-3β-ol; 4,4,14-trimethylcholesta-8,24-dien-3β-ol. | 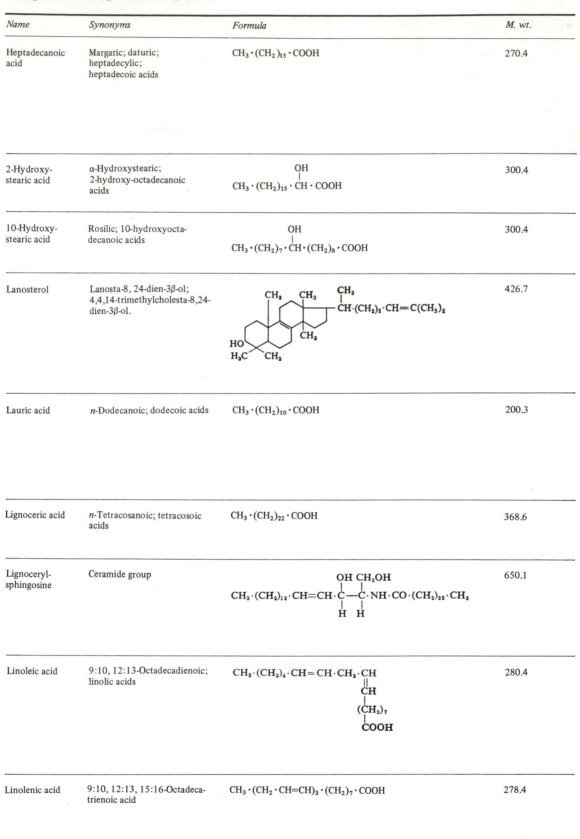 | 426.7 |
| Lauric acid | n-Dodecanoic; dodecoic acids | $CH_3 \cdot (CH_2)_{10} \cdot COOH$ | 200.3 |
| Lignoceric acid | n-Tetracosanoic; tetracosoic acids | $CH_3 \cdot (CH_2)_{22} \cdot COOH$ | 368.6 |
| Lignoceryl-sphingosine | Ceramide group | $CH_3 \cdot (CH_2)_{12} \cdot CH{=}CH \cdot \overset{OH}{\underset{H}{C}} {-} \overset{CH_2OH}{\underset{H}{C}} \cdot NH \cdot CO \cdot (CH_2)_{22} \cdot CH_3$ | 650.1 |
| Linoleic acid | 9:10, 12:13-Octadecadienoic; linolic acids | $CH_3 \cdot (CH_2)_4 \cdot CH{=}CH \cdot CH_2 \cdot CH$ $\underset{\displaystyle CH}{\overset{\displaystyle \|}{}}$ $(CH_2)_7$ $COOH$ | 280.4 |
| Linolenic acid | 9:10, 12:13, 15:16-Octadeca-trienoic acid | $CH_3 \cdot (CH_2 \cdot CH{=}CH)_3 \cdot (CH_2)_7 \cdot COOH$ | 278.4 |

| M.p | $[\alpha]_D^t$ | Solubility | General Remarks |
|---|---|---|---|
| 61.3 | | v.s. eth. At 20°C: 0.00042 $H_2O$, 9.23 benz., 2.5 MeOH, 4.17 95% EtOH, 4.28 acet., 0.12 gl. acetic | Col. plates. Traces found in many natural lipids, e.g. mutton fat, shark liver oil, butter-fat. |
| 91 | | i. $H_2O$; s. EtOH, eth.; v.s. hot benz. | Needles from $CHCl_3$. Occurs in wool wax and wheat flour cerebrosides. Me ester, M.p. 66. |
| 81–82 B.p. 213–17[4] | | i. $H_2O$; s. EtOH, eth. | Hex. plates. Present in faecal lipids. Me ester, M.p. 53–54. |
| 139 | + 60[25] (in $CHCl_3$) | i. $H_2O$; s. fat solvents | Found in small amounts in many natural lipids, e.g. wool wax, yeast, latex. Intermediate in biosynthesis of cholesterol. Acetate, M.p. 130. Benzoate, M.p. 194. |
| 44.2 B.p. 225[100] | | At 20°C: 0.0055 $H_2O$, 93.6 benz., 83 $CHCl_3$, 53 $CCl_4$, 120 MeOH, 105 EtOH, 60.5 acet., 297 gl. acetic, 52 Et acetate; v.s. eth. | Needles from EtOH. Widely distributed in animal, vegetable, and marine fats and oils. |
| 84·2 | | s. eth., EtOH, acet., benz., gl. acetic, $CS_2$ | Fine wh. crystals. Found in vegetable and marine oils. Methyl ester, M.p. 57. Ag, Pb salts, M.p. 117. |
| 94–95 | | s. eth., $CHCl_3$; sl. s. acet. | |
| −9 to −8 B.p. 230[16] | | i. $H_2O$; ∞ EtOH, eth., $CHCl_3$ | Col. or yel. oil. Takes up $O_2$ from the air forming hard glossy substance. Naturally occurring acid is the cis, cis-isomer. Found in vegetable oils, e.g. linseed. Precursor of arachidonic acid in animals. |
| α-, −17 to −16 | | α-, i. $H_2O$; s. EtOH, eth., $CHCl_3$ | Naturally occurring isomer is the α- or cis, cis, cis-form. Commonest fatty acid in green leaves and chloroplasts. |

# 8 Lipids and long-chain fatty acids

| Name | Synonyms | Formula | M. wt. |
|---|---|---|---|
| Lysolecithin ($\beta$) | 1-Acyl-sn-glycero-3-phospho-choline; lyso phosphatidyl-choline; lyso PC | $CH_2 \cdot O \cdot CO \cdot R$<br><br>$HO \blacktriangleright C \blacktriangleleft H$<br><br>$OH$<br>$CH_2 \cdot O \cdot P \cdot O \cdot CH_2 \cdot CH_2 \cdot \overset{+}{N}(CH_3)_3$<br>$\overset{\parallel}{O} \qquad OH^-$<br><br>R = fatty acid residue | Monostearoyl, 541.7; Mono-palmitoyl, 513.7 |
| 9,10-Methylene-hexadecanoic acid | | $CH_3 \cdot (CH_2)_5 \cdot CH—CH \cdot (CH_2)_7 \cdot COOH$<br>$\diagdown\diagup$<br>$CH_2$ | 268.4 |
| Monoglyceride | Monacylglycerol | $CH_2OCOR$ $\qquad$ $CH_2OH$<br><br>$CHOH$ $\qquad\quad$ $CHOCOR$<br><br>$CH_2OH$ $\qquad$ $CH_2OH$<br>1–monoglyceride $\quad$ 2–monoglyceride<br>($\alpha$) $\qquad\qquad\quad$ ($\beta$)<br><br>R =fatty acid residue | 119.1 + R<br>Monoolein 356.5<br>Monomyristin 302.3<br>Monopalmitin 330.4<br>Monostearin 358.5 |
| Myristic acid | n-Tetradecanoic; tetradecoic acids | $CH_3 \cdot (CH_2)_{12} \cdot COOH$ | 228.4 |
| Nervonic acid | 15:16- Tetracosenoic acid; selacholeic acid | $CH_3 \cdot (CH_2)_7 \cdot CH = CH \cdot (CH_2)_{13} \cdot COOH$ | 366.6 |
| Oleic acid | cis-9:10-Octadecenoic acid; trans-isomer, elaidic acid | $CH_3 \cdot (CH_2)_7 \cdot CH = CH \cdot (CH_2)_7 \cdot COOH$ | 282.5 |
| Oleoyl alcohol | cis-9:10-Octadecenol | $CH_3 \cdot (CH_2)_7 \cdot CH = CH \cdot (CH_2)_7 \cdot CH_2OH$ | 268.5 |
| Palmitaldehyde | Hexadecanal | $CH_3 \cdot (CH_2)_{14} \cdot CHO$ | 240.4 |
| Palmitic acid | n-Hexadecanoic; hexadecoic acids | $CH_3 \cdot (CH_2)_{14} \cdot COOH$ | 256.4 |
| Palmitoleic acid | 9:10-Hexadecenoic acid; zoomaric acid | $CH_3 \cdot (CH_2)_5 \cdot CH = CH \cdot (CH_2)_7 \cdot COOH$ | 254.4 |

| M.p | $[\alpha]_D^t$ | Solubility | General Remarks |
|---|---|---|---|
| Monopalmitoyl, 195—6; Mono-stearoyl, 257.5—8.5 | Mono-palmitoyl, $-2.2^{25}$; Mono-stearoyl, $-2.87^{25}$ (in MeOH/CHCl$_3$) | Emulsifies in H$_2$O; i. eth.; sp. s. acet.; s. EtOH, gl. acetic, CHCl$_3$, pyr. | Monostearoyl, needles. Labile in M-KOH at 37°C. Isolated enzymically with the fatty acid on the l-carbon atom of the glycerol. Shows detergent-like properties. |
| SYN. Me ester, B.p. 140$^{0.8}$ | | i. H$_2$O; s. fat solvents | Present in lipids of some bacteria together with other cyclopropane fatty acids, e.g. *E. coli*. Amide, M.p. (ISOL.) 70—72, (SYN.) 79—81. |
| 1-Monoolein 35 1-Monopalmitin 71—2 2-Monopalmitin 68.5 1-Monostearin 76—7 2-Monostearin 74.4 | $-4.4$ (in pyr.) $-3.58$ (in pyr.) | i. H$_2$O (disperses), sl. s. EtOH, MeOH, s. eth., CHCl$_3$, CCl$_4$ If residue (R) contains unsaturation generally more soluble in organic solvents. | Acyl migration can readily occur, with fall in optical rotation. Formed during intestinal digestion of fats (triglycerides). |
| 52—53 B.p. 249$^{100}$ | | At 20°C: 0.002 H$_2$O, 29.2 benz., 32.5 CHCl$_3$, 17.6 CCl$_4$, 17.3 MeOH, 23.9 EtOH, 15.9 acet., 10.2 gl. acetic, 15.3 Et acetate; sp. s. eth. | Waxy leaflets. Widely distributed in natural oils and fats. |
| cis, 39 trans, 61 | | s. EtOH, CHCl$_3$, acet. | *cis* Wh. needles. Occurs in marine oils and brain lipids; naturally occurring is *cis*-form. |
| cis, α, 13.4 β, 16.3 trans, 44.5 | | cis, trans, i. H$_2$O; s. EtOH, benz., CHCl$_3$, eth., MeOH, acet. | *cis* Col. needles, *trans* leaflets. *Cis-trans* conversion catalysed by nitrogen oxides, sulphurous acid, S, P, and Se. The cryst. form melting at 13.4 changes slowly to the stable form melting at 16·3. Dibromo compounds: oleic, M.p. 28.5—9; elaidic, M.p. 29—30. Ca salt, M.p. 83—84. Na salt, M.p. 230—5. |
| 2 B.p. 209$^{15}$ | | i. H$_2$O; s. EtOH, eth., CHCl$_3$ | Constituent of marine oils. |
| 34 | | i. H$_2$O; s. eth., acet., pet. eth., EtOH | Can be formed from plasmalogens on acid hydrolysis. Polymerizes on keeping to trimeride, M.p. 73. Oxime M.p. 88. Semicarbazone, M.p. 107. |
| 63.1 B.p. 211.5$^{10}$ | | i. H$_2$O; s. eth. At 20°C: 7.3 benz., 15.1 CHCl$_3$, 5.8 CCl$_4$, 3.7 MeOH, 7.21 EtOH, 5.4 acet., 2.1 gl. acetic, 6.1 Et acetate | Waxy needles. Widespread occurrence in plant and animal lipids. Ca salt, M.p. 153—6. Na salt, M.p. 270. |
| $-0.5$ to 0.5 (cis) | | s. CHCl$_3$, eth., benz. | A major component of many vegetable and animal fats. |

# 8 Lipids and long-chain fatty acids

| Name | Synonyms | Formula | M. wt. |
|---|---|---|---|
| Pelargonic acid | *n*-Nonanoic, nonylic acids | $CH_3 \cdot (CH_2)_7 \cdot COOH$ | 158.2 |
| Pentadecanoic acid | Pentadecylic acid | $CH_3 \cdot (CH_2)_{13} \cdot COOH$ | 242.4 |
| Phosphatidic acid | 1,2-Diacyl-*sn*-glycero-3-phosphate; L-α-phosphatidic acid. | $R_1.R_2 =$ fatty acid residues | $226.1 + R_1 + R_2$. Dimyristoyl, 592.5; Di-palmitoyl, 648.6; Distearoyl, 704.6 |
| Phosphatidyl-choline | PC; lecithin; 3-*sn*-phosphatidyl-choline; 1,2-diacyl-*sn*-glycero-3-phosphocholine | $R_1, R_2 =$ saturated or unsaturated fatty acid residues. | $329.3 + R_1 + R_2$ |
| Phosphatidyl-ethanolamine | PE; cephalin; 1,2-diacyl-*sn*-glycero-3-phospho-*O*-ethanolamine | $R_1, R_2 =$ fatty acid residues | $269.2 + R_1 + R_2$ |
| Phosphatidyl-glycerol | PG; 1,2-diacyl-*sn*-glycero-3-phospho-1'-*sn*-glycerol | $R_1, R_2 =$ fatty acid residues | $300.1 + R_1 + R_2$ |

| M.p | $[\alpha]_D^t$ | Solubility | General Remarks |
|---|---|---|---|
| 12–12.5<br>B.p. 180[100]<br>254[760] | | At 20°C: 0.026 $H_2O$;<br>∞ benz., hexane, acet.,<br>Et acetate, MeOH | Product of oxidative cleavage of oleic acid. |
| 52.3<br>B.p. 202–5[10] | | At 20°C: 0.0012 $H_2O$,<br>36.2 benz., 16.4 MeOH,<br>19.5 95% EtOH,<br>13.8 acet., 8.8 gl. acetic,<br>15.4 Et acetate,<br>22.3 Bu acetate | Cryst. waxy solid. Traces found in many natural lipids, e.g. butter-fat, mutton fat, shark liver oil. |
| | Dimyristoyl-<br>3-sn, + 4.4[24]<br>(in $CHCl_3$);<br>Dipalmitoyl-<br>3-sn, + 4.0[26]<br>(in $CHCl_3$);<br>Distearoyl-<br>3-sn, + 3.8[26]<br>(in $CHCl_3$) | ISOL. i. $H_2O$, EtOH;<br>s. acet., eth., $CHCl_3$.<br>SYN. i. $H_2O$; sl. s. EtOH;<br>sp. s. acet.; s. $CHCl_3$,<br>benz. | On acid hydrolysis α-phosphatidic acid yields α- and β- glycerophosphoric acid. On alkaline hydrolysis no migration of the phosphate group. Intermediate in the biosynthesis of phosphoglycerides but only traces present in tissues. |
| ISOL. (from lung),<br>sinters 75–80,<br>melts 237–8.<br>SYN. Di-<br>myristoyl-<br>sinters 90, melts<br>236–7;<br>Dipalmitoyl-<br>sinters 120, melts<br>235–6;<br>Distearoyl<br>sinters 120, melts<br>230–2 | All as 3-sn-<br>phosphatidyl<br>choline.<br>ISOL. (from<br>lung), + 6.25<br>(in MeOH/<br>$CHCl_3$).<br>Dipalmitoleoyl-<br>+ 6.6 ($CHCl_3$/<br>MeOH, 1:1)<br>SYN. Di-<br>myristoyl-<br>+ 7.0[24]<br>(in EtOH/<br>$CHCl_3$);<br>Dipalmitoyl-<br>+ 7.0[25]<br>(in $CHCl_3$);<br>Distearoyl-<br>+ 6.1 (in<br>MeOH/$CHCl_3$) | i. acet., Me acetate;<br>s. EtOH, eth., pet. eth.,<br>$CS_2$, $CHCl_3$, $CCl_4$, benz.<br>Dipalmitoleoyl,<br>i. pet. eth.<br>$R_1R_2$ both saturated.<br>i. eth.; sl. s. acet.;<br>s. EtOH, gl. acetic, $CHCl_3$ | Dipalmitoyl, needles from diisobutylketone. Hygr., waxy, plastic-like solid, turns brown in air. Solubility data depend on the absence of other lipids. Labile in M-alkali at 37°C and methanolic alkali at room temperature. Occurs naturally as L-α-isomer, i.e. 3-sn-phosphatidylcholine. |
| Dimyristoyl-<br>3-sn, sinters<br>86, melts 175–7;<br>Distearoyl-<br>3-sn, sinters<br>83 melts 173–5;<br>Dipalmitoyl-<br>3-sn, sinters<br>88, melts<br>172.5–5.0 | Dimyristoyl-<br>3-sn, + 6.0[26]<br>(in $CHCl_3$);<br>Distearoyl-<br>3-sn, + 6.0[24]<br>(in $CHCl_3$-<br>gl. acetic<br>9:1);<br>Dipalmitoyl-<br>3-sn, + 6.4[26]<br>(in $CHCl_3$) | ISOL. i. acet.; s. MeOH,<br>EtOH, $CHCl_3$,<br>benz., wet eth.,<br>pet. eth.<br>SYN. (saturated).<br>i. acet., eth., pet.<br>eth.; sl. s. EtOH,<br>benz., $CCl_4$; s. $CHCl_3$,<br>pyr. | Hygr.; isolated compound quickly becomes brown due to autoxidation. Solubility data depend on absence of other lipids. Labile in M-alkali at 37°C. Occurs naturally as L-α or 3-sn isomer. |
| Distearoyl-3-sn-<br>66.5–67.0 | Distearoyl-<br>3-sn, + 2.0[22]<br>(in $CHCl_3$);<br>Dioleoyl-<br>3-sn, + 2.0[21]<br>(in $CHCl_3$) | Emulsifies in $H_2O$;<br>s. EtOH, eth., $CHCl_3$,<br>acet., benz., MeOH | Found mainly in plants but traces in animal tissues. |

| Name | Synonyms | Formula | M. wt. |
|---|---|---|---|
| Phosphatidyl-1-inositol | Monophosphoinositide; PI; 1,2-diacyl-*sn*-glycero-3-phospho-1-*myo*-inositol | | $388.2 + R_1 + R_2$ |
| Phosphatidyl-serine | PS; 1,2-diacyl-*sn*-glycero-3-phospho-*O*-serine | | $313.2 + R_1 + R_2$ |
| Phytanic acid | 3,7,11,15-Tetramethyl-hexadecanoic acid | | 312.5 |
| Plasmalogens | Formerly called acetal phosphatides, phosphatidal-ethanolamine (-serine, -choline) EP, SP, CP (a) 1-alk-1'-enyl-2-acyl-*sn*-glycero-3-phospho-*O*-ethanolamine (-serine, -choline) | | (a) $267.2 + R + R'$ (b) $240.2 + R$ |

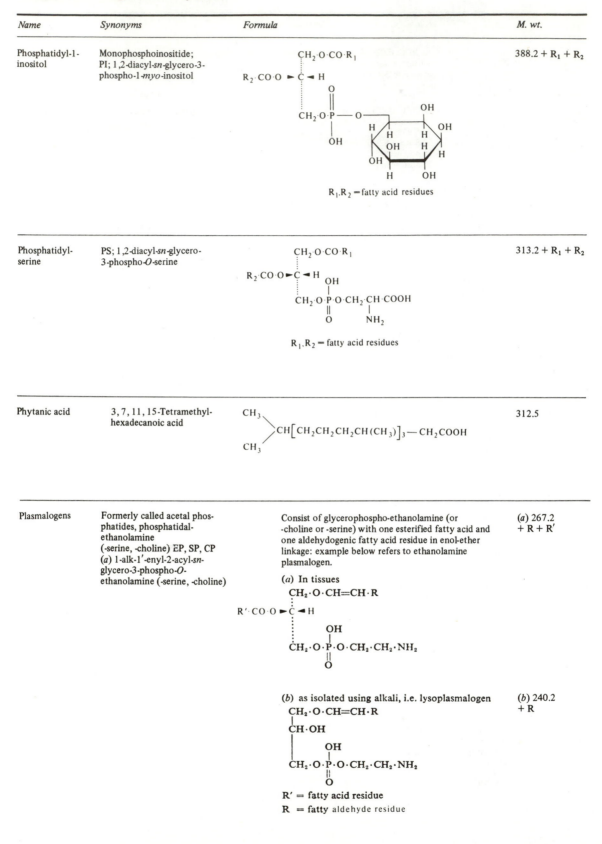

Phosphatidyl-1-inositol:
$$CH_2 \cdot O \cdot CO \cdot R_1$$
$$R_2 \cdot CO \cdot O \blacktriangleright C \blacktriangleleft H$$
$$CH_2 \cdot O \cdot P$$
$R_1, R_2 =$ fatty acid residues

Phosphatidyl-serine:
$$CH_2 \cdot O \cdot CO \cdot R_1$$
$$R_2 \cdot CO \cdot O \blacktriangleright C \blacktriangleleft H \quad OH$$
$$CH_2 \cdot O \cdot P \cdot O \cdot CH_2 \cdot CH \cdot COOH$$
$$O \qquad NH_2$$
$R_1, R_2 =$ fatty acid residues

Phytanic acid:
$$\begin{matrix} CH_3 \\ \quad \quad CH[CH_2CH_2CH_2CH(CH_3)]_3 - CH_2COOH \\ CH_3 \end{matrix}$$

Plasmalogens — Consist of glycerophospho-ethanolamine (or -choline or -serine) with one esterified fatty acid and one aldehydogenic fatty acid residue in enol-ether linkage: example below refers to ethanolamine plasmalogen.

(a) In tissues
$$CH_2 \cdot O \cdot CH{=}CH \cdot R$$
$$R' \cdot CO \cdot O \blacktriangleright C \blacktriangleleft H$$
$$OH$$
$$CH_2 \cdot O \cdot P \cdot O \cdot CH_2 \cdot CH_2 \cdot NH_2$$
$$O$$

(b) as isolated using alkali, i.e. lysoplasmalogen
$$CH_2 \cdot O \cdot CH{=}CH \cdot R$$
$$CH \cdot OH$$
$$OH$$
$$CH_2 \cdot O \cdot P \cdot O \cdot CH_2 \cdot CH_2 \cdot NH_2$$
$$O$$
R′ = fatty acid residue
R = fatty aldehyde residue

| M.p | $[\alpha]_D^t$ | Solubility | General Remarks |
|---|---|---|---|
| | Liver, + 5.60[25] | s. $H_2O$, $CHCl_3$, benz.; sl. s. MeOH, eth., pet. eth.; i. 95% EtOH, acet., Et acetate | Wh. amorph. solid. Cryst. Na salt. Ba salt insoluble in $H_2O$ but soluble in $CHCl_3$/MeOH (3:1 v/v). Occurs in most plant and animal membranes. |
| Distearoyl-3-sn, sinters 120, melts 159—61 | See *J B C* **212**, 25 (1955) | ISOL. (Na, K salt) emulsifies in $H_2O$; i. EtOH, MeOH, acet.; s. $CHCl_3$, eth., pet. eth. SYN. s. $CHCl_3$ only | Salt only stable when stored in $CHCl_3$ at $-72°$ C. Free acid more stable. Labile in methanolic M-NaOH at $37°$ C. Isolated lipid usually contains serine-containing plasmalogen. |
| −65 | | Similar to unsaturated fatty acids. i. $H_2O$; v.s. eth., $CHCl_3$, EtOH. | Review: *Progress in Chemistry of fats and other lipids* ed. R.T. Holman (1973) **14** part (1), p5. Found in ruminant fats, halobacteria, and accumulates in Refsum's disease. |
| | | (a) emulsifies in $H_2O$; s. $CHCl_3$, MeOH, eth. | (a) Converted to (b) structure by incubation in methanolic M-NaOH at $37°$C, but this deacylation is not so rapid as with diacyl phospholipids (*J. Neurochem.* **10**, 941 (1963)). The alk-1′-enyl grouping has the *cis*-configuration. |
| (b) muscle, 160—90 | (b) muscle, −8.6[26] (c = 4 in $CHCl_3$ : MeOH (1:1 v/v)) | (b) i. $H_2O$; sl. s. EtOH, eth., pet. eth., acet., benz.; s. hot MeOH, hot EtOH, $CHCl_3$ | (b) Stable in M-NaOH at $37°$ C. Labile in acids at room temp. Many early preparations produced the cyclic acetal. |

# 8 Lipids and long-chain fatty acids

| Name | Synonyms | Formula | M. wt. |
|---|---|---|---|
| Ricinoleic acid | 12-Hydroxy-*cis*-9:10-octa-decenoic acid; ricinolic acid | $CH_3 \cdot (CH_2)_5 \cdot CH \cdot CH_2 \cdot CH{=}CH$<br>     $\underset{OH}{\mid}$    $\underset{(CH_2)_7}{\mid}$<br>           $\underset{COOH}{\mid}$ | 298.5 |
| Sitosterols ($\alpha_1$-, $\beta$-) | | ($\alpha_1$) | $\alpha_1$, 412.7 |
| | $\beta$-, 22-Dihydrostigmasterol; $\Delta^5$-stigmastene-3$\beta$-ol | ($\beta$) | $\beta$, 414.7 |
| Sphingomyelin | Ceramide-1-phosphocholine; *N*-acyl-*erythro*-sphingosine-1-phosphocholine | $R \cdot CO \cdot NH{-}$<br>$CH_3 \cdot (CH_2)_{12} \cdot CH{=}CH \cdot CH(OH) \cdot CH \cdot CH_2$<br>$\underset{OH^-}{(CH_3)_3\overset{+}{N} \cdot (CH_2)_2 \cdot O \cdot \underset{OH}{\overset{O}{P}}{=}O}$<br>R = fatty acid residue | 509.6 + R |
| Sphingosine | 4-Sphingenine; *trans*-D-*erythro*-1,3-dihydroxy-2-amino-4:5-octadecene | $CH_3 \cdot (CH_2)_{12} \cdot CH{=}CH \cdot CH(OH)CHNH_2$<br>            $\underset{CH_2OH}{\mid}$ | 299.5 |
| —sulphate | | $C_{18}H_{37}NO_2 \cdot H_2SO_4$ | 397.6 |
| Squalene | Spinacene | | 410.7 |
| Stearaldehyde | Octadecanal | $CH_3 \cdot (CH_2)_{16} \cdot CHO$ | 268.5 |

| M.p | $[\alpha]_D^t$ | Solubility | General Remarks |
|---|---|---|---|
| *cis*, 5·5 (*trans*, 53) | $+6\cdot4^{22}$ (in acet.) | | Occurs in castor oil as the triglyceride triricinolein. Absolute configuration, see *Chem. Ind.* **1958**, 1554. |
| $\alpha_1$, 164—6 | $\alpha_1$, $-1.7^{28}$ (in $CHCl_3$) | $\alpha_1$, s. $CHCl_3$, eth. | $\alpha_1$, $\beta$ both needles from EtOH. Occurs in wheat germ and soya-bean oils. Precipitated by digitonin. $\alpha_1$-form: Acetate, M.p. 137. Benzoate, M.p. 172. |
| $\beta$, 136—8 | $\beta$, $-37.8^{25}$ (in $CHCl_3$) | $\beta$, s. $CHCl_3$ | $\beta$-form: Acetate, M.p. 123—4. Benzoate, M.p. 145—6. |
| 196—8 (209) | $+6$ to 7 (in $CHCl_3$/ MeOH) | i. eth., acet., $H_2O$; s. benz., $CHCl_3$, hot EtOH, hot Et acetate | Wh. cryst. Stable on incubation in M-NaOH at 37° C but hydrolyses at higher temperatures. Hydrolysed in methanolic HCl at 100° C producing phosphocholine and a little sphingosylphosphocholine. |
| 82·5—83 | Free base, $+3^{25}$ (26 mg in 2 ml pyr.) | i. $H_2O$; s. $CHCl_3$, EtOH, acet., MeOH. | Free base, needles from pet. eth. Sulphate, rosettes of needles from EtOH; v. hygr. Triacetyl deriv., M.p. 101—2. |
| Sulphate, 240—50 (149—52) | Sulphate, $-13.12^{20}$ (in $CHCl_3$) | Sulphate, s. $CHCl_3$, hot EtOH containing $H_2SO_4$ | |
| below $-20$ B.p. $213^1$ | | s. eth., $CHCl_3$; sp. s. EtOH, gl. acetic | Col. mobile oil. Intermediate in cholesterol biosynthesis. Found in many tissues in traces, but in appreciable amount in some marine liver oils. Hexahydrochlorides, M.p. 108—10, 144—5. |
| 63.5 (38), polymerizes very rapidly so M.p. unreliable | | i. $H_2O$; s. EtOH, eth., pet. eth., acet. | Scales from eth. Can be formed from plasmalogen on acid hydrolysis. Polymerizes very rapidly on keeping. |

# 8 Lipids and long-chain fatty acids

| Name | Synonyms | Formula | M. wt. |
|------|----------|---------|--------|
| Stearic acid | *n*-Octadecanoic; octadecoic acids | $CH_3 \cdot (CH_2)_{16} \cdot COOH$ | 284.4 |
| Triglyceride | Triacyl glycerol | 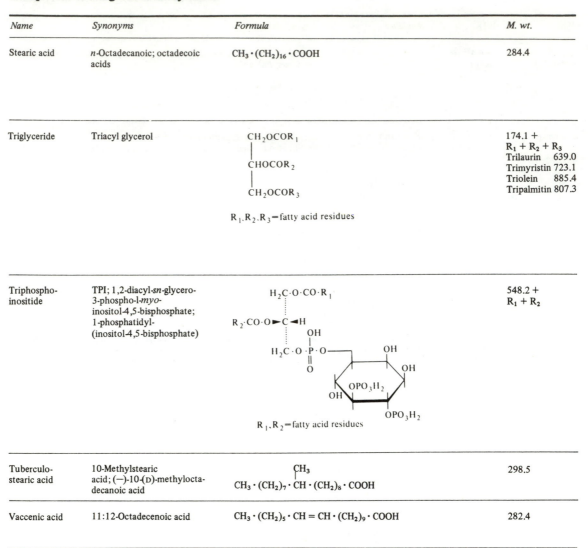 | 174.1 + $R_1 + R_2 + R_3$ <br> Trilaurin 639.0 <br> Trimyristin 723.1 <br> Triolein 885.4 <br> Tripalmitin 807.3 |
| Triphospho-inositide | TPI; 1,2-diacyl-*sn*-glycero-3-phospho-l-*myo*-inositol-4,5-bisphosphate; 1-phosphatidyl-(inositol-4,5-bisphosphate) | | 548.2 + $R_1 + R_2$ |
| Tuberculo-stearic acid | 10-Methylstearic acid; (−)-10-(D)-methylocta-decanoic acid | $CH_3 \cdot (CH_2)_7 \cdot \overset{\displaystyle CH_3}{CH} \cdot (CH_2)_8 \cdot COOH$ | 298.5 |
| Vaccenic acid | 11:12-Octadecenoic acid | $CH_3 \cdot (CH_2)_5 \cdot CH = CH \cdot (CH_2)_9 \cdot COOH$ | 282.4 |

For the Triglyceride structure:

$$CH_2OCOR_1$$
$$CHOCOR_2$$
$$CH_2OCOR_3$$

$R_1.R_2.R_3 = $ fatty acid residues

For the Triphospho-inositide structure:

$H_2C \cdot O \cdot CO \cdot R_1$
$R_2 \cdot CO \cdot O \blacktriangleright C \blacktriangleleft H$
OH
$H_2C \cdot O \cdot P \cdot O$
$\|$
$O$
OH
OH
$OPO_3H_2$
OH
$OPO_3H_2$

$R_1.R_2 = $ fatty acid residues

| M.p | $[\alpha]_D^t$ | Solubility | General Remarks |
|---|---|---|---|
| 69.6<br>B.p. 213.0[5] | | i. H$_2$O; s. eth. At 20°C:<br>2.5 benz., 6.0 CHCl$_3$,<br>2.4 CCl$_4$, 0.1 MeOH,<br>2.25 EtOH, 1.54 acet.,<br>0.12 gl. acetic,<br>0.5 Et acetate | Widely distributed in natural oils and fats; notably high content in depot fats of ruminants. Ca salt, M.p. 150—4. Na salt, M.p. 260. |
| Trimyristin<br>$\alpha$ 32<br>$\beta$ prime 44<br>$\beta$ 55.5<br>Triolein<br>$\alpha$ — 32<br>$\beta$ prime — 13<br>$\beta$ 3.8 (5.5)<br>Tripalmitin<br>$\alpha$ 44<br>$\beta$ prime 55.5<br>$\beta$ 65.5 | | i. H$_2$O,<br>sl. s. EtOH, MeOH;<br>s. eth., CHCl$_3$,<br>CCl$_4$, pet. eth.<br>If any residues<br>(R$_1$, R$_2$, R$_3$)<br>contain unsaturation<br>generally more soluble<br>in organic solvents. | Can exist in polymorphic forms.<br>Occurs widely in fat depots of animals and higher plants. |
| | | Free lipid, s. H$_2$O,<br>MeOH, EtOH, CHCl$_3$.<br>Na salt, s. H$_2$O,<br>wet CHCl$_3$; i. MeOH,<br>acet., eth. | Sodium salt (Na$_4$) stable when stored in moist CHCl$_3$ at −18° C, free acid slowly decomposes. Present in mammaliam nervous systems largely as stearoyl arachidonoyl species. PREP. *JBC* **239**, 1369 (1964). |
| 12.8—13.4<br>B.p. 175—8[0.7] | −0.08[19] | i. H$_2$O; s. fat solvents | Found in human and bovine tubercle wax and in leprosy bacilli.<br>Amide, M.p. 76·5—77. Tribromanilide, M.p. 93—94. |
| *cis*, 6.8<br>*trans*, 42.5 | | i. H$_2$O; s. CHCl$_3$, acet., eth. | *trans*-Isomer present in butter, beef fat. *cis*-Isomer present in lipids of many bacteria. |

## Retention volumes of methyl esters of the long-chain fatty acids relative to methyl palmitate

(From A. T. James, *Meth. Biochem. Anal.* 8, 1 (1960) with additions by J. H. Recourt, Unilever Research Laboratory, Vlaardingen, Holland.)

| | | Stationary phase | | | | |
|---|---|---|---|---|---|---|
| *Acid (chemical or trivial name)* | *Shorthand designation* | *Apiezon L at 197°C* | *Apiezon M at 197°C* | *Reoplex 400 at 197°C* | *Polyethylene glycol adipate at 180°C* | *Poly-diethylene glycol succinate at 203°C* |
| *n*-Pentanoic | 5:0 | 0·008 | .. | .. | .. | .. |
| *n*-Hexanoic | 6:0 | 0·013 | .. | .. | .. | .. |
| 4-Methylhexanoic | a.i.br. 7:0 | 0·017 | .. | .. | .. | .. |
| *n*-Heptanoic | 7:0 | 0·019 | .. | .. | .. | .. |
| 6-Methylheptanoic | a.i.br. 8:0 | 0·024 | .. | .. | .. | .. |
| *n*-Octanoic | 8:0 | 0·030 | .. | .. | 0·060 | .. |
| 6-Methyloctanoic | a.i.br. 9:0 | 0·041 | .. | .. | .. | .. |
| *n*-Nonanoic | 9:0 | 0·047 | .. | .. | 0·082 | .. |
| 8-Methylnonanoic | i.br. 10:0 | 0·061 | .. | .. | .. | .. |
| *n*-Decanoic | 10:0 | 0·073 | 0·069 | 0·179 | 0·134 | .. |
| 8-Methyldecanoic | a.i.br. 11:0 | 0·10 | .. | .. | .. | .. |
| *n*-Undecanoic | 11:0 | 0·117 | 0·112 | 0·232 | 0·183 | .. |
| 10-Methylundecanoic | i.br. 12:0 | 0·15 | .. | .. | .. | .. |
| *n*-Dodecanoic | 12:0 | 0·18 | 0·18 | 0·286 | 0·26 | 0·36 |
| 10-Methyldodecanoic | a.i.br. 13·0 | 0·242 | .. | .. | .. | .. |
| Undefined branched tri-decanoic | br. 13:0 | .. | 0·203 0·234 | .. | .. | .. |
| *n*-Tridecanoic | 13:0 | 0·250 | 0·267 | 0·388 | 0·362 | .. |
| *n*-Tetradecatrienoic | 14:3 | 0·291 | .. | .. | 0·90 | .. |
| *n*-Tetradecadienoic | 14:2 | .. | .. | .. | .. | .. |
| *n*-Tetradecenoic | 14:1 | 0·39 | 0·38 | 0·634 | 0·615 | .. |
| Undefined branched tetra-decanoic | br. 14:0 | .. | 0·37 | .. | .. | .. |
| *n*-Tetradecanoic | 14:0 | 0·42 | 0·416 | 0·555 | 0·51 | 0·60 |
| Undefined branched penta-decanoic | br. 15:0 | 0·55 | 0·548 | .. | .. | .. |
| 12-Methyltetradecanoic | a.i.br. 15:0 | 0·58 | .. | .. | .. | .. |
| Undefined branched penta-decanoic | br. 15:0 | .. | 0·52 | .. | .. | .. |
| *n*-Pentadecanoic | 15:0 | 0·66 | 0·65 | .. | 0·705 | .. |
| $\Delta^{6,9,12,15}$-Hexadecatetra-enoic | $16:4^{6,9,12,15}$ | .. | 0·74 | 1·97 | .. | .. |
| $\Delta^{6,9,12}$-Hexadecatrienoic | $16:3^{6,9,12}$ | .. | 0·77 | 1·59 | .. | .. |
| $\Delta^{9,12}$-Hexadecadienoic | $16:2^{9,12}$ | .. | 0·79 | 1·39 | .. | .. |
| $\Delta^{6,9}$-Hexadecadienoic | $16:2^{6,9}$ | .. | 0·86 | 1·28 | .. | .. |
| $\Delta^{9}$-Hexadecenoic | $16:1^{9}$ | .. | 0·89 | 1·13 | .. | .. |
| *cis*-$\Delta^{9}$-Hexadecenoic | *cis*-$16:1^{9}$ | 0·90 | 0·89 | 1·13 | 1·15 | 1·17 |
| *trans*-$\Delta^{9}$-Hexadecenoic | *trans*-$16:1^{9}$ | 0·92 | .. | .. | 1·15 | .. |
| *n*-Hexadecanoic | 16:0 | 1·0 | 1·0 | 1·0 | 1·0 | 1·0 |
| Dihydrohydnocarpic | .. | 1·43* | .. | .. | 1·66† | .. |
| *n*-Heptadecenoic | 17:1 | 1·31 | .. | .. | 1·62 | .. |
| 14-Methylheptadecanoic | a.i.br. 17:0 | 1·38 | .. | .. | .. | .. |
| *n*-Heptadecanoic | 17:0 | 1·51 | 1·55 | 1·32 | 1·40 | .. |
| $\Delta^{6,9,12,15}$-Octadecatetra-enoic | $18:4^{6,9,12,15}$ | .. | 1·72 | 3·48 | .. | .. |
| All-*cis*-$\Delta^{9,12,15}$-octadeca-trienoic | *cis*-$18:3^{9,12,15}$ | 1·93 | 1·84 | 2·95 | 3·51 | .. |

\* column at 205°C.          † column at 175°C.

| Acid (chemical or trivial name) | Shorthand designation | Stationary phase | | | | |
|---|---|---|---|---|---|---|
| | | Apiezon L at 197°C | Apiezon M at 197°C | Reoplex 400 at 197°C | Polyethylene glycol adipate at 180°C | Poly-diethylene glycol succinate at 203°C |
| All-cis-$\Delta^{6,9,12}$-octadeca-trienoic | cis-18:3$^{6,9,12}$ | 1·76* | .. | .. | 2·84† | .. |
| cis-trans-trans-$\Delta^{9,11,13}$-Octadecatrienoic | cis-trans-trans-18:3$^{9,11,13}$ | 3·82 | .. | .. | .. | .. |
| All-trans-$\Delta^{9,11,13}$-octa-decatrienoic | trans-18:3$^{9,11,13}$ | 4·44 | .. | .. | .. | .. |
| cis-cis-$\Delta^{9,12}$-Octadeca-dienoic | cis-18:2$^{9,12}$ | 1·9 | 1·81 | 2·38 | 2·69 | 2·40 |
| cis-trans-$\Delta^{9,11}$-Octadeca-dienoic | cis-trans-18:2$^{9,11}$ | 2·56 | .. | .. | .. | .. |
| trans-cis-$\Delta^{10,12}$-Octadeca-dienoic | trans-cis-18:2$^{10,12}$ | 2·56 | .. | .. | .. | .. |
| All-trans-$\Delta^{9,11}$-octadeca-dienoic | trans-18:2$^{9,11}$ | 3·09 | .. | .. | .. | .. |
| All-trans-$\Delta^{10,12}$-octadeca-dienoic | trans-18:2$^{10,12}$ | 3·09 | .. | .. | .. | .. |
| $\Delta^{6,9}$-Octadecadienoic | 18:2$^{6,9}$ | .. | 1·81 | 2·56 | .. | 1·93 |
| cis-$\Delta^{9}$-Octadecenoic | cis-18:1$^{9}$ | 2·03 | 2·08 | 2·02 | 2·21 | 1·93 |
| trans-$\Delta^{9}$-Octadecenoic | trans-18:1$^{9}$ | 2·12 | .. | .. | 2·21 | .. |
| cis-$\Delta^{6}$-Octadecenoic | cis-18:1$^{6}$ | 2·09 | .. | .. | 2·22 | .. |
| cis-$\Delta^{4}$-Octadecenoic | cis-18:1$^{4}$ | 2·12 | .. | .. | 2·23 | .. |
| trans-$\Delta^{4}$-Octadecenoic | trans-18:1$^{4}$ | 2·22 | .. | .. | .. | .. |
| n-Octadecanoic | 18:0 | 2·36 | 2·39 | 1·79 | 1·97 | 1·66 |
| Dihydrochaulmoogric | .. | 3·52* | .. | .. | 3·18† | .. |
| All-cis-$\Delta^{7,10,13}$-nona-decatrienoic | cis-19:3$^{7,10,13}$ | 2·62* | .. | .. | 3·85† | .. |
| All-cis-$\Delta^{10,13}$-nona-decadienoic | cis-19:2$^{10,13}$ | 2·92* | .. | .. | 3·48† | .. |
| n-Nonadecanoic | 19:0 | .. | .. | .. | .. | .. |
| $\Delta^{5,8,11,14,17}$-Eicosapenta-enoic | 20:5$^{5,8,11,14,17}$ | 3·48 | 3·48 | 6·64 | 8·5 | .. |
| $\Delta^{8,11,14,17}$-Eicosatetraenoic | 20:4$^{8,11,14,17}$ | .. | 3·48 | 5·35 | .. | .. |
| Arachidonic | 20:4$^{5,8,11,14}$ | 3·48 | 3·48 | 5·28 | 6·56 | .. |
| Undefined eicosatrienoic | 20:3 | 3·65 | 3·92 | 4·80 | 5·96 | .. |
| Undefined | 20:2 | .. | 4·5 | 3·88 | .. | .. |
| | 20:1 | .. | 4·75 | 3·57 | .. | .. |
| | 20:0 | 5·8 | 5·83 | 3·15 | 3·87 | .. |
| | 21:0 | .. | 8·72 | .. | .. | .. |
| | 22:6$^{4,7,10,13,16,19}$ | 7·15 | 7·15 | 13·5 | 18·2 | .. |
| | 22:5$^{5,8,11,14,17}$ | .. | 7·88 | 12·2 | .. | .. |
| | 22:1 | 10·9 | .. | .. | 8·15 | .. |
| | 22:0 | .. | 14·2 | 6·8 | .. | 4·67 |
| | 26:0 | .. | .. | .. | .. | 13·8 |

\* column at 205°C.　　　　† column at 175°C.

# 9 Steroids

## Nomenclature

'Rules for steroid nomenclature', *Pure Applied Chemistry* **31**, 283 (1972); *BJ* **113**, 5 (1969); *BJ* **127**, 613 (1972).

## Analytical methods

1. E. Heftmann (Ed.) *Modern methods of steroid analysis,* Academic Press (1973).
2. H. Breuer, D. Hamel, and H. R. Kruskemper (Eds.) *Methods of hormone analysis,* John Wiley (1976).
3. J. J. Ryan. Chromatographic analysis of hormone residues in food, *J. Chromatog.* **127**, 53–89 (1976).
4. S. Gorog and G. Szasz. *Analysis of steroid hormone drugs,* Elsevier (1978).

## Biological data

### General

Further details concerning the pharmacology of steroid hormones can be found in *The Merck index of chemicals and drugs,* Merck & Co. Inc., Rahway, NJ, USA, and in Martindale: *The extra pharmacopoeia,* The Pharmaceutical Press, London.

### Reference standards and isotope labelled steroids

1. A wide range of steroids are now available commercially. Two companies specializing in steroids are Steraloids Inc., Wilton, NH, 03086, USA, and IKapharm, PO Box 31, Ramat-Gan, Israel.
2. Small quantities of steroids are also available from the Medical Research Council Steroid Reference Collection. Requests should be made to Dr D. F. Johnson, Department of Health, Education and Welfare, NIH Bldg 4, Room 135, Bethesda, MD, 20014, USA.
3. A wide range of steroids labelled with radioactive isotopes are now available and may be purchased from Amersham International plc Bucks, UK; New England Nuclear Corporation, Boston, MA, USA; Centre d'Étude de L'Énergie Nucléaire, Mol-Donk, Belgium.

## Numbering of steroid carbon atoms

The carbon skeleton of a steroid is numbered according to the system given for cholestane below.

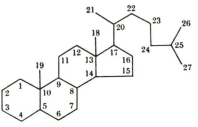

## Reviews

1. For structure–function relationships of androgens see *Androgens and anti-androgens* (Eds. L. Martini and M. Motta) Raven Press (1977).
2. For structure–function relationships of corticosteroids see *Glucocorticoid hormone action,* Monographs on endocrinology (Eds. V. D. Baxter and G. G. Rousseau) Springer-Verlag (1979).
3. For review of the physiological action of progesterone and the pharmacological effects of progestagens see *Postgrad. Med. J.* **54** (Supp 2), 11–24 (1978).

# 9 Steroids

| Name | Synonyms | Formula | M. wt. |
|------|----------|---------|--------|
| **Androgens (naturally occurring)** | | | |
| Aetiocholanolone | 3α-Hydroxy-5β-androstan-17-one | | 290.4 |
| Androstanediol | 5α-Androstan-3β,17β-diol | | 292.4 |
| Androstenedione | 4-Androstene-3,17-dione | | 286.4 |
| Androsterone | 3α-Hydroxy-5α-androstan-17-one | | 290.4 |
| Dehydroepiandro-sterone | 3β-Hydroxy-5-androsten-17-one; dehydroisoandrosterone; *trans*-dehydro-androsterone; dehydroandrosterone | | 288.4 |
| 5α-Dihydrotestosterone | 17β-Hydroxy-5α-androstan-3-one; androstanolone; stanolone; allodihydrotestosterone | | 290.4 |
| Epiandrosterone | *Trans*androsterone; 3β-Hydroxy-5α-androstan-17-one; isoandrosterone | | 290.4 |
| Testosterone | 17β-Hydroxy-4-androsten-3-one; 4-androsten-17β-ol-3-one | | 288.4 |

| Physical properties | Solubility | General remarks |
|---|---|---|
| needles from hexane | i. $H_2O$; s. organic solvents | Urinary metabolite of testosterone and androstenedione. Androgenic potency less than 1% of testosterone. |
| M.p. 117–118 | | Testosterone metabolite. Approximately 60% androgenic potency of testosterone. |
| cryst. from hexane; M.p. 170–4 | s. benz., EtOH, $CHCl_3$ | $\lambda_{max}$ 239 nm. Of gonadal and adrenal origin. Androgenic potency approx. 20% that of testosterone. |
| leaflets or needles from EtOH or acet. M.p. 183.5 | i. $H_2O$; s. organic solvents | Urinary metabolite of testosterone and androstenedione. Androgenic potency 10% that of testosterone. |
| dimorphous cryst. forms from benz.-pet. eth. M.p. 148 (needles) 152 (plates) | s. benz., eth., EtOH; sl. s. $CHCl_3$, pet. eth.; sp. s. $CCl_4$ | Mainly of adrenal origin (zona reticularis, secreted as sulphate). Androgenic potency approx. 10% that of testosterone. |
| M.p. 180–181 | i. $H_2O$; s. EtOH, eth., most organic solvents, veg. oils | Potent metabolite of testosterone, possibly the active androgenic principle within the target cell nucleus. Approximately equivalent androgenic potency to testosterone. 17-Valerate used clinically as anabolic, antioestrogenic androgen. |
| cryst. from EtOH | s. eth., benz., EtOH, MeOH | Urinary metabolite from gonadal and adrenal precursors. Androgenic potency 1% that of testosterone. |
| needles from acet. M.p. 155 | i. $H_2O$ ($1.3 \times 10^{-4}$ mol $l^{-1}$); s. EtOH, eth., most organic solvents, veg. oils; 6% rabbit serum ($3.3 \times 10^{-3}$ mol $l^{-1}$) | $\lambda_{max}$ 239 nm (log $\epsilon$ 4.23). Principal male sex steroid. Primarily of gonadal origin. Converted in man to androsterone, aetiocholanolone, and epiandrosterone. Available in esters for clinical use (e.g. propionate, phenylpropionate, isocaproate, oenanthate). |

# 9 Steroids

| Name | Synonyms | Formula | M. wt. |
|------|----------|---------|--------|

**Androgens and anabolic steroids (synthetic)**

| Ethylestrenol | 17α-Ethylestr-4-en-17β-ol. | | 288.5 |

| Fluoxymesterone | 9α-Fluoro-11β,17β-dihydroxy-17α-methyl-4-androsten-3-one | | 366.5 |

| Methandrostenolone | 17α-Methyl-17β-hydroxyandrosta-1,4-dien-3-one | | 300.4 |

| Methenolone | 17β-Hydroxy-1β-methyl-5α-androst-1-en-3-one | | 302.4 |

| Methyltestosterone | 17α-Methyltestosterone; 17α-methyl-4-androsten-3-one-17β-ol | | 302.4 |

| Nandrolone | 17β-Hydroxyestr-4-en-3-one | | 274.4 |

| Oxymetholone | 17β-Hydroxy-2-(hydroxymethylene)-17α-methyl-5α-androstan-3-one | | 332.5 |

**Oestrogens (naturally occurring)**

| Oestradiol-17α | 'β-Oestradiol' in old trivial nomenclature; 1,3,5-oestratriene-3,17α-diol | | 272.4; Hydrate, 281.4 |

| Physical properties | Solubility | General remarks |
|---|---|---|
| cryst.<br>M.p. 76–8 | | Orally active anabolic androgenic steroid. |
| cryst.<br>M.p. 270 d. | | $\lambda_{max}$ (EtOH) 240 nm (log $\epsilon$ 4.22). Anabolic-androgenic steroid. |
| cryst. from acet.-eth.<br>M.p. 163–4 | | $\lambda_{max}$ 245 nm (log $\epsilon$ 4.19). Anabolic steroid with some androgenic activity. |
| cryst. from iPr-eth.<br>M.p. 149–52 | | Acetate, enanthate used pharmacologically as orally active anabolic agent. |
| cryst.<br>M.p. 161–6 | i. $H_2O$; s. EtOH, acet., MeOH, benz.; sp. s. vegetable oils | $\lambda_{max}$ (EtOH) 241 nm (log $\epsilon$ 4.20). Orally active androgen. |
| dimorph. cryst.<br>M.p. 112 and 124 | s. EtOH, eth., $CHCl_3$ | $\lambda_{max}$ 241 nm (log $\epsilon$ 3.23). Cyclohexane propionate, cyclohexane carboxylate, and furyl propionate derivatives used pharmacologically as orally active anabolic agents. |
| cryst. from Et acetate.<br>M.p. 178–80 | | $\lambda_{max}$ 285 nm (log $\epsilon$ 3.99). Anabolic steroid; also available as enolacetate, Abs. max. 255 nm (log $\epsilon$ 4.09), enolpropionate (257 nm log $\epsilon$ 4.11) and enolbenzoate (230 nm, log $\epsilon$ 4.19). |
| needles from aq. EtOH with $\frac{1}{2}$ $H_2O$<br>M.p. Hydrate, 220–3 | i. $H_2O$; v.s. EtOH; s. acet. and most organic solvents | $\lambda_{max}$ 280 nm (log $\epsilon$ 3.31.) Minor metabolite in man but important in other species, no known biological activity. |

# 9 Steroids

| Name | Synonyms | Formula | M. wt. |
|------|----------|---------|--------|
| Oestradiol-17β | Dihydroxyoestrin; 17β-oestradiol; dihydroxyoestratriene; 'α-oestradiol' in old trivial terminology; 1,3,5-oestratriene-3,17β-diol; dihydrotheelin | | 272.4 |
| Oestriol | 1,3,5-Oestratriene-3,16α,17β-triol; trihydroxyoestrin; estriol; theelol | | 288.4 |
| Oestrone | 1,3,5-Oestratriene-3-ol-17-one; theelin; folliculin (oestrin) | | 270.4 |

**Oestrogens (synthetic)**

| Name | Synonyms | Formula | M. wt. |
|------|----------|---------|--------|
| Chlorotrianisene | Chlorotris (p-methoxyphenyl) ethylene | | 380.9 |
| Dienestrol | 4,4'-(Diethylideneethylene) diphenol | | 266.3 |
| Diethylstilboestrol | Stilboestrol; DES; trans-4,4'-dihydroxy-αβ-diethylstilbene | | 268.3 |
| Ethynyloestradiol | 19-Nor-17α-pregna-1,3,5(10)-triene-20-yne-3,17β-diol; 17α-ethynyloestra-1,3,5(10)-triene-3,17β-diol | | 296.4 |
| Mestranol | 3-Methoxy-19-nor-17α-pregna-1,3,5(10)-trien-20-yn-17-ol | | 310.4 |

| Physical properties | Solubility | General remarks |
|---|---|---|
| prisms<br>M.p. 173—9 | i. $H_2O$; s. aq. alkalis, EtOH, acet. | $\lambda_{max}$ 280 nm (log $\epsilon$ 3.28) and 225 nm. Principal female sex hormone also found in males. Available as esters for clinical usage. |
| cryst.<br>M.p. 282 (normal monocl.<br>form changes at 270—5) | sp. s. $H_2O$; s. EtOH, $CHCl_3$, eth., pyr., aq. alkali | $\lambda_{max}$ at 280 nm. Important oestrogen metabolite. Maternal blood and/or urinary levels used clinically to provide valuable index of foetal well being. |
| cryst.<br>M.p. 258—62<br><br>also 255 | 4.0 EtOH; 2.0 acet.; 1.0 $CHCl_3$; s. aq. alkali; i. $H_2O$ | $\lambda_{max}$ 280 nm (log $\epsilon$ 3.49). Ovarian product. Also formed in peripheral tissues (liver, fat) from circulating androstenedione. |
| cryst. from MeOH<br>M.p. 114—116 | i. $H_2O$; s. gl. acetic, acet, $CHCl_3$, benz., veg. oils | Potent oestrogen, active orally. |
| min. needles from EtOH—$H_2O$<br>M.p. 227—8, sublimes 130 at<br>1 mm Hg. | i. $H_2O$, acids; s. dil. alkalis; s. EtOH, eth., $CHCl_3$, warm veg. oils | Potent oestrogen. Available for clinical use as diacetate (M.p. 119), dipropionate (M.p. 99—102, sol. veg. oils), diisovalerate (M.p. 112—13), dibenzoate (M.p. 224), monomethylether (M.p. 142). |
| M.p. 169—72 | s. dil. aq. alkalis, acet., eth., $CHCl_3$, veg. oils; i. $H_2O$ | Oestrogen, active orally. |
| hemihydrate needles (from<br>MeOH—$H_2O$) M.p. 146; 183<br>(dehydrates after first M.p.) | i. $H_2O$; s. MeOH, EtOH, $CHCl_3$, acet., dioxan, eth. | Exists in two crystalline forms. $\lambda_{max}$ 248 nm. Orally active oestrogen. Available as 3-benzoate (M.p. 202) and 3-acetate (M.p. 153). |
| cryst. from MeOH or acet.<br>M.p. 150—1 | | Potent oestrogen, active orally. |

# 9 Steroids

| Name | Synonyms | Formula | M. wt. |
|------|----------|---------|--------|
| **Progestagens (naturally occurring)** | | | |

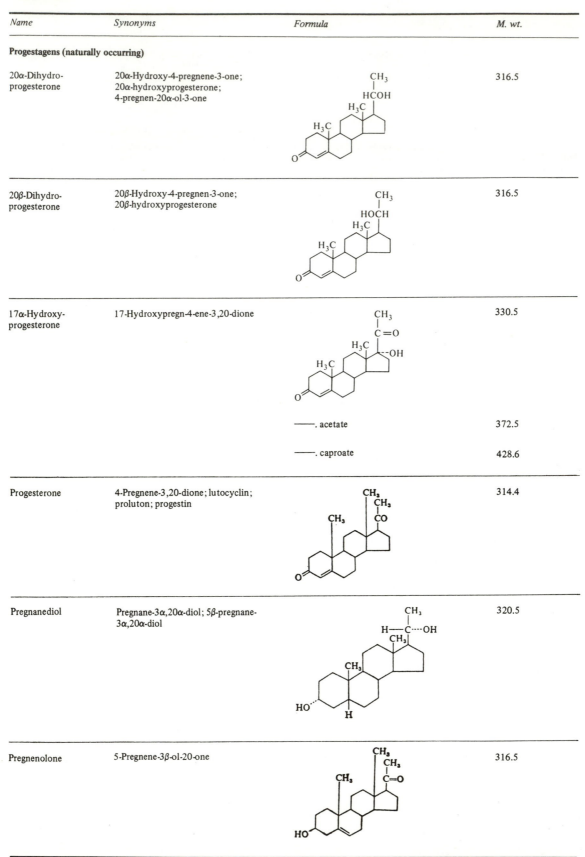

| Name | Synonyms | | M. wt. |
|------|----------|--|--------|
| 20α-Dihydro-progesterone | 20α-Hydroxy-4-pregnene-3-one; 20α-hydroxyprogesterone; 4-pregnen-20α-ol-3-one | | 316.5 |
| 20β-Dihydro-progesterone | 20β-Hydroxy-4-pregnen-3-one; 20β-hydroxyprogesterone | | 316.5 |
| 17α-Hydroxy-progesterone | 17-Hydroxypregn-4-ene-3,20-dione | | 330.5 |
| | ——. acetate | | 372.5 |
| | ——. caproate | | 428.6 |
| Progesterone | 4-Pregnene-3,20-dione; lutocyclin; proluton; progestin | | 314.4 |
| Pregnanediol | Pregnane-3α,20α-diol; 5β-pregnane-3α,20α-diol | | 320.5 |
| Pregnenolone | 5-Pregnene-3β-ol-20-one | | 316.5 |

| Physical properties | Solubility | General remarks |
|---|---|---|
| M.p. 166—7 | i. $H_2O$; s. EtOH, acet. | $\lambda_{max}$ 240 nm. Functionally important metabolite of progesterone. Progestagen with 20—33% potency of progesterone. Inhibitor of C-17,20-lyase activity ($K_i$ 9 $\mu$M). |
| M.p. 170—1 | i. $H_2O$; s. EtOH, acet. | $\lambda_{max}$ 240 nm. Progesterone metabolite of functional importance in some species. Progestagen with twice the potency of progesterone in Hooker—Forbes test. |
| cryst. from EtOH or acet. M.p. 222—3 (rapid heating) | | $\lambda_{max}$ 240 nm. Important intermediary in sex steroid biosynthesis. Hypertensive in sheep. Comp. inhibitor of 5α-reductase. |
| cryst. from $CHCl_3$-MeOH M.p. 239—240 (243—6 also reported) | | $\lambda_{max}$ 240 nm, (log $\epsilon$ 4.33). |
| cryst. from $CHCl_3$-MeOH M.p. 119—21 | s. sesame oil (25—29 mg /ml) | Caproate is long-acting progestagen used clinically by injection. |
| α, prisms from EtOH β, needles from pet. eth. M.p. α 127—31 β 121 | i. $H_2O$ (4.2 × $10^{-5}$ mols/l); s. EtOH, acet., conc. $H_2SO_4$; 6% rabbit serum (1.1 × $10^{-3}$ mols/l) | $\lambda_{max}$ 240 nm (log $\epsilon$ 4.25). Principal pregnancy-maintaining hormone produced by corpus luteum and placenta (1 mg = 1 I.U.). The two crystal types are polymorphic forms of single substance. |
| cryst. from EtOH or acet. M.p. 238 | sp. s. org. solv. | Not precipitated by digitonin. Principal urinary metabolite of progesterone in man, — excretion used as clinical index of progesterone production. |
| cryst. from EtOH M.p. 190—3 | v. sp. s. $H_2O$; s. EtOH, $CHCl_3$ | Important precursor in steroid biosynthesis in gonads, adrenal gland and placenta. |

# 9 Steroids

| Name | Synonyms | Formula | M. wt. |
|------|----------|---------|--------|
| **Progestagens (synthetic 19-nortestosterone derivatives)** | | | |
| Allylestrenol | 17-Allylestr-4-en-17β-ol; gestanon | | 300.5 |
| Chlormadinone | 17α-Acetoxy-6-chloropregna-4,6-diene-3,20-dione | | 404.9 |
| Dydrogesterone | 10α-Pregna-4,6-diene-3,20-dione; 9β,10α-pregna-4,6-diene-3,20-dione; duphaston | | 312.4 |
| Ethisterone | Anhydrohydroxyprogesterone; 17α-ethynyl-4-androsten-17β-ol-3-one; 17-ethynyltestosterone; pregneninolone | | 312.4 |
| Ethynodiol | 19-Nor-17α-pregn-4-en-20-yne-3β,17-diol | | 300.4 |
| Lynestrenol | 17α-Ethynylestr-4-en-17β-ol; orgametril | | 284.4 |
| Medroxyprogesterone | 17-Hydroxy-6α-methylpregn-4-ene-3,20-dione | | 344.5 |
| Megesterol acetate | 17α-Acetoxy-6-methylpregna-4,6-diene-3,20-dione | | 384.5 |

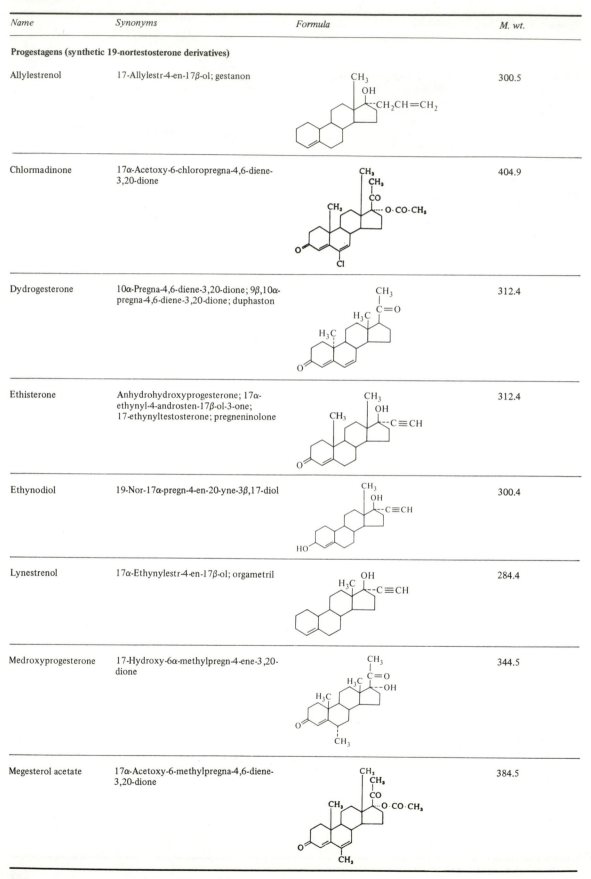

| Physical properties | Solubility | General remarks |
|---|---|---|
| cryst.<br>M.p. 79.5—80 | i. $H_2O$; s. EtOH, acet, eth, $CHCl_3$ | Sensitive to oxidising agents; orally active progestational agent. |
| cryst.<br>M.p. 210—11 | i. $H_2O$; s. EtOH, $CHCl_3$ | $\lambda_{max}$ (EtOH) 284—6 nm (log $\epsilon$ 4.30). Orally active progestational agent. |
| cryst. from acet. + hex.<br>M.p. 169—70 | i. $H_2O$; s. org. solv. | $\lambda_{max}$ 286.5 nm (log $\epsilon$ 4.42). Orally active progestational agent. |
| cryst.<br>M.p. 266—73 | i. $H_2O$; sl. s. EtOH, $CHCl_3$, acet. | $\lambda_{max}$ 241 nm ($A_{1\,cm}^{1\%}$ 513). Orally active progestational agent. |
| Diacetate cryst. from MeOH<br>M.p. 126—7 (diacetate) | i. $H_2O$; s. org. solv. | 3,17-Diacetate, orally active progestational agent. |
| M.p. 158—160 | i. $H_2O$; s. org. solv. | Orally active progestational agent. |
| cryst. from $CHCl_3$;<br>M.p. 220—223.5<br>acetate, cryst. from $CHCl_3$<br>M.p. 207—9 | i. $H_2O$; s. org. solv. | $\lambda_{max}$ (EtOH) 241 nm (log $\epsilon$ 4.20). 17-Acetate 240 nm (log $\epsilon$ 4.20). Orally active progestational agent (MAP, Provera). |
| cryst.<br>M.p. 218—20 | i. $H_2O$; s. $CHCl_3$, acet., benz.; sl. s. EtOH | $\lambda_{max}$ (EtOH) 287.5 nm (log $\epsilon$ 4.40). Orally active progestational agent. |

# 9 Steroids

| Name | Synonyms | Formula | M. wt. |
|------|----------|---------|--------|
| 19-Norethisterone | 17β-Hydroxy-19-nor-17α-pregn-4-en-20-yn-3-one; 19-nor-17α-ethynyl-testosterone | | 298.4 |
| | | —— . acetate | 340.5 |
| Norgestrel | | | 314.4 |

**Corticosteroids (naturally occurring)**

| Name | Synonyms | Formula | M. wt. |
|------|----------|---------|--------|
| Aldosterone | Electrocortin; 11β,21-dihydroxy-3,20-diketo-4-pregnen-18-al; 18-oxocorticosterone | | 360.4 |
| Corticosterone | 4-Pregnene-11β,21-diol-3,20-dione; 17β-(1-keto-2-hydroxyethyl)-4-androsten-3-one-11β-ol; 11,21-dihydroxy-progesterone; Compound B (Kendall) | | 346.4 |
| Cortisol | 4-Pregnene-11β,17α,21-triol-3,20-dione; Compound F (Kendall); hydrocortisone; 17-hydroxycorticosterone | | 362.4 |
| Cortisone | 4-Pregnene-17α,21-diol-3,11,20-trione; 17-hydroxy-11-dehydrocorticosterone; 17-(1-keto-2-hydroxyethyl)-4-androsten-3,11-dione-17-ol; Compound E (Kendall) | | 360.4 |
| Deoxycorticosterone | 4-Pregnene-21-ol-3,20-dione; 21-hydroxy-progesterone; 17α-(1-keto-2-hydroxyethyl)-4-androstene-3-one. DOCA = acetate | | 330.4 |

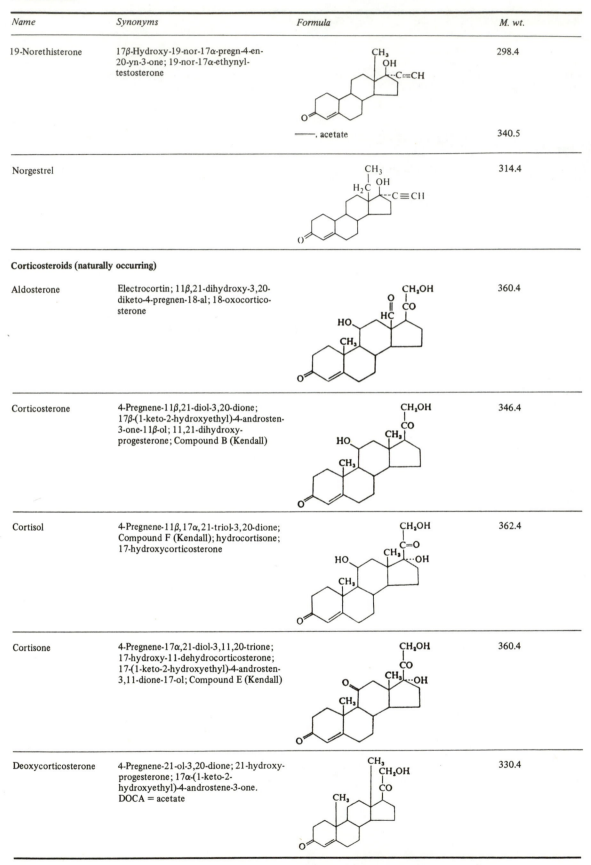

| Physical properties | Solubility | General remarks |
|---|---|---|
| cryst. <br> M.p. 203–4 | i. $H_2O$; s. $CHCl_3$, EtAc, EtOH | $\lambda_{max}$ (EtOH) 240 nm (log $\epsilon$ 4.38); acetate, 240 nm (log $\epsilon$ 4.28). Orally active progestational agent. |
| M.p. 161–2 | | |
| | i. $H_2O$; s. EtOH, acet. eth., $CHCl_3$ | Orally active progestational agent. |
| M.p. Anhyd., 164 <br> Monohydrate, 108–12 | s. $CHCl_3$, acet. | The form shown is in equilibrium with 11,18-semiacetal. Crystallizes with $1H_2O$ from acetone-water. Principal mineralocorticoid. Formed in outer zone of adrenal gland under the control of the renin–angiotensin system. Acts by stimulating Na transport across kidney tubule. |
| plates from acet.; needles +EtOH from EtOH <br> M.p. 182 | i. $H_2O$; s. EtOH, organic solvents | $\lambda_{max}$ at 240 nm. Active glucocorticoid with some mineralocorticoid activity; formed in the adrenal gland under the control of ACTH. |
| cryst. from EtOH <br> M.p. 217–20 | sl. s. $H_2O$; s. gl. acetic, dioxan, $CHCl_3$, MeOH | $\lambda_{max}$ 242 nm (log $\epsilon$ 4.20). Potent glucocorticoid. 21-(Dihydrogen phosphate) disodium salt, s. $H_2O$. |
| cryst. from EtOH <br> M.p. 215 | s. MeOH, EtOH, acet.; sl. s. eth., benz., $CHCl_3$; sp. s. $H_2O$ (0.028) | $\lambda_{max}$ at 237 nm (log $\epsilon$ 4.15). Glucocorticoid approx. 70% potency of cortisol. 21-(Dihydrogen phosphate) disodium salt, s. $H_2O$. |
| plates; cryst. from eth. <br> M.p. 141–2 | s. EtOH, acet., eth.; sp. s. $H_2O$ | $\lambda_{max}$ at 240 nm. Mineralocorticoid with about 5% sodium-retaining activity of aldosterone; acetate used clinically (M. wt. 372.5, M.p. 154–60; sl. s. MeOH, EtOH, acet., eth.). |

# 9 Steroids

| Name | Synonyms | Formula | M. wt. |
|------|----------|---------|--------|
| Tetrahydrocortisol | Pregnane-3α,11β,17α,21-tetrol-20-one | | 366.5 |
| Tetrahydrocortisone | Pregnane-3α,17α,21-triol-11,20-dione | | 364.5 |

**Corticosteroids (synthetic)**

| Name | Synonyms | Formula | M. wt. |
|------|----------|---------|--------|
| Betamethasone | 9-Fluoro-11β,17,21-trihydroxy-16β-methylpregna-1,4-diene-3,20-dione | | 392.5 |
| Dexamethazone | 9-Fluoro-11β, 17,21-trihydroxy-16α-methylpregna-1,4-diene-3,20-dione | | 392.5 |
| Fluocortolone | 6-α-Fluoro-11β,21-dihydroxy-16α-methylpregna-1,4-diene-3,20-dione | | 376.5 |
| 9α-Fluorohydro-cortisone | 9α-Fluoro-11β,17α,21-trihydroxy-4-pregnene-3,20-dione; 9α-fluorocortisol; fludrocortisone | | 380.5 |

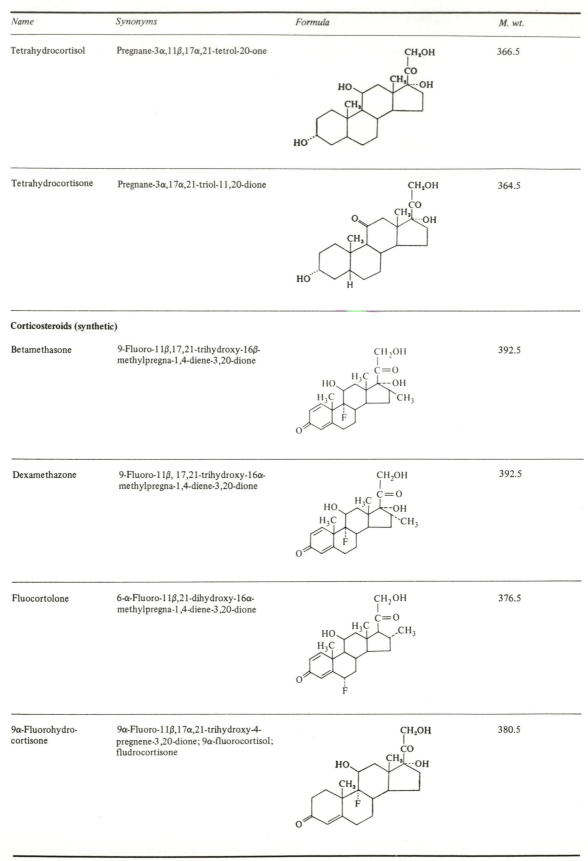

| Physical properties | Solubility | General remarks |
|---|---|---|
| cryst.<br>M.p. Diacetate 209—11 | s. acet., benz., CHCl$_3$ | Found as conjugate in human urine. Major metabolite of cortisol. |
| cryst.<br>M.p. Diacetate 232—4 | s. acet., benz., CHCl$_3$ | Major urinary metabolite of cortisol. |
| cryst. from Et acetate<br>M.p. 231—36d | | $\lambda_{max}$ 238 nm (log $\epsilon$ 4.18). Potent glucocorticoid, active orally. 21-(Dihydrogen phosphate) disodium salt, s. H$_2$O. |
| cryst.<br>M.p. 268—71 | sp. s. H$_2$O (0.01$^{25}$) | Potent glucocorticoid, active orally. Used in biochemical studies to induce liver tyrosine aminotransferase. 21-(Dihydrogen phosphate) disodium salt, s. H$_2$O. $\lambda_{max}$ 238—39 nm (log $\epsilon$ 4.15). |
| cryst.<br>M.p. 189—90 | sp. s. H$_2$O (0.029$^{37}$)<br>v. sl. s. EtOH (0.012$^{20}$)<br>sp. s. tol. (0.044$^{21}$) | $\lambda_{max}$ 242 nm (log $\epsilon$ 4.21). Anti-inflammatory corticosteroid. |
| cryst.<br>M.p. 261 d | 0.014 H$_2$O; s. MeOH, EtOH, CHCl$_3$, gl. acetic | $\lambda_{max}$ 239 nm, log $\epsilon$ 4.25 in EtOH. Orally active mineralocorticoid with some glucocorticoid effect. 21-(Dihydrogen phosphate) disodium salt, s. H$_2$O. |

## 9 Steroids

| Name | Synonyms | Formula | M. wt. |
|------|----------|---------|--------|
| Paramethasone | 6α-Fluoro-11β,17α,21-trihydroxy-16α-methyl-1,4,-pregnadien-3,20-dione | | 392.5 |
| Prednisolone | 11β,17α,21-Trihydroxy-1,4-pregnadiene-3,20-dione | | 360.5 |
| Prednisone | 17α,21-Dihydroxy-1,4-pregnadiene-3,11,20-trione | | 358.5 |
| Triamcinolone | 9α-Fluoro-11β,16α,17α,21-tetrahydroxy-1,4-pregnadiene-3,20-dione | | 394.4 |

**Miscellaneous steroids**

| Name | Synonyms | Formula | M. wt. |
|------|----------|---------|--------|
| Bromocriptine | CB154; 2-Bromo-α-ergocryptine; Parlodel (bromocryptine mesitylate) | | 654.6 |
| Calcitriol | 1,25-Dihydroxycholecalciferol; 9,10-seco (5Z, 7E) 5, 7, 10(19)-cholestatriene-1α,3β, 25-triol; 1,25-dihydroxyvitamin D₃ | | 416.6 |

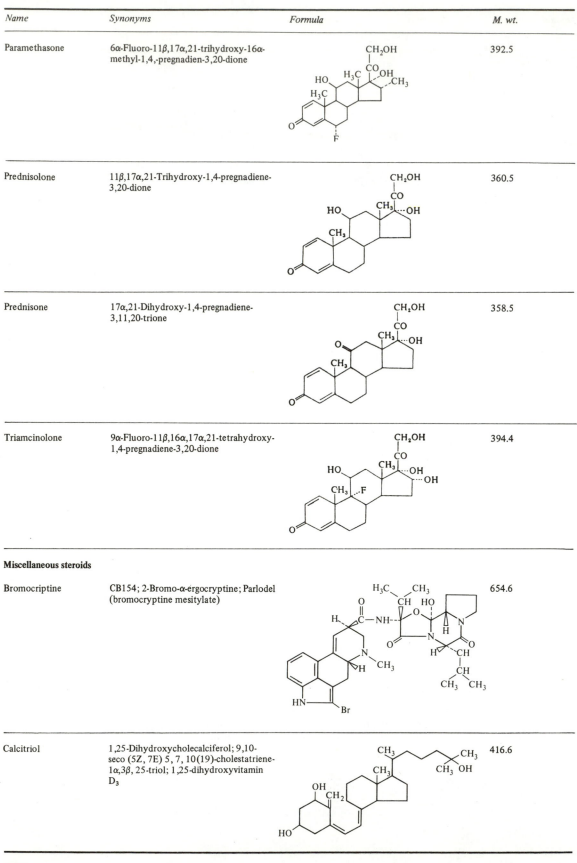

| Physical properties | Solubility | General remarks |
|---|---|---|
| | sp. s. $H_2O$ | Glucocorticoid. 21-(Dihydrogen phosphate) disodium salt, s. $H_2O$. |
| cryst.<br>M.p. 241 d | v. sl. s. $H_2O$; 3.3 EtOH;<br>0.55 $CHCl_3$; 2 acet. | $\lambda_{max}$ 242 nm (log $\epsilon$ 4.18 in MeOH). Potent glucocorticoid. 21-(Dihydrogen phosphate) disodium salt, s. $H_2O$ |
| cryst. from acet.-hexane<br>M.p. 234 d | sp. s. $H_2O$; 0.67 EtOH;<br>0.5 $CHCl_3$ | $\lambda_{max}$ 238 nm (log $\epsilon$ 4.18 in MeOH). Glucocorticoid. |
| solvated cryst.<br>M.p. 260–2 | s. Et acetate, acet.,<br>EtOH, $CHCl_3$ | $\lambda_{max}$ 238 nm (log $\epsilon$ 4.20). Potent glucocorticoid. 16,17-Acetonide used pharmacologically as topical anti-inflammatory agent. |
| | | Peptide ergot alkaloid active group. Dopamine receptor agonist. Used experimentally to suppress prolactin and $\alpha$-MSH secretion, *Acta Endocrinologica Supp. 216*, **88**, 111 (1978). Unstable in light. |
| | i. $H_2O$; s. org. solv. | Most active renal hormone in control of intestinal transport of calcium. Mucosal cells contain specific receptor in cytoplasm which is transported to cell chromatin. Used clinically to manage hypocalcaemic patients on chronic dialysis. |

# 9 Steroids

| Name | Synonyms | Formula | M. wt. |
|------|----------|---------|--------|
| Danazol | 17α-Pregna-2,4-dien-20-yno [2,3-d]-isoxazol-17-ol | | 337.5 |
| Digitonin | Digitin | R = 2 galactose + 2 glucose + 1 xylose | 1229.3 |
| Methyltrienolone | 17β-Hydroxy-17α-methylestra-4,9,11-trien-3-one; R 1881 | | 284.4 |
| Pregnenolone-16α-carbonitrile | 3β-Hydroxy-20-oxo-5-pregnene-16α-carbonitrile | | 341.5 |
| Promegestone | 17α-21-Dimethyl-19-norpregna-4,9-diene-3,20-dione; R 5020 | | 312.5 |

**Bile acids**

| | | | |
|------|----------|---------|--------|
| Chenodeoxycholic acid | 3α,7α-Dihydroxycholanic acid | | 392.6 |

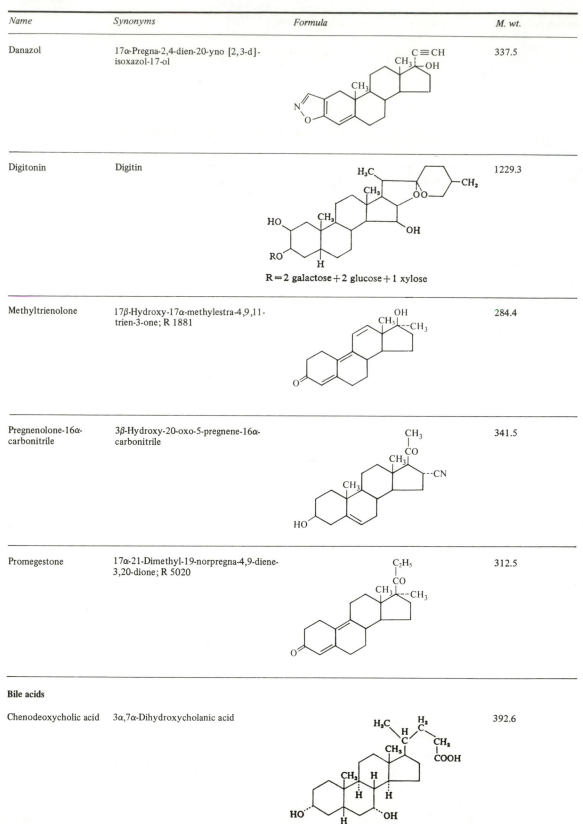

| Physical properties | Solubility | General remarks |
|---|---|---|
| cryst.<br>M.p. 225 | i. $H_2O$; s. $CHCl_3$, acet. | Antigonadotrophic compound devoid of oestrogenic and progestational activity. Used clinically in treatment of endometriosis. |
| cryst.<br>M.p. 235–40 | s. $H_2O$; 1.8 EtOH; i. $CHCl_3$ | Commonly obtained 80% pure. Forms equimolecular insoluble complex with free cholesterol. Also precipitates $\beta$-hydroxysteroids other than epi-$C_{10}$ compounds and is used for this purpose as an analytical reagent. The aglycone is digitogenin, M. wt. 448.6; for preparation see *JACS* **64**, 1843 (1942). Digitonin used as surface-active agent. |
| | | Synthetic ligand used in studies of androgen receptors. Also binds to progestin receptors in some tissues. *Steroids* **28**, 449 (1976) |
| | | Catatoxic steroid, inducer of hepatic drug metabolizing monooxygenase system, *Steroids* **31**, 849 (1978). |
| | | Synthetic ligand used in studies of progestin receptors, *Contraception* **10**, 457 (1974). |
| cryst. from Et acetate;<br>M.p. 140 | v. sl. s. $H_2O$; s. MeOH, EtOH, acetic acid | Found as glycine and taurine conjugates in bile |

| Name | Synonyms | Formula | M. wt. |
|------|----------|---------|--------|
| Cholic acid | 3α,7α,12α-Trihydroxycholanic acid; cholalic acid | | 408.6 Hydrate 426.6 |
| Deoxycholic acid | 3α,12α-Dihydroxycholanic acid | | 392.6 |
| Glycocholic acid | Cholylglycine | | 465.7 |
| Lithocholic acid | 3α-Hydroxycholanic acid | | 376.6 |
| Taurocholic acid | Cholyltaurine | $R\text{-}NH(CH_2)_2SO_3H$ (R = Cholyl; cf. glycocholic acid) | 515.8 |

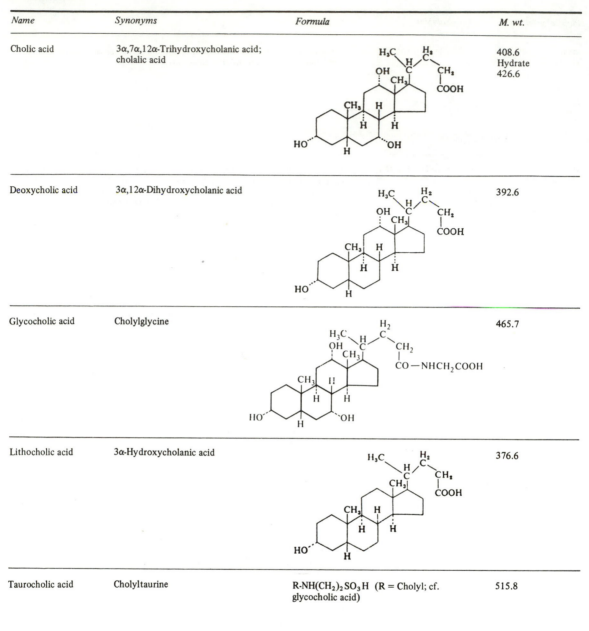

| Physical properties | Solubility | General remarks |
|---|---|---|
| Plates (+ $H_2O$) from $H_2O$; cryst. + EtOH from EtOH; M.p. anhyd. 196—8 | 0.028$^{20}$ $H_2O$; 3.0 EtOH; sl. s. eth.; s. acetic acid, acet., $CHCl_3$, alkalis | Found in bile of most animals chiefly as glycine or taurine conjugate. Not precipitated by digitonin. $pK_a = 6.4$. Can crystallize with 1 molecule of EtOH or $H_2O$ removable only by prolonged heating. Soluble in conc. $H_2SO_4$, giving yel. soln. with green fluorescence. |
| cryst. from EtOH or 60% aq. acetic; M.p. 172—6 | 0.02 $H_2O$; > 20 EtOH; v. sl. s. eth.; s. alkalis | Found in bile as glycine or taurine conjugate. Not precipitated by digitonin. $pK$ is approx. 6.6. Very stable coordination compounds, known as choleic acids, are formed with acids, esters, alcohols, ethers, phenols, hydrocarbons, and alkaloids. The choleic acid formed with stearic acid contains 8 molecules of deoxycholic acid to 1 of stearic acid. |
| | | Glycodeoxycholate also found in bile. |
| cryst from EtOH or gl. acetic M.p. 184—6 | s. hot EtOH, Et acetate, $CHCl_3$, gl. acetic, hot NaOH, $NaHCO_3$; sp. s. eth.; i. $H_2O$, ligroin | Found in bile as glycine or taurine conjugate. |
| | | Taurodeoxycholate also found in bile. |

# 10 Porphyrins and related compounds

## General references

Works of general importance are abbreviated where quoted as follows:

H. Fischer and H. Orth, *Die Chemie des Pyrrols*, vol. 2, Akademische Verlagsgesellschaft M.B.H., Leipzig (1937). Abbreviated as Fischer–Orth.
R. Lemberg and J. W. Legge, *Haematin compounds and bile pigments*, 1st ed., Interscience, New York (1949). Abbreviated as Lemberg–Legge.
J. E. Falk, *Porphyrins*, Elsevier, Amsterdam (1964). Abbreviated as Falk.
*Abderhalden's Handbuch der Biolog. Arbeitsmethoden*, Abt. **1**, Teil 11, p. 169 (1936). Abbreviated as Fischer–Abderhalden.

For abbreviations in chlorophyll section see p. 218.

## Additional literature

*Handbook of biological data*, ed. W. S. Spector, pp. 35–36, Table 26 III, Division of Biology and Agriculture, The National Academy of Sciences (1956).
*Handbook of respiration*, eds. D. S. Dittmer and R. M. Grebe, pp. 118–23, ibid. (1958).
*Porphyrins and metalloporphyrins* (Ed. K. M. Smith) Elsevier, Amsterdam (1978). Abbreviated as Smith.
*Porphyrins* (Ed. D. Dolphin) Academic Press, N.Y. (1978). Abbreviated as Dolphin.

## A. Bile pigments and related compounds

The common, naturally occurring bile pigments are all formally derived from protoporphyrin-IX (cf. porphyrins) by oxidative fission of the $\alpha$-methene linkage. They are therefore designated IX$\alpha$ and the arrangement of the side chains is thereby fixed. The side chains are either identical with those of protoporphyrin, or the vinyl groups are replaced by ethyl (giving *meso* compounds), or in the phycochromoproteins probably by an $\alpha$-substituted ethyl rather firmly linked to protein.

A ring written in the formulae in the lactim form [structure] can be present in the prototropic lactam form [structure] and a ring written in the formulae as $\alpha$-hydroxy-pyrrole [structure] in the tautomeric [structure] and [structure] forms. This enables compounds such as stercobilin, mesobilene, or biliverdin to form metal complexes in which one metal atom of, e.g., Cu or Zn, is bound to all four nitrogens of an approximately planar ring structure. This ring is probably stabilized by hydrogen bonds between the terminal $\alpha$ (> CO) and $\alpha'$ ($\geqslant$ COH) groups forming rings such as that shown below (Lemberg and Legge, p. 118).

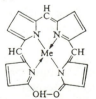

The bile pigments undergo a physiological hydrogenation from fully conjugated biliverdin to the colourless stercobilinogen which affects the tetrapyrrolic system as well as the vinyl side chains.

# 10 Porphyrins and related compounds

*General reference*

T. K. With, *Bile pigments*, Academic Press, New York (1978).


## B. Porphyrins (excluding chlorophyll porphyrins)

Porphyrins are derived formally from porphin

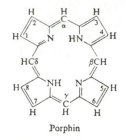

Porphin

by substitution of all or some of the eight $\beta$-hydrogens by side-chains which may be alkyl, hydroxyalkyl, vinyl, carbonyl, or carboxylic in character. Positional isomers are possible depending on the distribution of these side-chains around the macrocyclic ring. In porphyrins of natural origin no pyrrole ring contains two identical side-chains, so that for porphyrins with only two kinds of side-chains (aetioporphyrin, coproporphyrin, uroporphyrin) only four isomers (I–IV, of which type III is the normal biological isomer) are possible. With three different substituents fifteen isomers are possible. Every porphyrin and metalloporphyrin known to have a metabolic function (prosthetic groups of haemoproteins, chlorophylls, vitamin $B_{12}$) is modelled on this pattern of side-chain substitution and conforms to isomer 9 (systematically related to aetioporphyrin III).

Porphyrins can be regarded as being essentially planar (diameter 8.5 Å, thickness 4.7 Å) but deviations from planarity occur in metal complexes, which with Fe-porphyrins may be of significance in the further coordination of nitrogenous ligands. Apart from solubility aspects, the side-chains determine the electron distribution on the nitrogens and thus affect the redox potential of the Fe-porphyrin complexes.

Modification of the conjugation of double bonds of the tetrapyrrole can occur giving green compounds, either by hydrogenation of a pyrrole (chlorophylls) or by oxidation (protoporphyrin photo-oxide). Spectra of such compounds are characterized by an intense absorption band in the red; $\lambda_{max}$ and $\epsilon$ mM of the other visible bands are similar to the analogous porphyrin. Hydrogenation of the porphyrin nucleus at the two pyrrolenine nitrogens and all the methine bridge carbons yields porphyrinogens, intermediates in porphyrin biosynthesis; related partly hydrogenated porphyrins are also known. For extensive discussions of physical properties of porphyrins see Lemberg and Legge; Falk; Phillips, *Comprehensive Biochemistry*, vol. 9, pp. 34–72 (1963).


## Identification and Estimation

Spectra are of primary importance. The position ($\lambda_{max}$ nm) and intensity ($\epsilon$ mM) of absorption maxima are influenced by the degree of electrophilicity of the $\beta$-substituents (—CHO > —COCH$_3$ > —CH=CH$_2$ > alkyl) and their position relative to other electrophilic substituents: e.g. 4-monoformyldeuteroporphyrin III > IV > II > I, rhodotype (R); 2,4-diformyldeuteroporphyrin IV > III > II > I, aetiotype (A); 2-hydroxyalkyl-4-vinyl-8-formyl-8-desmethyldeuteroporphyrin III > II > IV > I, oxorhodotype (OR). Substitution at a methine bridge as in phylloporphyrin ($\gamma$-methyl) gives phyllotype (P) spectra IV > II > III > I. Solvent effects are marked.

The $\epsilon$ mM of the Soret band of porphyrin di-cations is much greater than that of the corresponding neutral porphyrin, providing a sensitive means of analysis. Equations for the analysis of polycarboxylic porphyrins in aq. HCl are available (*BJ* **75**, 620 (1960); Falk, p. 223).

Fluorometric assay though very sensitive requires strict control of experimental procedures because of other solutes and solvent effects.

### Solubility

Natural free porphyrins are ampholytes (isoelectric point 3.5–4.5), hence s. in mineral acids and aq. alkalis, particularly $NH_4OH$. Solubility is markedly influenced by impurities and there is little precise information on the solubilities of the pure substances. In general, the free porphyrins are v.s. gl. acet., Et acetate, pyr., cyclo-hexanone; s. gl. acetic-eth. (except uroporphyrins), conc. $H_2SO_4$, and conc. $NH_4OH$; moderately s. $CHCl_3$, eth. (except uroporphyrins); sl. s. or i. alcohols; i. $H_2O$, pet. ether. The methyl esters have greater solubility in the organic solvents generally, s. benz., v.s. $CHCl_3$. Solubility in alkali is abolished and in aq. media is diminished. Metal complexes of porphyrins in general have a lowered solubility in organic solvents. Fe-porphyrins, v.s. pyr., acet.-HCl; i. or sl. s. mineral acids. Methyl esters of metal complexes are generally s. in organic solvents. Non-ionic detergents, e.g. Tween 80, increase solubility in aq. media. Though having a similar effect anionic or cationic detergents are less used in biochemical experiments. See Falk, p. 142 for extensive discussion of solubilities.

HCl no. of a porphyrin is defined as that concentration in per cent (w/v) which, from an equal volume of an eth. solution of the porphyrin, extracts two-thirds of the porphyrin. Et acetate-HCl no. which is used for Me esters of polycarboxylic porphyrins is similarly defined, Et acetate replacing eth.

Porphyrin Me esters generally crystallize well from $MeOH–CHCl_3$; polycar-boxylic porphyrins from hot MeOH, porphyrins with carbonyl side-chains from $CHCl_3$-eth., metal complexes or porphyrins from benz. Double M.p. or poly-morphism may occur. Cu complexes of porphyrin Me esters are less subject to polymorphism and M.p.'s are sharper. X-ray powder diagnosis may distinguish between certain isomers.

Me esters can be prepared from free porphyrins using diazomethane, or MeOH containing 15 per cent (w/v) anhydrous HCl or 5 per cent (w/v) conc. $H_2SO_4$ (preferably at $0°C$). Diazomethane, though rapid, may react with formyl side chains and has the disadvantage that it cannot be used for haemins (*BBA* **71**, 150, 1963).

Paper chromatography is used extensively for identification of tetrapyrroles. (*See* Review, *J. Chromat.* **5**, 277, 1961; Smith p. 839). Lutidine-$H_2O$ solvent systems are used for determination of the number of free carboxyl groups. For this purpose paper electrophoresis is particularly useful for porphyrins with 4–8 carboxyls. Paper chromatography of the Me esters (*JBC* **190**, 643, 1951) is prefer-able for porphyrins with electrophilic groups and for distinguishing between iso-mers; thin layer chromatography is also used (*BBA* **237**, 356, 1971). High-pressure liquid chromatography is employed for separation and quantitation of porphyrins in biological fluids (*Chromatogr. Sci.* **10**, 103, 1979). For analysis and microprepara-tions electrophoresis on paper is an important technique (*Clin. Chim. Acta* **7**, 301, 1962).

Free haemins (*JBC* **233**, 743, 1958) and their Me esters (*JBC* **212**, 1, 1955) may be identified by paper chromatography.

Infra-red spectra, though used mainly to identify functional groups (*Aust. J. Scient. Res.* **4**, 519, 1951), may distinguish between isomeric forms, e.g. copro-porphyrin I and III (*BJ* **47**, 87, 1950; *JBC* **234**, 251, 1959).

## 10 Porphyrins and related compounds

### General

All solvents must be peroxide-free and copper-free. Excessive exposure of tetra-pyrroles to light should be avoided as photochemical alterations may occur.

### C. Iron porphyrins (Haems, Haematins)

#### Structure and nomenclature

The Fe atom of haems is coordinated to the four pyrrole nitrogens by bonds lying near the plane of the almost planar porphyrin ring. The fifth and sixth coordination positions of the Fe atom are directed perpendicularly to the porphyrin plane. The term 'haem' is preferred for generic use (e.g. haem-peptide, haemoprotein, ferro-haem, ferrihaem) irrespective of valency. A haematin is a ferric compound (e.g. alkaline haematin, neutral haematin (Lemberg & Legge, p. 170)). A haemin is a ferric compound in which an anion, usually a halogen, is coordinated to the iron atom in either the fifth or sixth coordination positions. Other nomenclature can be deduced from Table 1. Chlorins are derivatives of porphyrins in which the conjugation of the macro-ring is altered (*see* Porphyrin section). Their iron complexes are also termed haems, e.g. haem $a_2$ from cytochrome $a_2$ (*BJ* **64**, 626, 1956), Fe-chlorin (crystalline *Pseudomonas* oxidase, *BBA* **67**, 407, 1963). The general term 'haem' has sometimes been used also to describe the complexes of iron with non-porphyrin but closely related tetrapyrrolic compounds, e.g. verdohaem (*Proc. R. Soc.* **B138**, 386, 1951) or biliverdin haem (*Rev. pure appl. Chem.* **6**, 1, 1956).

#### Functional structure

The Fe atom of haems is conjugated with the conjugation of the macro-ring. Thus, alteration of the macro-ring conjugation as in haem $a_2$ or variation in conjugated $\beta$-pyrrole substituents affects the reactions of the Fe atom. This effect may be upon the redox potential as in haem *a* or haem $a_2$ (*Haematin enzymes*, eds. J. E. Falk, R. Lemberg and R. K. Morton, p. 361, Pergamon Press, 1961) or upon reactivity, e.g. oxygen affinity in artificial haemoglobins (*Arch. B.B.* **85**, 37, 1959). Other changes in the properties of the haem prosthetic group may be imposed by the nature and spatial arrangement of iron-protein bonds.

*In vivo* haems are coupled to proteins and have high- or low-spin E.S.R. characteristics. For ligand interactions see *Adv. Biophysics* **11**, 153, 1978.

A key property of haems is the oxidation–reduction poise (Em). For an extensive list of the oxidation–reduction potentials of Fe-porphyrins and haemoproteins see *Handbook of Biochemistry* (Ed. H.A. Sober) Chemical Rubber Co. Ohio; Section J. 35. For a review of electronic aspects of haems see *Adv. Biophys.* **11**, 13 (1978).

#### Assay of haems

Most commonly from extinction of the α-band of ferrohaemochrome. Also by differential ferro-ferrihaemochromes (*BJ* **87**, 181 (1963)), provided ferrihaemochrome is fully oxidized. Haemochromes electrophilically substituted are difficult to maintain in the fully oxidized state.

#### Aqueous solution of haems

Haems are soluble in alkaline solutions or at physiological pH in aqueous detergents (*BJ* **87**, 181 (1963)).

#### Characterization of haem prosthetic groups—haemochromes

As a first approach to the identification of substituents at the β-pyrrole positions the spectrum of the dipyridine ferrohaemochrome (pyridine haemochromogen) is of value. The data in Table 1 apply to compounds having the same macro-ring conjugation as in protohaem. An electrophilic substituent moves the α-absorption maximum of the haemochrome towards the red; a second or third strong electrophilic group has much less effect in this respect than the first. Electrophilic substituents on opposite pyrroles (but not adjacent pyrroles) tend to abolish the β-band. Pyridine (20–30% v/v) is the standard base; for haemoproteins, alkali (0.01M–0.1M-NaOH) may be required to disrupt completely the Fe-protein bonds but can give erroneous or different band positions; for formylhaems (*Nature, Lond.* **193**, 373 (1962)), haems with side-chains labile to alkali (e.g. milk peroxidase, *BBA* **71**, 157 (1963)), and haems substituted with unesterified carboxyls conjugated to the porphyrin conjugation (*Nature, Lond.* **192**, 750, 1961), $Na_2S_2O_4$ is the usual reducer.

For a review of new methods for the isolation and characterization of haems see *Meth. Enzymol.* **52**, 421, 1978.

TABLE 1

| Pyridine ferrohaemochrome | α-band (nm) | β-band (nm) | Δ α-band (nm) (ref. deutero-haemochrome) |
|---|---|---|---|
| Deuterohaemochrome (2:4-dihydro-compound) | 545 | 513 | .. |
| Mesohaemochrome (2:4-diethyldeutero-) | 547 | 518 | + 2 |
| From cytochrome *c* (2:4-di(-CH(SR)CH₃)) | 550 | 522 | + 5 |
| Protohaemochrome (2:4-divinyldeutero-) | 557 | 525 | + 12 |
| 2-Acetyldeuterohaemochrome | 571 | 530 | + 26 |
| From milk peroxidase (? structure) | 565–71 | | + 20–26 |
| 4-Formyldeuterohaemochrome | 578 | 548 | + 33 |
| From chlorocruorin (2-formyl-4-vinyldeutero-) | 580 | 545 | + 35 |
| Cryptohaemochrome *a* (formyl, vinyl, or vinylogue-) | 581 | (*BBA* **35**, 496, 1959) | + 36 |
| Oxorhodohaemochrome ester (2-acetyl-6-carboxylic ester-) | 582 | none | + 37 |
| 2:4-Diformyldeuterohaemochrome | 584 | 549 | + 39 |
| From cytochrome oxidase-haemochrome *a* (2-hydroxylalkyl-4-vinyl-8-formyl-) | 587 | none | + 42 |
| From myeloperoxidase (? structure) | 590 | none | + 45 |

## D Chlorophylls and related pigments

### Nomenclature

The chlorophyll pigments are magnesium complexes of various tetrapyrroles (see formulae). They can be considered as derivatives of protoporphyrin, a porphyrin which has two carboxylic acid groups; these may be free or esterified. Thus chlorophyll *a* has a carboxymethyl group at $C_{10}$ and the phytol ester of propionic acid at $C_7$. Removal of magnesium, which is readily effected by mild acid treatment, yields a product known as a phaeophytin. Hydrolysis of the phytol ester bond of a chlorophyll yields a chlorophyllide: the metal-free chlorophyllide is known as a phaeophorbide.

All these compounds are highly coloured and fluoresce strongly except when dissolved in organic solvents under very strictly anhydrous conditions. Their characteristic absorption spectra are useful in the identification and determination of the pigments. The solubility of these compounds in HCl is often used, particularly as a guide to the presence or absence of esterifying alcohols. The HCl number is defined as that concentration of HCl (in % w/v) which, from an equal volume of an ether solution of a pigment, extracts two-thirds of the pigment. The *phase test* is carried out by underlaying an ether solution of a chlorophyll with an equal volume of a 30% solution of KOH in MeOH. A coloured ring is formed at the interface of the two phases (Smith & Benitez, p. 192, listed below). The use of *thin layer chromatography* (e.g. *Planta,* **58**, 564 (1962)) permits rapid detection of chlorophylls in crude extracts. See also Holden in *Plant Pigments* (listed below).

The chlorophylls are unstable in light; they may undergo oxidation to allomerized chlorophylls if allowed to stand in air in methanolic or ethanolic solution.

Chlorophylls are complexed to proteins *in vivo* and may be isolated as such (*Rev. Photochem. Photobiol.* **29**, 203 (1979)). In complexed form their absorption spectra are significantly different from those of free chlorophylls in organic solvents.

Chlorophylls may be crystallized, addition of $H_2O$ or $Ca^{2+}$ to the organic solvent assisting the process.

*References for further information*

H. Fischer and A. Stern, *Die Chemie des Pyrrols*, vol. 2, pt. ii, Akademische Verlagsgesellschaft M.B.H., Leipzig (1940). Cited in this section as Fischer & Stern.

J. H. C. Smith and A. Benitez, *Modern methods of plant analysis*, eds. K. Paech and M. V. Tracey, vol. 4, p. 142, Springer-Verlag, Berlin (1955). Cited in this section as Smith & Benitez.

C. S. French, *Handb. PflPhysiol.* **5**, 252 (1960).

H. H. Strain, *Chloroplast pigments and chromatographic analysis*, Pennsylvania State University (1958).

L. P. Vernon and G. R. Seely, *The chlorophylls*, Academic Press, New York and London (1966). Cited in this section as Vernon & Seely.

*Chemistry and Biochemistry of plant pigments* (Ed. T. W. Goodwin) 2nd Edn. Academic Press, London (1976).

# 10 Porphyrins and related compounds

## A. BILE PIGMENTS AND RELATED COMPOUNDS

| Name | Synonyms | Structure | M. wt | Absorption spectrum | |
|------|----------|-----------|-------|---------------------|---|
| | | | | Solvent | $A_{max}$ nm ($\epsilon$ mM) |
| Bilirubin | Biladiene (a,c)-IX$\alpha$ | (M, V, P, see Biliverdin) | 584.7 | CHCl$_3$ | 450 (56–61) |
| | | | | serum | 460 (42–57) |
| Biliverdin | Dehydro-bilirubin, bilatriene-IX$\alpha$ | (a) (b) (c) (M = CH$_3$, V = CH=CH$_2$, P = CH$_2\cdot$CH$_2\cdot$CO$_2$H) | 582.7 | MeOH | 392 (25)   640 (10.4) |
| | | ———. HCl | 619.1 | MeOH | 377 (48)   680 (28) |
| | | | | 5% HCl | 372 (47)   665–70 (23.5) |
| Meso-bilane-IX$\alpha$ | Uro-bilinogen, mesobili-rubinogen | (M, P, see Biliverdin, E = C$_2$H$_5$) | 592.7 | colourless | |
| Mesobilene-(b)-IX$\alpha$ | Urobilin, Urobilin-IX$\alpha$ | | 590.7 | dioxan | 330 (3.6)   452 (26) |
| | | ———. HCl | 627.2 | dioxan | 380 494 (6.6) (45) |
| | | | | EtOH | 232 378 490 (17) (7.2) (50) |
| | | | | MeOH–HCl | (rev. spect.) 494–5 |
| Meso-biliviolin | Meso-biladiene (2'a,5'b) | | 588.7 | CHCl$_3$ | 570 |

| Physical form | M.p. | Solubility | General remarks |
|---|---|---|---|
| yellow to red-brown cryst. | Blackens | s. alkalis, hot $CHCl_3$; sl. s. gl. acetic; v. sl. s. EtOH, eth.; i. $H_2O$, acids | Present in bile, gallstones (Ca salt). In bile mainly as diglucuronide; path. in tissues, serum, urine in jaundice. Van den Bergh and Gmelin reactions positive. $Zn–I_2$ as biliverdin. Determination 'direct' and 'indirect': *Clin. Chim. Acta* **8**, 149 (1978). Conjugated and free bilirubin separated by h.p.l.c. *J. Liq. Chromat.* **2**, 37 (1979). Prep. *JBC* **202**, 305 (1953). Dry solid stable, $CHCl_3$ soln. stable in dark, alk. soln. rapidly oxidizes. Dimethyl ester m.p. 198–200. Mesobilirubin has ethyl instead of vinyl – Prep. *ZPC* **268**, 225 (1941). |
| blue-green needles (MeOH) | Blackens | v.s. alkalis, hot gl. acetic, hot MeOH; sl. s. $CHCl_3$, eth. (extr. from eth. in 2% HCl) | Present in bile of birds, amphibia, dog placenta (uteroverdin), egg shells (oocyan), human meconium in path. conditions, tissues and fluids. Gmelin reaction positive; Van den Bergh and Ehrlich negative. Zn acetate and $I_2$, blue-green colour ($A_{max}$ 637 nm) with intense red fluorescence. Prep. *JCS* **1961**, 2264, Est. *BJ* **35**, 363 (1941). Dimethyl ester mp. 216–33; Prep. *Bull. Soc. Chim. Biol.* **27**, 621 (1945). Mesobiliverdin has ethyl instead |
| green cryst. | | s. hot MeOH, gl. acetic; sl. s. dil. HCl | of vinyl. Occurs as prosthetic groups of green–blue chromoproteins of insect integuments and haemolymph. Free in some invertebrates. Prep. *BJ* **45**, 199 (1945). |
| | 197–203 | v.s. alkalis, $NH_4OH$; s. eth., benz., ethyl acetate sl. s. $H_2O$, pet. eth. | Smaller part of 'stercobilinogen' and 'urobilinogen' of faeces and path. urine. Unstable; crystals darken even in absence of $O_2$ and light. In soln. oxidizes in air to mesobilene-(b)-IXα. Ehrlich aldehyde reaction positive, van den Bergh and Gmelin reactions negative. $FeCl_3$ oxidizes to mesobiliverdin. Prep. Fischer–Orth, 692. |
| orange-red cryst. | 190 SYN. 177 (darkens 158, sinters 171) | v.s. MeOH, EtOH, gl. acetic, alkali; s. $CHCl_3$, acet.; sl. s. eth. (extracted from eth. by dil. acetic) | Smaller part of 'stereobilin' and 'urobilin' of faeces and path. urine. Unstable, readily dehydrogenated to mesobiliviolin and mesobiliverdin, e.g. by $FeCl_3$. Crystals retain $CHCl_3$, ? compound. Combines readily with Zn, Cu. Zn complex with Zn acetate in EtOH, strong green fluorescence, max 509 nm. Pentdyopent reaction positive. Optically inactive. Syn. *ZPC* **242**, 101 (1936). Prep. Fischer–Orth, 685. |
| | 191–200 ($CHCl_3$) M. p. not sharp, retains $CHCl_3$ | v.s. MeOH, EtOH, gl. acetic; s. $CHCl_3$; sl. s. acet., benz., $H_2O$ | |
| amorph. | | v.s. alcohols, $CHCl_3$, gl. acetic, alkalis; s. eth. (extracted from eth. 0.1м-HCl), acids; i. $H_2O$, dil. acetic | See remarks in Phycocyanobilin. Unstable. Characteristic Zn complex in EtOH, strong red fluorescence, max 625 (575) nm. Prep. *Biochemistry* **2**, 375 (1963). |

# 10 Porphyrins and related compounds

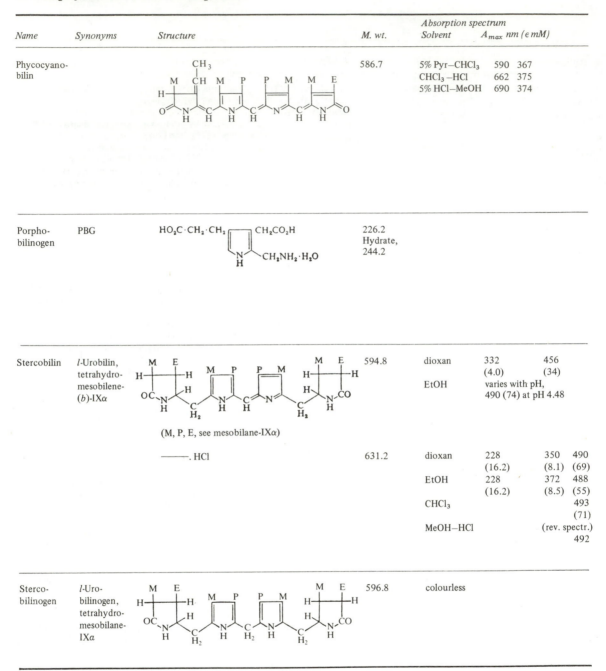

| Name | Synonyms | Structure | M. wt. | Absorption spectrum Solvent | $A_{max}$ nm ($\epsilon$ mM) |
|------|----------|-----------|--------|---------|-------|
| Phycocyano-bilin | | | 586.7 | 5% Pyr–CHCl₃ | 590  367 |
| | | | | CHCl₃ –HCl | 662  375 |
| | | | | 5% HCl–MeOH | 690  374 |
| Porpho-bilinogen | PBG | HO₂C·CH₂·CH₂ ⌐ CH₂CO₂H ... CH₂NH₂·H₂O | 226.2 Hydrate, 244.2 | | |
| Stercobilin | l-Urobilin, tetrahydro-mesobilene-(b)-IXα | (M, P, E, see mesobilane-IXα) | 594.8 | dioxan | 332  456 (4.0)  (34) |
| | | | | EtOH | varies with pH, 490 (74) at pH 4.48 |
| | | ——— . HCl | 631.2 | dioxan | 228  350  490 (16.2) (8.1) (69) |
| | | | | EtOH | 228  372  488 (16.2) (8.5) (55) |
| | | | | CHCl₃ | 493 (71) |
| | | | | MeOH–HCl | (rev. spectr.) 492 |
| Sterco-bilinogen | l-Uro-bilinogen, tetrahydro-mesobilane-IXα | | 596.8 | colourless | |

## B. PORPHYRINS (EXCLUDING CHLOROPHYLL PORPHYRINS)

| Name | Structure | M. wt. | Absorption spectrum Solvent | $A_{max}$ nm ($\epsilon$ mM) | | | | |
|------|-----------|--------|---------|-----|-----|-----|-----|-----|
| Chlorocruoro-porphyrin (*Spirographis* porphyrin) | 1:3:5:8-Tetramethyl-2-formyl-4-vinylporphin-6:7-dipropionic acid | 564.6 | eth. | 642 592.5 | 583 | 555 | 514.5 | |
| | | | dioxan | 639 (2.3) | 581 (7.9) | 553 (12.4) | 514 (10.3) | |
| | | | 4% HCl | 614 | 565 | | | 418 |
| | | | 20% HCl | 616 | 565 | | | 421 |

| Physical form | M.p. | Solubility | General remarks |
|---|---|---|---|
| s. $H_2O$ , polar org. solv. | | | Chromophore of *allo*phycocyanin, C and R-phycocyanin of blue-green algae and accompanying pigments of red algae; also in cryptophyta. Chromophore of higher plant phytochrome has related structure. Prep. *Am. J. Bot.* **55**, 314 (1968); *BJ* **105**, 903 (1967); *Phytochemistry* **5**, 993 (1966). Pigment converts to mesobiliviolin or biliverdin in some isolation procedures. Phycoerythrobilin is a structural isomer covalently bound to protein of C and R-phycoerythrin. Prep. *Biochem. Soc. Symp.* **28**, 110 (1968); *J. Biochem.* **51**, 89 (1962); *JACS* **89**, 5976 (1967); *BJ* **80**, 25P (1961); Synth. *JACS* **100**, 5928 (1962). |
| col. cryst. | Darkens 120–30; decomp. 170–80 | s. dil. alkalis, $NH_4OH$, pyr.; almost i. $H_2O$, common organic solvents | Not a bile pigment. Intermediate in porphyrin biosynthesis. Found in urine in acute porphyria. Aq. soln. unstable, forms porphobilin in light, uroporphyrin on boiling. $pK' = 3.70$, 4.95, 10.1. Hydrochloride monohydrate, needles from 2м-HCl; m.p. 165–70 d. Red colour with Ehrlich aldehyde reagent. i. Hg salt. Lactam, m.p. 281–4, Prep. *BJ* **57**, 476 (1954); Est. *JBC* **219**, 435 (1956). |
| yel. cryst. | 236 | v.s. EtOH, MeOH, gl. acetic, alkalis, $NH_4OH$, pyr.; s. $CHCl_3$, acet.; sl. s. $H_2O$, dil. acid, eth.; i. pet. eth. | Greater part of 'stercobilin' and 'urobilin' of faeces and path. urine. Stable. From $CHCl_3$ narrow prisms, M.p. 234–6, $[\alpha]_{6560}^{20} - 824$ (in gl. acetic). Zn complex in EtOH strong green fluorescence, max 507 nm. Gmelin, Van den Bergh, pentdyopent and $FeCl_3$ reactions negative. Prep. *JBC* **114**, 47 (1936); *Chem. Ind.* **1955**, 652; Est. *J. Lab. Clin. Med.* **54**, 1 (1959). |
| yel. prisms ($CHCl_3$) | 120–65 not sharp, decomp. | v.s. EtOH; s. $CHCl_3$, acet.; sl. s. ethyl acetate, dil. HCl; i. eth., pet. eth. | |
| amorph. | | s. alcohols, alkalis, $NH_4OH$, $CHCl_3$; sl. s. eth.; i. $H_2O$ | Greater part of 'stercobilinogen' and 'urobilinogen' of faeces and path. urine. Readily oxidizes to stercobilin. Prep. *ZPC* **238**, 59 (1936). |

| Type | Physical form | M.p. | General remarks |
|---|---|---|---|
| (R) | fine needle-prisms (eth.) | | HCl no. = 4.6. Tween 80 solubilizes in aqueous buffers. Present as chlorocruorohaem, prosthetic group of chlorocruorin of *Spirographis sabella*. |
| (R) | | | Prep. *ZPC* **242**, 139 (1936). |

| Name | Structure | M. wt. | Solvent | Absorption spectrum $A_{max}$ nm($\epsilon$ mM) | | | | | |
|------|-----------|--------|---------|--------------------------------------------------|---|---|---|---|---|

**Chlorin $a_2$** — M. wt. 582.6

| Solvent | | | | | | |
|---------|---|---|---|---|---|---|
| eth. | 653 | 598 | 573 | 534 | 503 | 405 |
| Ratio of intensities | 3.3 | 0.3 | | | 1 | 12 |
| 10% HCl | | 630 | | 536 | | 405 |
| 20% HCl | | 647 | | 530 (diffuse) | | 412 |

---

**Coproporphyrin I (copro I)** — M. wt. 654.7

1:3:5:7-Tetramethylporphin-2:4:6:8-tetrapropionic acid

| Solvent | | | | | |
|---------|---|---|---|---|---|
| eth. | 623.5 | 567.5 | 528 | 495 | 398 |
| 25% HCl | 593 | 550 | | | 406 |
| | (5.5) | (16.2) | | | |
| 1M-HCl | 591 | 548 | | | 401 |
| | (6.1) | (17.5) | | | (470) |
| 0.1M-HCl | | | | | 399.5 |
| | | | | | (489) |

---

**Coproporphyrin III (copro III)** — 1:3:5:8-Tetramethylporphin-2:4:6:7-tetrapropionic acid — M. wt. 654.7

| Solvent | Absorption spectrum |
|---------|---------------------|
| eth. | Spectroscopically identical with copro I (q.v.) |
| 0.1M-HCl | |
| 1M-HCl | |

---

**Cryptoporphyrin $a$, dimethyl ester** — M. wt. 761–793

(R = $C_{12}H_{25}$ to $C_{15}H_{31}$)

| Solvent | | | | | |
|---------|---|---|---|---|---|
| CHCl$_3$ | 642.5 | 584 | 559 | 519 | 416 |
| $A^{1\%}_{1cm}$ | | 31 | 127 | 194 | 148 |
| 10% HCl | 613.5 | 563.5 | | | |
| Pyridine haemochrome, max 582, 533 | | | | | |

---

**Deuteroporphyrin 9 (Schumm's co-pratoporphyrin)** — 1:3:5:8-Tetramethylporphin-6:7-dipropionic acid — M. wt. 510.6

| Solvent | | | | | |
|---------|---|---|---|---|---|
| eth. | 621.5 | 567 | 526 | 494 | |
| pyr. | 621 | 566 | 530 | 497 | |
| 25% HCl | 591 | 548 | | | 404 |
| 0.1M-HCl | 588 | 548 | | | 398 |
| | (5.34) | (13.7) | | | (433) |

| Type | Physical form | M.p. | General remarks |
|------|---------------|------|-----------------|
| | | | As haemin prosthetic group of cytochrome $a_2$ in bacteria (*A. aerogenes, E. coli*). Structure not definitive. HCl no. = 10. Conversion to a porphyrin may occur during removal of iron from the ferrochlorin. The ferrochlorin is best est. as the chloroferrochlorin (the haemin) $A_{max}$ 603–4 nm; the pyridine haemochrome ($A_{max}$ 613–4 nm) is extremely unstable; obtained associated with lipid. Prep. *BJ* **64**, 626 (1956). |
| (A) | prisms (from pyr.-gl. acetic) | | Traces in normal serum (esp. foetal), amniotic fluid, meconium. Normal human adult excretes 40–160 μg per 24 hr. Urine excretion increased in pathological conditions. Hedgehog spikes. Shell of mollusc *Pinctada vulgaris*. Micro-organisms, yeasts, plants. HCl no. = 0.09. Et acetate–HCl no. = 0.35. Not extracted from dil. HCl by $CHCl_3$. Colloidal solution in $H_2O$. Zn complex $A_{max}$ 575, 539, 408 nm. Cu complex $A_{max}$ 561, 524, 400 nm. Na, K salts s. $H_2O$ and strong alkalis. Dihydrochloride, violet-red double pyramids, colloidal soln. in $H_2O$, ether, $CHCl_3$. Best source: meconium. Conveniently prepared by decarboxylation of uroporphyrin I. Prep. *JBC* **227**, 505 (1957), Est. *Meth. Biochem. Anal.* **8**, 221 (1960). |
| | cryst. with difficulty; globular aggregates | | Traces in normal erythrocytes, urine (normal human adults excrete 20–80 μg/day). Increase in porphyrias and toxic states (sulphonamides). Owl feathers, legume root nodules, and other plants, yeast and bacteria esp. in Fe deficiency. Prep. *Biochem. Prep.* **7**, 36 (1960); *JCS* **1958**, 1430. Est. *Clin. Chim. Acta* **89**, 25 (1978). Latter ref. also for spectra of cations. HCl no. = 0.09. Na, K salts, s. $H_2O$, strong alkalis. Dihydrochloride, red prisms, v.s. $H_2O$. Ethyl acetate–HCl no. = 3.5. Differentiated from copro I by thin-layer chromatography (*J. Chromat.* **10**, 236 (1963)). $pK_3$ 7.2, 20°; $pK_2$ 4.2, 20°. |
| (R) | prisms<br>leaflets<br>plates (pentag) | 254–7<br>259–60<br>256–60 | Present in ox heart-muscle, liver; pigeon breast muscle. Yeasts and bacteria (*S. lutea*), as haemin; *BBA* **54**, 573 (1961). Found in crude porphyrin *a* preps. as free porphyrin. HCl no. = 4.0. As haemin from ox-heart muscle preps. (*JBC* **233**, 743 (1958)). M. wt. calculated from specific extinction. |
| (A) | cryst. (pyr-gl. acetic) | | Present in faeces, putrefying blood, decaying meat. HCl no. = 0.3. Ether/0.45% HCl, $K$ = 0.36. Na salt, insol. in $H_2O$. Dihydrochloride, s. $CHCl_3$; extracted into $CHCl_3$ from 0.2% HCl. Cu complex from $CHCl_3$–acetic in needles; m.p. 335. Key compound in structure determination and preparation of model compounds of biochemical interest. Prep. *JBC* **202**, 781 (1953); *JACS* **74**, 6276 (1952). Est. *JBC* **208**, 537 (1954); *BJ* **49**, 157 (1951). |

# 10 Porphyrins and related compounds

| Name | Structure | M. wt. | Solvent | $A_{max}$ nm($\epsilon$mM) | | | | | | |
|---|---|---|---|---|---|---|---|---|---|---|
| Harderoporphyrin | Porphin-2-vinyl-1:3:5:8-tetramethyl-4:6:7-tripropionic acid | 608.7 | CH$_2$Cl$_2$ (trimethyl ester) | 630 (5.37) | 574 (10.2) | 540 (13.0) | 507 (17.4) | 405 (178) | | |
| Porphyrin a (cytoporphyrin) | | 798.0 | eth. | 647 (1.3) | 582 (10.9) | 558 (21) | 518 (8.86) | 414 (160) | | |
| | | | CHCl$_3$ | 646 | 584.5 | 563.5 | 520 | 418.5 | | |
| | | | 5% HCl | 614.8 | 559.1 | | | | | |
| | | | 25% HCl | 619.0 | 564.2 | | | | | |
| | | | Dimethyl ester in eth. | 647 | 584 | 560 | 577 | 412 | | |
| | | | Abs. ratios | | 2.28:1 | | | | | |
| Protoporphyrin 9; Schumm's haematoporphyroidin; Kammerer's porphyrin; Snapper's porphyrin; ooporphyrin | 1:3:5:8-Tetramethyl-2:4-divinylporphin-6:7-dipropionic acid | 562.7 | eth. | 633 | 576 | 538 | 503 | | | |
| | | | dioxan | 631 (5.2) | 576 (6.5) | 538 (10.8) | 504 (14.8) | | | |
| | | | 25% HCl | 602 (5.9) | 557 (16.4) | | | 411 (278) | | |
| | | | 2.7M-HCl | 598 (5.75) | 554 (13.5) | | | 408 (262) | | |
| Sirochlorin (sirohydrochlorin) | | 862.8 | MeOH + tr. H$_2$SO$_4$ | 618 1 | 575 0.52 | 523 0.45 | 492 0.45 | 403 3.6 | 383 3.2 | 373 3.2 |
| | | | CHCl$_3$ | 638 | 588 | 545 | 510 | 480 | 378 | 362 |
| | | | Cu deriv. | 585 (2) | 545 | 397 | | | | |
| | | | Zn deriv. | 605 (3) | 560 | 408 | | | | |
| Uroporphyrin I (urinporphyrin, uro I) | Porphin-1:3:5:7-tetraacetic acid-2:4:6:8-tetrapropionic acid | 830.7 | 25% HCl | 597 | 554 | | | 410 | | |
| | | | 0.5M-HCl | 594 (6.52) | 552 (18.3) | | | 405 (541) | | |

226

| Type | Physical form | M.p. | General remarks |
|------|---------------|------|-----------------|
| (A) | | | Found in harderian glands of rat; precursor of protoporphyrin 9. Prep. *FEBS Lett.* **6**, 9 (1970); **7**, 205 (1970); Smith p. 52, H.p.l.c. *JCS Perkin* **7**, 1188 (1974). |
| (OR) | | (Dimethyl ester) | As haem, prosthetic group of cytochrome oxidase (cytochrome $a + a_3$) and of cytochrome $a_1$ (bacteria, e.g. *E. coli*). Native porphyrin $a$ ($\alpha$ form), HCl no. = 15. |
| (OR) | | 128–130 | Transition to spectrally identical porphyrin $a\beta$, HCl no. = 5, occurs on standing porphyrin $a\alpha$ in aq. HCl or acidified organic solvents. Alteration products may form during removal of iron from the haemin. Highly photosensitive. Cu complex $A_{max}$ 598, 550 nm. A second, more polar component of undetermined structure present in equal amount in preps. Prep. *BJ* **78**, 793 (1961). |
| (A) | cryst. from MeOH–KOH, | | Occurs as protohaem (q.v.) in Harderian glands of rat, egg shells, immature |
| (A) | pyr., eth. | | erythrocytes, mutants of bacteria and yeasts deprived of iron. As monomethyl ester in algae, yeasts, and photosyn. bacteria. HCl no. = 2.5. Unstable in soln. esp. in light. Na salt, sl. s. $H_2O$, precipitates from strong alkalis. Tween 80 assists sol. in $H_2O$. K salt may be crystallized. Dihydrochloride, s. $CHCl_3$. Readily hydrated in dil. HCl. Prep. *BJ* **63**, 87 (1956). Est. *Clin. chim. acta* **89**, 25 (1978). |
| | | | Occurs as haem—prosthetic group of $SO_3^{2-}$ and $NO_2^-$ reductases of spinach, *E. coli*, sulphur bacteria. As free *iso*-bacteriochlorin in *Propionibacterium shermanii*; precursor of vit. $B_{12}$. Prep. *Tetrah. Lett.* 2217 (1977); *JBC* **248**, 6911 (1973). Chromatographic and electrophoretic properties resemble uroporphyrin. Fluoresc. 2м-HCl; 628 (660 shoulder). Piperidine 596 > 639. $CHCl_3$ 597 > 640. |
| | needles | | Traces in normal urine, increased excretion in pathological conditions (esp. |
| | (pyr.-gl. acetic) | | congenital porphyria). Molluscan shells. Readily yields coproporphyrin I by partial decarboxylation. Ethyl acetate HCl no. = 0.1; i. eth. Prep. *JBC* **233**, 501 (1958); *BJ* **57**, 476 (1954); **50**, 202 (1952). Est. *J. chromat.* **10**, 141 (1963); *BJ* **75**, 620 (1960); *Br. J. Ind. Med.* **35**, 61 (1978); *S. afr. J. lab. clin. med.* **45**, 221 (1971); *Z. anal. chem.* **252**, 104 (1970); *BJ* **55**, 105, 109, 867 (1953); *Clin. chem. Acta* **7**, 301 (1962). |

# 10 Porphyrins and related compounds

| Name | Structure | M. wt. | Absorption spectrum Solvent | $A_{max}nm(\epsilon mM)$ |
|------|-----------|--------|---------|--------------------------|
| Uroporphyrin III (uro III) | Porphin-1:3:5:8-tetraacetic acid-2:4:6:7-tetrapropionic acid | 830.7 | 0.5M-HCl | Quantitatively identical with uro I (q.v.) |
| Uroporphyrin-ogen III (Hexahydrouroporphyrin, urospectrin, urogen III) | | 836.8 | water | 202 (50) |

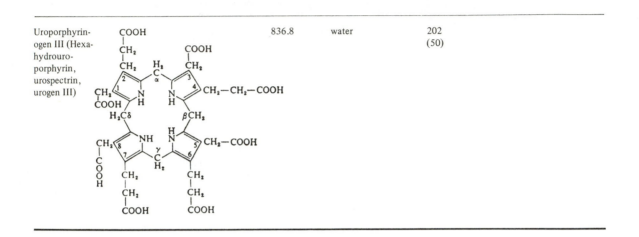

## C. IRON PORPHYRINS (HAEMS, HAEMATINS)

| Name | Synonyms | Structure | M. wt. |
|------|----------|-----------|--------|
| Chlorocruoro-haemin | Ferrochloro-cruoroporphyrin; *Spirographis* haem | | 657.2 |
| Haem | Ferroprotohaem IX, protohaem, ferro-protoporphyrin, reduced haematin | | 616.5 |

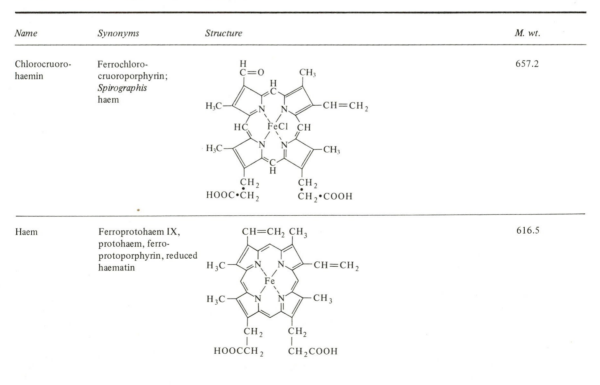

| Type | Physical form | M.p. | General remarks |
|------|---------------|------|-----------------|
| | | | Traces in normal urine, increased excretion in pathological conditions (esp. acute porphyria) and in experimental porphyria (e.g. Sedormid induced). As Cu complex, turacin, in *Turacos* feathers, *BJ* **50**, 194 (1951). Ethyl acetate— HCl no. = 9.4. Readily yields coproporphyrin III by partial decarboxylation. Paper-electrophoresis a valuable method in the preparation of this and other polycarboxylic porphyrins, *Clinica chim. Acta* **7**, 301 (1962). Cu complex, turacin, thin needles; s. dil. alkalis: i. eth., CHCl$_3$, EtOH, gl. acetic. $A_{max}$ at 562.5, 526 nm (alkali) and 583, 542 nm (acid). Prep. *JBC* **227**, 505 (1957) *BJ* **55**, 109, 867 (1953). Spectra of cations and est. *Clin. chim.* **25**, 71 (1979). |
| | | | Present in urine esp. path. conditions. *J. Lab. clin. Med.* **37**, 831 (1951); *Aust. J. exp. Biol. med. Sci.* **31**, 457 (1953). Intermediate in porphyrin biosynthesis. Readily oxidized by iodine to uroporphyrin, tetrahydro- ($A_{max}$ 500 nm) and dihydro- ($A_{max}$ 737, 440 nm) uroporphyrin as intermediates. Photocatalytically autooxidized. For other porphyrinogens see *JBC* **236**, 1173 (1961); Falk, p. 8. Prep. *JBC* **232**, 1141 (1958). Est. *Nature* **181**, 1592 (1958). |

| Absorption spectrum | | | | | |
|---------------------|---|---|------|------------|-----------------|
| Solvent | $A_{max}$ nm($\epsilon$ mM Fe) | | Type | Solubility | General remarks |
| Pyr. | 573.5 | 547.5 | 425.5 | | | Prosthetic group of chlorocruorin, oxygen carrier of some polychaete worms (*Spirographis, Sabella, Branchiomma*). Forms Schiff bases with denatured proteins at pH > 10 with blue shift of $A_{max}$. |
| abs. ratios | 1 : | 0.41 : | 5.4 | | | |
| 20% Pyr–0.08 M NaOH | .580 | 412.5 | | | | |
| abs. ratios | 1 : | 5.4 | | | | |
| pH 7–12 borate or phosphate buffer | 570–80 (5.5–6.5) | | | | i. H$_2$O, dil. acids; sl. s. dil. alkalis; s. EtOH–eth. | Prosthetic groups of de-oxygenated vertebrate haemoglobins, erythrocruorins, myoglobins, reduced cytochromes *b*, ? cytochrome *ć* peroxidase, ? tryptophan pyrrolase. Rapidly autoxidizes, Fe removed by HCl (e.g. *Aust. J. exp. Biol. med. Sci.* **34**, 211, 1956). Exists as dimer in solution. Ligands at co-ordination positions 5 and 6 = H$_2$O, H$_2$O. Prep. *Experientia* **28**, 1396 (1972). Readily forms ferrohaemochromins with bases. Pyridine– haemochrome $A_{max}$ (0.2 M-NaOH–25% pyr.) 557, 525 nm ($\epsilon$ mM Fe 31–35, 16–17.5); *JBC* **140**, 373 (1941); *Acta chim. scand.* **7**, 1284 (1953). |

# 10 Porphyrins and related compounds

| Name | Synonyms | Structure | M. wt. |
|------|----------|-----------|--------|
| Haem a | Cytohaem | | 851.8 |
| Haematin | Ferriprotohaem IX; hydroxyferriproto-porphyrin; alkaline haematin | | 633.5 |
| Haemin | Protohaemin IX; chlorohaemin, chloro-ferriprotoporphyrin | | 652.0 |
| Erythrocyte green haem | | Formyl-haem of uncertain structure; one or more hydroxyl functions and possibly 3 carboxyl groups | ? |

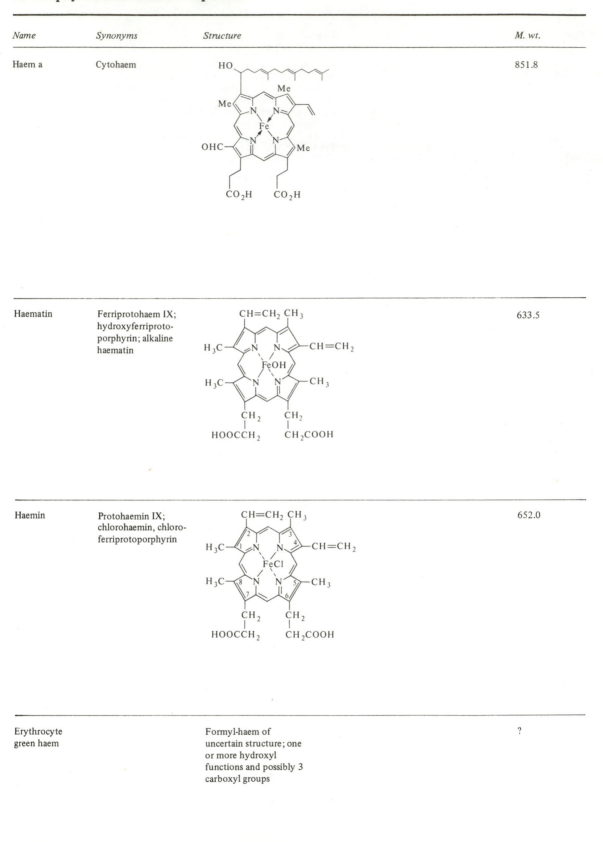

| Absorption spectrum Solvent | $A_{max}$ nm ($\epsilon$ mM Fe) | | | | | Type | Solubility | General remarks |
|---|---|---|---|---|---|---|---|---|
| ·Fe$^{2+}$ haem, pH 7.5 | 598 (9.7) | 410 (69) | | | | | s. eth, CHCl$_3$, acet; i.H$_2$O, dil. acids | Prosthetic group of cytochrome oxidases $a + a_3$, $a_1$, $a$. Forms Schiff bases with denatured protein with blue shift of $A_{max}$. Prep. *BJ* **78**, 793 (1961), *JBC* **250**, 7602 (1975). Forms complexes with $-OH$, $O_2$, H$_2$O$_2$, pyr, CO, $-CN$. |
| pyr–0.1M-NaOH | 587 (30) | 430 (117) | | | | | | |
| Fe$^{2+}$–CO, pH 7.5 | 607 (18.9) | 428 (79) | | | | | | |
| Fe$^{2+}$–CN + 0.1M-NaOH | 598 (23.0) | 534 (10.9) | 446 (10.1) | | | | | |
| Fe$^{3+}$–CN + 0.1M-NaOH | 635 (9.0) | 405 (60) | | | | | | |
| Fe$^{3+}$ pH 7.5 | 635 (79) | 400 (67) | | | | | | |
| borate, pH 10.0 | 600 (4.5) | | | | | | i. H$_2$O, dil. acids, EtOH, eth., CHCl$_3$, acet.; sl. s. gl. acetic; s. dil. alkalis. | Hydroxy-derivative of prosthetic group of methaemoglobins, meterythrocruorin, metmyoglobin, plant peroxidases, catalases, cytochromes $b$, methaemalbumin. In urine in pathological conditions, in erythrocytes in malaria. Reduced to haem by Na$_2$S$_2$O$_4$. Ligands at co-ordination positions 5 and 6 = H$_2$O, OH; both displaced by bases to form ferrihaemochromes. |
| 0.1 M-aq. NaOH | 610 (4.6) | 385 (58.44) | | | | | | |
| $5 \times 10^{-4}$ M-aq. NaOH | | 385 (49) | | | | | | |
| $5 \times 10^{-4}$ M-NaOH in 99% EtOH | | 403 (80) | | | | | | |
| eth.-acetic (as ester) | 638 (*BBA* **71**, | 540 165 (1963)) | 512 | 407 | 381 | | i. H$_2$O, dil. acids; s. dil. alkalis, NH$_4$OH; s. org. bases; sl. s. gl. acetic, 70–80% EtOH; i. EtOH, eth., acet., CHCl$_3$; s. aq. HCl–EtOH, aq. HCl–acetic | Removal of Fe requires conc. H$_2$SO$_4$ (cf. haem). Dimethyl ester, s. gl. acetic, CHCl$_3$; sl. s. MeOH; absorption bands in CHCl$_3$, 625, 565, 515 nm. Est. *JBC* **140**, 373, 387 (1941); *Acta chem. Scand.* **7**, 1284 (1953); *J. gen. Microbiol.* **15**, 404 (1956). Stable form. Prep. *JBC* **228**, 123 (1957); *BBA* **76**, 437 (1957). Recrystallization tends to alter vinyl side chains. Mono- and di-hydroxyethyl derivatives are by-products of prep. and crystallization. |
| gl. acetic-75% EtOH | 635 | 510 | 400 (90) | | | | | |
| pyr.–Fe$^{3+}$ | 579 | 538 | 432 | | | (A) | s. polar solv., H$_2$O | Prosthetic group of green haemoprotein of human erythrocytes. Haem dissociates on electrophoresis at pH 9.5. Usual methods for Fe removal cause degradation. Unstable in acids, stable in alkalis. Prep. *JBC* **251**, 3927 (1976). |
| acetic acid | 549 | 518 | 412 | | | | | |
| CHCl$_3$ (Me ester) | 647 | 590 | 561 | 518 | 423 | | | |

# 10 Porphyrins and related compounds

| Name | Synonyms | Structure | M. wt. |
|---|---|---|---|
| Sirohaem | | 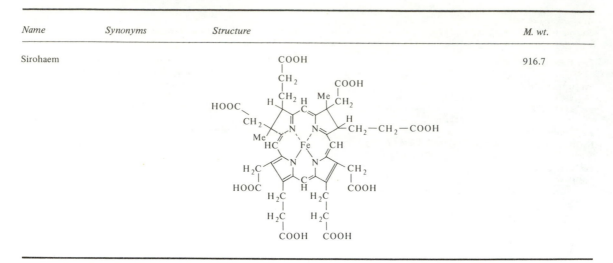 | 916.7 |

## D. CHLOROPHYLLS AND RELATED PIGMENTS

| Name | Structure | M. wt. | Absorption spectrum $A_{max}$ nm($\epsilon$ mM) | | | | | |
|---|---|---|---|---|---|---|---|---|
| Chlorophyll *a* (and derivatives) | $CH_2$ ... R = $C_{20}H_{39}$(phytyl) $C_{55}H_{72}O_5N_4Mg$ | 893.5 | eth: 662 (91.2) acet: 663 (75.05) | 615 (13.8) 615 (14.03) | 578 (7.6) 580 (7.75) | 533.5 (3.7) 535 (3.47) | 430 (121) 430 (94.71) | 410 (76.1) 410 (68.9) |
| Phaeophytin *a* | As chlorophyll *a* without Mg. | 871.2 | eth.: 667 (55.5) | 609.5 (8.5) | 560 (3.1) | 534 (11.0) | 505 (12.7) | 471 (4.4) 408.5 (115.8) |
| Chloro-phyllide *a* | As chlorophyll *a* except R = H | 614.9 | As chlorophyll *a* | | | | | |
| Protochloro-phyll | As chlorophyll *a*, except bond between C atoms 7, 8 is unsaturated: $C_{55}H_{70}O_5N_4Mg$ | 891.5 | eth: 623 (35.6) | 571 (13.3) | 535 (6.4) | 432 (289.7) | | |
| Chlorphyll *b* (and derivatives) | As chlorophyll *a*, except 3, —CHO instead of —CH$_3$ $C_{55}H_{70}O_6N_4Mg$ | 907.5 | eth: 644 (51.5) acet.: 645 (47.0) | 595 (9.89) 595 (10.3) | 549 (5.62) .. | 455 (155) 455 (133.3) | 430 (53.1) .. | |
| Phaeophy-tin *b* | As phaeophytin *a*, except 3, —CHO instead of —CH$_3$: $C_{55}H_{72}O_6N_4$ | 885.2 | eth.: 655 (37.3) | 599 (8.4) | 555 (7.7) | 525.5 (12.6) | 434 (191) | 412.5 (73.5) |

*Absorption spectrum*

| Solvent | $A_{max}$ nm($\epsilon$ mM Fe) | | | Type | Solubility | General remarks |
|---|---|---|---|---|---|---|
| acetic−0.015 M -HCl | 594 | 547 | 376 | | s. pyr., MeOH, EtOH, | Prosthetic group of sulphite and nitrite |
| abs. ratio | 1 : | 3.5 | | | $H_2O$ | reductases. $Fe^{2+}$ removed by HCl. Prep. *JBC* |
| pyr. | 557 | 520 | 401 | | | **248**, 251 (1973); *PNAS* **71**, 612 (1974). |
| abs. ratio | 1 : | 2.7 | | | | Forms complexes with −OH, CO, −CN, pyr. |
| 0.1 M -NaOH | 567 | 385 | | | | Rev. *Meth. Enzymol.* **52**, 436 (1978). |
| abs. ratio | 1 : | 3.6 | | | | |
| 0.1 M -NaOH + 1 mM KCN | 580 | 403 | | | | |
| abs. ratio | 1 : | 3.2 | | | | |
| 0.1 M -NaOH + 1 mM KCN + $Na_2S_2O_4$ | 566 | 408 | | | | |
| abs. ratio | 1 : | 3.3 | | | | |
| 0.1 M -NaOH + $Na_2S_2O_4$ | 603 | 564 | 406 | | | |
| abs. ratio | 1 : | 4.3 | | | | |

| Solubility | General remarks |
|---|---|
| s. EtOH, acet., benz., eth., CHCl₃ ; sl. s. pet. eth.; i. $H_2O$ | Present in all photosynthetic organisms evolving oxygen in photosynthesis, i.e. higher plants, green, red, and brown algae, diatoms, etc. Fluorescence max. (eth.) 668, 723 nm. Phase test: yel. → green. Unstable, especially in light. Spectra affected by addition of $H_2O$ to org. solv. Review of spectra *Spectrochim. Acta* **21**, 1835 (1965); $A_{max}$ shifts of 4−26 nm when complexed to proteins *in vivo*; *Photochem. Photobiol.* **26**, 319 (1977). Prep. *BBA* **58**, 486 (1962); **75**, 306 (1963); *BBRC* **83**, 501 (1978). Isomerization of *a* and *b* occurs in hot $H_2O$. Est. H.p.l.c. separations. *J. Chromat.* **152**, 247 (1978); **154**, 73 (1978); *J. Agric. Food. Res.* **263**, 67 (1978). Est. *Planta* **78**, 200 (1968); Smith and Benitez p. 143; *BBA* **253**, 222 (1971). |
| s. eth., acet., benz., CHCl₃ ; sl. s. EtOH, pet. eth.; i. $H_2O$ | Occurrence as for chlorophyll *a*, possibly due to decomposition of chlorophyll *a*. Fluorescence max. (eth.) 672.5, 715 nm. Phase test: positive. HCl no. ≈ 29. Unstable, especially in light. Prep. *Bot. Gaz.* **102**, 463 (1941); *BBA* **58**, 486 (1962). Est. *Planta* **29**, 114 (1938−9). |
| s. Et acetate | Formed by photo-conversion of protochlorophyllide. Phase test positive. Ethyl chlorophyllide *a* (R = $C_2H_5$) usually present in EtOH extracts of leaves due to chlorophyllase action; *Am. J. Bot.* **41**, 710 (1954). Found in etiolated seedlings; *JBC* **183**, 713 (1950). |
| s. EtOH, acet., benz., eth.; i. pet. eth., $H_2O$ | Found in etiolated leaves of seedlings. A similar, but not identical pigment found in inner seed coats of Curcurbitaceae. |
| s. EtOH, acet., benz., eth.; sl. s. MeOH; i. $H_2O$, pet. eth. | Present in all higher plants and many green algae. Fluorescence max. (eth.) 646, 704. −79 K° fluorescence (EtOH) 658, 720; Phase test: red → brown → green. Prep. *BBA* **58**, 486 (1962). Smith and Benitez, p. 143; Est. Smith and Benitez, p. 154; *Photochem. Photobiol.* **1**, 259 (1962). |
| s. eth., acet., CHCl₃ , benz.; sl. s. MeOH, pet. eth.; i. $H_2O$ | Occurrence as for chlorophyll *b*. Possibly due to decomposition of chlorophyll *b*. Prep. as for chlorophyll *a*. HCl no. ≈ 35. |

| Name | Structure | M. wt. | Absorption spectrum $A_{max}$ nm($\epsilon$ mM) |
|---|---|---|---|
| Ethyl chloro-phyllide $b$ | As chlorophyll $a$, except 3, —CHO instead of —CH$_3$ R = C$_2$H$_5$: C$_{37}$H$_{36}$O$_6$N$_4$Mg | 657.0 | As chlorophyll $b$ |

| Name | Structure | M. wt. | Absorption spectrum $A_{max}$ nm($\epsilon$ mM) |
|---|---|---|---|
| Chlorophyll c$_1$ | (R = CH$_2$CH$_3$) | 610.9 | acet. + 1% pyr.: $\epsilon_{sp}$ 629.1 577.9 446.1 (39.2) (28.6) (348.0) 90% acet + 1% pyr.: $\epsilon_{sp}$ 630.6 579.4 443.2 (44.8) (26.0) (318.0) pyr.: $\epsilon_{sp}$ 639.6 593.2 461.5 (35.0) (30.4) (346.0) MeOH: 663 584 445 eth.: 626 576 444 |
| Phaeophor-bide c$_1$ (phaeopor-phyrin c$_1$) | As chlorophyll c$_1$ without Mg | 588.6 | acet.: 648 590 574 550 abs. ratios 0.1 : 0.98 : 1.0 : 0.64 eth. (Me ester): 666 590 570 525 424 abs. ratios 0.78 : 0.94 : 0.97 : 1 : 7.6 |

| Name | Structure | M. wt. | Absorption spectrum $A_{max}$ nm($\epsilon$ mM) |
|---|---|---|---|
| Chlorophyll c$_2$ (and deriva-tives) | as chlorophyll c$_1$ except R = —CH$_2$=CH$_2$ | 608.9 | acet. + 1% pyr.: $\epsilon_{sp}$ 629.6 581.3 444.6 (37.2) (35.7) (321.0) acet. 90% + 1% pyr.: $\epsilon_{sp}$ 630.9 581.2 443.8 (40.4) (30.7) (374.0) pyr.: $\epsilon_{sp}$ 641.5 597.3 466.0 (31.8) (42.0) (459.0) |
| Phaeophor-bide c$_2$ (phaeopor-phyrin c$_2$) | As chlorophyll c$_2$ without Mg | 586.6 | acet.: 651 596 574 532 abs. ratios 0.1 : 0.9 : 1.0 : 0.9 eth. (Me ester): 665 595 573 530 428 abs. ratios 0.57 : 0.95 : 0.97 : 1.0 : 8.87 |

| Name | Structure | M. wt. | Absorption spectrum $A_{max}$ nm($\epsilon$ mM) |
|---|---|---|---|
| Chlorophyll $d$ | As chlorophyll $a$ except 2—CHO instead of —CH=CH$_2$ | 892.5 | eth.: $A_{max}$: 688 643 595 548.5 512 447 392 $\epsilon_{sp}$: 110.4 14.3 9.47 4.03 1.98 97.8 58.9 |

| Name | Structure | M. wt. | Absorption spectrum $A_{max}$ nm($\epsilon$ mM) |
|---|---|---|---|
| Bacteriochloro-phyll $a$ | R = C$_{20}$H$_{39}$(phytyl) C$_{55}$H$_{74}$O$_6$N$_4$Mg | 911.5 | eth.: 773 577 391.5 358.5 (697) (530) 91.1 20.8 48.1 73.3 (9.1) (2.7) MeOH: 772 608 .. 365 (685) 42.0 15.4 .. 53.9 (8.6) |

| Solubility | General remarks |
|---|---|
| sl. s. eth., v. sl. s. EtOH | Usually present in alcoholic extracts of leaf tissue, due to chlorphyllase action. Prep. *Am. J. Bot.* **41**, 710 (1954). |
| s. MeOH, $CH_2Cl_2$, pyr. | Crystallized as green plates. Isolated from *Sorgassum, BBA* **279**, 15 (1972); *Fucus, Tetrahedron* **27**, 1447 (1971). Fluorescence max. 20°C (acet.) 633, 694 nm. |
| s. MeOH, $CH_2Cl_2$, pyr. | Formed by acid treatment of chlorophyll $c_1$. Prep. *Tetrahedron* **27**, 1447 (1971). Fluorescence max. 20°C (acet.) 717 > 652 nm. |
| s. MeOH, EtOH, EtAc, pyr. | Found in brown algae, diatoms, dinoflagellates and *Vaucheria*. Est. *Biochem. Physiol. Pflanzen* **167**, 191 (1975). Fluorescence $A_{max}$ 20°C (acet.) 635, 696 nm; (EtOH) 638, 700 nm. |
| as phaeophorbide $c_1$ | Prep. and Est as phaeophorbide $c_1$. Fluorescence max. 20°C (acet.) 725 > 655 nm. |
| s. EtOH, eth., acet., benz.; v. sl. s. pet. eth. | Found in red algae (*Gigartina papillata*). Prep. *Can. J. Bot.* **39**, 327 (1961); **37**, 507 (1959). Fluorescence max. (eth) 696, 752 nm. HCl no. > 32. Forms dimethyl acetal reversibly. |
| s. eth., acet., MeOH, benz., pyr.; i. pet. eth. | Found in purple and brown photosynthetic bacteria, some green sulphur bacteria. Phase test: yel. → brown → green. HCl no. ≈ 25. Fluorescence max. (EtOH) 805 nm. More stable when pure than in crude extracts. Prep. *ABB* **53**, 228 (1954); *Am. J. Bot.* **41**, 718 (1954). Phaeophorbide prepared by acid treatment of chlorophyll; not reported to occur naturally. |

| Name | Structure | M. wt. | Absorption spectrum $A_{max}$ nm ($\epsilon mM$) |
|---|---|---|---|

*Chlorobium* chlorophyll c; (660) (Bacteriochlorophyll c; bacterioviridin)

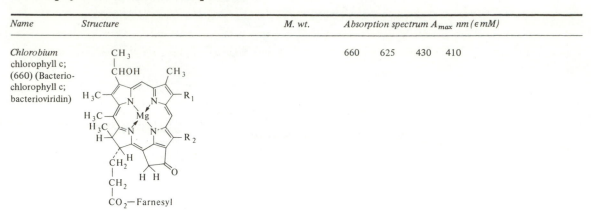

$R_1$, $R_2$ — see general remarks

660  625  430  410

---

*Chlorobium* chlorophyll (650) (Bacteriochlorophyll d)

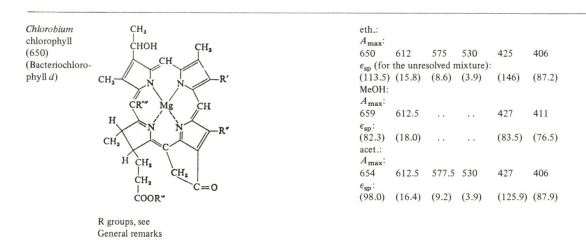

R groups, see General remarks

eth.:
$A_{max}$:
650    612    575    530    425    406
$\epsilon_{sp}$ (for the unresolved mixture):
(113.5) (15.8)  (8.6)  (3.9)  (146)  (87.2)
MeOH:
$A_{max}$:
659    612.5   ..     ..     427    411
$\epsilon_{sp}$:
(82.3) (18.0)   ..     ..     (83.5) (76.5)
acet.:
$A_{max}$:
654    612.5  577.5  530    427    406
$\epsilon_{sp}$:
(98.0) (16.4)  (9.2)  (3.9)  (125.9) (87.9)

| *Solubility* | *General remarks* |
|---|---|
| | Found in *Chlorobium limicola, Chloroflexus aurantiacus* (in latter farnesyl replaced by stearyl or other groups; *Ann.* **1979**, 408). $R_1$, $R_2$ are Et, Et (71%); Pr. Et (18%); Et, Me (10%); Bu, Et (1%); *Can. J. Chem.* **48**, 88 (1966). Structure *JCS Perkin* I 845 (1978). Fluorescence max. (eth.) 667 nm. Negative phase test. For methyl phaeophorbide lacking Mg and farnesyl replaced by methyl see *JCS Perkin* I, 850 (1978). |
| s. eth., acet., MeOH; i. pet. eth. | Found in green sulphur bacteria. Negative phase test. Fluorescence max. (eth.) 653 nm. The corresponding phaeophorbides, but not the chlorophylls themselves, have been separated into six components $R' = C_2H_5$, $C_3H_7$ or *iso*-$C_4H_{10}$; $R'' = CH_3$ or $C_2H_5$; $R''' = $ *trans-trans*-farnesyl ($C_{15}H_{25}$); $R'''' = H$. See Vernon & Seely, p. 112; *Plant Cell Physiol. Tokyo* **4**, 49 (1963). Prep. *BBA* **41**, 478 (1960). |

# 11 Carotenoids

A selection of the most commonly occurring carotenoids is given here. The order of presentation in the table is approximately that of the sequence on chromatograms, the least strongly adsorbed members being at the beginning.

## Solubility

Most carotenoids are soluble in acetone, benzene, and $CS_2$ but insoluble in water. Those at the top of the table are more soluble in hexane and other hydrocarbons, less soluble in alcohols, while those with hydroxyl groups and further down in the table are more soluble in alcohols.

*The formula* for β-carotene is:

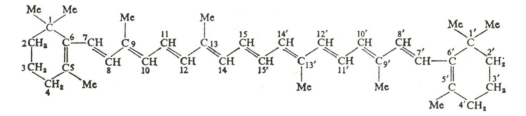

Since all carotenoids are related to β-carotene, only condensed formulae are shown in the table.

## Nomenclature

Tentative rules for the nomenclature of carotenoids are given in *BJ* **127**, 741 (1972); *EJB* **25**, 397 (1972).

| Name | Formula | M. wt. | Spectral absorption maxima (nm) | | |
|------|---------|--------|------|------|------|
| Phytoene | 7,8,11,12,12',11',8',7'-Octahydrolycopene $C_{40}H_{64}$ | 545.0 | Hexane | 298 | 286 | 275 |
| Phytofluene | 7,8,12',11',8',7'-Hexahydrolycopene $C_{40}H_{62}$ | 542.9 | Pet. eth. $A_{1\,cm}^{1\%}$ | 367–8 | 348 1350 (cis) 1540 (all-trans) | 332 |
| α-Carotene | $C_{40}H_{56}$ | 536.9 | Hexane $A_{1\,cm}^{1\%}$ | 475 | 445 2710 | 420 |
| | | | CS$_2$ $A_{1\,cm}^{1\%}$ | 509 | 477 2180 | |
| β-Carotene (carotin) | $C_{40}H_{56}$ | 536.9 | Hexane $A_{1\,cm}^{1\%}$ | 482 | 451 2550 | 425 |
| | | | CS$_2$ $A_{1\,cm}^{1\%}$ | 520 | 485 1940 | 450 |
| δ-Carotene | $C_{40}H_{56}$ | 536.9 | Hexane | 486 | 456 | 430 |
| γ-Carotene | $C_{40}H_{56}$ | 536.9 | Pet. eth. $A_{1\,cm}^{1\%}$ | 495 | 462 2720 | 431 |
| | | | CS$_2$ | 533.5 | 496 | 463 |
| Lycopene | $C_{40}H_{56}$ | 536.9 | Hexane $A_{1\,cm}^{1\%}$ | 506 | 474 3470 | 446 |
| | | | CS$_2$ | 547 | 507 | 477 |
| β-Cryptoxanthin (cryptoxanthol) | 3-Hydroxy-β-carotene $C_{40}H_{56}O$ | 552.9 | Hexane $A_{1\,cm}^{1\%}$ | 483 | 451 2460 | 425 |
| | | | CS$_2$ $A_{1\,cm}^{1\%}$ | 518 | 483 2040 | 453 |
| Spirilloxanthin (rhodoviolascin) | $C_{42}H_{60}O_2$ | 596.9 | Benz. $A_{1\,cm}^{1\%}$ | 548 | 511 2470 | 482 |
| | | | CS$_2$ $A_{1\,cm}^{1\%}$ | 573.5 | 534 1965 | 496.5 |
| Lutein (luteol, xanthophyll) | 3,3'-Dihydroxy-α-carotene $C_{40}H_{56}O_2$ | 568.9 | Hexane | 477 | 447 | 420 |
| | | | CS$_2$ $A_{1\,cm}^{1\%}$ | 508 | 475 2160 | 445 |
| | | | MeOH | 474 | 444 | 418 |

| Physical properties | Occurrence and General remarks |
|---|---|
| Colourless viscous oil | Small quantities in many leaves and fruits. Autoxidizes rapidly when pure. Optically inactive. |
| Colourless fluorescent oil | Small amounts in many green plant tissues, fruits, and some flowers. *Cis*-form from tomatoes readily isomerizes to the more stable all-*trans*-form when illuminated. With $SbCl_3$ in $CHCl_3$ gives transient blue colour changing to purple. |
| Violet prisms and clusters from benz.-MeOH; M.p. 187—8 | Leaf and root of *Daucus carota*. Fruit of red palm. Often reported in other materials without distinction from geometric isomers of $\beta$-carotene. $[\alpha]_{Cd}$ + 385 (in benz.). With $SbCl_3$ in $CHCl_3$ gives a blue colour absorbing maximally at 542 nm. Half the vitamin activity of $\beta$-carotene. |
| Dark violet hexagonal prisms from benz.-MeOH; M.p. 183 | Major carotenoid in green plant tissues and brown seaweeds. Widely distributed in plants and animals. Exceptionally concentrated in flower of *Narcissus*. Optically inactive. Vitamin A active. With $SbCl_3$ in $CHCl_3$ gives blue colour ($\lambda_{max}$ 590 nm). |
| Long red needles from $CS_2$-hexane-EtOH; M.p. 140.5 | Fruits of *Lycopersicum esculentum*. $[\alpha]$ + 317 (in $CS_2$, using Corning filters nos. 242 and 244). |
| Dark red prisms from benz.-MeOH; M.p. 131—78 | Leaf of *Cuscuta salina*, and of *Juniperis virginiana* infected with fungus. Some fruits and flowers. Many fungi. Major carotenoid in *Chlorobium* sp. Variations in M.p. from natural sources ascribed to different proportions of all-*trans*-$\gamma$-carotene and pro-$\gamma$-carotene. |
| Long red needles from $CS_2$-EtOH; M.p. 175 | Major pigment in fruit of *Lycopersicum esculentum*, *Rosa canina*, and others. Isomeric with $\beta$-carotene, but has no vitamin A activity. |
| Prisms from benz.-MeOH; M.p. 169 | Seed of *Zea mais*, fruit of *Physalis* sp., and small quantities in other fruits, some green tissues and a few flowers. Also eggs, butter, and blood. When prefix omitted, $\beta$-form is understood. Half the vitamin A activity of $\beta$-carotene. Occurs esterified. Dark blue colour ($\lambda_{max}$ 590 nm) with $SbCl_3$ in $CHCl_3$. Monoacetyl deriv., M.p. 117—18. Phase test as for $\alpha$-crytoxanthin. |
| Deep red, spindle-shaped crystals from benz; M.p. 218 | Major carotenoid of red and purple photosynthetic bacteria. Some fungi, e.g. *Neurospora crassa*. Blue colour ($\lambda_{max}$ 642 nm) with $SbCl_3$ in $CHCl_3$. |
| Violet prisms + 1 MeOH from MeOH; M.p. 193 | Major carotenol (xanthophyll) of green plant tissues. Extensively distributed in fruits, seeds, flowers. In eggs and many animal fats. $[\alpha]_{Cd}$ + 160 ($CHCl_3$). No vitamin A activity. Intense dark blue colour with $SbCl_3$ in $CHCl_3$. Green colour in conc. $H_2SO_4$ turning blue. Diacetyl deriv., M.p. 170. |

# 11 Carotenoids

| Name | Formula | M. wt. | Spectral absorption maxima (nm) | | | |
|------|---------|--------|------|------|------|------|
| Zeaxanthin (zeaxanthol) | 3,3'-Dihydroxy-$\beta$-carotene $C_{40}H_{56}O_2$ | 568.9 | Hexane $A_{1\,cm}^{1\%}$ CS$_2$ $A_{1\,cm}^{1\%}$ | 483 517 | 451 2480 482 2230 | 423 450 |
| Lutein epoxide (eloxanthin) | Lutein-5,6-epoxide $C_{40}H_{56}O_3$ | 584.9 | Pet. eth. CS$_2$ | 471 501.5 | 442 472 | |
| Flavoxanthin | 5,8-Epoxylutein $C_{40}H_{56}O_3$ | 584.9 | Hexane CS$_2$ | 450 479 | 421 449 | |
| Violaxanthin | 5,6,5',6'-Diepoxyzeaxanthin $C_{40}H_{56}O_4$ | 600.9 | Hexane CS$_2$ | 472 501 | 443 470 | 417.5 440 |
| Auroxanthin | 5,8,5',8'-Diepoxyzeaxanthin $C_{40}H_{56}O_4$ | 600.9 | EtOH $A_{1\,cm}^{1\%}$ CS$_2$ | 428 454 | 403 1850 423 | 382 |
| Astacene (astacin) | $C_{40}H_{48}O_4$ | 592.8 | CS$_2$ | 500 | | |
| Astaxanthin | $C_{40}H_{52}O_4$ | 596.9 | CS$_2$ Pyr. | 502 513 | 493 | 476 |
| Fucoxanthin | 3'-Acetyloxy-6',7'-didehydro-5,6-epoxy-5,5',6,6',7,8-hexahydro-3,5'-dihydroxy-8-oxo-$\beta$-carotene $C_{42}H_{58}O_6$ | 658.9 | Hexane $A_{1\,cm}^{1\%}$ CS$_2$ | 469 510 | 451 760 477 | 438 445 |

| Physical properties | Occurrence and General remarks |
|---|---|
| Yellow plates from MeOH; M.p. 215.5 | Fruit, seeds, and some flowers. Traces in green leaves, egg yolk. $[\alpha]_D$ −40 to −45.2 (CHCl$_3$). Diacetyl deriv., M.p. 154—5. |
| Reddish-yellow crystals from benz.-MeOH; M.p. 192 | Flowers and leaves. Very unstable towards acids, even in traces, being converted to flavoxanthin and chrysanthemaxanthin. Diacetyl deriv., M.p. 184—5. |
| Golden, clustered prisms from MeOH; M.p. 184 | Flower of *Ranunculus acer*, *Taraxacum officinale*, and a few others. Small quantities in green tissues and some fruits. Isomer of chrysanthemaxanthin. May be formed from lutein epoxide during extraction. $[\alpha]_{Cd}^{20}$ +190 (in benz.). Unstable blue colour with conc. HCl. Blue colour with SbCl$_3$ in CHCl$_3$. Diacetyl deriv., M.p. 157. |
| Yellow-orange prisms from MeOH; M.p. 200 (208) | Flower of *Viola tricolor* and many others. A few fruits. Important carotenol of green leaves. $[\alpha]_{Cd}$ + 35 (in CHCl$_3$). Very unstable to acids. Soln. in conc. H$_2$SO$_4$ is indigo blue, in gl. acetic acid is green. Deep blue with SbCl$_3$ in CHCl$_3$. Dibenzoyl deriv., M.p. 217. |
| Yellow needles from MeOH; M.p. 203 | Flower of *Viola tricolor*. Formed when violaxanthin is treated with dil. HCl. Very stable blue colour with 15% HCl. |
| Violet needles from pyr.-H$_2$O; M.p. 240—3 | Many animal tissues especially Crustacea shells, sometimes with astaxathin. Found esterified (astacein) in shells of lobster and crabs. Astacin is formed from ovoverdin, the astaxanthin-protein complex; thus some reported isolation of astacin may be in error. Optically inactive. Blue-green colour with SbCl$_3$ in CHCl$_3$. Diacetyl deriv., M.p. 235 d; dipalmitoyl, M.p. 121. |
| Violet plates from pyr.; M.p. 215—16 d | Characteristic carotenoid of many animal tissues, especially crustaceans. Some green algae, incl. *Haematococcus pluvialis*. Occurs in chromoproteins, e.g. ovoverdin from lobsters, from which it is released by acids, organic solvents, and heat. In absence of air gives blue colour with alkalis. Optically inactive. Diacetyl deriv., M.p. 203—5; dipalmitoyl, M.p. 71.5—72.5. |
| Brown-red prisms + 3 MeOH from MeOH; needles from ether-pet. eth.; M.p. 166—8 | Characteristic carotenoid of Phaeophyceae, Chrysophyceae, and diatoms. With conc. H$_2$SO$_4$ gives deep blue colour. Hydrochloride, C$_{42}$H$_{58}$O$_6$ · 4HCl, M.p. 215. Pure compound optically inactive in benz. (also given as $[\alpha]_D^{18}$ + 72 ± 9 (CHCl$_3$)). Deep blue colour with 25% HCl. |

# 12 Plant growth regulators

This Table includes natural phytohormones, synthetic growth substances, anti-hormones, and those herbicides which are used to induce specific beneficial changes in agriculture such as enhanced yields, improved quality, or easier harvesting. Other herbicides may be found under Inhibitors of mitochondrial and chloroplast function, p. 302.

## Phytohormones

D. S. Letham, P. B. Goodwin, and T. J. V. Higgins (eds.) *Phytohormones and related compounds. Vol. 1, The biochemistry of phytohormones and related compounds. Vol. II, Phytohormones and the development of higher plants.* Elsevier/North-Holland, Amsterdam (1978).

Recent volumes of *Annual Review of Plant Physiology* include chapters on abscisic acid (**31**, 453, 1980); auxins (**25**, 487, 1974 and **28**, 439, 1977); cytokinins (**24**, 415, 1973 and **34**, 163, 1983); ethylene (**30**, 533, 1979); gibberellins (**24**, 571, 1973 and **29**, 149, 1978). Other chapters deal with regulation of ribonucleic acid metabolism by plant hormones (**28**, 537, 1977); hormone binding in plants (**27**, 267, 1976 and **32**, 569, 1981); rapid responses to plant hormones (**25**, 195, 1974); and analytical methods for growth substances (**32**, 511, 1981).

*The encyclopedia of plant physiology* (N.S.) Vol. 4, (1976). *Physiological plant pathology* (A. Pirson *et al.*, eds.); and Vol 9 (1980) *Hormonal regulation of development, 1. Molecular aspects of plant hormones* (J. MacMillan, ed.) have chapters on natural growth regulators in healthy and diseased plants.

## Growth regulators in horticulture and agriculture

A. J. Weaver, *Growth substances in agriculture*. W. H. Freeman, San Francisco (1972).

L. G. Nickell, *Plant growth regulators: agricultural uses*. Springer-Verlag, Berlin (1982).

T. H. Thomas (ed.), *Plant growth regulator potential and practice*. BCPC Publications, Croydon (1982).

## Herbicides

L. G. Audus (ed.), *Herbicides − physiology, biochemistry, ecology*. Vols. I, II. Academic Press, London (1976).

D. E. Moreland, Mechanism of action of herbicides. *Ann. Rev. Plant Physiol.* **31**, 597, 1980.

C. Fedtke, *Biochemistry and physiology of herbicide action*. Springer-Verlag, Berlin (1982).

## Growth regulators in plant tissue culture

J. Reinert and Y. P. S. Bajaj (eds.), *Applied and fundamental aspects of plant cell, tissue, and organ culture*. Springer-Verlag, Berlin (1977).

H. E. Street (ed.), *Plant tissue and cell culture*, 2nd edn, Blackwell, Oxford (1977).

J. F. Reynolds and T. Murashige, Plant Cell lines, *Meth. Enzymol.* **58**, 478 (1979).

| Name | Synonyms | Formula | M. wt. |
|------|----------|---------|--------|
| Abscisic acid | ABA; dormin; abscisin II; 5-(1-hydroxy-2,6,6-trimethyl-4-oxo-2-cyclohexen-1-yl)-3-methyl-2,4-pentadienoic acid | | 264.3 |
| AMO 1618 | 2-Isopropyl-4-dimethylamino-5-methylphenyl-1-piperidinecarboxylate methyl chloride | | 354.9 |
| Ancymidol | α-Cyclopropyl-α-(*p*-methoxyphenyl)-5-pyrimidinemethanol; EL-531; A-rest | | 256.3 |
| Benzimidazole | | | 170.5 |
| $N^6$-Benzyladenine | 6-Benzylaminopurine; BA | | 225.3 |
| CCC | Chlormequat; (2-chloroethyl) trimethyl-ammonium chloride; Cycocel; chlorocholine chloride | | 158.1 |
| 2,4-Dichlorophenoxy-acetic acid | 2,4-D | | 221.0 |

| Physical properties | Solubility | General remarks |
|---|---|---|
| $\lambda_{max}$(MeOH) 252 nm ($\epsilon$ 25 200). Naturally occurring form (+)-2-*cis* | 0.06 $H_2O$; s. aq. $NaHCO_3$, acet., $CHCl_3$; sp. s. pet. eth. | Natural growth inhibitor causing dormancy of leaves and buds, abscission of fruit and leaves, senescence, delayed seed germination and flowering, stomatal closure. Linear response in stomatal aperture bioassay (in citrate, pH 5.5) given over range $10^{-10}$–$10^{-7}$M. Used as defoliant and growth inhibitor. $LD_{50}$ orally in rats: $>400$ mg/kg. |
| M.p. 179 | | Anti-gibberellin growth retardant. Inhibits GA biosynthesis by blocking cyclization of $C_{20}$ geranylgeranyl diphosphate to (−)-kaurene; in pathway for microsomal cholesterol biosynthesis inhibits squalene-2,3-oxide cyclase causing accumulation of squalene-2,3-epoxide, *JBC* **250**, 1571 (1975); also inhibits desmethylsterol biosynthesis, *Phytochem.* **17**, 705 (1978). |
| M.p. 110–1. Unstable in solution $\leqslant$ pH 4 | 0.065 $H_2O$; s. acet., MeOH, $CHCl_3$ | Anti-gibberellin. At $10^{-4}$M inhibits normal internode growth; effect overcome by $GA_3$, *Plant Physiol.* **48**, 537 (1971). Inhibitor of *ent*-kaur-16-ene oxidation in microsomal preps. $K_i \sim 2 \times 10^{-9}$M. Specific for plant tissues. Similarity in behaviour to metyrapone as an inhibitor of liver microsomes. Both bind to Cyt P450, *Plant Physiol.* **62**, 571 (1978). |
| Weak base, $pK_a$: 5.48 at 25°C; M.p. 170.5 | s. EtOH; sp. s. cold $H_2O$, more s. hot; sp. s. eth.; i. benz., pet. eth. | Shows some activity as a cytokinin in leaf senescence and pigment production bioassays ($5 \times 10^{-4}$M) but not in stimulating cell division or mobilisation of metabolites. |
| $pK_a$: 10.9. M.p. 232; $\lambda_{max}$ (EtOH): 270 nm ($\epsilon$ 18 000); (0.1 M-HCl): 274 (16 500) (0.1M-NaOH): 275 (17 000) | 0.006 $H_2O$; $<0.001$ hexane; 0.37 acet.; 0.68 MeOH; 13.3 DMSO | Synthetic cytokinin. At $10^{-8}$M stimulates cell division in undifferentiated tissue in culture, in the presence of auxin; increases formation of secondary plant products ($10^{-6}$M); causes cell enlargement in cotyledons, promotes seed germination, retards senescence, promotes movement of metabolites ($10^{-6}$–$10^{-4}$M). Used as dormancy breaker and growth promoter, *Anal. Meth. Pestic. Plant Growth Regul.* **10**, 545 (1978). |
| Decomp. 245. Aqueous solutions stable but corrosive to metals | $74^{20}$ $H_2O$ | Anti-gibberellin growth retardant. Analogue of choline. Used as a height shortener in wheat and poinsettias, a sugarcane ripener and to reduce 'lodging' in cereal grains. |
| $pK_a$: 2.64. $\lambda_{max}$: 201 nm ($\epsilon$ 38 000), 230 (7500), 283 (1900), 291 (1600) M.p. 140.5 | $0.06^{25}$ $H_2O$; $60^{31}$ EtOH; $45^{33}$ acet. | Synthetic auxin and selective weed killer. Selectivity partly due to poor translocation in grasses as compared to broad leaf weeds, and to greater leaf surface area for collecting spray in dicots. Abnormal accumulation of coumarin derivatives, more toxic to broad leaf plants than grasses, may contribute to death. Used as herbicide and fruit-drop controller. $LD_{50}$ orally in rats: 0.3–1 g/kg. Other important chlorinated phenoxy compounds are (2,4,5-trichlorophenoxy)acetic acid (2,4,5-T), ((4-chloro-*O*-tolyl)oxy) acetic acid (MCPA) and 4-(2,4-dichlorophenoxy)-butyric acid (2,4-DB). The latter (and other phenoxy acids with even no. of C atoms in chain) in sensitive plants, is converted by $\beta$-oxidation to 2,4-D; alfalfa is resistant, lacking this pathway. 2,4,-D used in cell culture ($10^{-7}$–$10^{-5}$M) in preference to IAA which is quickly metabolized. |

| Name | Synonyms | Formula | M. wt. |
|------|----------|---------|--------|
| Diquat | 1,1′-Ethylene-2,2′-bipyridylium dibromide | | 344.1 |
| N,N′-Diphenylurea | DPU; 1,3-diphenylurea; diphenylcarbamide; carbanilide | | 212.3 |
| Ethephon | 2-Chloroethylphosphonic acid; Ethrel; Cepha | $ClCH_2 CH_2 PO_3 H_2$ | 144.5 |
| Ethylene | Ethene | $CH_2{=}CH_2$ | 28.1 |
| Gibberellic acid | $GA_3$; 2,4a,7-trihydroxy-1-methyl-8-methylenegibb-3-ene-1,10-carboxylic acid-1,4-lactone | | 346.4 |
| Glyphosine | N,N-Bis (phosphonomethyl) glycine; Polaris | $HOOC \cdot CH_2N(CH_2PO_3H_2)_2$ | 263.1 |
| 3-Indoleacetic acid | IAA; auxin | | 175.2 |
| 3-Indolebutyric acid | IBA | | 203.2 |
| $N^6$-($\Delta^2$-Isopentenyl)-adenine | IPA; 2iP; $i^6$Ade; 6-(3-methyl-2-butenylamino) purine; $N^6$-($\gamma\gamma$-dimethylallyl) adenine | | 203.2 |

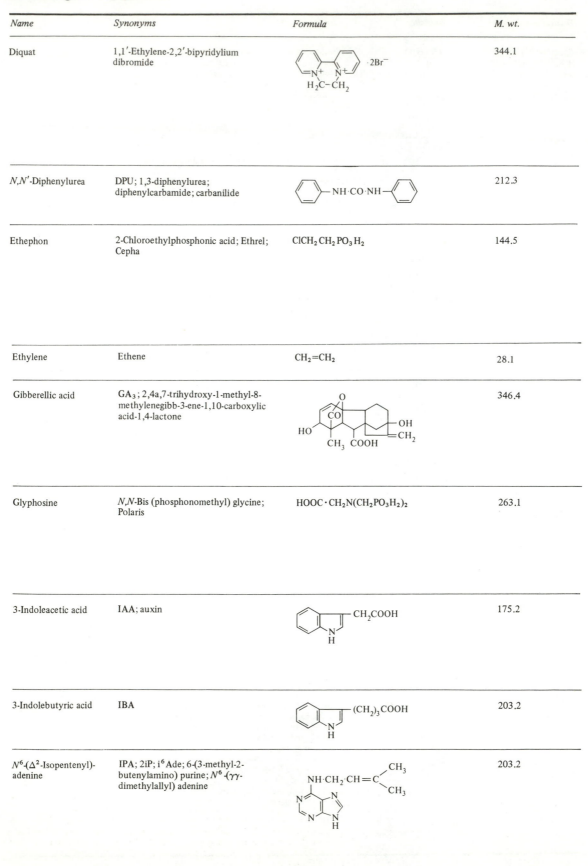

| Physical properties | Solubility | General remarks |
|---|---|---|
| $E_0'$ $-0.349$ V. $\lambda_{max}$ 308.3 nm ($\epsilon$ 18 000). Stable in acid or neutral soln. | $70^{20}$ $H_2O$ | Used as redox indicator, contact herbicide and sugar cane flowering suppressant. Most effective bipyridylium herbicides are quaternary salts derived from $2,2'-$ (e.g. diquat) and $4,4'-$ (e.g. paraquat) $-$ bipyridyl. Confined to compounds with redox potentials between $-300$ and $-500$ mV in which the two pyridine rings are in the same plane. Exception is benzyl viologen possibly due to slower penetration into plant. See also paraquat (methyl viologen) and benzyl viologen. Proposed mode of action: destruction of cell membranes following breakdown of unsaturated fatty acids, due to $O_2^-$ produced from reoxidation of bipyridylium. $LD_{50}$ orally in rats, mice, rabbits: 231, 125, 101 mg/kg. Summers, L. A. *The bipyridinium herbicides*. Academic Press, London (1980). |
| M.p. 238 B.p. 260d | 0.015 $H_2O$; s. eth., gl. acetic; sp. s. EtOH, acet., $CHCl_3$; 6.9 pyr. | A number of substituted phenylureas show cytokinin activity in delaying leaf senescence, promoting lateral bud development, stimulating germination and cell division, *Proc. Roy. Soc. B,* **165**, 245 (1966). |
| v. hygr. needles from benzene; M.p. 74–5 | v.s. $H_2O$, MeOH, acet., ethylene glycol; sl. s. benz., toluene; i. pet. eth. | Ethylene generator. Aq. solns. stable $<$ pH 3.5. Releases ethylene at pHs $>$ 4.1, *Plant Physiol* **63**, 474 (1979). Induces abscission of leaves, flowers, and fruit, promotes flowering and fruit ripening, causes epinasty of leaves, breaking of dormancy, and induction of enzyme synthesis. Inhibits mitosis, DNA synthesis, polar and lateral auxin transport. Used at $2-200$ $\mu l/l$. Used as stimulator of latex flow in rubber, sugarcane ripener, flowering agent for pineapple, color enhancer. Treatment before or after harvesting accelerates maturation of many fruit. $LD_{50}$ orally in rats: 4.2 g/kg. Spray formulations are $\sim$ pH 1.0; may be irritating to exposed skin or eyes or if inhaled. |
| Col. gas; B.p. $-102.4$ | v.s. EtOH; s. eth.; i. $H_2O$ | See ethephon for action. Triple pea test bioassay linear for 0.025–0.1 p.p.m. $HgClO_4$ used to adsorb and remove ethylene from air. |
| M.p. 227d | v.s. EtOH, acet.; s. pet. eth., eth.; sl. s. $H_2O$ | Natural phytohormone involved in elongation of internode growth, flower induction, sub-apical cell division, reversal of dwarfism, induction of parthenocarpy, stimulation of amylase synthesis. Linear response in bioassays given over range $10^{-5}-10^{-2}$ $\mu g/ml$ (barley endosperm), 0.001–10 $\mu g$/plant (dwarf maize), 0.025–125 $\mu g/ml$ (pea internode). Mode of action through induction of specific mRNAs and control of membrane biosynthesis and function. Used as stimulator of amylase content of malting barley, seedless grape enlarger, flower initiator (replaces long day/or low temp. requirements), shoot growth stimulator. |
| M.p. 200d | $24.8^{20}$ $H_2O$ | Chemical ripener. Increases sucrose content of sugar cane. $LD_{50}$ orally in mammals: 3.9 g/kg. Glyphosate ($N$-(phosphonomethyl)glycine isopropylamine salt, Roundup) used as herbicide. In sub-lethal conc. ($7.5 \times 10^{-5}$ M) induces tillering in sorghum, wheat. Inhibits basipetal auxin transport, *Plant Physiol.* **63**, 882 (1979). At $10^{-3}$ M stimulates phenylalanine lyase of roots of dark-grown maize seedlings, *Plant Sci. Lett.* **11**, 185 (1978). At $6 \times 10^{-4}$ M uncouples corn mitochondria, enhances mitochondrial ATPase activity, *FEBS Lett.* **97**, 279 (1979). Primary effect on aromatic amino acid biosynthesis, *Plant Physiol.* **66**, 823, 830 (1980). |
| M.p. 165d (162–70); $pK_a$ 4.54. Aq. solns are decomposed by u.v. but are stable to visible light | 0.16 $H_2O$; v.s. EtOH; s. acet., eth.; sl. s. benz., dichloroethane; i. $CHCl_3$ | Natural phytohormone involved in cell enlargement esp. in coleoptiles, initiation of root formation but inhibition of root growth, apical dominance and bud inhibition, abscission of leaves and fruit, differentiation, and fruit growth parthenocarpy. Activates proton extrusion and $K^+$ uptake in sensitive cells; the hydrogen ions either directly or indirectly (through effect on enzymes) increase plasticity of cell walls, allowing cell expansion in response to cell turgor pressure. Auxins also act at the level of gene expression. |
| M.p. 123–5 | s. EtOH, acet., eth.; i. $H_2O$, $CHCl_3$ | Synthetic auxin, used as a root initiator in cuttings. $LD_{50}$ i.p. in mice 100 mg/kg. Hypoglycaemic and tumorigenic in rats. |
| M.p. 212–4. $\lambda_{max}$ (pH 7) 269 nm ($\epsilon$ 19 400); (pH 1): 273 (18 600); (pH 13): 275 (18 100); $pK_a$: 3.4, 10.4 | | Naturally-occurring cytokinin. See benzyladenine for action. Occurs in tRNA (adjacent to the 3'-OH end of the anticodon, in yeast (0.05–0.17 mole/100 mole tRNA). In bacteria it is largely replaced by the 2-methylthio derivative, and in plant tissues by the hydroxy derivative, $N^6$-(*cis*-4-hydroxyisopentenyl) adenine and the corresponding 2-methylthio-compound. These modified bases always occur in tRNA species that respond to a codon starting with U, *PNARMB* **10**, 57 (1970); **12**, 49 (1972). Riboside: $N^6$-($\Delta^2$-isopentenyl) adenosine (6-(3-methyl-2-butenylamino)9-$\beta$-D-ribofuranosylpurine; 2iPA; $i^6$ A), M. wt. 335.4. M.p. 145–147. $\lambda_{max}$ (pH 7): 269 nm ($\epsilon$ 20 000); (pH 1): 265 (20 400); (pH 13): 269 (19 800). |

# 12 Plant growth regulators

| Name | Synonyms | Formula | M. wt. |
|------|----------|---------|--------|
| Kinetin | $N^6$-Furfuryladenine; 6-furfurylamino-purine | | 215.2 |
| Maleic hydrazide | 1,2-Dihydro-3,6-pyridazinedione; MH | | 112.1 |
| 3-Methyl-7-(3-methylbutylamino)-pyrazolo {4,3-d}-pyrimidine | | | 218.3 |
| Morphactin | CFL; IT3299; 2-chloro-9-hydroxy-fluorene-9-carboxylate; Chlorflurenol Methyl derivative, IT 3456 | | 260.7 |
| 1-Naphthaleneacetic acid | NAA; napthylacetic acid | | 186.2 |
| $N$-1-Napthylphthalamic acid | NPA; naptalam; Alanap | | 291.3 |
| $N$-Phenyl-$N'$-(4-pyridyl)-urea | NC 5392 | | 213.2 |
| Phosphon D | Chlorphonium chloride; 2,4-dichlorobenzyltributylphosphonium chloride | | 397.8 |
| $n$-Propyl gallate | Tenox PG | | 212.2 |
| Rhizobitoxine | L-2-Amino-4-(2'-amino-3'-hydroxypropoxy)-trans-3-butenoic acid; Ro | | 190.2 |

| Physical properties | Solubility | General remarks |
|---|---|---|
| M.p. 266–7 (sealed tube) sublimes 220. p$K_a$: 2.7, 9.9. $\lambda_{max}$ (EtOH): 268 nm ($\epsilon$ 18 650); (0.1 M-HCl): 274 (16 900); (0.1 M-NaOH): 273 (17 400) | sl. s. $H_2O$, MeOH, EtOH; s. dil. aq. HCl or NaOH; can be extracted from neutral aq. solns. by shaking with eth. | Synthetic cytokinin. See benzyladenine for action. Originally isolated from autoclaved DNA. Used as a dormancy breaker. Can detect $5 \times 10^{-9}$ M in soybean callus bioassay. Linear response in bioassays given over range $5 \times 10^{-8} - 5 \times 10^{-6}$ M (radish leaf disc expansion), $5 \times 10^{-7} - 5 \times 10^{-5}$ M (*Xanthium* leaf senescence) $2 \times 10^{-8} - 5 \times 10^{-5}$ M (soybean callus), $5 \times 10^{-9} - 5 \times 10^{-7}$ M (carrot root tissue). |
| Decomp. 260 | $0.6^{25}$ $H_2O$; sl. s. hot EtOH | Synthetic growth inhibitor, herbicidal at high conc. An analogue of uracil. General inhibitor of meristematic activity. As diethanolamine salt, used as a turf growth retardant, to prevent sprouting of potato tubers and of onions and suckering of tobacco. $LD_{50}$ orally in rats: 4 g/kg. |
| M.p. 184–8 $\lambda_{max}$ (pH 1): 311 nm (sh 327) ($\epsilon$ 12 700); (pH 7): 295 (sh 288) (12 100); (pH 12): 245 (sh 265) (14 700) | | Cytokinin antagonist, *Phytochem.* **12**, 25 (1973), *Biochem. Soc. Symp.* **38**, 195 (1973). At 0.003 $\mu$M IPA, in tobacco bioassay, inhibition detected at 0.1 $\mu$M, lethal at 0.73 $\mu$M. |
| M.p. 152 | $0.0018^{20}$ $H_2O$ | Anti-auxin, probably acting by influencing auxin transport and metabolism. Inhibits geo- and phototropisms at $6 \times 10^{-5}$ M. Stimulates abscission of flowers and fruit, probably via an increase in $C_2H_4$ production. Auxin counteracts. Inhibits fusion of Golgi into cell plate. Weed killer at higher conc. *Ann. Rev. Plant Physiol.* **21**, 499 (1970). |
| M.p. 134–5 | $0.04^{17}$ $H_2O$; s. 30% EtOH; v.s. acet., eth., $CHCl_3$ | Synthetic auxin. Used in plant cell culture ($10^{-7} - 10^{-5}$ M) in preference to IAA which is quickly metabolized. Used as a fruit thinner, flowering agent for pineapple, preventer of pre-harvest drop and a root inducer on cuttings. $LD_{50}$ orally in rats: 1 g/kg. |
| M.p. 203. Hydrolysed by strong acids and bases | $< 0.02$ $H_2O$; s. alk. soln., decomp. $> $ pH 9.5; sl. s. EtOH, acet., benz. | Anti-auxin; inhibits polar auxin transport, probably by competing for an auxin binding protein. Used as a pre-emergence herbicide. $LD_{50}$ orally in mammals: $> 8.5$ g/kg. |
| M.p. 162–3 | $> 0.01$ $H_2O$ | Synthetic cytokinin, especially in promotion of shoot formation, *Physiol. Plant.* **38**, 35 (1976). Structure–function study of derivatives shows the most active in tobacco callus bioassay are $N$-(2-chloro-4-pyridyl)-$N'$ (substituted or unsubstituted phenyl) ureas, *Phytochem.* **17**, 1201 (1978). |
| M.p. 114–20 | s. $H_2O$ | Anti-gibberellin, growth retardant. Subapical meristem dwarfed without affecting meristem. |
| M.p. 150 | $0.35^{25}$ $H_2O$; $103^{25}$ EtOH; $83^{25}$ eth. | Inhibitor of ethylene synthesis (1mM), *Plant Physiol.* **60**, 794 (1977); inhibitor of lipoxygenase and of 'alternate respiration' in soybean (0.5mM), *Plant Physiol.* **62**, 470 (1978). In latter is × 10 more effective than salicylhydroxamic acid. Used in food as an anti-oxidant. Darkens in the presence of iron salts. $LD_{50}$ orally in rats: 2.5–4 g/kg. |
| | | Anti-ethylene phytotoxin produced by certain strains of soybean nodule bacterium, *Rhizobium japonicum*. At $10^{-4} - 10^{-3}$ M inhibits ethylene production, *Plant Physiol.* **61**, 886 (1978). Inhibits $\beta$-cystathionase; reversed by pyridoxal phosphate, *BBA* **227**, 671 (1971). Related amino acid analogues, *Ann. Rev. Plant Physiol.* **30**, 544 (1979). |

# 12 Plant growth regulators

| Name | Synonyms | Formula | M. wt. |
|------|----------|---------|--------|
| SADH | B-9; Alar; B-995; daminozide; succinic acid-2,2-dimethylhydrazide | $HOOC \cdot CH_2 \cdot CH_2 \cdot CO \cdot NHN(CH_3)_2$ | 160.0 |
| Silver nitrate | | $Ag^+NO_3^-$ | 169.9 |
| Tetrahydropyranyl-benzyladenine | SD 8339; PBA; 6-benzyl-amino-9-(tetrahydropyran-2-yl) purine | | 227.3 |
| 2,3,5-Triiodobenzoic acid | TIBA | | 499.8 |
| Zeatin | $t$-io[6] Ade; 6-(4-hydroxy-3-methyl-*trans*-2-butenylamino) purine | | 219.2 |

| Physical properties | Solubility | General remarks |
|---|---|---|
| M.p. 145–6 | $10^{25}$ $H_2O$ | Inhibits IAA synthesis. Used as a growth retardant, and a multiple flower stimulator. |
| | | Anti-ethylene. Silver ions, used at $10^{-4}$–$10^{-3}$ M to inhibit response of plants to both endogenous and exogenous ethylene, *Plant Physiol.* **63**, 169 (1979). Anionic complex silver thiosulphate, $Ag(S_2O_3)_2^{3-}$, is less phytotoxic; mobile in plant transport system, *Scientia Hortic.* **20**, 211 (1983) |
| | | Synthetic cytokinin of high activity. See benzyladenine for action. |
| M.p. 224–6 | sl.s. $H_2O$; s. acet., eth., toluene | Anti-auxin. Less endogenous auxin available. May block auxin transport, increase IAA degradation or cause auxin immobilisation. Used as a growth retardant and to increase pod set in soybean. |
| | | Naturally-occurring cytokinin. Can detect $5 \times 10^{-11}$ M in soybean callus bioassay. Occurs in *cis*-form in tRNA from plant tissues (0.01–0.075 mole/100 mole tRNA). See isopentenyladenine for ref. Riboside:ribosylzeatin; (6-(4-hydroxy-3-methyl-*trans*-2-butenylamino)-9-$\beta$-D-ribofuranosylpurine; *t*-io$^6$ A), M. wt. 351.4. |

# 13 Antimetabolites, antibacterial agents, and enzyme inhibitors

## A. COMPOUNDS AFFECTING NUCLEIC ACIDS

This Table includes inhibitors of nucleoside, nucleotide, DNA and RNA synthesis, mutagens and carcinogens, and antimitotic drugs.

### General references

Purine analogues and pyrimidine analogues, in *Metabolic inhibitors*, eds. R.M. Hochster and J.H. Quastel, vol. 1, pp. 215, 239, Academic Press, New York (1963). ATP analogues, *Adv. Enzymol.* **43**, 1 (1975).

Nucleoside and nucleotide antibiotics, *PNARMB* **22**, 193 (1979).

Mechanism of action of inhibitors of DNA synthesis, *ARB* **46**, 641 (1977).

The chemical effects of nucleic acid alkylation and their relation to mutagenesis and carcinogenesis, *PNARMB* **15**, 219 (1975).

Chemical carcinogenesis, *ARB* **44**, 79 (1975).

Use of inhibitors in the study of hormone mechanisms in cell culture, *Meth. Enzymol.* **40**, 273 (1975).

Cell cycle specific agents, *BBA* **458**, 243 (1976); **516**, 389 (1978).

*The molecular basis of antibiotic action*, 2nd edition, E.F. Gale *et al.*, Wiley-Interscience, London (1981).

*Antibiotics,* vol. 1. *Mechanism of action*, eds. D. Gottlieb and P.D. Shaw, Springer-Verlag, Berlin (1967).

*Antibiotics*, vol. 3. *Mechanism of action of antimicrobial and antitumour agents*, eds. J.W. Corcoran and F.E. Hahn, Springer-Verlag, Berlin (1975).

*Antibiotics,* vol. 5. *Mechanism of action of antieukaryotic and antiviral compounds*, ed. F.E. Hahn, Springer-Verlag, Berlin (1979).

| Name | Synonyms | Formula | M. wt. |
|------|----------|---------|--------|
| Actinomycin | | | D, 1255.5 |
| ADP-$\beta$-S | Adenosine 5′-O-(2-thiodiphosphate) | | 443.2 |
| Adriamycin | | as Daunomycin except R = CO·CH$_2$OH | 543.5 |
| Aflatoxin B$_1$ | | | 312.3 |
| $\alpha$-Amanitin | | | 903.0 |
| Amethopterin | Methotrexate; 4-amino-$N^{10}$-methylpteroyl-glutamic acid | [R = benzoylglutamic acid] | 454.5 |

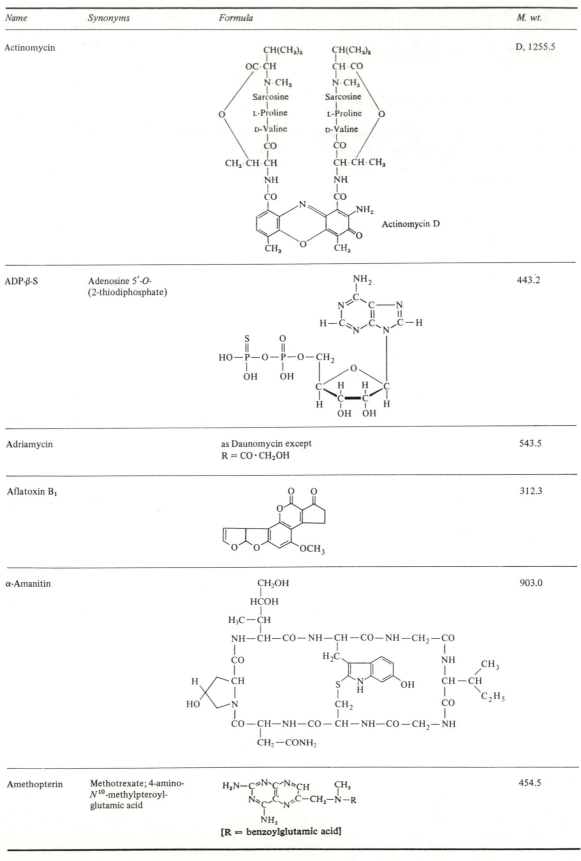

| Physical properties | Solubility | General remarks |
|---|---|---|
| red cryst.; $\epsilon_{260}$ (pH 7) 24 600. Store dry, $-20\,^\circ$C in dark | v.s. acet., benz., $CHCl_3$, gl. acetic; s. ethyl acetate, MeOH, EtOH; sl. s. eth., $H_2O$; i. pet. eth.; s. dil. mineral acids; i. alkalis | Inhibits DNA-primed RNA polymerase by complexing with DNA, via deoxyguanosine residues. At higher concentrations DNA polymerase inhibited. $0.25-0.75\,\mu$g/ml inhibits growth of *S. aureus* whereas $100\,\mu$g/ml is required to inhibit *E. coli* due to permeability differences. Active in mammalian systems – potent antitumour agent. Obtained as mixtures of closely related compounds, formed in different proportions by different strains of *Streptomyces*. The various actinomycins have the same chromophore but different peptide side chains. Actinomycin D is the most widely used of the group. |
| | | Competitive inhibitor of *E. coli* alkaline phosphatase, $K_i = 6.6 \times 10^{-5}$ M. Substrate for polynucleotide phosphorylase (*Micrococcus lysodeikticus*). Translocated by mitochondrial ATP/ADP translocase. Not phosphorylated in oxidative phosphorylation but potent inhibitor of State 3 respiration, indicating firm binding to ATP-synthesis complex. Li$_3$ salt, $C_{10}H_{12}N_5O_9P_2SLi_3$, m. wt. 461.0. |
| p$K_a$ 8.22 | | Action as for daunomycin (q.v.). Hydrochloride, m. wt. 580.0, s. $H_2O$, MeOH. |
| M.p. 268–9; $\lambda_{max}$ (EtOH) 223, 265, 362 nm $\epsilon$ 25 600, 13 400, 21 800 | | Caution: extremely toxic and carcinogenic. One of several aflatoxins produced by *Aspergillus flavus*. Metabolized by liver microsomal systems yielding products which bind covalently to DNA, *BBA* **585**, 134 (1979). |
| | s. $H_2O$, MeOH, EtOH | Handle with extreme care – extremely dangerous; toxic by mouth, skin, or inhalation. Inhibits eukaryote RNA polymerase II (polymerase B) at $10^{-8}-10^{-9}$ M, polymerase III (C) at $10^{-4}-10^{-5}$ M but not polymerase I (A) or bacterial polymerase. Produced by mushroom, *Amanita phalloides*. Review on *Amanita* toxins: *Critical Revs. in Biochem.* **5**, 185 (1978). |
| yel. cryst.; M.p. 185–204 | s. dil. HCl | Folic acid antagonist. Reversed by FA itself, and by 5-formyltetrahydrofolic acid. Inhibits dihydrofolate reductase. Various halogenated derivatives act similarly, *J. Pharmac. Exp. Ther.* **128**, 419 (1960). Action, *BBA* **458**, 264 (1976). Used to control leukaemia; dosage more readily controlled than aminopterin. See *Adv. Cancer Res.* **7**, 192 (1963) for mechanisms of resistance. |

# 13A  Compounds affecting nucleic acids

| Name | Synonyms | Formula | M. wt. |
|------|----------|---------|--------|
| Aminopterin | 4-Aminopteroyl-glutamic acid | | Hydrate + 2H$_2$O, 476.4; Anhyd., 440.4 |
| AMP-PCP | Adenylyl ($\beta, \gamma$-methylene)-diphosphonate; adenosine 5'-($\beta, \gamma$-methylene)-triphosphate | | 505.2 |
| AMP-PNP | Adenylyl imidodiphosphate; adenosine 5'-($\beta, \gamma$-imido)-triphosphate | | 506.2; Li$_4$ salt, 529.9; Na$_4$ salt + 4H$_2$O, 666.2 |
| AMP-S | Adenosine 5'-O-thiophosphate | | 363.2; Li$_2$ salt, 375.1 |
| Ap$_5$A | $P^1,P^5$-Bis-(adenosine-5') pentaphosphate | | 916.4; Li$_3$ salt, 934.2 |

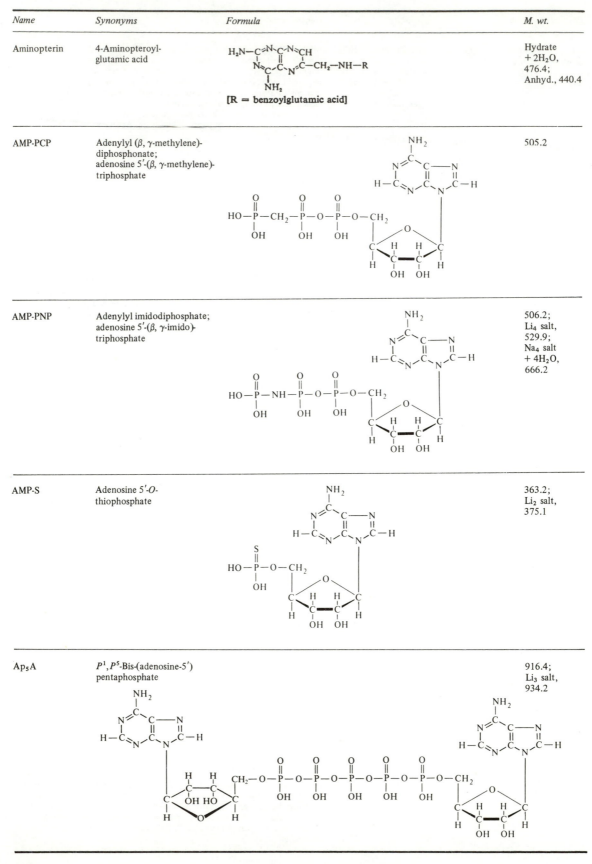

| Physical properties | Solubility | General remarks |
|---|---|---|
| yel. needles | s. aq. NaOH; sl. s. $H_2O$ | Folic acid antagonist, similar in action to amethopterin (q.v.). Used to control leukaemia. |
| | s. $H_2O$ | ATP analogue ($-CH_2-$ in place of $-O-$ between the $\beta,\gamma$-phosphates). Used in study of ATP-dependent reactions; C–P bond resistant to phosphorylation and transphosphorylation reactions. Hydrolysed by alkaline phosphatase. Replaces ATP in atractyloside-sensitive transport across mitochondrial membrane. Does not support $Na^+$, $K^+$ transport and prevents ouabain binding to $(Na^+ + K^+)$ ATPase. Can replace ATP (30–50% as effective) in RNA polymerase systems. Inhibits polynucleotide phosphorylase. $Li_4$ salt, $C_{11}H_{14}N_5O_{12}P_3Li_4$, m. wt. 528.9, stable at $+4\,^\circ C$. |
| $\epsilon_{260}$ (pH 7) 15 000 | s. $H_2O$ | ATP analogue ($-NH-$ between the $\beta, \gamma$-phosphates instead of the oxygen). Interacts strongly with heavy meromyosin, myosin and actomyosin. Potent competitive inhibitor of heavy meromyosin ATPase. Phosphodiesterase from venom splits AMP-PNP into AMP and imidodiphosphate; alkaline phosphatase (*E. coli*) splits the P–N bond to give $ADP-NH_2$ and $P_i$. Not hydrolysed by ATPases but is converted to cyclic AMP by adenylate cyclase. AMP-PNP hydrolyses in acid medium to corresponding phosphoramidate and inorganic phosphate. |
| | | Substrate and inhibitor for AMP-dependent enzyme systems, *Biochem.* **7**, 4023 (1968). |
| | | Strong competitive inhibitor of myokinase (adenylate kinase), *JBC* **248**, 1121 (1973). |

| Name | Synonyms | Formula | M. wt. |
|------|----------|---------|--------|
| AraATP | Adenine-β-D-arabinofuran-oside 5′-triphosphate | | 507.2 |
| Arabinosyl-adenine | 9-β-D-Arabinofuranosyl-adenine; spongo-adenosine; vidarabine; adenine arabinoside; adenine-β-D-arabinofuranoside; AraA | | 267.2 |
| Arabinosyl-cytosine | 1-β-D-Arabinofuranosyl-cytosine; cytabarine; cytosine-β-D-arabinofuranoside; cytosine arabinoside; AraC | | 243.2 |
| AraCTP | Cytosine-β-D-arabinofuranoside 5′-triphosphate | | 483.2; Ba salt, 618.5 |
| ATP-γ-S | Adenosine 5′-O-(3-thiotriphosphate) | | 523.2; Li₄ salt, 547.0 |
| 8-Azaguanine | Guanazole; 5-amino-7-hydroxy-1-v-triazolo-[d]-pyrimidine | | 152.1 |
| Azaserine | O-Diazoacetyl-L-serine | | 173.1 |

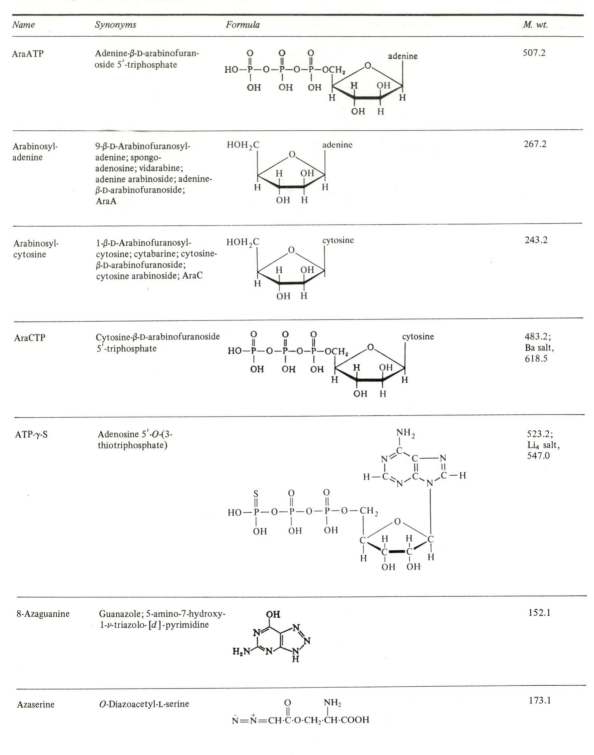

| Physical properties | Solubility | General Remarks |
|---|---|---|
| | | Acts as chain terminator in DNA synthesis — has been used in DNA sequencing instead of dideoxynucleoside triphosphates (q.v.), *PNAS* **74**, 5463 (1977). However certain DNA polymerases will extend chains ending in ara-nucleotide, *J. Virol.* **15**, 759 (1975). *See also* araCTP. |
| $\lambda_{max}$(pH 1) 257.5 nm $\epsilon$ 13 400; (pH 13) 259 nm $\epsilon$ 14 000; M.p. 257 | sl. s. $H_2O$ | Natural antibiotic; for action see arabinosylcytosine. Review on nucleoside antibiotics, *PNARMB* **22**, 193 (1979). Hydrate $+\frac{1}{2}$ $H_2O$, m. wt. 276.3. |
| M.p. 212–3; $\lambda_{max}$ (pH 2) 281, 212.5 nm $\epsilon$ 13 171, 10 230; (pH 12) 272.5 nm $\epsilon$ 9259 | | Selectively inhibits DNA synthesis in mammalian cells (L-cells, 97% at $4 \times 10^{-7}$ M without effect on RNA synthesis); bacteria generally insensitive. Triphosphate may act as competitive dCTP analogue and also incorporation may cause slow chain extension. Review, *PNARMB* **22**, 193 (1979). |
| | | *See* araATP *entry.* Still used in DNA sequencing to resolve certain ambiguities in dideoxy-method, *Meth. Enzymol.* **65**, 568 (1980). |
| | | Inhibitor of alkaline phosphatase. Substrate for *E. coli* DNA-dependent RNA polymerase ($K_m = 3.8 \times 10^{-5}$ M). Hydrolysed by snake-venom phosphodiesterase. No reaction with hexokinase. Translocated by mitochondrial ATP/ADP translocase. Potent inhibitor of ATP-driven reverse electron transport. |
| col. cryst.; decomp. $> 300$ | s. dil. acids | Guanine analogue incorporated into RNA; causes translation errors from messenger RNA to protein. |
| orthorhombic pale yel. to green cryst. from 90% EtOH; Decomp. 146–62; $pK_a$ 8.55; $\epsilon$ at 250.5 nm 19730 | v.s. $H_2O$; s. aq. EtOH; sl. s. MeOH, EtOH, acet. | A glutamine analogue, like DON, prevents transfer of amide group from glutamine to formylglycinamide ribotide in purine synthesis (inactivates phosphoribosylformylglycineamidine synthetase irreversibly by covalent attachment to —SH group). Active against several *Clostridium* sp., *Mycobacterium tuberculosis*, and *Rickettsiae*. Also possesses antitumour activity. A few fungi including several yeasts are inhibited by this compound. Bacteria in minimal medium show greater sensitivity than in complex medium (*E. coli* inhibited by 0.02 and 5.0 µg/ml and *B. subtilis* 1.0 and 6.6 µg/ml in minimal and complex medium, respectively). Aqueous solns. most stable at pH 8, stability rapidly falls off above and below this pH, can be heated at $100\,^{\circ}$C in neutral aqueous soln. for 5 min. |

| Name | Synonyms | Formula | M. wt. |
|------|----------|---------|--------|

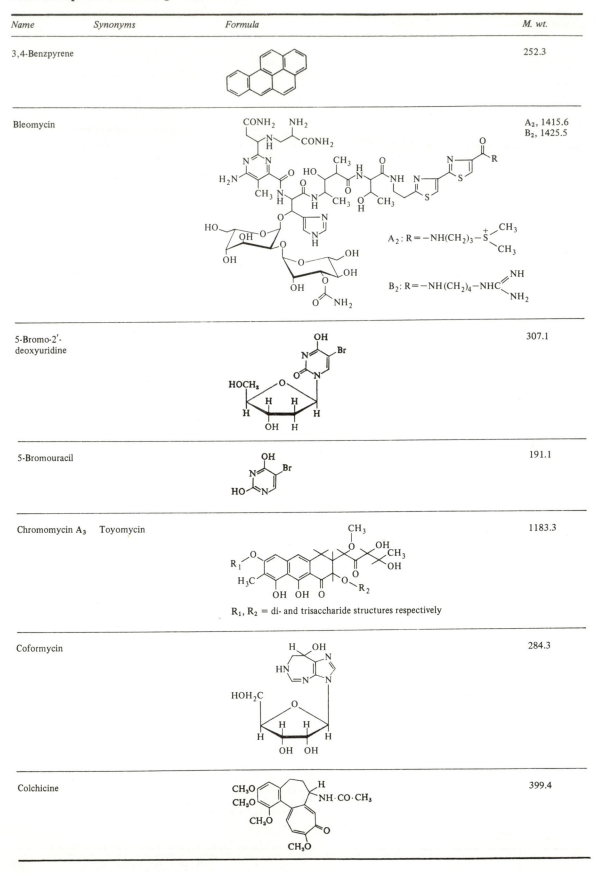

| | | | |
|---|---|---|---|
| 3,4-Benzpyrene | | | 252.3 |
| Bleomycin | | | A₂, 1415.6<br>B₂, 1425.5 |
| 5-Bromo-2′-deoxyuridine | | | 307.1 |
| 5-Bromouracil | | | 191.1 |
| Chromomycin A₃ | Toyomycin | R₁, R₂ = di- and trisaccharide structures respectively | 1183.3 |
| Coformycin | | | 284.3 |
| Colchicine | | | 399.4 |

$$A_2 : R = -NH(CH_2)_3 - \overset{+}{S} \begin{matrix} CH_3 \\ CH_3 \end{matrix}$$

$$B_2 : R = -NH(CH_2)_4 - NHC \begin{matrix} NH \\ NH_2 \end{matrix}$$

| Physical properties | Solubility | General remarks |
|---|---|---|
| yel. plates and needles; M.p. 179; Fluor. in conc. $H_2SO_4$, A 521 nm (470 nm) F 548 nm (493 nm) | s. benz., toluene, xylene; sp. s. EtOH, MeOH; i. $H_2O$ | Carcinogenic agent, the important factor in carcinogenesis by polycyclic hydrocarbons being the relative rate of synthesis and breakdown of carcinogenic intermediates, *BBA* **473**, 149 (1978). Hydroxylated in positions 5, 8 and 10. Some metabolites excreted in the bile. |
| col. or yel. powder; $pK_a$ 7.3, 4.7, 2.9 | v.s. $H_2O$; sl. s. EtOH; i. acet., eth. | Family of antibiotics differing in terminal R groups. Inhibits DNA synthesis $>$ RNA; causes single strand scission of DNA *in vivo* and *in vitro*, enhanced by reducing agents and $Fe^{2+}$; requires $O_2$ and reducing agent. Effects on L-cells at 0.1 $\mu$g/ml. Many modified bleomycins prepared; preps. usually contain copper. For mechanism see *BBRC* **77**, 1150 (1977). Review, *PNARMB* **20**, 21 (1977). Revised structure, *J. Antibiotics (Japan)* **31**, 801 (1978). Mechanism of action involves generation of hydroxyl free radicals, leading to cleavage of *N*-glycosidic bonds and base elimination (mainly T) followed by phosphodiester bond scission. Streptonigrin has similar action. Review of bleomycin and closely related phleomycin, *Antibiotics* **5**, 124 (1979). |
| $\lambda_{max}$ (pH 2) 280 nm $\epsilon$ 9250; $pK_a$ 8.1 | s. $H_2O$ | Thymidine analogue, *see* 5-bromouracil. |
| | s. $H_2O$ | Thymine analogue. Mutagen (induces GC $\rightarrow$ AT transition mutants). Density marker for DNA. Anabolized to bromodeoxyuridylic acid and to BUdR triphosphate. Incorporated into DNA where it may lead to blocking of further DNA synthesis in some organisms. Pox viruses particularly sensitive. |
| yel. powder | v.s. $H_2O$, MeOH | Inhibits RNA synthesis $>$ DNA (in mammalian cells 100 $\mu$g/ml and 10 $\mu$g/ml inhibited RNA synthesis 55% and 30% respectively while DNA synthesis scarcely affected; in *B. subtilis* 0.1 $\mu$g/ml inhibited both about 75%). Binds to G:C pairs of helical DNA, does not intercalate. Mithramycin (different sugars) and olivomycin (different sugars and sl. modified chromophore) have similar action. Review, *ARB* **40**, 775 (1971). |
| | | Extremely effective adenosine deaminase inhibitor ($K_i = 1 \times 10^{-11}$ M); 2'-deoxy derivative (covidarabine, pentostatin) also ($K_i = 2.5 \times 10^{-12}$ M). Potentiates effects of formycin, arabinosyladenine, and cordycepin by preventing deamination. 2'-Deoxyadenosine, non-toxic at low concentrations, may become toxic to cells in presence of coformycin. Due to tight binding of latter, effect can persist after removal of coformycin from medium. Other inhibitors such as *erythro*-9-(2-hydroxy-3-nonyl) adenine bind less tightly ($K_i$ 1.6 $\times$ $10^{-9}$ M), *Biochem. Pharmacol.* **26**, 359 (1977). Review, *PNARMB* **22**, 193 (1978). |
| pale yel. powder; darkens in light; M.p. 142–50 | 4 $H_2O$; v.s. EtOH, $CHCl_3$; s. eth. | Mitotic arrest (plants and animals); uricosuric. Effect is on metaphase. Interferes with microtubule organisation at $10^{-8}$–$10^{-7}$ M, in particular those of the mitotic spindle. Effect on transport, *see* vinblastine. Less toxic than cinchophen. Aurichloride only salt. Forms cryst. compounds with $CHCl_3$, decomposed at 60 °C. |

## 13A Compounds affecting nucleic acids

| Name | Synonyms | Formula | M. wt. |
|------|----------|---------|--------|
| Cordycepin | 3′-Deoxyadenosine | 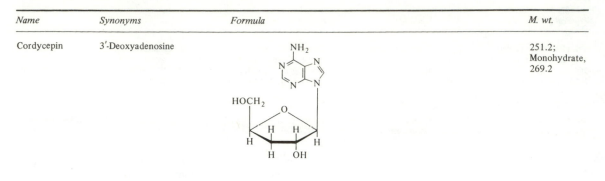 | 251.2; Monohydrate, 269.2 |
| Coumermycin A₁ | | 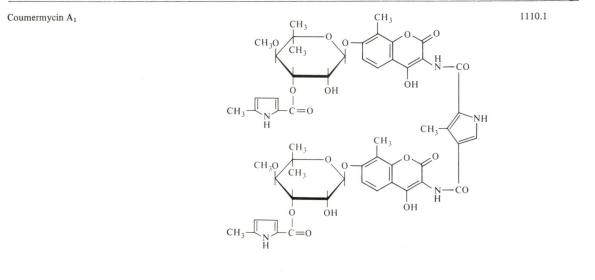 | 1110.1 |
| Daunomycin | Daunorubicin | 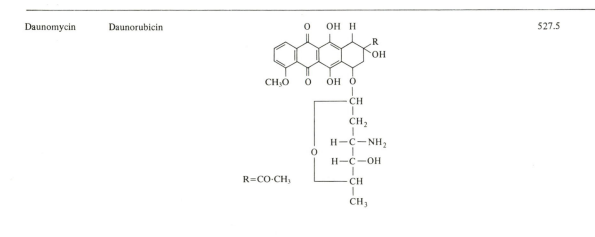 | 527.5 |
| 2,6-Diaminopurine | |  | 150.2 |

R=CO·CH₃

| Physical properties | Solubility | General remarks |
|---|---|---|
| $\lambda_{max}$ (EtOH) 260 nm $\epsilon$ 14 600 | s. $H_2O$ | Selectively inhibits poly-adenylation of Hn-RNA in HeLa cells at 50 $\mu$g/ml; also inhibits 45 S rRNA synthesis, antitumour, cytostatic agent in eukaryote cells. Reversed by adenosine, not 2'-deoxyadenosine. Natural antibiotic. Review, *PNARMB* **22**, 193 (1979). |
| | | Inhibits bacterial DNA gyrase > 90% at 0.3 $\mu$g/ml. Inhibits *Staphylococcus aureus* growth at 0.004 $\mu$g/ml. In *E. coli* inhibits DNA and RNA synthesis at 30 $\mu$g/ml. Has similar action to novobiocin (q.v.) but 10-fold higher concentration of latter needed to inhibit gyrase, *PNAS* **73**, 4474 (1976). Site of action on gyrase different from that of nalidixic acid (q.v.), *PNAS* **74**, 4772 (1977). Structurally virtually a dimer of novobiocin. Reacts with $\beta$-subunit of gyrase, *PNAS* **75**, 4838 (1978); *Science* **207**, 953 (1980). Stock soln. of Na salt (40 mg/ml) in DMSO stable at $-20°$C. |
| $\lambda_{max}$ (MeOH) 234, 252 nm $A_{1\,cm}^{1\%}$ 665, 462 | HCl: s. $H_2O$, MeOH; i. $CHCl_3$, eth. Red soln. turns blue at alk. pH. | Inhibits DNA and RNA synthesis to about same extent; cytotoxic antitumour agent; intercalates into DNA (but derivatives with low affinity for DNA still antimitotic – see *BBA* **512**, 254 (1978)). Store solid in dark in desiccator at 4 °C; solns. prepared in buffer immediately before use, *BBA* **277**, 489 (1972). Adriamycin (q.v.) closely related. This and adriamycin best known of antibiotic family including nogolamycin, cinerubin, rhodomycins and rubomycins. Hydrochloride, m. wt. 563.5, red cryst. |
| $pK_a$ < 1, 5.09, 10.77 | $0.24^{25}$, $0.59^{100}$ $H_2O$ | Purine antagonist, especially of adenine-containing cofactors of 1 carbon transfer reactions. Sulphate, $(C_5H_6N_6)_2 \cdot H_2SO_4 \cdot H_2O$, m. wt. 416.4, wh. needles. |

## 13A  Compounds affecting nucleic acids

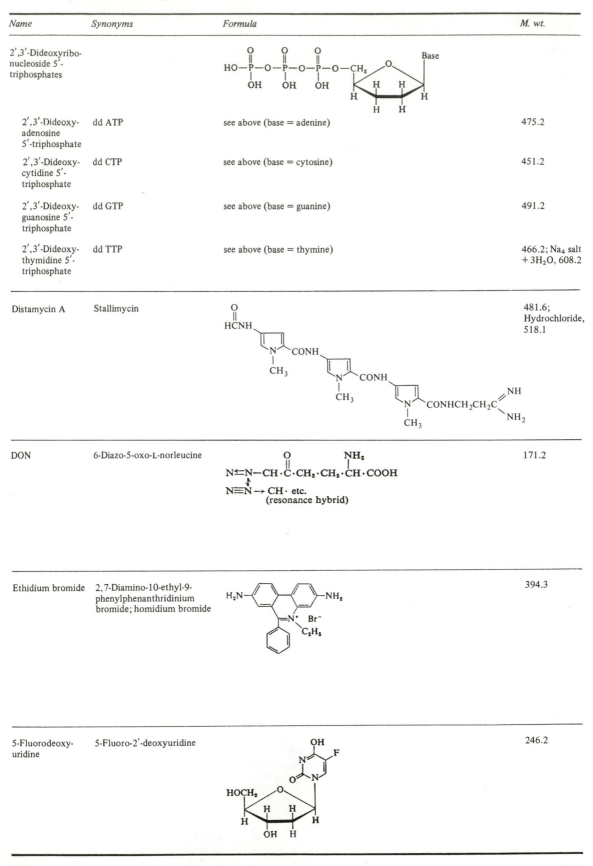

| Name | Synonyms | Formula | M. wt. |
|------|----------|---------|--------|
| 2',3'-Dideoxyribo-nucleoside 5'-triphosphates | | | |
| 2',3'-Dideoxy-adenosine 5'-triphosphate | dd ATP | see above (base = adenine) | 475.2 |
| 2',3'-Dideoxy-cytidine 5'-triphosphate | dd CTP | see above (base = cytosine) | 451.2 |
| 2',3'-Dideoxy-guanosine 5'-triphosphate | dd GTP | see above (base = guanine) | 491.2 |
| 2',3'-Dideoxy-thymidine 5'-triphosphate | dd TTP | see above (base = thymine) | 466.2; Na$_4$ salt + 3H$_2$O, 608.2 |
| Distamycin A | Stallimycin | | 481.6; Hydrochloride, 518.1 |
| DON | 6-Diazo-5-oxo-L-norleucine | | 171.2 |
| Ethidium bromide | 2,7-Diamino-10-ethyl-9-phenylphenanthridinium bromide; homidium bromide | | 394.3 |
| 5-Fluorodeoxy-uridine | 5-Fluoro-2'-deoxyuridine | | 246.2 |

| Physical properties | Solubility | General remarks |
|---|---|---|
| | | Act as chain terminators in DNA synthesis by *E. coli* polymerase I. Used in DNA sequencing as more satisfactory than the 'plus and minus' method, *PNAS* **74**, 5463 (1977). Synthesis, *ibid.* |
| $\lambda_{max}$ (−HCl, in 0.02 M-NaCl) 303, 237−8 nm $\epsilon$ 34 000, 29 000 | s. $H_2O$ | Inhibits DNA and RNA synthesis; active against DNA viruses (at 100 $\mu$g/ml prevents T-series viruses infecting *E. coli* without effect on host cell growth); antitumour activity. Action similar to netropsin (q.v.). Aq. solns. decompose in hours giving yellow colour. Review, *PNARMB* **15**, 285 (1975). Binds to A:T regions of helical DNA. Inhibits various DNA and RNA polymerases *in vitro*. |
| pale yel. cryst. from dil. EtOH; Decomp. 145−55; $A_{1cm}^{1\%}$ at 274 nm 683 | v.s. $H_2O$; s. aq. solns. of MeOH, EtOH, acet.; sl. s. abs. alcohols | Inhibits purine synthesis in bacterial and mammalian systems. Glutamine analogue, interferes with the transfer of amide group from glutamine to formylglycinamide ribotide (phosphoribosylformylglycineamidine synthetase irreversibly inhibited). At high conc. other glutamine-requiring reactions inhibited. Prevents the growth of exptl. tumours but toxic to animals. Of 57 strains of bacteria tested only 6 were sensitive to 12.5 $\mu$g/ml or less and of 104 fungi and yeasts examined only 5 yeasts inhibited by 50 $\mu$g/ml or less. Aqueous solutions should be kept at pH 4.5−6.5. Compd. rapidly destroyed in neutral aq. soln. at 100 °C. |
| dark red cryst. or powder; M.p. 247−9 | s. $H_2O$, EtOH, MeOH | Potent inhibitor of DNA synthesis *in vivo*; inhibits DNA synthesis by cell-free DNA polymerase and RNA synthesis by cell-free DNA-dependent RNA polymerase. Intercalates with DNA (binding intensifies fluorescence − useful to stain DNA). Reverses supercoiling of circular DNA. Has selective effect on extraction of DNA (bacterial plasmids, trypanosome kinetoplasts, mitochondrial DNA of yeasts). 'Cures' bacteria of plasmids. Propidium (− $CH_2 \cdot CH_3$ group replaced by − $(CH_2)_3 \cdot N^+{\overset{Et}{\underset{Et}{\diagdown Me}}}$) shows similar intercalating properties, *Antibiotics* **3**, 141 (1975). Review on intercalating agents as probes of chromatin structure, *Meth. Cell Biol.* **18**, 351 (1978). **WARNING:** Ethidium bromide is a powerful mutagen and should be handled with great care. |
| wh. cryst.; p$K_a$ 7.6 | s. $H_2O$ | Inhibits DNA synthesis by blocking thymidylic acid synthetase when metabolized to fluorodeoxyuridylic acid. Thymidylate synthetase as a target enzyme in cancer chemotherapy, review: *BBA* **473**, 73 (1977). |

## 13A  Compounds affecting nucleic acids

| Name | Synonyms | Formula | M. wt. |
|------|----------|---------|--------|
| 5-Fluorouracil | 5-Fluoro-2,4-dihydroxy-pyrimidine | | 130.1 |
| Formycin A | Formycin; 8-aza-9-deaza-adenosine | | 267.2 |
| Formycin B | 8-Aza-9-deazainosine | | 268.2 |
| GMP-PCP | Guanylyl ($\beta$, $\gamma$-methylene)-diphosphonate; guanosine 5'-($\beta$, $\gamma$-methylene)-triphosphate | | 521.2; Li$_4$ salt, 544.9; Na$_4$ salt + 1 H$_2$O, 627.1 |
| GMP-PNP | Guanylyl imidodiphosphate; guanosine 5'-($\beta$, $\gamma$-imido)-triphosphate | | 522.2; Li$_4$ salt, 545.9; Na$_4$ salt + 2H$_2$O, 646.2 |
| GTP-$\gamma$-S | Guanosine 5'-$O$-(3-thiotriphosphate) | See ATP-$\gamma$-S; adenine residue replaced by guanine | 539.2; Li$_4$ salt, 563.0 |

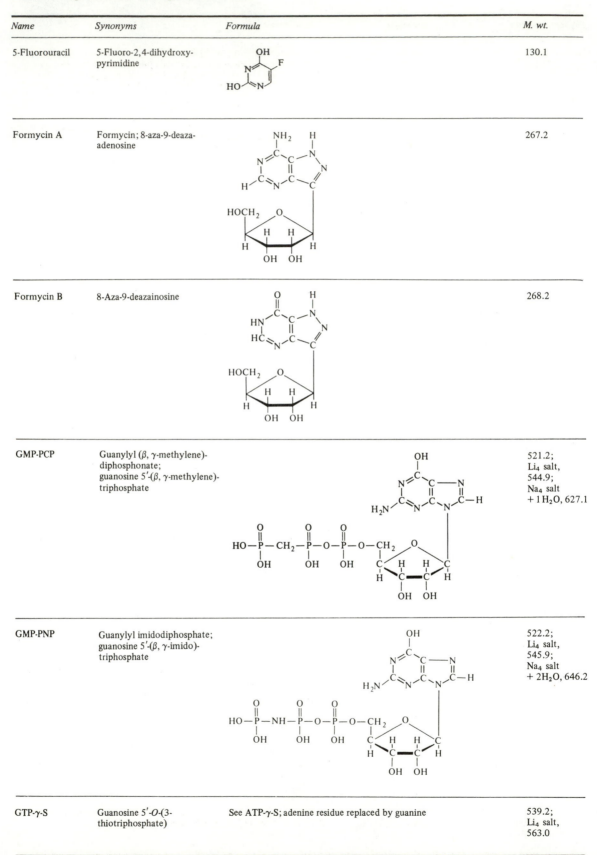

| Physical properties | Solubility | General remarks |
|---|---|---|
| wh. powder; M.p. 282–3 d.; p$K_a$ 8.0 | s. $H_2O$ | Metabolized to fluorodeoxyuridylic acid which inhibits thymidylic acid synthetase and to fluorouridine triphosphate which is incorporated into RNA in the place of UTP. Inhibits DNA synthesis; causes translation errors from messenger RNA to protein; causes transition mutations in RNA organisms. Used in cancer chemotherapy. |
| | s. $H_2O$, MeOH; sl. s. EtOH; i. eth., acet. | Inhibits *de novo* purine biosynthesis in tumour cells; incorporated into RNA; interferes with normal processing of 4S tRNA probably by inducing abnormal degradation of the precursor. Rapidly deaminated to formycin B in erythrocytes. |
| | s. $H_2O$: v. sl. s. organic solvents | Competitive inhibitor of NAD in poly(ADP-ribose) polymerase; inhibits tumour cell growth 50% at 16 $\mu$M. Inhibits purine nucleoside phosphorylase and is not itself a substrate. Review, *PNARMB* **22**, 193 (1979). |
| | | GTP analogue (methylene —$CH_2$— group between the $\beta$, $\gamma$-phosphate). Used for study of GTP-dependent systems as AMP-PCP is for ATP-dependent systems. Competitive inhibitor of the GTP reaction (translocation step) of protein synthesis. Less effective than GTP-PNP (q.v.). |
| $\epsilon_{260}$ (pH 7) 11 800 | | GTP analogue (imido group —NH— between the $\beta$, $\gamma$-phosphate). Similar hydrolysis characteristics to AMP-PNP. Competitive inhibitor of the ribosome-dependent GTPase, inhibiting the translocation step in protein synthesis. |
| | | Activation of adenyl cyclase, *JBC* **250**, 867 (1974). Hydrolysed at much slower rate than ATP by myosin fragment S-1 ATPase. |

| Name | Synonyms | Formula | M. wt. |
|------|----------|---------|--------|
| Hadacidin | N-Formylhydroxyamino-acetic acid | | 119.1 |
| Hydroxyurea | N-Hydroxyurea | | 76.1 |
| 5-Iodo-2'-deoxy-uridine | | | 354.1 |
| 6-Mercaptopurine | Purinethiol | | 152.2; Hydrate, 170.2 |
| Methyl-cholanthrene | | | 268.3 |
| 9-Methylfolic acid | | | 455.4 |
| N-Methyl-N'-nitro-N-nitroso-guanidine | NNG; MNG; NTG; NG; MeNNG | | 147.1 |
| Mitomycin C | | | 334.3 |

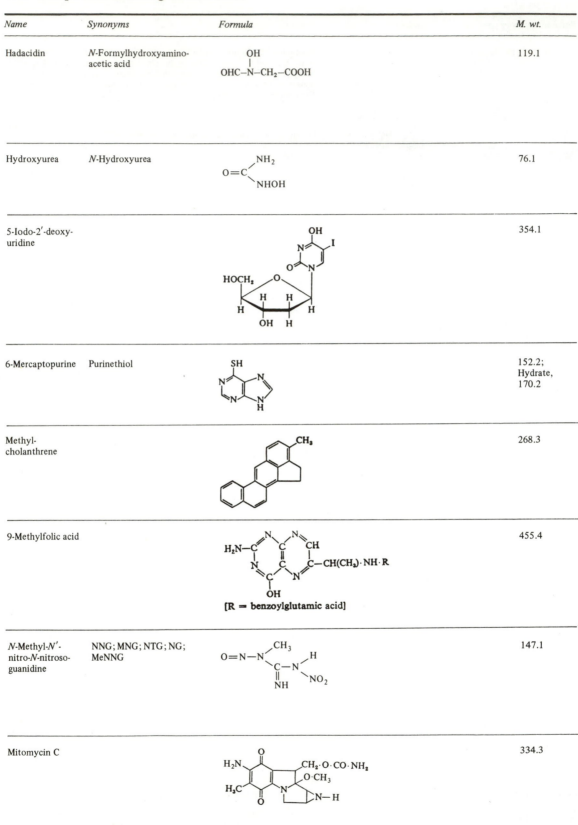

| Physical properties | Solubility | General remarks |
|---|---|---|
| Free acid: unstable cryst.; M.p. 119–20; p$K_a$ 3.5, 9.1 Na salt: cryst.; decomp 205–10 | Cryst. acid: s. $H_2O$, MeOH, EtOH, acet., eth. Monosodium salt: s. $H_2O$, MeOH; i. EtOH | Inhibits purine biosynthesis in bacterial and mammalian systems. Inhibits growth of human adenocarcinoma-1 in embryonated egg. Stops biosynthesis of AMP and dAMP; acts as analogue of L-aspartate, which can reverse the inhibition. Acts by inhibiting adenylosuccinate synthetase, involved in conversion of IMP to adenylosuccinic acid; competes effectively with aspartic acid, *JBC* **237**, 1932, 1937 (1962). The free acid is unstable and in soln. hydrolyses to give formic acid and hydroxyaminoacetic acid. |
| wh. cryst. powder; M.p. 140 | v.s. $H_2O$ | Specific inhibitor of DNA synthesis *in vivo*; RNA and protein synthesis not affected. Mechanism may be via inhibition of deoxyribonucleotide synthesis from ribonucleotides; antiviral and antineoplastic; causes chromosome breakage. DNA repair synthesis not inhibited. Actions reversible. |
| col. cryst.; $\lambda_{max}$ (pH 2) 288 nm $\epsilon$ 7770 | s. $H_2O$ | Thymidine analogue. Chemotherapy of herpes simplex keratitis. |
| yellow prisms + 1$H_2O$, lost at 140; M.p. 313–14 d. | s. $H_2O$ | Interferes with purine interconversion; the nucleoside 5′-triphosphate interferes with NAD synthesis. Used in cancer chemotherapy; treatment of leukaemia. |
| pale yel. cryst.; M.p. 179–80 | s. benz., toluene, xylene; sl. s. amyl alcohol; i. $H_2O$ | Carcinogenic. Protect skin when working with this substance. Water-soluble derivative is methylcholanthrene choleic acid. |
|  |  | Folic acid antagonist. Probably causes a block at folic reductase level. |
|  | s. $H_2O$ | Extreme care in handling! One of most potent mutagens known; carcinogenic. Used as bacterial mutagen (for optimum conditions with *E. coli*, see *BBRC* **18**, 788 (1965)). Usually gives > 1 mutation per cell. Solid may decompose generating explosive pressure in sealed containers. For other mutagenizing procedures using 2-aminopurine, diethyl sulphate, 5-BUdR, ICR191, and u.v. light, see *Meth. Enzymol.* **17A**, 1 (1970). For a review of alkylating agents on DNA, see *PNARMB* **15**, 219 (1975). |
| purple or deep violet cryst.; M.p. > 360 d. | s. $H_2O$ | Inhibits DNA synthesis. Broad spectrum antitumour activity and strong bactericidal action against gram + ve and gram − ve organisms and acid-fast bacilli. Group of compounds of which C is most widely used since the least toxic and with most potent antitumour activity. Antibiotic is reduced metabolically (or with dithionite) to hydroquinone derivative, yielding bifunctional alkylating agent. This covalently links DNA strands, inhibits DNA synthesis before RNA and DNA degradation occurs. Complete inhibition of net DNA synthesis in *E. coli* by 10 $\mu$g/ml. Drug stable in aq. soln. pH 6–9, can be stored at +5 °C for 1 week with little loss of activity. Readily decomposed by light. |

## 13A Compounds affecting nucleic acids

| Name | Synonyms | Formula | M. wt. |
|------|----------|---------|--------|
| Mustard gas | Sulphur mustard; bis-(2-chloroethyl)sulphide | | 159.1 |
| Nalidixic acid | 1-Ethyl-1,4-dihydro-7-methyl-4-oxo-1,8-naphthyridine-3-carboxylic acid; NAL | | 232.2 |
| Netropsin | Congocidine | | 430.5; Disulphate, 626.7 |
| Novobiocin | | | 612.6; Na salt, 634.6 |
| Oxolinic acid | 1-Ethyl-6,7-methylenedioxy-4-quinolone-3-carboxylic acid | | 261.2 |
| Phenethyl alcohol | 2-Phenylethanol | $C_6H_5 \cdot CH_2 \cdot CH_2OH$ | 122.2 |
| Proflavin | 3,6-Diaminoacridine | | 209.3; Dihydrochloride + 2H$_2$O, 318.2; Sulphate, 307.3 |
| Psicofuranine | 6-Amino-9-D-psicofurano-sylpurine | | 296.3 |

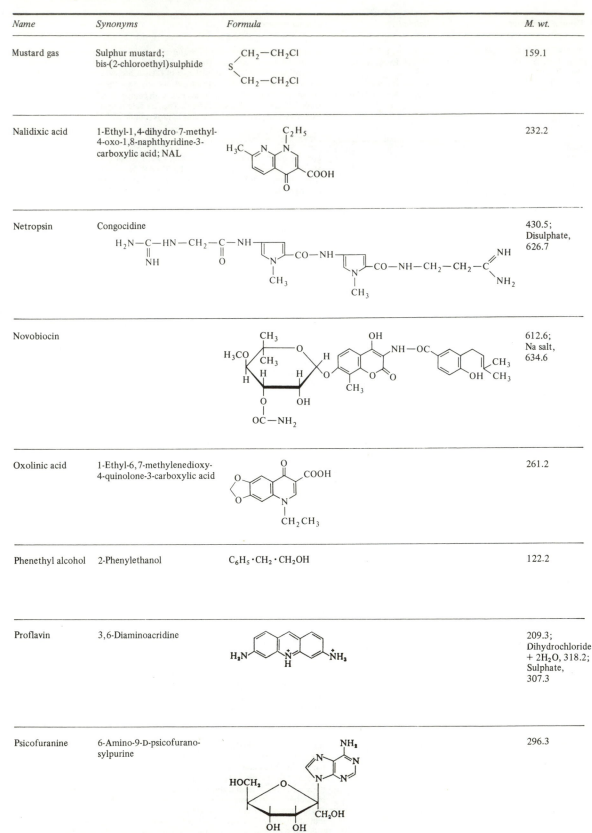

272

| Physical properties | Solubility | General remarks |
|---|---|---|
| col. oily liq. or cryst.; M.p. 13. | s. EtOH, eth., CHCl$_3$, benz. | Dangerous vesicant to be handled with extreme care. Antitumour agent; cross links and mono-alkylates DNA; reaction also with protein —SH. Nitrogen mustard (NH(CH$_2$CH$_2$Cl)$_2$) similar action. Review of DNA alkylating reagents, *PNARMB* **15**, 219 (1975). |
| M.p. 229–30 | sl. s. H$_2$O; s. alkali solns.; v. sl. s. EtOH, MeOH | Inhibits subunit A of bacterial DNA gyrase; 2–10 $\mu$g/ml inhibits *E. coli* growth, 50 $\mu$g/ml inhibits replicative DNA synthesis in toluenized cells, no effect on repair DNA synthesis. Oxolinic acid (q.v.) similar but ten times more potent on gyrase. Site of action on gyrase different from that of coumermycin A$_1$ (q.v.), *PNAS* **74**, 4772 (1977); *Science* **207**, 953 (1980). |
| $\lambda_{max}$(—HCl in 0.02M-NaCl) 295–6, 235 nm $\epsilon$ 21 000, 20 000 | Disulphate: sl. s. H$_2$O (0.5 mg/ml at 25 °C); i. organic solvents | Inhibits DNA and RNA synthesis; *E. coli* growth inhibited at approx. 10 $\mu$g/ml. Binds to helical DNA at A-T rich regions (not by intercalation) with spectral shift from 296 nm to 325 nm. Aq. solns. stable 3 days at 4 °C. Similar in action to distamycin (q.v.). Review, *PNARMB* **15**, 285 (1975). |
| yel. cryst.; p$K_a$ 4.3, 9.1; $\lambda_{max}$ (0.1M-NaOH) 307 nm $A_{1cm}^{1\%}$ 600; (0.1M-MeOH—HCl) 324 nm $A_{1cm}^{1\%}$ 390; (pH7, phosphate buffer) $A_{1cm}^{1\%}$ 350 | i. acids; s. > pH 7.5; s. organic solvents Na salt: s. H$_2$O, acet., MeOH, EtOH | Inhibits bacterial DNA gyrase, *PNAS* **73**, 4474 (1976); inhibits *E. coli* growth 50% at 20 $\mu$M; *in vivo* inhibits replicative, not repair, DNA synthesis and RNA almost as much; *in vitro* replicative DNA synthesis 90% inhibited by 1 $\mu$g/ml, RNA synthesis less so. Solns. stable long periods at 4 °C; at 25 °C decompose 50% in 30 days. Site of action on DNA gyrase different from that of nalidixic and oxolinic acids (q.v.), *PNAS* **74**, 4772 (1977). Coumermycin is virtually a dimer of novobiocin. See former for mechanism of action and references. |
|  | s. dil. KOH | Inhibits subunit A of DNA gyrase 10 times more effectively than nalidixic acid (q.v.). Site of action on gyrase different from that of coumermycin A$_1$ and novobiocin (q.v.), *PNAS* **74**, 4772 (1977); *Science*, **207** 953 (1980). |
| col. liq.; B.p. 219–21 | s. EtOH, eth.; 1.6$^{20}$ H$_2$O | Inhibits DNA synthesis without affecting protein and RNA synthesis at 0.25%. At higher conc. protein and RNA synthesis inhibited and cells no longer elongate. Bacteriostatic to a wide variety of bacterial species (exception: *Streptococci*). Gram —ve susceptible at 0.27%, gram +ve at 0.5%. |
| orange red cryst; p$K_a$ 9.65 | Hydrochloride; s. H$_2$O; v. sl. s. EtOH; i. CHCl$_3$, eth. | Mutagen (on *E. coli* at about 4 $\mu$g/ml); intercalates into double helical DNA and inhibits DNA synthesis *in vivo* > RNA synthesis. Selective effect on extrachromosomal DNA, cures cells of plasmids, selectively affects kinetoplasts of trypanosomes and mitochondrial DNA of yeasts (giving respiration deficient yeasts). Binding quenches drug fluorescence. 0.1% soln. of hydrochloride is acid; soln. unstable in light becoming turbid. Acriflavin is a mixture of proflavin and the 10-methylacridinium chloride derivative. |
| needle-shaped cryst., M.p. 212–14 d. |  | Inhibits purine synthesis, possesses antitumour in addition to antibacterial properties. Structural analogue of adenosine; acts by inhibiting the conversion of xanthosine 5′-phosphate (XMP) to GMP by XMP aminase. Inhibition of growth of *S. aureus* by drug reversed by guanine, guanosine, and GMP. Inhibition is non-competitive with adenosine but acts at nucleoside level probably by allosteric inhibition. Review: *PNARMB* **22**, 193 (1979). |

# 13A  Compounds affecting nucleic acids

| Name | Synonyms | Formula | M. wt. |
|------|----------|---------|--------|
| Pyrimethamine | 2,4-Diamino-5-p-chlorophenyl-6-ethylpyrimidine | | 248.7 |
| Rifampicin | Rifampin | | 823.0 |
| Streptolydigin | Portamycin | | 600.7; Na salt, 622.7 |
| 6-Thioguanine | 2-Amino-6-mercaptopurine | | 167.2 |
| Thiouracil | 2-Mercapto-4-hydroxypyrimidine | | 128.2 |
| Vinblastine sulphate | | | 909.0 |

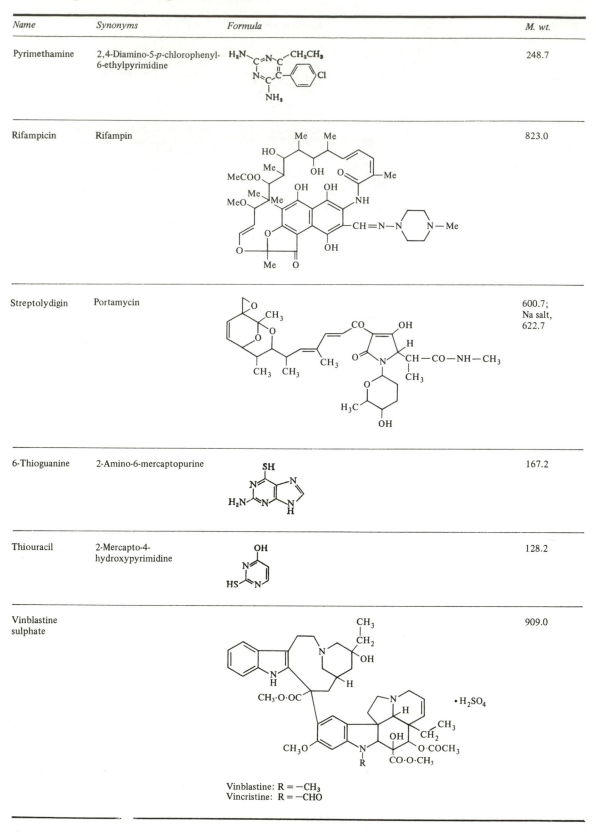

Vinblastine: R = —CH₃
Vincristine: R = —CHO

| Physical properties | Solubility | General Remarks |
|---|---|---|
| cryst. | sl. s. EtOH; i. $H_2O$ | Folic acid antagonist. Has antimalarial activity and used in control of toxoplasmosis. |
| $pK_a$ 1.7, 7.9; $\lambda_{max}$(pH 7.4) 237, 255, 334, 475 nm $\epsilon$ 33 200, 32 100, 27 000, 15 400 | v. sl. s. $H_2O$; v.s. dimethylsulphoxide; sl. s. MeOH | Semisynthetic derivative of rifamycin B; inhibits transcription in bacteria at extremely low concns. (0.01 $\mu$g/ml). No effect on eukaryote RNA polymerases at 10 000 times level needed for inhibiting bacterial enzyme (mitochondrial and chloroplast enzymes may be inhibited at 1 $\mu$g/ml). Binds to $\beta$ subunit of bacterial RNA polymerase and inhibits chain initiation, not elongation once initiated. Streptovaricin structurally related and similar action but higher concs. needed (> 20 $\mu$g/ml). Rifampicin is stable when dry at 4 °C in absence of light. |
| $\lambda_{max}$(0.01M-KOH–EtOH) 261, 291, 336 nm $A_{1cm}^{1\%}$ 223.6, 270.7, 331.0 | s. EtOH, eth., $CHCl_3$; v. sl. s. $H_2O$ Na salt: s. $H_2O$, organic solvents except hydrocarbons | Inhibits RNA synthesis (in *Bacillus megaterium* 80% at $1.4 \times 10^{-4}$ M); binds to bacterial RNA polymerase and inhibits chain polymerization, not initiation (cf. reverse with rifampicin (q.v.)). Rifampicin inhibits RNA synthesis at 100 × lower concs. |
| col. needles | s. dilute alkalis; v. sl. s. EtOH; i. $H_2O$, $CHCl_3$ | Incorporated into DNA and to lesser extent into RNA. Inhibits DNA synthesis after incorporation. Inhibits growth of neoplasms and microorganisms. |
| col. prisms; M.p. 340 d. | s. alkalis; 0.06 $H_2O$; v. sl. s. EtOH, eth., acids | Uracil analogue. Incorporated into RNA, but not into DNA. Causes translation errors from messenger RNA to protein. |
| cryst.; M.p. 284–5 | s. $H_2O$ | Antineoplastic alkaloid isolated from *Vinca rosea*, inhibits karyokinesis and secretion. Interferes with microtubule organization at $4.3 \times 10^{-7}$ M. Effect on transport of leucine, uridine, deoxyglucose in cultured cells depends on nutritional state of cells. With serum starvation uptake stimulated greatly; in rapidly growing cells, sl. decrease shown. Inhibits RNA synthesis. Effects not easily reversible. Vincristine has similar antimicrotubule effects but used differently clinically (vinblastine for Hodgkin's disease, vincristine for leukaemias). See P. Dustin, *Microtubules*, Springer-Verlag, Berlin (1978). |

# B. PROTEIN SYNTHESIS INHIBITORS AND AMINO ACID ANALOGUES

## General references

D. Vázquez, *Inhibitors of protein biosynthesis*. Molecular Biology and Biophysics 30. Springer-Verlag, Berlin (1978).

*Antibiotics 3*, eds. J.W. Corcoran and F.E. Hahn, Springer-Verlag, Berlin (1975).

*FEBS Letts.* **40**, S63 (1974).

*Metabolic inhibitors*, eds. R.M. Hochster, M. Kates, and J.H. Quastel, vol. 4, p. 107. Academic Press (1973).

| Name | Synonyms | Formula | M. wt. |
|---|---|---|---|
| α-Amino-β-chlorobutyric acid | | $CH_3 \cdot CH(Cl) \cdot CH(NH_2) \cdot COOH$ | 137.6 |
| Aurintricarboxylic acid | ATA | (structure) | 422.4 |
| 7-Azatryptophan | α-Amino-β-(7-aza-3-indolyl)-propanoic acid | (structure) $-CH_2 \cdot CH(NH_2) \cdot COOH$ | 205.2; Hydrate, 223.2 |
| Azetidine-2-carboxylic acid | | (structure) $CH \cdot COOH$ | 101.1 |
| Canavanine | α-Amino-γ-guanidinooxy-*n*-butyric acid | $\begin{array}{c} HN \\ H_2N \end{array}\!\!C \cdot NH \cdot O \cdot CH_2 \cdot CH_2 \cdot CH(NH_2) \cdot COOH$ | 176.2 |
| Chloramphenicol | CAP; chloromycetin | $O_2N-$(ring)$-CH \cdot CH \cdot NH \cdot C \cdot CHCl_2$ with $OH$, $CH_2OH$, $O$ | 323.1 |
| Cycloheximide | Actidione | (structure) | 281.3 |
| Emetine | 6′,7′,10,11-Tetramethoxyemetan | (structure) | 480.6; Dihydrochloride, 553.6 (anhyd.) |

| Physical properties | Solubility | General remarks |
|---|---|---|
| col. cryst.; M.p. 246d. | sl. s. $H_2O$; s. acids | Valine analogue. Inhibits valine incorporation into haemoglobin. Competitive inhibition of valine activating enzyme. |
| | | In low concs. (50–100 $\mu$M), reported to be a relatively specific inhibitor of initiation of protein synthesis, at higher concs. elongation is affected, *ABB* **183**, 228 (1977). Other effects reported; rat liver RNA polymerases inhibited at 3–5 $\mu$g/ml, if added at start of reaction – less effective if added later. DNA synthesis 90% inhibited in permeable ascites cells at 100 $\mu$M, purified DNA polymerase at 10 $\mu$M. *E. coli* RNA polymerase inhibited at 10 $\mu$M apparently by blocking initiation of synthesis. Proposed that ATA affects all nucleic acid binding proteins – effect on protein synthesis is to inhibit binding of mRNA to small ribosomal subunit. For refs. see *BBRC* **79**, 179 (1977). |
| fluffy needles; M.p. Hydrate, 257–9 d. | v. sl. s. $H_2O$; sl. s. acids | Tryptophan analogue. Inhibits phage multiplication in *E. coli*. Incorporated into bacterial protein and into phage coat protein. Can be activated by pancreatic tryptophan activating enzyme. |
| col. cryst.; darkens above 200 d. | v.s. $H_2O$ | Proline analogue. Can replace proline in protein of *E. coli* and mung-bean (*Phaseolus aureus*). |
| col. cryst.; M.p. 184 d.; $pK_a$ 2.50 (COOH), 6.60 (guanidinooxy), 9.25 ($\alpha$-NH$_2$) | v.s. $H_2O$ | Arginine analogue. Growth inhibitory to some strains of *S. aureus* and *E. coli*. May be incorporated into protein of Walker sarcocarcinoma and *S. aureus*. Acts as substrate to most enzymes normally acting on arginine. |
| yel. powder | 0.25 $H_2O$; v.s. MeOH, EtOH | Inhibits bacterial protein synthesis by blocking peptidyl transferase reaction, *JMB* **28**, 161 (1967). Inhibits mitochondrial and chloroplast protein synthesis. Irreversible toxicity to animal cells and humans at very high concs. may be due to inhibition of DNA synthesis, *Molec. Pharm.* **13**, 504 (1977). Chloramphenicol inhibits ribosomal formation of (p)ppGpp thus de-repressing rRNA transcription and RNA accumulates. |
| cryst. | s. $H_2O$, $CHCl_3$, EtOH, MeOH | Inhibits cytoplasmic eukaryote protein synthesis but not prokaryote. 75% inhibition in liver cell-free system at 1 mg/ml, 95% in intact reticulocytes at 0.03 mg/ml. Confusing reports on action but proposed that it inhibits initiation, elongation, and termination, the most affected step varying with concentration of drug, *ABB* **182**, 171 (1977). Unstable in alkali. |
| wh. powder; M.p. 74 | v. sl. s. $H_2O$; s. EtOH, eth., $CHCl_3$, acet. Dihydrochloride: v.s. $H_2O$ | Selectively inhibits protein synthesis in eukaryote cells and extracts. Acts on 40S ribosomal subunit site and inhibits translocation, *Biochem.* **16**, 4727 (1977). 50% inhibition of HeLa cell growth at $4 \times 10^{-8}$ M in media but cells concentrate it. Effect irreversible. DNA synthesis also affected. Cell-free yeast system inhibited 80% by 0.1 mM. Store in dark. Alkaloid tubulosine has similar action. Dihydrochloride has variable water of crystallization. |

## 13B Protein synthesis inhibitors and amino acid analogues

| Name | Synonyms | Formula | M. wt. |
|------|----------|---------|--------|
| Erythromycin | Ery | 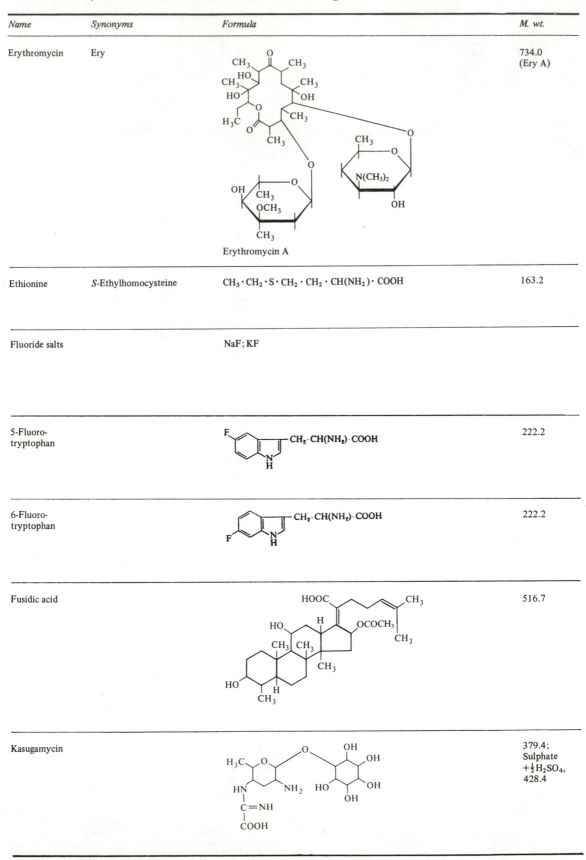  Erythromycin A | 734.0 (Ery A) |
| Ethionine | *S*-Ethylhomocysteine | $CH_3 \cdot CH_2 \cdot S \cdot CH_2 \cdot CH_2 \cdot CH(NH_2) \cdot COOH$ | 163.2 |
| Fluoride salts | | NaF; KF | |
| 5-Fluoro-tryptophan | | | 222.2 |
| 6-Fluoro-tryptophan | | | 222.2 |
| Fusidic acid | | | 516.7 |
| Kasugamycin | | | 379.4; Sulphate $+\frac{1}{2}H_2SO_4$, 428.4 |

| Physical properties | Solubility | General remarks |
|---|---|---|
| $\lambda_{max}$ (pH 6.3) 280 nm $\epsilon$ 50; p$K_a$ 8.8 | v.s. MeOH, EtOH; s. eth.; slowly s. H$_2$O (2 mg/ml) | Inhibitor of bacterial protein synthesis. *B. subtilis* growth 50% inhibited at 0.04 μg/ml. One of the macrolide group which includes spiramycin and carbomycin. Soln., basic reaction. |
| col. plates; M.p. 272 d. | s. H$_2$O | Methionine analogue. Growth of *E. coli* inhibited; effect reversed by methionine. May be incorporated into protein of mammals and bacteria in place of methionine. Activated by methionine activating enzymes. |
| | | KF or NaF inhibits translation in mammalian cells and cell-free systems. 30 mM-KF inhibits initiation of protein synthesis in reticulocyte lysates, with much less effect on chain elongation, *JBC* **250**, 3443 (1971). Proposed that it prevents 60S subunit joining 40S initiation complex. No reports on similar actions in prokaryote systems. |
| col. cryst.; M.p. 264—5 d. | v. sl. s. H$_2$O; s. acids, alkalis | Tryptophan analogue. Probably inhibits same reaction as 6-fluorotryptophan (q.v.). Can be activated by pancreatic tryptophan activating enzyme. |
| col. cryst. | v. sl. s. H$_2$O; s. acids, alkalis | Tryptophan analogue. Inhibits synthesis of *N-o*-carboxyphenyl-D-ribosylamine 1-phosphate from anthranilic acid and phosphoribosyl diphosphate in tryptophan biosynthetic pathway. Can be activated by pancreatic tryptophan activating enzyme. |
| p$K_a$ 5.35; $\lambda_{max}$ 204 nm $\epsilon$ 9900 | sl. s. H$_2$O; s. EtOH, acet., CHCl$_3$ | Inhibits protein synthesis in bacteria, bacterial lysates, eukaroyte cell lysates (but not intact cells, presumably due to non-permeability). In *E. coli* cell-free system, 60% inhibition at approx. 0.2 mM. Forms stable fusidic acid-GDP-ribosome-EFG (or EF$_2$) complex; prevents aminoacyl-tRNA from binding. Reported inhibition of translocation in cell-free systems due to binding all available EFG or EF$_2$ rather than inhibiting translocation reaction, *EJB* **57**, 431 (1975). |
| Sulphate: wh. cryst. | Sulphate: s. H$_2$O; sl. s. EtOH | Inhibits bacterial protein synthesis. Antifungal agent at pH 4—5. In *E. coli* cell-free system directed by f2 mRNA, 95% inhibition at $2 \times 10^{-4}$ M, *BBRC* **43**, 196 (1971). Interacts with 30S subunit and prevents binding of fMet-tRNA and hence protein synthesis initiation. Does not cause misreading. Eukaryote cell-free protein synthesis reported to be inhibited though most eukaryote cells insensitive. Almost all studies on prokaryote systems. |

## 13B Protein synthesis inhibitors and amino acid analogues

| Name | Synonyms | Formula | M. wt. |
|------|----------|---------|--------|
| 7-Methylguanosine 5'-monophosphate | m$^7$G$^{5'}$p | | 377.3 |
| ω-Methyllysine | α, ε-Diaminoheptanoic acid; ε-C-methyllysine | $CH_3 \cdot CH(NH_2) \cdot (CH_2)_3 \cdot CH(NH_2) \cdot COOH$ | 160.2 |
| O-Methylthreonine | | | 133.2 |
| 5-Methyltryptophan | | | 218.3 |
| Negamycin | | $H_2N \cdot CH_2 \cdot \overset{OH}{CH} \cdot CH_2 \cdot \overset{NH_2}{CH} \cdot CH_2 \cdot CO \cdot NH \cdot \overset{CH_3}{N} \cdot CH_2 \cdot COOH$ | 248.3 |
| Norleucine | α-Aminocaproic acid | $CH_3 \cdot CH_2 \cdot CH_2 \cdot CH_2 \cdot CH(NH_2) \cdot COOH$ | 131.2 |
| Pactamycin | | | 558.6 |
| Puromycin | Stylomycin | | 471.5 |
| Selenomethionine | | $CH_3 \cdot Se \cdot CH_2 \cdot CH_2 \cdot CH(NH_2) \cdot COOH$ | 196.1 |

| Physical properties | Solubility | General remarks |
|---|---|---|
| | | Inhibits the translation of mRNAs with $m^7G(5)-$ as the 5′-terminal sequence. Prevents mRNA interaction with the 40S ribosomal subunit at approx. 0.25 mM. Completely inhibits translation of rabbit globin mRNA in a wheat germ system, *PNAS* **73**, 19 (1976). |
| col. cryst.; M.p. 191 (as di–HCl) | s. $H_2O$ | Lysine analogue. Growth inhibition of *S. faecalis* and *L. mesenteroides*; reversed by lysine. Incorporated in place of lysine in *S. aureus* cell wall. |
| col. cryst. | s. $H_2O$ | Isoleucine analogue. Competitive inhibition of leucine incorporation into Ehrlich ascites tumour cells. Allo-*O*-methylthreonine not active. |
| col. leaflets; M.p. 264 d. | sl. s. $H_2O$; s. acids | Tryptophan analogue. Not incorporated into protein. Competitive inhibition of tryptophan activating enzyme in liver and bacteria, but not itself activated. Inhibits synthesis of anthranilic acid from shikimic acid 5-phosphate and glutamate in *E. coli* by 'false' feedback inhibition. Completely inhibits phage synthesis. |
| $pK_a$ 3.55, 8.1, 9.75; M.p. 110d. | s. $H_2O$; i. org. solvents | Inhibitor of bacterial protein synthesis and causes misreading (latter uniquely for non-aminosugar antibiotic). Bactericidal and effective, amongst others, against *Pseudomonas* and multiple-drug resistant gram-negatives. Claimed to selectively inhibit chain termination, *BBA* **442**, 251 (1976), but may have multiple effects on ribosome. |
| col. leaflets; M.p. 301 d.; $pK_a$ 2.39, 9.76 | s. $H_2O$ | Methionine analogue. May be incorporated into protein of *E. coli* in place of methionine. Competitive inhibition of methionine activation in *E. coli*. |
| | s. EtOH, $CHCl_3$, dil. acids and alkalis | Inhibits protein synthesis in bacteria and prokaryotes. Inhibits initiation but reported not to affect elongation since it does not prevent polysome break-down, *BBA* **294**, 118 (1973). At $10^{-4}$ M inhibits protein synthesis in reticulocycles by 88%. Unstable. |
| wh. cryst.; M.p. 175–7; $pK_a$ 6.8, 7.2 | Free base, sp. s. $H_2O$ as well as organic solvents. Dihydrochloride and monosulphate, readily s. $H_2O$ | Inhibits protein synthesis. Prevents growth of bacteria, algae, protozoa, and mammalian cells. Causes premature release of partially formed protein chains from ribosomes by acting as analogue of acceptor aminoacyl-tRNA. |
| col. cryst. | s. $H_2O$ | Methionine analogue. Can replace methionine completely in protein of *E. coli*. Also found in protein of animals grazing in pastures rich in selenium compounds. |

# 13B  Protein synthesis inhibitors and amino acid analogues

| *Name* | *Synonyms* | *Formula* | *M. wt.* |
|---|---|---|---|
| Sparsomycin | | | 361.4 |

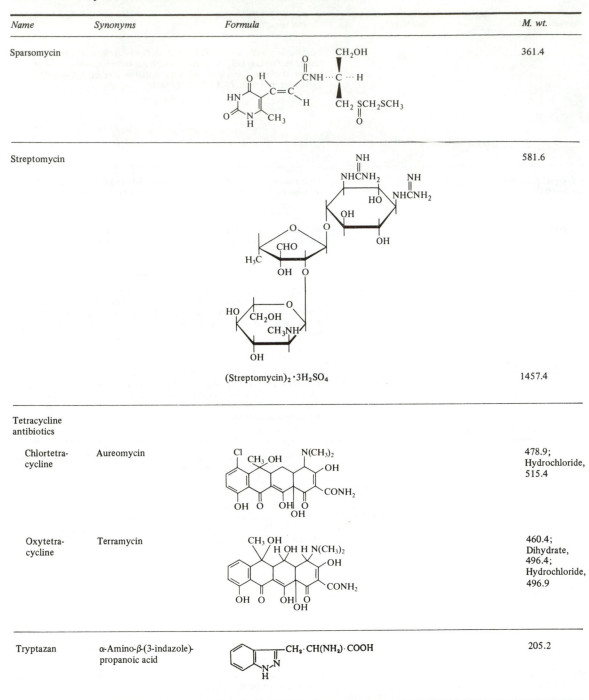

| Streptomycin | | | 581.6 |

(Streptomycin)$_2 \cdot 3H_2SO_4$       1457.4

**Tetracycline antibiotics**

| Chlortetra-cycline | Aureomycin | | 478.9; Hydrochloride, 515.4 |
| Oxytetra-cycline | Terramycin | | 460.4; Dihydrate, 496.4; Hydrochloride, 496.9 |
| Tryptazan | α-Amino-β-(3-indazole)-propanoic acid | | 205.2 |

| Physical properties | Solubility | General remarks |
|---|---|---|
| | | One of the most effective inhibitors of protein synthesis in pro- and eukaryotes and widely used as a biochemical tool. Inhibits peptide bond formation, probably acting at acceptor site on large ribosomal sub-unit. Has no effect on intact reticulocytes even at high concs. but in cell-free systems inhibits 84% at $0.8 \times 10^{-4}$ M, *BBA* **119**, 109 (1966). $K_i$ for peptidyl puromycin synthesis is $2 \times 10^{-7}$ M for bacterial polysomes and $10^{-6}$ M for rat liver polysomes. |
| Base, sulphate and hydrochloride all hygroscopic wh. powders | s. $H_2O$ | Inhibits initiation, elongation and termination of protein synthesis in prokaryotes and induces misreading. Binds to small ribosomal subunit. In *E. coli*, inhibits protein synthesis completely at concs. $> 20 \,\mu g/ml$. Low concs. ($2 \,\mu g/ml$) cause phenotypic suppression of mutations due to misreading. Related aminoglycoside antibiotics, kanamycin and neomycin, also cause misreading. Streptomycin sulphate used to precipitate nucleic acids in enzyme purification. |
| | v.s. $H_2O$; i. EtOH | |
| yel. cryst.; $\lambda_{max}$ (0.1M-HCl) 230, 262.5, 367.5 nm | sl. s. $H_2O$ (0.5 mg/ml); v.s. $> pH 8.5$. Hydrochloride: s. $H_2O$ (8.6 mg/ml), MeOH | Inhibitors of protein synthesis in pro- and eukaryotes; preferentially accumulated by bacteria conferring therapeutic value. Chlortetracycline inhibits 50% in cell-free systems at $30 \,\mu M$ (*E. coli*) and $125 \,\mu M$ (rat liver). Inhibits binding of aminoacyl-tRNA to ribosomes, *JBC* **244**, 5680 (1969). Ribosomal (p)ppGpp synthesis inhibited in bacteria. |
| Dihydrate: cryst. from $H_2O$. Hydrochloride: yel. cryst. from $H_2O$; $\lambda_{max}$ (0.1M-phosphate pH 4.5): 249, 276, 353 nm $A_{1cm}^{1\%}$ 240, 322, 301 | s. $H_2O$ (1.1 mg/ml pH 7; 39.6, pH 9); s. EtOH. Hydrochloride: v.s. $H_2O$ (1 g/ml) | Aq. solns. of hydrochloride stable 4 weeks, pH 3–9, at 5 °C. |
| col. needles; M.p. 249–50 d. | sl. s. $H_2O$; s. acids | Tryptophan analogue. Incorporated in protein of *E. coli* in place of tryptophan. May be activated by pancreatic tryptophan activating enzyme. |

# C. COMPOUNDS AFFECTING MEMBRANE FUNCTION

This Section includes surface-active agents, lectins, transport inhibitors, and iono-phores and related channel formers. However the selection is necessarily subjective and the Section on inhibitors of mitochondrial and chloroplast function, p. 302, should also be consulted for further compounds affecting membrane function.

## Surface-active compounds

## General references

Properties of detergents, *Meth. Enzymol.* **56**, 734 (1979).
*Solubilization by surface-active agents and its application in chemistry and the biological sciences*, P. H. Elworthy *et al.*, Chapman & Hall, London (1968).
Selective release from microsomes without membrane disassembly, *Meth. Enzymol.* **31**, 215 (1974).

| Name | Synonyms | Formula | M. wt. |
|---|---|---|---|
| **Anionic surfactants** | | | |
| Bile Salts | | | |
| Dioctyl sodium sulphosuccinate | Aerosol OT; bis(2-ethylhexyl) sodium sulphosuccinate | $H_2C\cdot CO\cdot O\cdot CH_2\cdot CH\cdot(CH_2)_3\cdot CH_3$ ($C_2H_5$); $NaO_3S\cdot\underset{H}{C}\cdot CO\cdot O\cdot CH_2\cdot CH\cdot(CH_2)_3\cdot CH_3$ ($C_2H_5$) | 444.6 |
| Diosgenin | (25R)-Spirost-5-en-3β-ol; nitogenin | | 414.6 |
| Sarkosyl | N-Laurylsarcosine, Na salt | | 293.4 |
| SDS | Sodium dodecyl sulphate; sodium lauryl sulphate; Irium | $\left[CH_3\cdot(CH_2)_{10}\cdot CH_2-O-\overset{O}{\underset{O}{\overset{\|}{\underset{\|}{S}}}}-O\right]Na$ | 288.4 (see general remarks) |
| **Cationic surfactants** | | | |
| Cetylpyridinium chloride | 1-Hexadecylpyridinium chloride; Ceepryn chloride; Cepacol chloride; Cetamium | | 358.0 |

Use of detergents for nuclei isolation, *Meth. Enzymol.* **31**, 254, 558 (1974); *Meth. Cell Biol.* **15**, 223 (1977).

Solubilization of membranes, *BBA* **415**, 29 (1975); **733**, 210 (1983); **737**, 285 (1983).

Effect of hydrophile–lipophile balance (HLB) and critical micellar concentration (CMM) as factors in the solubilization of membrane proteins, *JBC* **251**, 4442 (1976); *BBA* **455**, 796 (1976); *BBA* **553**, 40 (1979).

Characterization of membrane proteins in detergent solutions, *BBA* **457**, 133 (1976).

Polyacrylamide gel electrophoresis following solubilization with detergents, *Meth. Enzymol.* **32**, 82 (1974).

Preparation and characterization of mammalian plasma membranes, W. H. Evans in *Laboratory techniques in biochemistry and molecular biology*, eds. T. S. Work and E. Work, vol. 7, North-Holland, Amsterdam (1979).

| Physical properties | HLB | CMM (µM) | General remarks |
|---|---|---|---|
| | | | See bile acids, p. 208. Sodium salts of cholic, deoxycholic, taurocholic, and taurodeoxycholic acids are widely used as surface active agents (CMM: 13–15, 4–6, 10–15, 2–6 mM, respectively). |
| waxy solid; s. $H_2O$ (18 g/l. at 30°C), $CCl_4$, acet., benz., MeOH | | | Anionic detergent. Slightly hygroscopic, stable in acid and neutral solution, hydrolyses in alkaline solutions. Bactericidal activity increases as pH falls, active only against gram +ve bacteria at neutral pH but active against gram +ve and −ve at pH **4** (*Bull. Int. Ass. Milk Deal.* **33**, 491 (1941)). |
| needles or plates from acet.; M.p. 204–7; s. most organic solvents | | | Steroidal sapogenin isolated from extract of *Dioscorea tokoro*, Makino. Forms insoluble digitonide. Saponin, dioscin = diosgenin bis-α-L-rhamnopyranosyl-(1 → 3, 1 → 4)-β-D-glucopyranoside, $C_{45}H_{72}O_{16}$, M. wt. 869.1. |
| $\lambda_{max}$ 220, 265 nm $\epsilon_{280}$ 3 | | | Anionic detergent. |
| wh. or creamy wh. powder or cryst.; s. $H_2O$, EtOH | | 8200($H_2O$) 520(0.5M-NaCl) | Anionic detergent, commercial product is a mixture of alkyl sulphates. Bactericidal activity is greatest at low pH and at pH 4 it is active against gram +ve and −ve organisms. Causes disaggregation of cell walls of gram −ve bacteria (*J. Gen. Microbiol.* **23**, 137 (1960)). Used to separate nucleic acid from protein: RNA (*JACS* **75**, 4041 (1953)); DNA (*JBC* **190**, 165 (1951)). Solubilizes proteins and confers strong negative charge on them; widely used in electrophoresis. |
| wh. powder; M.p. 77–83; v.s. $H_2O$, EtOH, $CHCl_3$; v. sl. s. benz., eth. | | | Cationic detergent. Bactericidal, active at alkaline pH against both gram +ve and −ve organisms. Denatures proteins (*Adv. Protein Chem.* **4**, 79 (1948)) and disorganizes bacterial cell membranes in a manner similar to CTAB. Has been used to modify cell permeability. Reverses the surface charge on bacteria (*J. Bacteriol.* **51**, 149 (1946)). |

285

# 13C Compounds affecting membrane function

| Name | Synonyms | Formula | M. wt. |
|------|----------|---------|--------|
| Cetyltrimethyl-ammonium bromide | Cetavlon; Cetrimide; CTAB; Cetylamine; Quamonium | $(CH_3)_3 \cdot \overset{+}{N} \ Br^-$<br>$C_{16}H_{33}$ | 364.5 (see general remarks) |

**Zwitterionic surfactants**

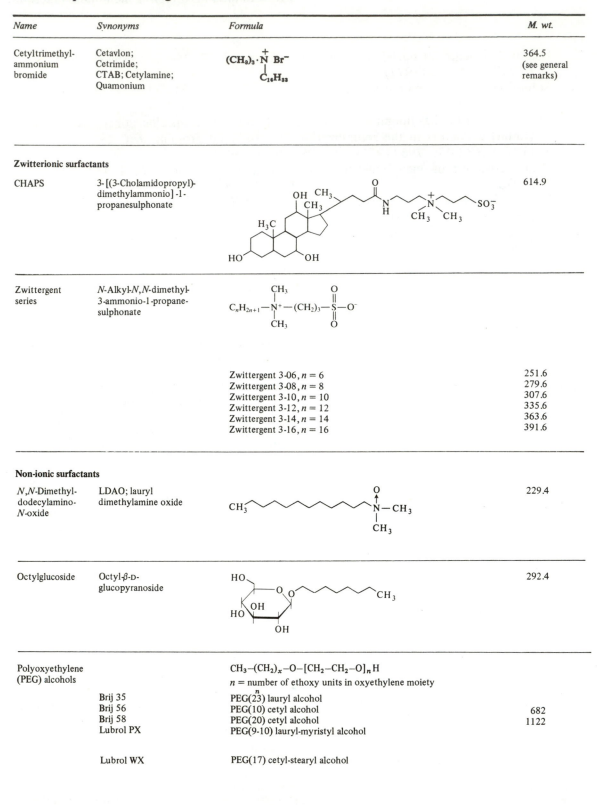

| CHAPS | 3-[(3-Cholamidopropyl)-dimethylammonio]-1-propanesulphonate | | 614.9 |
|-------|-----|--|-------|
| Zwittergent series | N-Alkyl-N,N-dimethyl-3-ammonio-1-propane-sulphonate | | |

| | | |
|--|--|--|
| Zwittergent 3-06, $n = 6$ | | 251.6 |
| Zwittergent 3-08, $n = 8$ | | 279.6 |
| Zwittergent 3-10, $n = 10$ | | 307.6 |
| Zwittergent 3-12, $n = 12$ | | 335.6 |
| Zwittergent 3-14, $n = 14$ | | 363.6 |
| Zwittergent 3-16, $n = 16$ | | 391.6 |

**Non-ionic surfactants**

| N,N-Dimethyl-dodecylamino-N-oxide | LDAO; lauryl dimethylamine oxide | | 229.4 |
|------|------|--|-------|
| Octylglucoside | Octyl-β-D-glucopyranoside | | 292.4 |

| Polyoxyethylene (PEG) alcohols | | $CH_3-(CH_2)_x-O-[CH_2-CH_2-O]_n H$<br>$n$ = number of ethoxy units in oxyethylene moiety | |
|------|------|------|------|
| | Brij 35 | PEG(23) lauryl alcohol | |
| | Brij 56 | PEG(10) cetyl alcohol | |
| | Brij 58 | PEG(20) cetyl alcohol | 682 |
| | Lubrol PX | PEG(9-10) lauryl-myristyl alcohol | 1122 |
| | Lubrol WX | PEG(17) cetyl-stearyl alcohol | |

| Physical properties | HLB | CMM (μM) | General remarks |
|---|---|---|---|
| creamy wh. powder; v.s. EtOH, MeOH; 10 $H_2O$ | | | Cationic detergent. Commercial product a mixture of alkyl ammonium bromides (c. 80% CTAB). Bactericidal, activity annulled by soaps and anionic detergents, active at alkaline pH against both gram +ve and gram −ve organisms. Disorganizes cell membranes, releasing amino acids, purines, pyrimidines, and other small molecules (*J. Gen. Microbiol.* **5**, 391 (1951)). Used to render cells permeable to substrates in enzyme assays and to accelerate enzyme action (*BJ* **45**, 325 (1949)). Denatures protein (*Adv. Protein Chem.* **4**, 79 (1948)). |
| M.p. 117 d. | | | Zwitterionic detergent, combining useful properties of both the sulphobetaine type and the bile acid detergents. |
| | | | Sulphobetaine zwitterionic detergents; 3-10 and 3-12 recommended as most effective in releasing proteins from membrane-bound compartments without denaturing them, *BBA* **733**, 210 (1983). Sulphobetaines have no net charge between pH 2 and 12, useful in isoelectric focusing. |
| | | Large<br>Large<br>1.2%<br>0.12%<br>0.012%<br>0.0012% | |
| | | | Non-ionic detergent |
| | | 25 000 | Non-ionic detergent with no absorption at 228 nm, best suited for solubilization and isolation of membrane proteins. |
| | | | Non-ionic. Polyoxyethylene detergents with simple alkyl chains are subject to autoxidation especially in light, leading to formation of u.v.-absorbing products. A small amount of antioxidant (*e.g.* butylated hydroxytoluene) can be added to stabilize. |
| | 12.9<br>15.7 | 2<br>77 | Superior to Triton X-100 in solubilizing membrane-bound adenyl cyclase, *BBRC* **38**, 86 (1970). |
| waxy wh. solid; s. $H_2O$, EtOH | 14.9 | 20–66 | Effective solubilizer of NaK-activated ATPase of cerebral microsomes, *JBC* **246**, 531 (1971).<br>Used in conjunction with deoxycholate as 0.5% soln. in 0.25 M-sucrose to fractionate proteins from mammalian microsomes and to prepare ribonucleo-protein particles (*BJ* **70**, 254 (1958); *Exp. Cell Res.* **23**, 517 (1961)). A 0.05% solution in buffers facilitates the separation of serum proteins by paper electrophoresis (*Clin. Chem.* **6**, 413 (1960)). |

| Name | Synonyms | Formula | M. wt. |
|---|---|---|---|

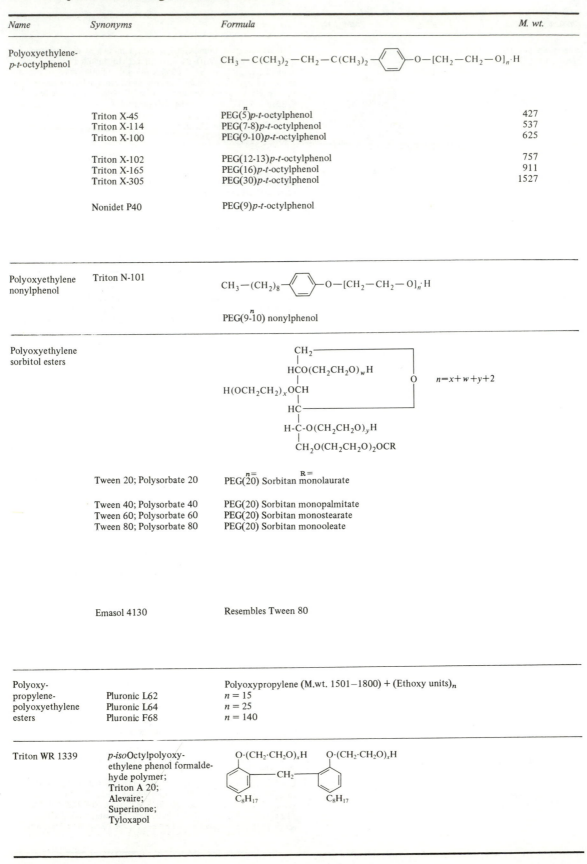

**Polyoxyethylene-*p-t*-octylphenol**

$$CH_3-C(CH_3)_2-CH_2-C(CH_3)_2-\text{⟨benzene⟩}-O-[CH_2-CH_2-O]_n \cdot H$$

| Name | Synonyms | Formula | M. wt. |
|---|---|---|---|
| | Triton X-45 | PEG($\overset{n}{5}$)*p-t*-octylphenol | 427 |
| | Triton X-114 | PEG(7-8)*p-t*-octylphenol | 537 |
| | Triton X-100 | PEG(9-10)*p-t*-octylphenol | 625 |
| | Triton X-102 | PEG(12-13)*p-t*-octylphenol | 757 |
| | Triton X-165 | PEG(16)*p-t*-octylphenol | 911 |
| | Triton X-305 | PEG(30)*p-t*-octylphenol | 1527 |
| | Nonidet P40 | PEG(9)*p-t*-octylphenol | |

**Polyoxyethylene nonylphenol** — Triton N-101

$$CH_3-(CH_2)_8-\text{⟨benzene⟩}-O-[CH_2-CH_2-O]_n \cdot H$$

PEG($\overset{n}{9}$-10) nonylphenol

**Polyoxyethylene sorbitol esters**

$$n=x+w+y+2$$

| | Tween 20; Polysorbate 20 | PEG($\overset{n=}{20}$) Sorbitan monolaurate $\overset{R=}{}$ |
| | Tween 40; Polysorbate 40 | PEG(20) Sorbitan monopalmitate |
| | Tween 60; Polysorbate 60 | PEG(20) Sorbitan monostearate |
| | Tween 80; Polysorbate 80 | PEG(20) Sorbitan monooleate |
| | Emasol 4130 | Resembles Tween 80 |

**Polyoxy-propylene-polyoxyethylene esters**

Polyoxypropylene (M.wt. 1501–1800) + (Ethoxy units)$_n$

| | Pluronic L62 | $n = 15$ |
| | Pluronic L64 | $n = 25$ |
| | Pluronic F68 | $n = 140$ |

**Triton WR 1339** — *p-iso*Octylpolyoxyethylene phenol formaldehyde polymer; Triton A 20; Alevaire; Superinone; Tyloxapol

$O \cdot (CH_2 \cdot CH_2O)_x H$      $O \cdot (CH_2 \cdot CH_2O)_x H$

$C_8H_{17}$      $C_8H_{17}$

| Physical properties | HLB | CMM (μM) | General remarks |
|---|---|---|---|
| | | | Polyoxyethylene detergents with alkylphenyl hydrophobic groups absorb UV and interfere with spectrophotometric determination of proteins. Detergents should be stored in glass containers at 0 °C after opening to retard peroxidation, *Meth. Enzymol.* **52**, 145 (1978). NaBH$_4$ can be used to destroy peroxides, *Anal. Biochem.* **83**, 274 (1977). |
| | 10.4 | 100 | |
| Cloud pt. 22 °C | 12.4 | 210 | |
| Cloud pt. 65 °C | 13.5 | 250 | Triton X-100 often reagent of choice to maximize qualitatively and quantitatively variety and yield of soluble membrane components recovered under non-denaturing conditions. The extent of solubilization increases with increasing detergent up to plateau of 0.5–1, detergent/ protein ratio, *BBA* **553**, 40 (1979). |
| Cloud pt. 88 °C | 14.6 | 330 | |
| Cloud pt. 100 °C | 15.8 | 430 | |
| Cloud pt. 100 °C | 17.3 | 650 | |
| pale yel. viscous liq.; ∞ H$_2$O; s. EtOH, *iso*PrOH, eth., acet., benz. | 13.1 | 290 | Used as a 1.5% (v/v) solution in 0.2 M-phosphate buffer at pH 7.2, containing 0.006M-MgCl$_2$, to solubilize lipid material and allow the isolation of endosperm protoplasts (*Aust. J. Biol. Sci.* **16**, 375 (1963); **17**, 102 (1964)). |
| | 13.5 | 85 | |
| | 16.7 | 60 mg/l | Weak non-ionic detergent sometimes used for preextraction of membranes to remove peripheral proteins, *BBA* **455**, 796 (1976). |
| | 15.6 | 29 mg/l | |
| | 14.9 | 27 mg/l | |
| amber, viscous liq.; v.s. H$_2$O; s. EtOH, MeOH, Et acetate, toluene | 15.0 | 13 mg/l | Non-ionic detergent. Little or no antibacterial activity. Used to promote submerged growth of tubercle bacilli (opt. conc. 0.1%) (*J. Exp. Med.* **83**, 409 (1946)). May be metabolized to release oleic acid which is growth inhibitory to some bacteria (*Annls Inst. Pasteur, Paris* **85**, 277 (1953)). Induces a change from smooth to rough forms in some bacteria (*C.R. Séanc. Soc. Biol. Paris* **146**, 820 (1952)). Used in fractionation of tissue culture cells (*Proc. R. Soc.* **B 156**, 521 (1962)). |
| amber coloured viscous liquid; v.s. H$_2$O; s. EtOH | 16.5 | | Used extensively as a 1% solution in 0.1M-tris or phosphate buffer at pH 7.4 for extraction and solubilization of cytochrome *a* from mammalian tissues (*J. Biochem., Tokyo* **46**, 917 (1959); *JBC* **235**, 845 (1960)). |
| col. liq.; v.s. H$_2$O | | | Non-ionic detergent. Anti-tuberculous activity *in vivo* (*Nature, Lond.* **168**, 150 (1951)). REVIEW: Influence of certain surface-active agents on the host-parasite relationship in experimental tuberculosis in *CIBA Foundation Symposium on Experimental Tuberculosis*, p. 299 (1955). Corrects hepatic and serum lipid changes caused by ethynyloestradiol treatment, *PNAS* **75**, 4130 (1978). Inhibitor of hepatic microsomal cholesterol–acyl-CoA transferase, *BJ* **174**, 45 (1978). Used in isolation of modified lysosomes (tritonsomes), *Meth. Enzymol.* **31**, 323 (1974). |

| Name | General remarks |
|---|---|
| **Miscellaneous** | |
| Chaotropic agents | Order of effectiveness in extracting proteins from membranes: $CCl_3COO^- > SCN^- >$ guanidine $> ClO_4^- > Br^- > NO_3^- >$ urea Chaotropic anions increase solubility in water of apolar moieties, *PNAS* **62**, 1129 (1969). Some proteins are dissociated from membranes by chaotropic agents. Yield may be low but selectivity can make them useful agents. Guanidine-HCl and urea have similar effects. Urea has greater solubilizing effect at 0 °C than at 25 °C. Antichaotropic anions (large polyvalent or small monovalent anions such as $SO_4^{2-}$, $PO_4^{3-}$, and $F^-$) are useful in reconstituting membrane components detached by chaotropic anions. |

## Lectins

Lectins are cell-agglutinating and sugar-specific proteins found in plants — usually seeds — (phytohaemagglutinins), and in invertebrates and lower vertebrates. Binding of lectins to surface plasma membrane of cells has a broad range of effects on the structural and functional state of the membranes, e.g. changes in the arrangement of surface proteins and glycoproteins, physical state of membrane lipid, permeability of the membrane to a variety of substances, and activities of membrane enzymes. Certain of the individual changes are key events responsible for further changes in the membrane and within the cell, e.g. mitogenic lectins induce replication of nucleic acids and proliferation of lymphocytes.

## General references

N. Sharon and H. Lis, Lectins: cell-agglutinating and sugar-specific proteins, *Science* **177**, 949 (1972).

H. Lis and N. Sharon, The biochemistry of plant lectins (phytohaemagglutinins), *ARB* **42**, 541 (1973).

I.E. Liener, Phytohaemagglutinins (phytolectins), *Ann. Rev. Plant Physiol.* **27**, 291 (1976).

J. C. Brown and R. C. Hunt, Lectins, *Int. Rev. Cytology* **52**, 277 (1978).

Purification and properties of carbohydrate—binding proteins, *Meth. Enzymol.* **28**, 313 (1972).

Agglutination and binding assays, *Meth. Enzymol.* **32**, 615 (1974).

Group-specific separation of glycoproteins, *Meth. Enzymol.* **34**, 331 (1974).

| Name | Formula | M. wt. | General remarks |
|---|---|---|---|
| Concanavalin A | Protein of 2 identical sub-units, each of 237 amino acids; 2 $Ca^{2+}$ binding sites; 2 transition-metal binding sites; 2 saccharide-binding sites (when both kinds of metal-binding sites are occupied) | Sub-unit, 26 000; tetramer at pH > 7 | Haemagglutinin from jack bean (*Canavalia ensiformis*); forms insoluble complexes with biopolymers containing multiple α-D-glucopyranosyl (or its 2-acetamido-2-deoxy deriv.), α-D-mannopyranosyl or β-D-fructofuranosyl residues as non-reducing termini. May also bind mannose residues in interior of molecule. Mitogenic. |
| *Helix pomatia* lectin | | Hexamer, 79 000 | Lectin from snails, specific for *N*-acetyl-D-galactosamine residues. Binds to T-lymphocytes treated with neuraminidase but not to B-cells so treated. Specific for Group A human erythrocytes. |

| Name | Formula | M. wt. | General remarks |
|------|---------|--------|-----------------|
| Lentil lectin | | | From *Lens esculenta*. Affinity for α-D-mannopyranosyl and α-D-glucopyranosyl residues; haemagglutinating; mitogenic towards untreated lymphocytes. |
| Phytohaem-agglutinin (Leuco-agglutinin) | See *Ann. Rev. Plant Physiol.* **27**, 291 (1976) | Tetramer, 126 000; L and R sub-units, 31 000 — 34 000 | Crude preparation from red kidney bean (*Phaseolus vulgaris*) widely used as mitogen. Different biological activities by family of 5 heterogeneous proteins, each consisting of isomeric non-covalently bound tetramers made up of two different types of sub-unit, L (conferring leucoagglutinating activity) and R (haemagglutinating). Hybrid molecules are mitogenic. |
| Protein A | Single polypeptide | 42 000 | From cell wall of *Staphylococcus aureus*. Binding specific for Fc fragment of IgG molecules of several species. Widely used in immunological precipitation work since it removes need for optimum antigen/antibody ratios, *Anal. Biochem.* **97**, 24 (1979); *J. Immunol.* **115**, 1617 (1975). |
| Ricin | Dimer of 493 amino acid residues. A- and B-chains joined by disulphide bridge | Dimer, 66 000; A-chain, 32 000; B-chain, 34 000 | Extremely toxic glycoprotein from seeds of castor oil plant, *Ricinus communis*. Entry into cell is in two stages, (a) toxin becomes linked by B-chain to terminal galactose of receptor on cell surface, (b) disulphide bond cleaved, releasing A-chain to enter cell where it binds to 60S ribosomal subunit, apparently in the region where $EF_1$ and $EF_2$ bind. Abrin, M. wt. 65 000, is a similar toxin from seeds of *Abrus pecatorius*. |
| Soybean lectin | Tetramer over wide range of pH | 120 000 | From *Glycine max*. Specific for *N*-acetyl-D-galactosamine residues. Mitogenic for neuraminidase-treated lymphocytes. |
| Wheat germ lectin | | | From *Triticum vulgare*. Binding site complementary to sequence of three β(1-4)-linked *N*-acetyl-D-glucosamine residues; does not agglutinate normal cells except under certain conditions (e.g. after protease treatment), while transformed cells are agglutinated. |

## 13C Compounds affecting membrane function

### Transport inhibitors

### General references

R. M. Hochster and J. H. Quastel, eds., *Metabolic Inhibitors*, vol. 3, ch. 1–3, 10 (1972).

| Name | Synonyms | Formula | M. wt. |
|---|---|---|---|
| 1,8-Anilino-naphthalene-sulphonic acid | ANS | | 229.4 |
| Atractyloside | Potassium atractylate | Atractyloside: R = H<br>Carboxyatractyloside (Gummiferin): R = COOH | Atractyloside $K_2$ salt, 803.0; Carboxy-atractyloside, 770.8; Carboxy-atractyloside $K_2$ salt + $1H_2O$, 865.0 |
| Bongkrekic acid | | | 486.6 |
| α-Bungarotoxin | | Polypeptide of 74 amino acids, *ZPC* **353**, 243 (1972) | 7983 |
| β-Bungarotoxin | | Protein with two sub-units, M. wt. 7000 and 13 500 | 20 500 |
| Cycloleucine | 1-Aminocyclopentane-carboxylic acid | | 129.2 |

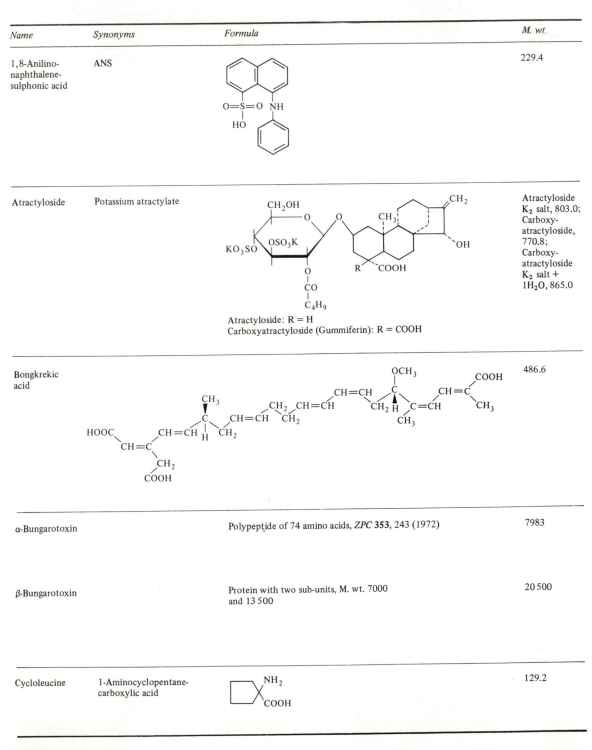

| Physical properties | Solubility | General remarks |
|---|---|---|
| fluorescence emission max. 480 nm (in EtOH). | | Fluoresces strongly in organic solvents but not in aqueous solns. Used as hydrophobic probe in membranes and protein studies. Best known of family of probes. Review, *Meth. Enzymol.* **32**, 234 (1974). Inhibits anion permeability in red cell membranes, *J. Mem. Biol.* **5**, 154 (1971). |
| col. cryst. | s. EtOH; i. $H_2O$ | Prevents movement of adenine nucleotides across inner mitochondrial membrane by displacing nucleotides from translocase protein in the membrane. 50% inhibition at less than 1 nmole/mg of protein. Carboxyatractyloside is also a specific inhibitor of adenine nucleotide transport but non-competitive towards nucleotides. Plant mitochondria relatively insensitive to atractyloside but not to carboxy derivative. Review, *BBA* **456**, 1 (1976). *See also* bongkrekic acid. |
| | s. dil. alk. | Prevents movement of adenine nucleotides across inner mitochondrial membrane by preventing release of nucleotides from carrier protein (translocase) on the matrix side. 50% inhibition at less than 1 nmole/mg protein. Bongkrekic acid is *trans*-isomer at dicarboxylic end; isobongkrekic acid (*cis*-isomer) has a similar action, *Biochem.* **15**, 2323 (1976); Review, *BBA* **456**, 1 (1976). |
| | | Neurotoxin from snake venom, acting postsynaptically via blockade of the acetylcholine receptor, *ARB* **42**, 235 (1973). Extremely toxic. Handle with great care. $LD_{50}$ i.p. in mice: 0.15 mg/kg. |
| | | Neurotoxin from snake venom. Modifies release of neurotransmitter from mammalian motor-nerve terminals; inhibits $Ca^{2+}$ accumulation in subcellular fractions of brain, *BBRC* **58**, 475 (1974). Has $Ca^{2+}$ dependent phospholipase $A_2$ activity, *PNAS* **73**, 178 (1976). Extremely toxic. Handle with great care. $LD_{50}$ s.c. in mice: 89 µg/kg. |
| cryst. from EtOH–$H_2O$; M.p. 330 (decomp) | 5 $H_2O$ | Non-metabolizable synthetic amino acid; valine antagonist. Inhibits amino acid transport, *Can. J. Physiol. Pharm.* **53**, 1027 (1975). |

# 13C Compounds affecting membrane function

| Name | Synonyms | Formula | M. wt. |
|------|----------|---------|--------|
| Cytochalasin | | 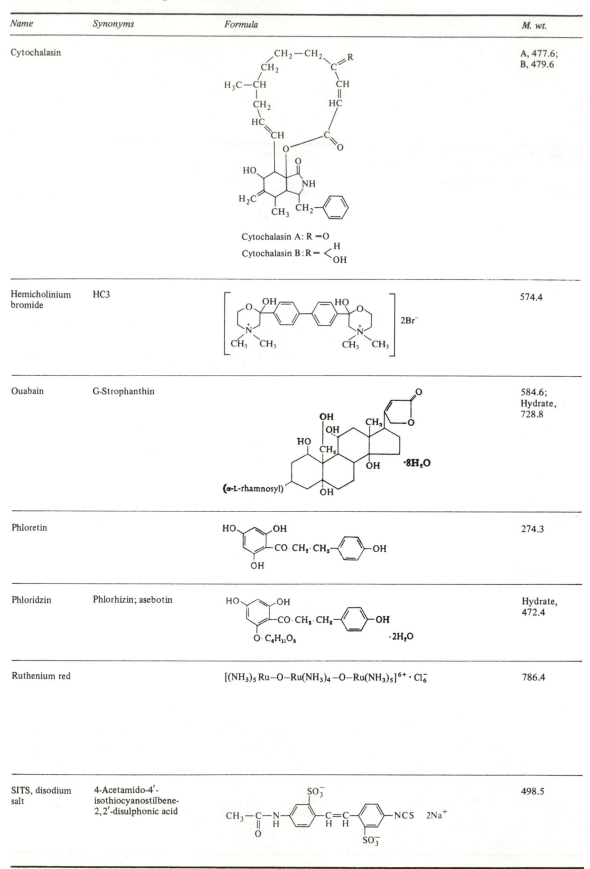 Cytochalasin A: R =O<br>Cytochalasin B: R = <H, OH | A, 477.6;<br>B, 479.6 |
| Hemicholinium bromide | HC3 | | 574.4 |
| Ouabain | G-Strophanthin | (α-L-rhamnosyl) ·8H₂O | 584.6;<br>Hydrate,<br>728.8 |
| Phloretin | | HO, OH, CO·CH₂·CH₂─OH, OH | 274.3 |
| Phloridzin | Phlorhizin; asebotin | HO, OH, CO·CH₂·CH₂─OH, O·C₆H₁₁O₅ ·2H₂O | Hydrate,<br>472.4 |
| Ruthenium red | | $[(NH_3)_5 Ru-O-Ru(NH_3)_4-O-Ru(NH_3)_5]^{6+} \cdot Cl_6^-$ | 786.4 |
| SITS, disodium salt | 4-Acetamido-4'-isothiocyanostilbene-2,2'-disulphonic acid | CH₃·C·NH─ SO₃⁻ C=C ─NCS  2Na⁺ SO₃⁻ | 498.5 |

| Physical properties | Solubility | General remarks |
|---|---|---|
| B: M.p. 218–21 | i. $H_2O$; s. dimethyl sulphoxide, acet. | Inhibits cell motility, phagocytosis and the division of cytoplasm; causes nuclear extrusion; modifies, reversibly, cell microfilaments at $0.5–3.0\,\mu g/ml$; actin bundle patterns rapidly disorganised by B while microtubules are not affected, *Cell motility*, eds. T. Pollard, J. Rosenbaum, Cold Spring Harbour Lab. (1976) pp. 403–18. Cytochalasin A inhibits tubulin and actin assembly *in vitro* and decreases the colchicine binding of tubulin, through an irreversible action on -SH groups of proteins, *J. Supramol. Struct.* **5**, 81 (1976). At lower conc. ($10^{-8}–10^{-6}$ M) A inhibits transport of small molecules (e.g. hexoses and nucleosides). At $10^{-6}–10^{-4}$ M affects all motility and morphology. Binding sites, *JBC* **252**, 5464 (1977); glucose transport, *JBC* **252**, 5456 (1977). |
| wh. cryst. powder | s. $H_2O$ | Respiratory paralysant. Blocks cholinergic transmission by interfering with ACh synthesis. Inhibits choline uptake and choline kinase. |
| shiny plates of octahydrate; M.p. anhyd., 190; Hydrate, 130 | s. $H_2O$, EtOH | Inhibits cation transport. Classical inhibitor of $Na^+/K^+$ ATPase ($10^{-6}$ M). |
| col. needles; M.p. 264–71d. | s. EtOH, acet., acetic acid; i. $H_2O$, eth. | Inhibits muscle phosphorylase and also uptake of glucose by erythrocytes. Mechanism of action on erythrocytes not clear. |
| silky wh. needles; M.p. 108; solidifies 138; remelts 170 | v.s. hot $H_2O$; s. EtOH; v. sl. s. eth. | Non-comp. inhibition of muscle, but not potato, phosphorylase. Inhibits phosphatases and UDPG-glycogen transglucosylase. Causes glucosuria by prevention of glucose reabsorption in renal tubules. |
| red powder, exists as tetrahydrate | s. $H_2O$ | Inhibits $Ca^{2+}$ transport into mitochondria 50% at 4 nmoles/mg protein. Inhibition is non-competitive in contrast to compet. inhibition by $La^{3+}$, (*Curr. Topics in Bioenergetics* **6**, 259 (1977)). Reacts with mucopolysaccharides and is used as stain, *J. Cell Biol.* **57**, 874 (1973). Another compound which reacts with mucopolysaccharides, hexamine cobaltichloride, also specifically inhibits $Ca^{2+}$ transport. Ruthenium red needs to be purified prior to use; prone to oxidation under mildly acid conditions; absorbs strongly to glass and quartz raising contamination problems between experiments. |
| | | Anion transport inhibitor, *JBC* **255**, 1113 (1980); non-penetrating membrane probe reacting with amino, sulphydryl and possibly imidazole groups. Removed by albumin wash, *J. Mem. Biol.* **10**, 311 (1972); **15**, 207 (1974). DIDS = 4,4'-diisothiocyano-2,2'-stilbenedisulphonate. |

# 13C Compounds affecting membrane function

| Name | Synonyms | Formula | M. wt. |
|------|----------|---------|--------|
| Tetrodotoxin | TTX | 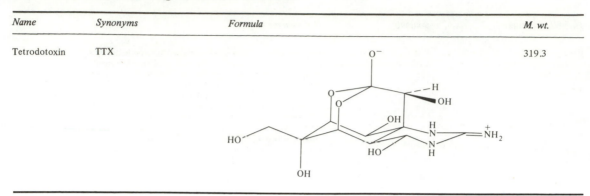 | 319.3 |

## Ionophores and related channel formers

### General references

The use of ionophores and channel formers in the study of the function of biological membranes, *Current Topics in Bioenergetics* **6**, 221 (1977).
Biological applications of ionophores, *ARB* **45**, 501 (1976).

| Name | Synonyms | Formula | M. wt. |
|------|----------|---------|--------|
| A 23187 | | 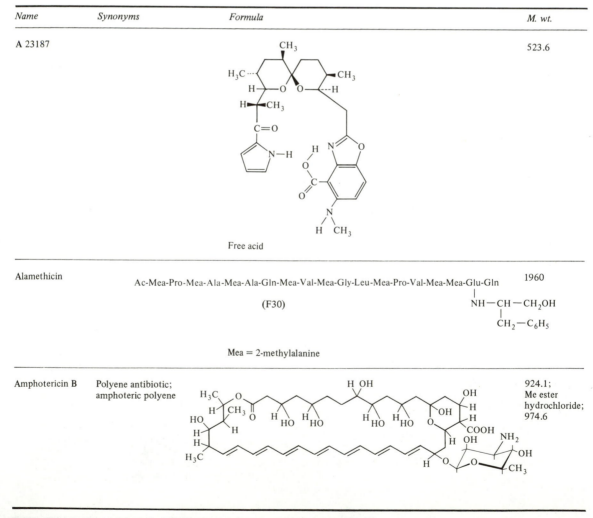 Free acid | 523.6 |
| Alamethicin | | Ac-Mea-Pro-Mea-Ala-Mea-Ala-Gln-Mea-Val-Mea-Gly-Leu-Mea-Pro-Val-Mea-Mea-Glu-Gln (F30) NH—CH—CH₂OH CH₂—C₆H₅ Mea = 2-methylalanine | 1960 |
| Amphotericin B | Polyene antibiotic; amphoteric polyene | | 924.1; Me ester hydrochloride; 974.6 |

296

| Physical properties | Solubility | General remarks |
|---|---|---|
| col. cryst.; darkens 220 °C without melting; $[\alpha]_D^{25} - 8.64$ (in dilute acetic acid); $pK_a$ 8.7 | sp. s. $H_2O$, eth., EtOH; s. dil. acetic acid | Neurotoxin inhibiting the action potential of nerve membranes at $10^{-9} - 10^{-7}$ M. It blocks the early transient inward flow of Na ions necessary for the initial depolarization of the nerve membrane. Occurs in certain fishes (e.g. puffer) and amphibia (e.g. newts). In puffer fishes it mainly occurs in liver and ovaries. Stable in solution when at pH 4–5 and 0 °C. Unstable in acid and alkaline solutions; rapidly destroyed by boiling at pH 2 and below. The weak base is converted into hemilactal on protonation. Extremely toxic. Handle with great care. $LD_{50}$ i.v. in mice: 8 $\mu g/kg$. |

| Physical properties | Solubility | General remarks |
|---|---|---|
| $\lambda_{max}$ (EtOH) 378, 278, 225, 204 nm $\epsilon$ 8200, 18 200, 26 200, 28 200; $pK_a$ 6.9 | s. EtOH ($> 200\,\mu M$); i. $H_2O$ | Ionophore; catalyses exchange of protons for $Ca^{2+}$ and $Mg^{2+}$ (relative affinities $Ca^{2+}:Mg^{2+} = 2.6:1$); used as $Ca^{2+}$ ionophore; high selectivity for divalent over monovalent cations. Review, *ARB* **45**, 501 (1976). In presence of EDTA depletes mitochondria of $Ca^{2+}$ and $Mg^{2+}$ in $<30$ s at 0.3 nmole/mg protein, *JBC* **247**, 6970 (1972). Potentially most useful of divalent ionophores since max. affinity is for physiological ions (cf. X537A (q.v.) with max. divalent affinity for Ba). |
| | Na salt; s. $H_2O$ | Channel forming antibiotic; catalyses exchanges of protons for monovalent cations with little difference in affinities ($H^+ > Cs^+ \cong Rb^+ \cong K^+ \cong Na^+ \cong Li^+$). Interaction of antibiotic with membrane voltage-dependent. Review, *Curr. Topics in Bioenergetics* **6**, 221 (1977). Previously thought to be cyclic molecule; alamethicin is mixture of several components; main ones $F_{30}$ (85%) and $F_{50}$ (12%); latter differs only in terminal Gln–COOH being $\alpha$-amidated. Structure: *BJ* **153**, 181 (1976); mechanism, *Ann. N.Y. Acad. Sci.*, **264**, 247 (1977). Suzukacillin is closely related peptide, *BBA* **433**, 164 (1976). |
| $\lambda_{max}$ (MeOH) 318.5, 304, 291, 230 nm $A_{1cm}^{1\%}$ 800, 870, 580, 300 (values depend on conc., mode of solution, age of stock soln. in DMSO, vigour of mixing aq. soln). | v. sl. s. $H_2O$ at pH 7; sl. s. DMF (2–4 mg/ml), DMSO (30–40 mg/ml); s. pH 2 and 11. Me ester HCl: s. $H_2O$ ($> 75$ mg/ml). | Induces loss of small M.wt. substances from cells with low selectivity; probably forms channels by complexing with membrane cholesterol; mitochondria not affected; lyses red blood cells; effective at low concs. ($10^{-6}$ M). Candidin, nystatin, and fungichromin have similar activities. Review, *Adv. Lip. Res.* **14**, 127 (1976). Stock solns. made in DMSO or DMF; may be diluted in $H_2O$ giving concs. of 50–100 $\mu g/ml$. Stock solns. stable if light and $O_2$ carefully excluded. Methyl ester HCl has full antifungal activity of parent antibiotic and is water soluble. Methyl ester aspartate commonly available, also water soluble. Ester hydrochlorides of other zwitterionic polyenes also retain full activity, *J. Antibiotics* **25**, 256, 259, 261 (1972). No effect on prokaryotic cells. |

## 13C Compounds affecting membrane function

| Name | Synonyms | Formula | M. wt. |
|------|----------|---------|--------|

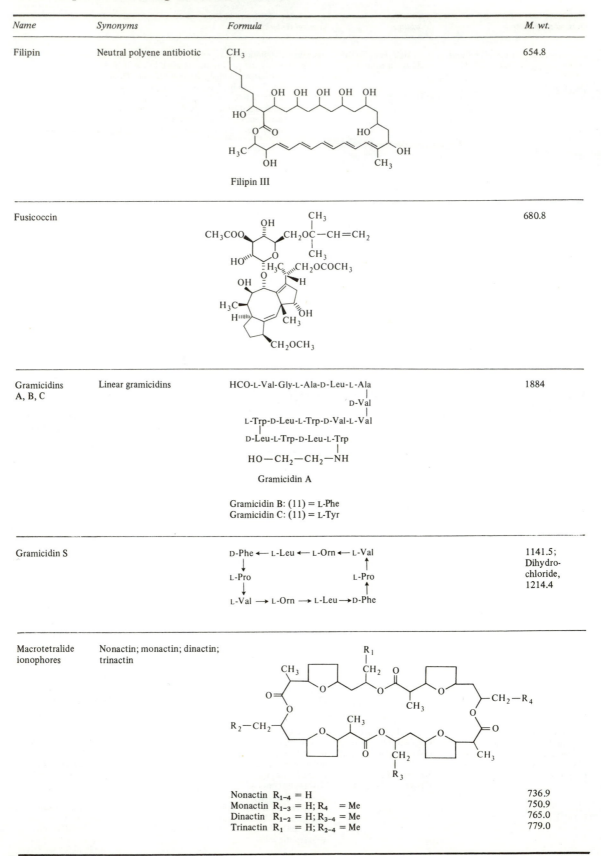

**Filipin** — Neutral polyene antibiotic — Filipin III — 654.8

**Fusicoccin** — 680.8

**Gramicidins A, B, C** — Linear gramicidins

HCO-L-Val-Gly-L-Ala-D-Leu-L-Ala
|
D-Val
|
L-Trp-D-Leu-L-Trp-D-Val-L-Val
D-Leu-L-Trp-D-Leu-L-Trp
|
HO—CH$_2$—CH$_2$—NH

Gramicidin A

Gramicidin B: (11) = L-Phe
Gramicidin C: (11) = L-Tyr

1884

**Gramicidin S**

D-Phe ← L-Leu ← L-Orn ← L-Val
↓                  ↑
L-Pro            L-Pro
↓                  ↑
L-Val → L-Orn → L-Leu → D-Phe

1141.5; Dihydrochloride, 1214.4

**Macrotetralide ionophores** — Nonactin; monactin; dinactin; trinactin

Nonactin R$_{1-4}$ = H — 736.9
Monactin R$_{1-3}$ = H; R$_4$ = Me — 750.9
Dinactin R$_{1-2}$ = H; R$_{3-4}$ = Me — 765.0
Trinactin R$_1$ = H; R$_{2-4}$ = Me — 779.0

| Physical properties | Solubility | General remarks |
|---|---|---|
| $\lambda_{max}$ (MeOH) 355, 338, 322 nm<br>$A_{1cm}^{1\%}$ 1330, 1360, 910 | v.s. DMF; s. 95% EtOH, MeOH; almost i. $H_2O$ | Filipins II, III and IV have 8, 9 and 9-OH groups respectively. Filipin III is isomeric with filipin IV. Filipin I is a mixture of components. For action, properties and refs. *see* Amphotericin B entry. |
| | | Phytotoxic compd. Isolated from *Fusicoccum amygdali* Del., fungus causing canker of peach and almond trees. Used at $10^{-5}-10^{-7}$ M. Binds to plant cell membranes, enhances energy-linked net $H^+$ efflux, $K^+$ influx, and cell membrane potential. No effect on passive transport of solutes, nor electric conductance (basal or valinomycin-activated) in artificial phospholipid membranes, *Plant Sci. Lett.* **10**, 75 (1977). Review, *Ann. Rev. Plant Physiol.* **30**, 273 (1979). |
| | | Channel forming antibiotics, rendering membranes permeable to protons and alkali metal cations; haemolyse red blood cells at 0.5–1 $\mu$g/ml; cause $K^+-H^+$ exchange in mitochondria. Not voltage dependent (cf. alamethecin q.v.): action and structure probably unrelated to gramicidin S (q.v.).<br>Occurs as mixture of A (85%), B, and C. Review, *EJB* **94**, 321 (1979). |
| | s. EtOH; i. $H_2O$ | Uncouples oxid. phosphorylation in mitochondria, 50% at 0.01 $\mu$M. Structure and action resembles tyrocidins (q.v.) rather than linear gramicidins A, B, and C (q.v.). |
| | s. EtOH; i. $H_2O$ | Neutral ionophores, selectively transport $K^+$ in presence of other alkali metal cations at equal concs. Selectivity pattern: $NH_4^+ > K^+ > Rb^+ > Cs^+ > Na^+ > Li^+$. Uncouple oxidative phosphorylation at $10^{-7}$M. Review, *ARB* **45**, 501 (1976); *Curr. Topics in Bioenergetics* **6**, 221 (1977). |

# 13C Compounds affecting membrane function

| Name | Synonyms | Formula | M. wt. |
|------|----------|---------|--------|

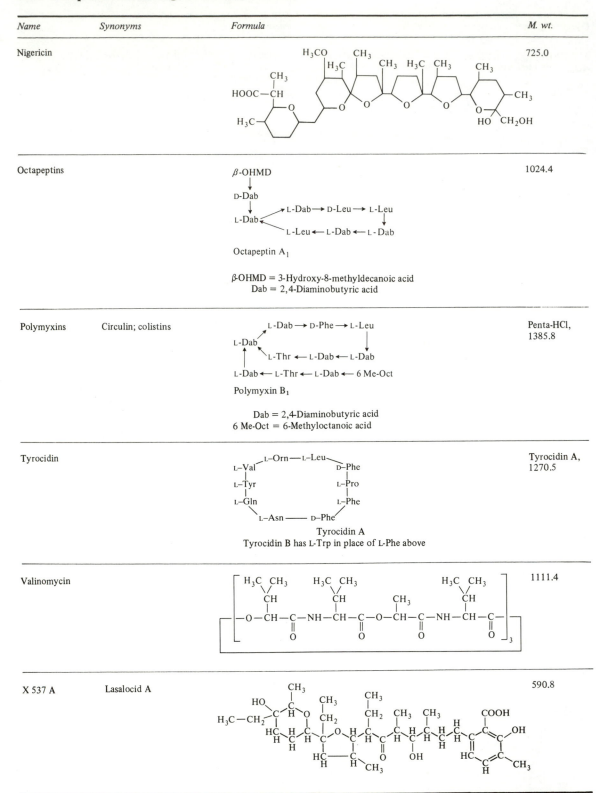

**Nigericin** — 725.0

**Octapeptins** — 1024.4

β-OHMD
↓
D-Dab
↓
L-Dab ← → L-Dab → D-Leu → L-Leu
        ↓
        L-Leu ← L-Dab ← L-Dab

Octapeptin A₁

β-OHMD = 3-Hydroxy-8-methyldecanoic acid
Dab = 2,4-Diaminobutyric acid

**Polymyxins** — Circulin; colistins — Penta-HCl, 1385.8

L-Dab → D-Phe → L-Leu
L-Dab
  ↑   L-Thr ← L-Dab ← L-Dab
L-Dab ← L-Thr ← L-Dab ← 6 Me-Oct

Polymyxin B₁

Dab = 2,4-Diaminobutyric acid
6 Me-Oct = 6-Methyloctanoic acid

**Tyrocidin** — Tyrocidin A, 1270.5

L–Orn — L–Leu
L–Val            D–Phe
L–Tyr            L–Pro
L–Gln            L–Phe
  L–Asn — D–Phe

Tyrocidin A
Tyrocidin B has L-Trp in place of L-Phe above

**Valinomycin** — 1111.4

**X 537 A** — Lasalocid A — 590.8

| Physical properties | Solubility | General Remarks |
|---|---|---|
| p$K_a$ 8.45 | s. EtOH; i. $H_2O$ | Carboxylic ionophore; catalyses exchange of $K^+$ for $H^+$. Selectivity pattern $K^+ > Rb^+ > Na^+ > Cs^+ \gg Li^+$. Effects on mitochondria at $10^{-7}$ M. Review, *Curr. Topics in Bioenergetics* **6**, 221 (1977), *Fed. Proc.* **32**, 1698 (1973). Monensin and dianemycin are related open chain macrotetralides with differing ion affinities. |
| | | Family of 7 octapeptides varying in acyl group and in residues 6 and 7. Disrupt normal membrane permeability to small molecules. Octapeptin mixture is 3–10-fold more effective against gram-positive bacteria than is polymyxin (q.v.). Review, *ARB* **46**, 723 (1977). |
| | HCl: v.s. $H_2O$, MeOH. Free base: sl. s. $H_2O$; v. sl. s. EtOH; i. organic solvents | Family of 7 decapeptides varying in amino acid composition, all with 5 or 6 Dab residues; acyl group 6 Me-Oct or 6-Me-heptanoic acid; inhibit growth of microorganisms (*E. coli* at 2 µg/ml); gram-negative generally more sensitive than gram-positive. Polymyxins combine with cell membrane and disrupt normal permeability to small molecules. Polymyxin B (sulphate) is a mixture of $B_1$ and $B_2$; also known as aerosporin. Polymyxins $E_1$ and $E_2$ also called colistin A and B resp. See also octapeptin entry. Review, *ARB* **46**, 723 (1977). |
| Hydrochloride of tyrocidin complex obtained as fine needles from MeOH or EtOH + HCl; Complex hydrochloride, M.p. 240 d. | Complex hydrochloride, s. 95% EtOH, gl. acetic, pyr.; sl. s. $H_2O$, acet., EtOH; i. eth., hydrocarbons, $CHCl_3$ | Surface active agent. Effective against gram + ve and gram − ve bacteria. 'Tyrocidin' is a family of basic homeomeric peptides, certain of which are cyclic, related to each other and characterized by the possession of ornithine. Three major components have been separated, A, B, and C; A has been studied in the most detail. Disorganizes cell membrane permeability. Gramicidin S is closely related. |
| cryst. | s. $CHCl_3$, acet.; v. sl. s. $H_2O$ | Neutral ionophore; acts effectively as relatively specific $K^+$ ionophore; selectivity pattern $Rb^+ > K^+ > Cs^+ > NH_4^+ > Na^+ \cong Li^+$ (stability of $K^+$ complex is $10^3$–$10^4$ fold higher than $Na^+$ complex). Induces $K^+$ conductivity in cell membranes at concentrations down to $10^{-8}$ M. Review, *EJB* **94**, 321 (1979). |
| p$K_a$ 5.8; $\lambda_{max}$ (50% *iso*PrOH: $H_2O$) 248, 318 nm $\epsilon$ 6750, 4200 | i. $H_2O$; s. organic solvents | Carboxylic ionophore of broad complexing spectrum. Catalyses exchange of divalent or monovalent cations for protons. Monovalent cations transported 10 times more effectively than divalent cations in bulk phases in conc. dependent process. Transports catecholamines. Review, *ARB* **45**, 501 (1976); *Fed. Proc.* **32**, 1698 (1973). A 23187 (q.v.) more specific for $Ca^{2+}$ and $Mg^{2+}$. |

## D. INHIBITORS OF MITOCHONDRIAL AND CHLOROPLAST FUNCTION

### General references

J. L. Webb, *Enzyme and Metabolic Inhibitors*, 4 volumes, Academic Press, New York (1963).

R. M. Hochster and J. H. Quastel, eds., *Metabolic Inhibitors*, 2 volumes, Academic Press, New York (1963), vol. 3 (1972), vol. 4 (1973).

W. G. Hanstein, Uncoupling of oxidative phosphorylation, *BBA* **456**, 129 (1976).

S. Izawa, Inhibitors of electron transport, Ch. 16 in *Encyclopedia of plant physi-*

| Name | Synonyms | Formula | M. wt. |
|------|----------|---------|--------|
| 3-Amino-1*H*-1,2,4-triazole | Amitrole; Amizol | | 84.1 |
| Amytal, Na salt | Na 5-ethyl-5-isoamyl-barbiturate; amobarbital; Somnal | | 248.3 |
| Antimycin | | Antimycin A$_1$; R = *n*-hexyl <br> Antimycin A$_3$; R = *n*-butyl | A$_1$ 548.6 <br> A$_3$ 520.6 |
| Arsenic acid, Na salt | Sodium arsenate | $Na_2HAsO_4 \cdot 7H_2O$ | Hydrate, 312.0 |
| Arsenious acid | Arsenic trioxide; arsenolite | $As_2O_3 (As_2O_3 + 3H_2O \rightleftharpoons 2As(OH)_3)$ | 197.8 |
| ——, Na salt | Sodium meta-arsenite | $NaAsO_2$ | 129.9 |
| Atebrin hydro-chloride | Atabrine; mepacrine; quinacrine; SN390 | | Hydrate + 2H$_2$O, 508.9 |
| Atrazine | 2-Chloro-4-ethylamino-6-isopropylamine-*s*-triazine; Gesaprim | | 215.7 |

*ology* (N.S) vol. 5, *Photosynthesis I*, eds. A. Trebst and M. Avron, Springer-Verlag, Berlin (1977).

S. Izawa and N. E. Good, Inhibition of photosynthetic electron transport and photophosphorylation, Ch. 32 in *Meth. Enzymol.* 24, Photosynthesis and Nitrogen Fixation, Part B, ed. A. San Pietro, Academic Press, New York (1972).

Substances shown as inhibiting electron transport will consequently inhibit oxidative phosphorylation, photosynthesis, and photophosphorylation. Certain substances (e.g. dinitrophenol) which uncouple or inhibit phosphorylation, or inhibit the oxygen evolving step of photosynthesis, may have no effect on, or even stimulate electron transport.

| *Physical properties* | *Solubility* | *General remarks* |
|---|---|---|
| col. cryst. from EtOH; M.p. 159 | $28^{23}$ $H_2O$; s. EtOH, MeOH, $CHCl_3$; i. eth., acet. | Irreversible inhibitor of catalase in presence of $H_2O_2$ at $2 \times 10^{-2}$ M; no action on peroxidase. Inhibits $\delta$-aminolaevulinate synthetase, cyclization reactions leading to $\beta$-carotene ($\delta$-carotene accumulates). At $10^{-4}$ M causes chlorosis, disorganization of chloroplast membranes; blocks 18S Fraction I protein and chloroplast DNA formation; blocks formation of 70S ribosomes. Inhibits riboflavin biogenesis. Commercial grade, used as herbicide and cotton defoliant; generally contains catalase anti-inhibitory impurity. |
| wh. hygr. powder | v.s. $H_2O$; v. sl. s. eth. | Inhibits $NADH_2$ oxidizing enzymes and some other flavoproteins at $10^{-3}$ M, and succinic dehydrogenase at $10^{-2}$ M. Acts at same site as rotenone and piericidin A (q.v.), but much higher conc. needed compared with latter two agents. Not specific. Review, *Adv. Enzymol.* 34, 79 (1971). May also inhibit energy transfer reactions at NAD-flavoprotein phosphorylation site. |
| col. cryst. | ($A_1$), v.s. acet., eth., EtOH; almost i. $H_2O$. ($A_3$), v.s. acet., $CHCl_3$; s. EtOH, MeOH; almost i. $H_2O$ | Inhibits mitochondrial electron transport specifically between cytochromes $b$ and $c$, 50% inhibition at approx. 0.5 $\mu$M. Antimycin has 4 components, all apparently with same activity. |
| col. monocl. cryst.; M.p. 120–30; $pK_a$ 2.25, 6.77, 11.53 | s. $H_2O$; sl. s. EtOH | Uncouples substrate level and oxidative phosphorylation at $10^{-2}$ M; uncoupling increases with time and is not complete. Phosphorolysis replaced by arsenolysis. |
| wh. powder; sublimes 193; $pK_a$ 9.22 | s. acids, alkalis; sl. s. $H_2O$ ($2^{25}$, $11.5^{100}$); sl. s. EtOH, eth. | Inhibits dehydrogenases containing dithiols, e.g. $\alpha$-ketoglutaric dehydrogenase, at $10^{-4}$ M. Also uncouples oxidative phosphorylation. Dissolve in alkali to prepare arsenite solution. Weedicide, pesticide. |
| wh. hygr. powder | s. $H_2O$; sl. s. EtOH | Commercial salt not satisfactory; *see above*. |
| yel. needles; M.p. 248d.; $pK_a$ 7.7, 10.3. | HCl, s. $H_2O$, MeOH, EtOH; i. eth., acet. Base, sl. s. $H_2O$ | Intercalates with DNA. Inhibits some flavoprotein enzymes at $10^{-4}$ M. Uncouples oxidative and photophosphorylation at $10^{-3}$ M. Inhibits ATPase. Antimalarial. |
| solid; M.p. 171–4 (173–5); stable in sl. acidic or basic media | $0.007^{25}$ $H_2O$; 1.2 eth.; $1.8^{27}$ MeOH | Selective herbicide for control of broad leaf and grassy weeds. Corn rapidly detoxifies, by conjugation with glutathione; *Rec. Adv. Phytochem.* 5, 239 (1972). Inhibits photosynthesis (50% at $5 \times 10^{-7}$ M) on the reducing side of PS II, at same sites as phenylureas and HOQNO, probably between Q and cyt. $b_{559}$. Low concs. (1 $\mu$M) increase nitrate reductase, *Phytochem.* 17, 1021 (1978). $LD_{50}$ orally in rats: 3 g/kg. Formulations usually contain simazin, 2-chloro-4,6-bis(ethylamine)-s-triazine, M. wt. 201.7. Simazin, prac. i. $H_2O$ ($\sim 3 \times 10^{-5}$ M). Atrazine is $\sim$10x more soluble. |

## 13D Inhibitors of Mitochondrial and Chloroplast Function

| Name | Synonyms | Formula | M. wt. |
|------|----------|---------|--------|
| Aurovertin B | | | 460.5 |
| Carbon monoxide | | CO | 28.0 |
| CCP | Carbonylcyanide phenyl-hydrazone; phenylhydrazone malononitrile | | 170.1 |
| CCCP | Carbonylcyanide *m*-chlorophenylhydrazone | 3–Cl–CCP | 204.6 |
| 3-(*p*-Chloro-phenyl)-1,1-dimethylurea | CMU; Monuron | Cl—⟨ ⟩—NH·CO·N(CH₃)₂ | 198.7 |
| Chlorpromazine | Largactil | | Hydrochloride, 355.3; Free base, 318.9 |
| CIPC | Chloro-IPC; isopropyl-*N*-(3-chlorophenyl)carbamate; Chlorpropham | | 213.7 |
| DBMIB | 2,5-Dibromo-3-methyl-6-isopropyl-*p*-benzoquinone; dibromothymoquinone | | 322.0 |
| DCCD | *N*,*N*'-Dicyclohexylcarbodi-imide | | 206.3 |
| 3-(3,4-Dichloro-phenyl)-1,1-dimethylurea | DCMU; Diuron | | 233.1 |

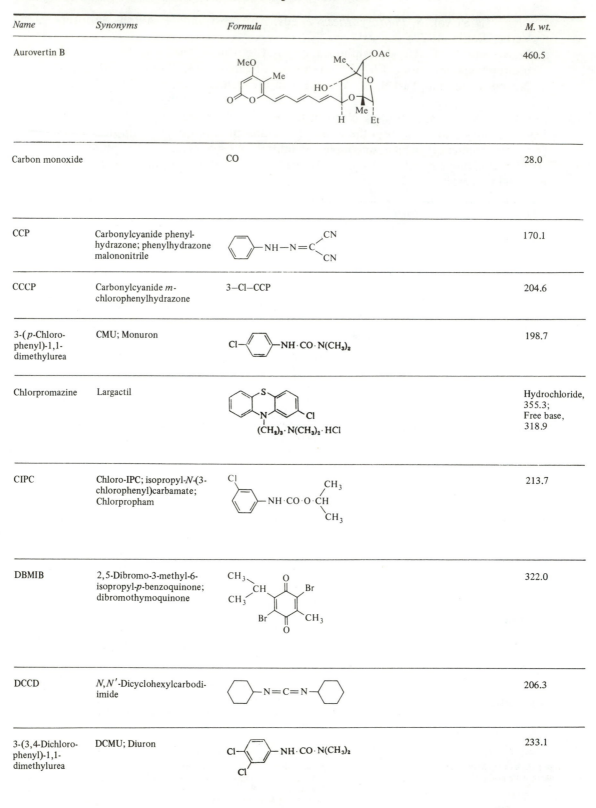

| Physical properties | Solubility | General remarks |
|---|---|---|
| pale yel. cryst. | s. EtOH; i. $H_2O$ | Binds to mitochondrial ATPase, preventing phosphoryl group transfer and thereby oxidative phosphorylation; effective on isolated enzyme. *Not* as potent a mitochondrial inhibitor as oligomycin (q.v.), *Biochem.* **3**, 1961 (1964); *Fed. Proc.* **34**, 1707 (1975); *Adv. Enzymol.* **49**, 223 (1979). For determination of conc. in stock EtOH solutions, see *BBA* **462**, 422 (1977) (value for abs. at 367.5 nm reported at 28.5 mM$^{-1}$ cm$^{-1}$). Structure, *JCS Chem Comm.* 874 (1974). Aurovertin D differs from B only in replacement of sec. alcohol hydroxyl by H. |
| col. gas; B.p. −190 | s. benz., $Cu_2Cl_2$ soln.; sl. s. $H_2O$ ($\alpha = 0.02$ at 20 °) | Inhibits wide range of metalloenzymes, including hydrogenase and haemoglobins, at low concs., and cytochrome oxidase at 50–95% (in gas phase). Light-reversible CO inhibition is characteristic of cytochrome oxidase and other haem proteins. $Cu^+$ and other metal carbonyls not light-sensitive. CAUTION: CO is respired by many tissues and micro-organisms. |
| $pK_a$ 6.55 | s. EtOH, MeOH; sp. s. $H_2O$ ($< 10^{-4}$ M) | Uncouples oxidative phosphorylation (50% at 0.4 $\mu$M), and photophosphorylation. |
| M.p. 175-7d.; $pK_a$ 6.0 | | 50% uncoupling at 0.06 $\mu$M (mitochondria); $10^{-6}$ M–$10^{-5}$ M (max. effect) in chloroplasts. Higher conc. strongly inhibitory to electron transport. |
| wh. prisms from MeOH; M.p. 171 (176) | $5^{27}$ EtOH; s. MeOH, acet.; $0.023^{25}$ $H_2O$ | Inhibits $O_2$ evolution step of photosynthesis at $10^{-6}$–$10^{-7}$ M. Herbicide, sugar cane flowering suppressant. $LD_{50}$ orally in rats: 3.6 g/kg. See DCMU. |
| wh. cryst.; M.p. 179−80d. | v.s. $H_2O$; s. MeOH, EtOH; i. eth. | Uncouples and inhibits oxidative phosphorylation at $10^{-3}$–$10^{-4}$ M, *BJ* **72**, 204; **73**, 16 (1959). Sedative, *see* p. 340. Interaction of phenothiazine antipsychotics with calmodulin, *Biochem. Pharmacol.* **31**, 2217 (1982); see also B.D. Roufogalis, Specificity of trifluoperazine and related phenothiazines for calcium-binding proteins, in *Calcium and cell function*, vol. 3, (ed. W. Y. Cheung), Academic Press, New York (1982). |
| wh. solid; M.p. 41−4 (38−40); Decomp. 150 | $0.01^{25}$ $H_2O$; s. eth. | Inhibitor of photosynthesis on the reducing side of PS II; similar action to phenylureas (q.v.). Mitotic poison with an effect like colchicine, *Plant and Cell Physiol.* **8**, 613 (1967). Used as a potato sprout suppressant and, at higher conc., a herbicide. Other phenylurethanes so used are IPC (isopropyl-*N*-phenylcarbamate), barban [4-chloro-2-butyryl-*N*-(3-chlorophenyl)carbamate], BCPC [*sec*-butyl-*N*-(3-chlorophenyl)carbamate]. $LD_{50}$ (CIPC) orally in rats: 5−7.5 g/kg. |
| | | Specific inhibitor (50% at $2–3 \times 10^{-7}$ M) of plastoquinol oxidation, blocking electron flow from PS II to PS I. No inhibition of reduction of indophenol or ferricyanide through PS II. No inhibition of cyclic photophosphorylation through phenazine methosulphate. DBMIB inhibition reversed by adding plastoquinone. Inhibits oxidation of ubiquinol; reversed by addition of more ubiquinone. Inhibits succinate and NADH oxidation in mitochondria. Prevents cyt. $b_{522}$ reduction. No effect on cyt. $c_1$ or $c$ or $aa_3$, *ARB* **46**, 439 (1977). |
| M.p. 34−5 | s. EtOH, $CH_2Cl_2$ | Inhibitor of membrane-bound ATP-ase, *BBA* **233**, 521 (1971); **241**, 334 (1971). Peptide condensing agent. Reagent for spectrophotometric determination of carboxylic acids, *Anal. Chem.* **47**, 34 (1975). Irritant. |
| wh. cryst.; M.p. 158−9; Decomp. 180−90 | v. sl. s. $H_2O$ (42 ppm); v. sl. s. hydrocarbon solvents; 5.3 acet. | Potent and specific inhibitor of Hill reaction; 50% inhibition of electron transport in isolated chloroplasts by $5 \times 10^{-8}$–$10^{-7}$ M; intact algal cells need 10× conc. Inhibition (completely reversible) most pronounced at rate-determining (low) light intensities. Inhibition site closely associated with electron acceptor Q. At higher conc. ($> 10^{-4}$ M) secondary effect − inhibition of PS I-independent cyclic photophosphorylation (probably through an uncoupling action). Many structurally related compds. such as chlorophenyl-carbamates (CIPC, q.v.) and acylchloroanilides [*Plant Physiol.* **36**, 788 (1961)] potent inhibitors at same site. Herbicide. Detoxification by *N*-demethylation, *Rec. Adv. Phytochem.* **5**, 225 (1972). |

| Name | Synonyms | Formula | M. wt. |
|---|---|---|---|
| Dicoumarol | Bishydroxy-coumarin; dicoumarin | 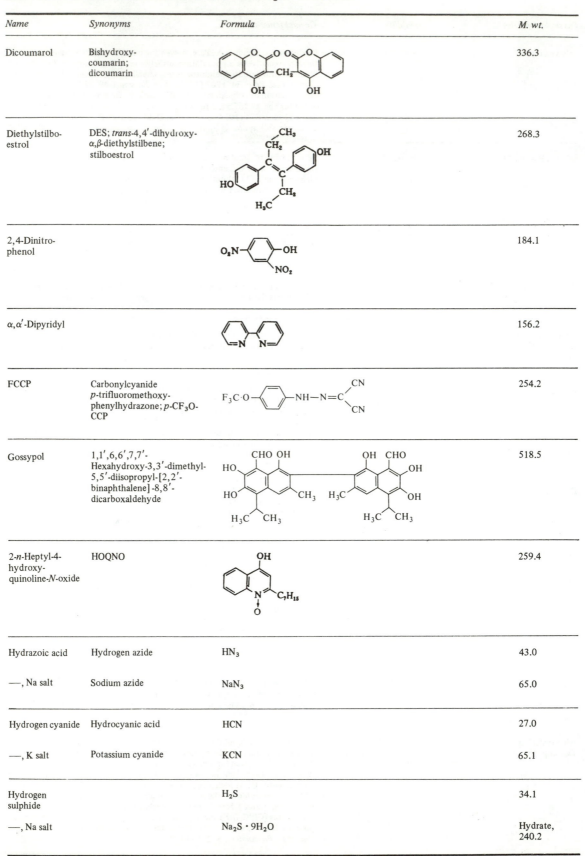 | 336.3 |
| Diethylstilbo-estrol | DES; *trans*-4,4'-dihydroxy-α,β-diethylstilbene; stilboestrol | | 268.3 |
| 2,4-Dinitro-phenol | | | 184.1 |
| α,α'-Dipyridyl | | | 156.2 |
| FCCP | Carbonylcyanide *p*-trifluoromethoxy-phenylhydrazone; *p*-CF$_3$O-CCP | | 254.2 |
| Gossypol | 1,1',6,6',7,7'-Hexahydroxy-3,3'-dimethyl-5,5'-diisopropyl-[2,2'-binaphthalene]-8,8'-dicarboxaldehyde | | 518.5 |
| 2-*n*-Heptyl-4-hydroxy-quinoline-*N*-oxide | HOQNO | | 259.4 |
| Hydrazoic acid | Hydrogen azide | HN$_3$ | 43.0 |
| —, Na salt | Sodium azide | NaN$_3$ | 65.0 |
| Hydrogen cyanide | Hydrocyanic acid | HCN | 27.0 |
| —, K salt | Potassium cyanide | KCN | 65.1 |
| Hydrogen sulphide | | H$_2$S | 34.1 |
| —, Na salt | | Na$_2$S · 9H$_2$O | Hydrate, 240.2 |

| Physical properties | Solubility | General remarks |
|---|---|---|
| wh. cryst.; M.p. 287—93 | s. alkalis; sl. s. $CHCl_3$; i. $H_2O$, EtOH, eth. | Uncouples oxidative phosphorylation at $2 \times 10^{-5}$ M; inhibits cellulose synthesis by blocking transfer of oligosaccharide from dolichol-P-P-oligosaccharide to a protein acceptor, *FEBS Lett.* **86**, 259 (1978); inhibits vit. K reductase. Medical use as anticoagulant. Acts by compet. interference with hepatic utilisation of vit. K in prothrombin synthesis. Other hepatic functions unaffected. |
| wh. cryst. powder; M.p. 169—72 | s. dil. aq. alkalis, acet., eth., $CHCl_3$, vegetable oils; i. $H_2O$ | Uncouples oxidative phosphorylation, *ABB* **117**, 573 (1966). Inhibits Na K-ATPase, *Metabolic Inhibitors*, vol. III. Inhibits plasma membrane ATPase in plants, *Plant Sci. Lett.* **10**, 319 (1977). Synthetic oestrogen. Used in replacement therapy. Not stored in fat. Readily absorbed G.I.T. About 20% excreted in urine (conjugated). |
| yel. plates; M.p. 111; $pK_a$ 4.1 | s. benz.; sl. s. EtOH, eth.; $0.56^{18}$ $H_2O$ | Uncouples oxidative phosphorylation at $10^{-5}$—$10^{-4}$ M by mediating proton conductance across inner mitochondrial membrane; stimulates mitochondrial ATPase. Even at $10^{-3}$ M only slight uncoupling of chloroplasts at pH 6. Does not uncouple substrate-level phosphorylation. Comparison of 28 phenols as uncouplers, *EJB* **21**, 565 (1971). |
| M.p. 70 | v.s. EtOH, eth., $CHCl_3$; sl. s. $H_2O$. | May inhibit $Fe^{2+}$ enzymes at $10^{-8}$ M. *See also* data in Chelating Agents (p. 402). |
| M.p. 173; $pK_a$ 5.8; stable at 4 °C | s. EtOH, MeOH; sp. s. $H_2O$ ($<10^{-4}$ M) | 50% uncoupling given by 0.04 μM. At site II and site III, 1 mole FCCP bound, at site I, 14 moles bound. Increases electrical conductivity of model phospholipid membranes. Inactivated *in vitro* by vicinal aminothiols (e.g. cysteamine or free cysteine) and dithiols (dimercaprol). |
| yel. pigment | s. MeOH, EtOH, eth., $CHCl_3$; v. sl. s. pet. eth.; i. $H_2O$. Freely sol. (with slow decomp.) in dil. aq. soln. $NH_3$ and $Na_2CO_3$ | Toxic to non-ruminant animals. $LD_{50}$ orally in rats: 2.6g/kg. Developed as male contraceptive. Uncouples beef heart mitochondria 50% at $2 \times 10^{-5}$ M. 100% inhibition succinoxidase (soy-bean) at $2.5 \times 10^{-4}$ M; succinic dehydrogenase at $7.5 \times 10^{-3}$ M; cytochrome oxidase at $2 \times 10^{-3}$ M, *Plant Physiol.* **41**, 787 (1966); **43**, 1996 (1968). |
| wh. cryst. from EtOH; M.p. 158—60; $\epsilon_{253}$ ($10^{-3}$ M-NaOH) 24000; $\epsilon_{346}$ ($10^{-3}$ M-NaOH) 9500 | s. EtOH; v. sl. s. $H_2O$. Make stock soln. in 0.01M-NaOH, 50 μg/ml.; sol. in $H_2O$ $10^{-5}$ M at pH 7, $2.5 \times 10^{-4}$ M at pH 9 | Inhibits cytochrome systems at or near cytochrome *b*, at $10^{-5}$—$10^{-8}$ M. In chloroplasts $10^{-5}$ M inhibits electron transport 50%; action similar to DCMU. Active against some bacterial systems not inhibited by antimycin. |
| col. liq.; $pK_a$ 4.72<br><br>col. cryst. | Free acid, ∞ $H_2O$; s. EtOH<br><br>Salt, s. $H_2O$; i. eth. | Inhibits catalase, Fe enzymes at $10^{-3}$ M; uncouples phosphorylation at $10^{-4}$ M; inhibits $O_2$ evolution in photosynthesis. Not effective at alkaline pH. (Use HCN or $H_2S$ at alkaline pH.) |
| col. liq. or gas; M.p. —14; B.p. 26; $pK_a$ 9.14<br><br>col. deliq. cryst. | Free acid, ∞ $H_2O$, EtOH; sl. s. eth.<br><br>Salt, v.s. $H_2O$; s. EtOH | Inhibits by complexing with metals in metallo-enzymes, e.g. cytochrome oxidase, at $10^{-3}$—$10^{-5}$ M; or by forming cyanhydrins with carbonyl groups. Check metal inhibition activity with azide, CO or hydrogen sulphide. High concs. cyanide may be respired. Active form is undissoc. acid. |
| col. gas; B.p. —62; $pK_a$ 7.04, 14.9<br><br>col. deliq. cryst. | Gas, s. $CS_2$; sl. s. $H_2O$<br><br>Na salt, s. $H_2O$; i. eth. | Inhibits metallo-enzymes at $10^{-3}$ M. Not a carbonyl reagent. Sulphide is respired by some tissues and microorganisms. |

## 13D Inhibitors of Mitochondrial and Chloroplast Function

| Name | Synonyms | Formula | M. wt. |
|---|---|---|---|
| Hydroxamic acids | | | |
| —, mCLAM | m-Chlorobenzhydroxamic acid | R = | 171.6 |
| —, mIBM | m-Iodobenzhydroxamic acid | R = | 263.0 |
| —, SHAM | Salicylhydroxamic acid; N,2-dihydroxybenzamide | R = | 153.1 |
| Hydroxylamine hydrochloride | Hydroxyammonium chloride | $NH_2OH \cdot HCl$ | 69.5 |
| 2-n-Nonyl-4-hydroxy-quinoline-N-oxide | NOQNO | | 287.4 |
| Oleic acid | | $CH_3 \cdot (CH_2)_7 \cdot CH=CH \cdot (CH_2)_7 \cdot COOH$ | 282.5 |
| Oligomycin B | | | 805.1 |
| Pentachloro-phenol | PCP | | 266.4 |
| Pentenylguani-dine sulphate | Galegine sulphate; 4-methyl-3-butenyl-guanidine sulphate | $(NH_2)_2 \cdot C:N \cdot CH_2 \cdot CH=C(CH_3)_2 \cdot H_2SO_4$ | 225.3 |
| 1,10-Phenan-throline | o-Phenanthroline | | Hydrate + 1H_2O, 198.2 |

| Physical properties | Solubility | General remarks |
|---|---|---|
| | | Specific inhibitors for CN-insensitive pathway, *Plant Physiol*. **47**, 124 (1971) (50% inhibition at 0.03 mM (*m*CLAM), 0.02 mM (*m*IBM), and 0.06 mM (SHAM) in mung bean mitochondria); also inhibit peroxidase, *JBC* **248**, 502 (1973), tyrosinase, *Plant Physiol*. **59**, 60P (1977) and lipoxygenase, *Plant Physiol*. **62**, 470 (1978). |
| M.p. 177d. | | |
| col. cryst.; M.p. 151; p$K_a$ 6.2 | v.s. $H_2O$, EtOH; i. eth. | Inhibits catalase; also inhibits $O_2$ evolution in photosynthesis at $10^{-4}$ M. Also inhibits alcohol dehydrogenases and vitamin $B_6$ enzymes; carbonyl reagent forming oximes. |
| wh. cryst. from EtOH; M.p. 148–9 | s. EtOH; v. sl. s. $H_2O$. Make stock soln. in 0.001M-NaOH 5 $\mu$g/ml. | As HOQNO, although 3–10 times more active. In chloroplasts, $10^{-6}$ M inhibits electron transport 50%. Commercially available; less soluble than HOQNO ($\times \frac{1}{10}$). |
| col. needles; M.p. 14 | $\infty$ EtOH, eth.; s. benz.; i. $H_2O$ | Uncouples oxidative phosphorylation. Inhibits 2,4-dinitrophenol-stimulated ATPase. Active at 120 $\mu$moles/g protein. Action reversed by adding serum albumin. *See also* data in Lipids. |
| $\lambda_{max}$ (EtOH) 225 nm $\epsilon$ approx. 20 000 | 0.002 $H_2O$; s. EtOH | Inhibits mitochondrial ATPase ($F_1$) preventing phosphoryl group transfer; inhibits only membrane bound, not isolated, form. 50% inhibition at less than approx. 1 $\mu$g/mg protein. Inhibits $Na^+/K^+$ ATPase (*JBC* **243**, 1993 (1968)). Review. *Fed. Proc.* **34**, 1707 (1975). Rutamycin is 26-demethyl-28-deoxy-oligomycin B. |
| needle-like cryst.; M.p. 190–1; p$K_a$ 4.89 | 0.008 $H_2O$; s. EtOH, eth.; sl. s. cold pet. eth. | Uncouples at 2 $\mu$M at pH 6, *EJB* **21**, 565 (1971). At $10^{-5}$ M strong electron transport inhibitor. $LD_{50}$ orally in rats: 0.2 g/kg. Used as pre-harvest defoliant, general herbicide. |
| col. cryst. | s. EtOH; sl. s. $H_2O$ | Inhibits oxidative phosphorylation at the site between NAD and cytochrome *b*. Inhibitory action of related alkyl guanidines increases with chain length of the alkyl group. |
| wh. cryst. powder; M.p. 93–4, Anhyd. M.p. 117; p$K_a$ 4.96 | s. EtOH, eth.; sl. s. $H_2O$, benz. | Inhibits $O_2$ evolution in photosynthesis (50% at $10^{-5}$ M), possibly by Zn or Mn chelation; inhibits some Fe enzymes at $10^{-8}$ M; inhibits glutamic dehydrogenase. Inhibits ubiquinol-cyt. *c* reductase only 28% at 0.5mM; inhibition not affected by uncouplers, *ARB* **46**, 452 (1977). *See also* data in Chelating Agents. |

## 13D  Inhibitors of Mitochondrial and Chloroplast Function

| Name | Synonyms | Formula | M. wt. |
|---|---|---|---|
| Phenylurethane | Phenylethyl carbamate; ethylcarbanilate | $C_6H_5 \cdot NH \cdot COO \cdot C_2H_5$ | 165.2 |
| Piericidin A | | | 400.6 |
| Quinine | | | 324.4 |
| Rotenone | | | 394.4 |
| SF 6847 | 3,5-Di-*tert*-butyl-4-hydroxybenzylidene malononitrile | | 282.4 |
| Thyroxine | | | 776.9 |
| Tributyltin chloride | | $[CH_3(CH_2)_3]_3\,Sn^+Cl^-$ | 325.5 |
| TTFB | 4,5,6,7-Tetrachloro-2-trifluoromethyl-benzimidazole | | 323.9 |

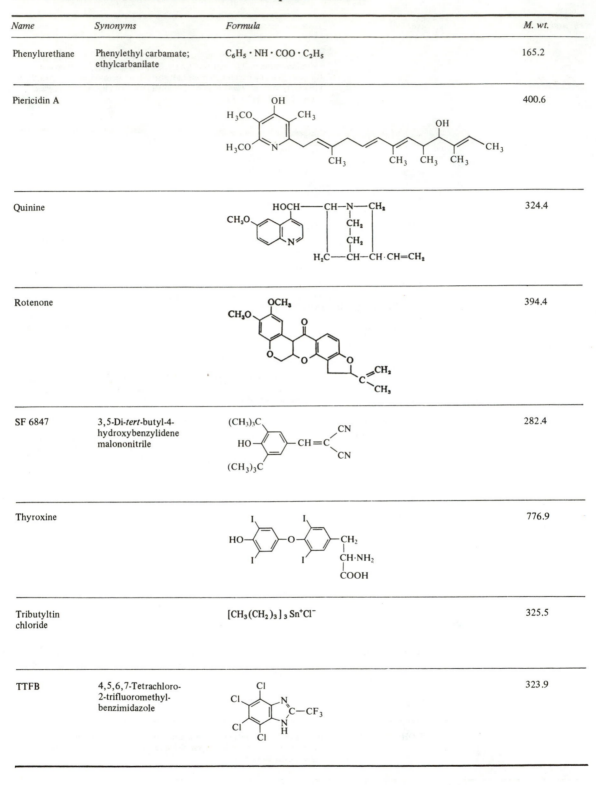

| Physical properties | Solubility | General remarks |
|---|---|---|
| wh. cryst.; M.p. 52–3 | s. EtOH, eth.; sl. s. H$_2$O | Inhibitor of O$_2$ evolution in photosynthesis, at $10^{-3}$–$10^{-4}$ M; *see* CIPC. |
|  | s. EtOH | Structural analogue of ubiquinone. Inhibits NAD-linked substrate oxidation by mitochondria at same site as rotenone (q.v.); 50% inhibition at about 10 pmol/mg protein. Insecticide. Action, *JBC* **243**, 834 (1968); Review, *Adv. Enzymol.* **34**, 79 (1971). |
| triboluminescent wh. needles from EtOH; M.p. 177d.; p$K_a$ 4.13, 8.3 | v.s. EtOH; sl. s. eth.; v. sl. s. H$_2$O. Hydrochloride, v.s. H$_2$O | Inhibits some flavoprotein enzymes at $10^{-3}$ M. Also inhibits choline esterases. Antimalarial. |
| col. plates; M.p. 165 | s. EtOH, acet., eth.; almost i. H$_2$O | Inhibits NAD-linked substrate oxidation by mitochondria at oxygen side of NADH dehydrogenase; 50% inhibition at about 10 pmol/mg protein. Insecticide from derris root. Decomposed by light and exposure to air; solutions in organic solvents oxidize with colour formation. Acts at same site as piericidin (q.v.). Action, *JBC* **243**, 834 (1968); Review, *Adv. Enzymol.* **34**, 79 (1971). |
|  |  | Uncouples at 0.03 $\mu$M (less than 0.2 molecules per respiratory chain), *BBA* **387**, 507 (1975). |
| wh. needles; M.p., DL-, 231-3 d.; L-, 235–6 d. | s. dil. alkali; i. H$_2$O, EtOH and org. solvents. | Uncouples mitochondrial oxidative phosphorylation at $5 \times 10^{-5}$ M. Requires preincubation with particles, may affect their structure. *See also* data in Amino Acids. |
| B.p. 171–3 (25 mm) |  | 50% uncoupling at 0.8 $\mu$M. Blocks respiration in some systems but gives maximum respiration and uncoupling in presence of NAD$^+$. Trialkylleads have similar properties. In chloroplasts, at $10^{-7}$ M, inhibits phosphorylating electron transport. ATPases not affected. |
| p$K_a$ 5.6 |  | 100% uncoupling at 0.03 $\mu$M in rat heart mitochondria, *BJ* **98**, 284 (1966). Inhibits chloroplast electron transport in area around PS II. |

# E. INHIBITORS OF STEROID SYNTHESIS AND FUNCTION

| Name | Synonyms | Formula | M. wt. |
|------|----------|---------|--------|
| Aminogluteth-imide | 2-(*p*-Aminophenyl)-2-ethyl-glutarimide | | 232.2 |
| Amphenone B | 3,3-Bis(*p*-aminophenyl)-butan-2-one | | 254.3 |
| Cyproterone | 6-Chloro-17-hydroxy-1α,2α-methylenepregna-4,6-diene-3,20-dione | | 374.9 |
| *o*,*p*′-DDD | 1,1-Dichloro-2-(*o*-chloro-phenyl)-2-(*p*-chlorophenyl)-ethane; mitotane | | 320.1 |
| 4-Hydroxyandr-ostene-3,17-dione | | | 302.4 |
| MER 25 | 1-[*p*-(2-Diethylamino-ethoxy)-phenyl]-1-phenyl-2-(*p*-methoxyphenyl)-ethanol; ethamoxytriphetol | | 419.6 |
| Metyrapone | Metopirone; 2,3-bis(3-pyridyl)-2-methylpropan-3-one; SU 4885 | | 226.3 |

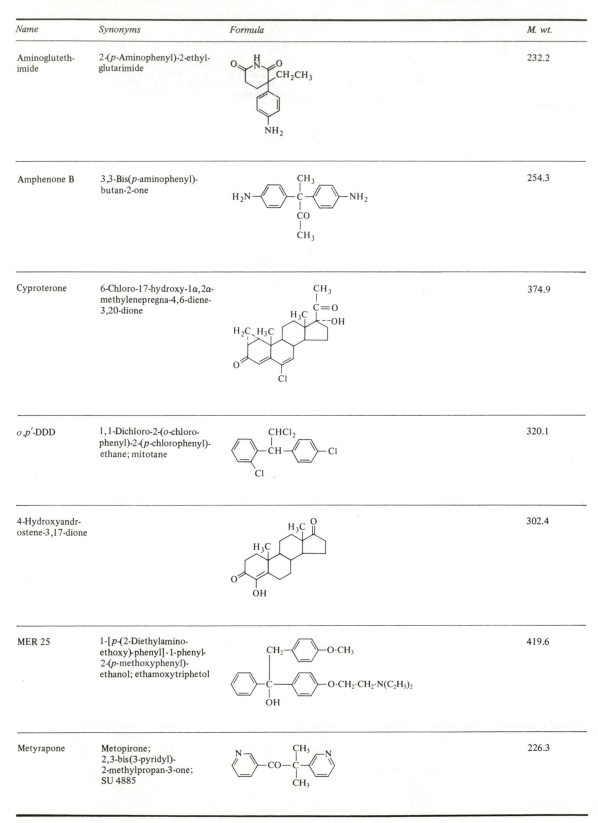

| Physical properties | Solubility | General remarks |
|---|---|---|
| cryst. from MeOH or Et acetate; M.p. 149–50 | Hydrochloride, s. $H_2O$ | Inhibits conversion of cholesterol to pregnenolone and other steroid hydroxylase activities (20, 21, 22, 19, 18, 11$\beta$). Clinically in limited use as inhibitor of corticoid secretion. |
| cryst.; M.p. 138 | Di-HCl, s. $H_2O$, EtOH | Inhibits hydroxylation reactions and so corticoid production by adrenal cortex. Many side reactions *in vivo*. |
| cryst. from Et acetate; M.p. 237.5–240; $\lambda_{max}$ 281 nm (log $\epsilon$ 4.24 in MeOH) | | Acetate, cryst. from diisopropyl ether, M.p. 200–1. Potent antiandrogen. |
| cryst. from pentane or MeOH; M.p. 76–78 | i. $H_2O$; s. EtOH, isooctane, $CCl_4$ | Inhibitor of adrenocortical function. |
| | i. $H_2O$; s. organic solvents | Aromatase inhibitor. Other effective aromatase inhibitors are androst-1,4,6-triene-3,17-dione-5$\alpha$-dihydrotestosterone, 7$\alpha$-$p$-aminothiophenylandrostenedione, testosterone acetate and 4-acetoxy-4-androstene-3,17-dione, *Biology of Reproduction* **18**, 365 (1978). |
| M.p. 104–6 | i. $H_2O$; s. EtOH, $CHCl_3$ | Strongly inhibits *in vivo* the action of steroid and non-steroid oestrogens. |
| cryst. from eth.-pentane; M.p. 50–1 | | Inhibits 11$\beta$-hydroxylation *in vivo* by adrenal cortex and so alters corticoid production. Many side effects on other endocrine glands. |

# 13E  Inhibitors of steroid synthesis and function

| Name | Synonyms | Formula | M. wt. |
|------|----------|---------|--------|
| RMI 12 936 | 17β-Hydroxy-7α-methylandrost-5-en-3-one | | 302.4 |
| Spironolactone | 17-Hydroxy-7-mercapto-3-oxo-17α-pregn-4-ene-21-carboxylic acid γ-lactone 7-acetate | | 416.6 |
| Tamoxifen | 1-(p-β-Dimethylaminoethoxy-phenyl)-trans-1,2-diphenylbut-1-ene; ICI 46 474 (citrate) | | 371.5 |
| Triparanol | MER 29; 1-[p-(2-diethyl-aminoethoxy)-phenyl]-1-(p-tolyl)-2-(p-chloro-phenyl)-ethanol | | 438.0 |

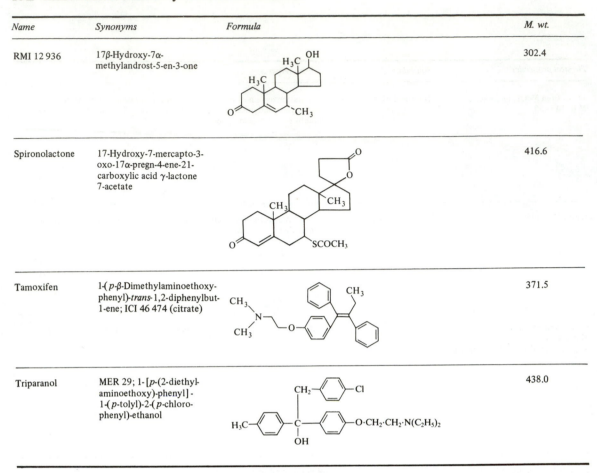

| Physical properties | Solubility | General remarks |
|---|---|---|
| | i. $H_2O$; s. organic solvents | Competitive inhibitor of $\Delta^5$, 3-oxo-steroid isomerase activity, *Acta Endocrinol.* **88**, 157 (1978). Other effective inhibitors include 6-dehydrotestosterone, cyanoketone and trilostane, *Steroids* **32**, 257 (1978). |
| cryst. from MeOH; M.p. 134–5; $\lambda_{max}$ 238 nm (log $\epsilon$ 4.30) | i. $H_2O$; s. organic solvents | Competitive antagonist to the action of aldosterone. Widely used as K-conserving diuretic and antihypertensive agent. |
| cryst.; M.p. 96–8 | | Antioestrogen of triphenylethylene type. Forms complex with oestrogen receptor which competes for nuclear acceptor sites, *Molec. Cell Endocr.* **7**, 177 (1977). |
| cryst.; M.p. 102–4 | | *In vivo* causes a block in cholesterol synthesis from mevalonate with an accumulation of desmosterol. |

# F. OTHER ENZYME INHIBITORS

This section includes some vitamin analogues with as yet undefined mechanism of action.

| Name | Synonyms | Formula | M. wt. |
|------|----------|---------|--------|
| Acetazolamide | 5-Acetamido-1,3,4-thiadiazole-2-sulphonamide; Diamox | | 222.3 |
| N-Acetylglucos-aminonolactone | 2-Acetamido-2-deoxy-gluconolactone | | 219.2 |
| Adenosine 5′-monosulphate, Ba salt | | | 830.0 |
| α-Amino-methoxyphenyl-methanesulphonic acid | 1-Amino-1-(p-methoxyphenyl)methane-sulphonic acid; AMPS | $CH_3 \cdot O$—⬡—$CH(NH_2) \cdot SO_3H$ | 217.2 |
| 2-Amino-2-methylpropanol | | | 89.1 |
| α-Amino-oxyacetic acid | O-(Carboxymethyl)-hydroxylamine | $H_2NOCH_2COOH$ | 91.1; Hydrochloride + $\frac{1}{2}$HCl, 109.3 |
| Aminophylline | (Theophylline)$_2$ ethylenediamine; 3,7-dihydro-1,3-dimethyl-1H-purine-2,6-dione compd. with 1,2-ethanediamine | $(\text{Theophylline})_2 \cdot C_2H_4(NH_2)_2$ | 420.4; Dihydrate, 456.5 |
| p-Amino-salicylic acid | PAS | | 153.1 |
| Antabuse | Tetraethylthiuram-disulphide | $(H_5C_2)_2 \cdot N \cdot \overset{\text{S}}{\overset{\|}{C}} \cdot S \cdot S \cdot \overset{\text{S}}{\overset{\|}{C}} \cdot N \cdot (C_2H_5)_2$ | 296.5 |

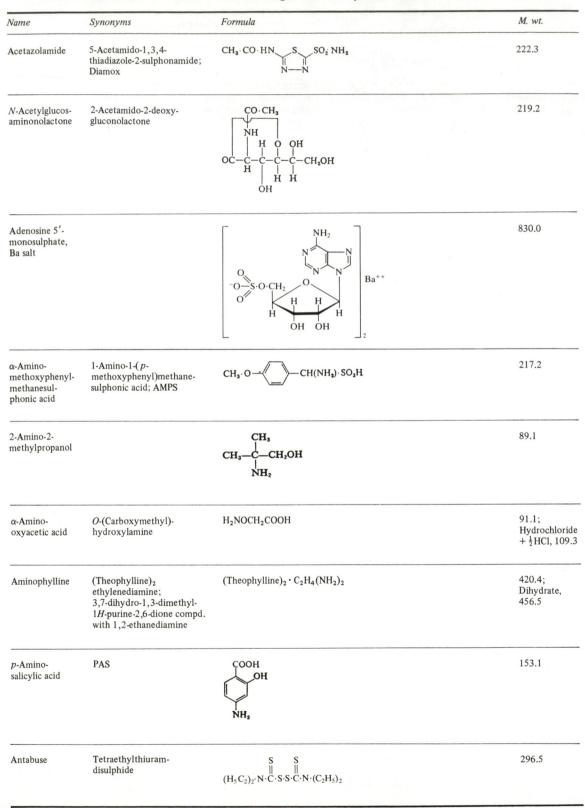

| Physical properties | Solubility | General remarks |
|---|---|---|
| wh. cryst. from $H_2O$; M.p. 258 d.; p$K_a$ 7.2; $\lambda_{max}$ 270 nm $\epsilon$ 7900 | sl. s. $H_2O$ | Non-competitively inhibits carbonic anhydrase at $10^{-8}$ M. Used as a diuretic. |
| wh. powder; v. deliq. | s. $H_2O$ | Competitively inhibits $\beta$-$N$-acetylglucosaminidase at $10^{-5}$ M. In general, aldonolactones competitively inhibit corresponding glycosidases, *BJ* **65**, 389 (1957); **82**, 225 (1962). |
| col. cryst. | s. $H_2O$ | Inhibits amino acid oxidase at $10^{-3}$ M by competing with adenylic acid moiety of FAD. |
|  |  | Inhibits uptake of influenza virus by chorioallantoic cells. |
| cryst. (or viscous oil); M.p. 30 | $\infty$ $H_2O$; s. EtOH | Choline antagonist in rats, as judged by kidney changes. Inhibits choline oxidase *in vitro*. |
| HCl: cryst.; M.p. 156 |  | General inhibitor of pyridoxal phosphate-dependent enzymes (amino acid transaminases and decarboxylases), *BJ* **171**, 771 (1978). At 0.5 mM inhibits anthocyanin production in plants, *Phytochem.* **18**, 585 (1979). |
| Dihydrate, wh. or sl. yel. granules or powder | 20 $H_2O$; i. EtOH, eth. | Methylxanthine, inhibits cAMP phosphodiesterase. See theophylline. Keep tightly closed; gradually absorbs $CO_2$ from air and becomes incompletely soluble due to formation of theophylline. Solutions may become turbid on standing. $LD_{50}$ orally in mice: 0.5 g/kg. |
| wh. powder; M.p. 150 | s. EtOH; sl. s. $H_2O$ | *p*-Aminobenzoic acid antagonist in tubercle bacillus. Can replace this factor in some strains of *E. coli*. May be incorporated into a folic acid-like molecule. |
| col. cryst.; M.p. 70 | s. EtOH, $CHCl_3$ | Inhibits oxidation of acetaldehyde *in vivo* probably by inhibiting glyceraldehyde dehydrogenase. Inhibits yeast alcohol dehydrogenase. Used in treatment of alcoholism. |

## 13F  Other enzyme inhibitors

| Name | Synonyms | Formula | M. wt. |
|------|----------|---------|--------|

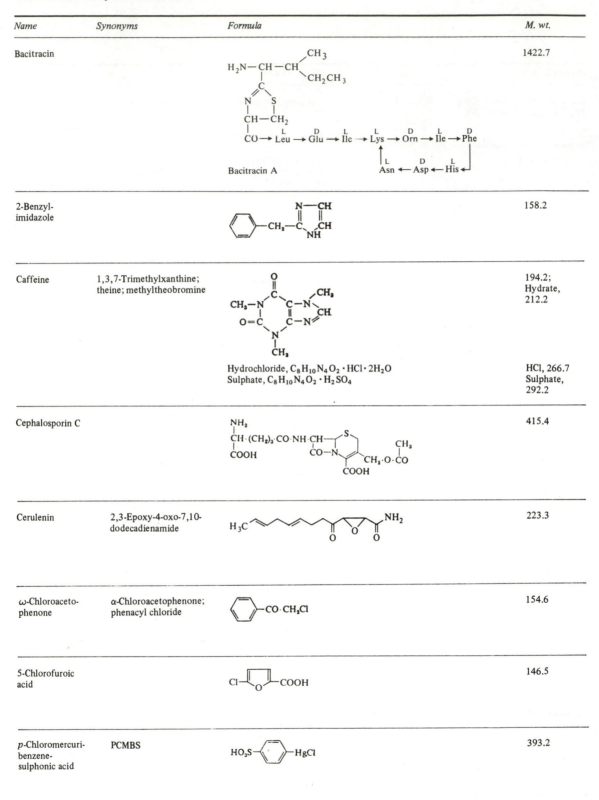

**Bacitracin** — 1422.7

Bacitracin A

**2-Benzyl-imidazole** — 158.2

**Caffeine** — 1,3,7-Trimethylxanthine; theine; methyltheobromine — 194.2; Hydrate, 212.2

Hydrochloride, $C_8H_{10}N_4O_2 \cdot HCl \cdot 2H_2O$
Sulphate, $C_8H_{10}N_4O_2 \cdot H_2SO_4$

HCl, 266.7
Sulphate, 292.2

**Cephalosporin C** — 415.4

**Cerulenin** — 2,3-Epoxy-4-oxo-7,10-dodecadienamide — 223.3

**ω-Chloroaceto-phenone** — α-Chloroacetophenone; phenacyl chloride — 154.6

**5-Chlorofuroic acid** — 146.5

**p-Chloromercuri-benzene-sulphonic acid** — PCMBS — 393.2

| Physical properties | Solubility | General remarks |
|---|---|---|
| grey-wh. powder | v.s. $H_2O$, MeOH; s. EtOH; sl. s. acet., benz., eth.; i. $CHCl_3$ | The bacitracins are a family of cyclic polypeptides of which bacitracin A is the main component. Inhibits cell wall synthesis. Resembles penicillin in causing protoplast formation and accumulation of cell wall precursors. Inhibits dephosphorylation of the pyrophosphate derivative of $C_{55}$-isoprenol alcohol, *PNAS* **57**, 767 (1967). Rel. stable in acid soln.; unstable above pH 9. Revised structure, *Adv. Appl. Microbiol.* **24**, 187 (1978). |
| col. needles; M.p. 125 | s. $H_2O$, EtOH | Inhibits penicillinase at $10^{-3}$ M. |
| wh. needles from EtOH; prisms by sublimation; M.p. Anhyd. 237; sublimes above 178 | s. hot $H_2O$, EtOH, acet., $CHCl_3$, benz.; sl. s. cold $H_2O$; sp. s. eth. | Inhibits cAMP phosphodiesterase (*see* theophylline). Stimulates CNS. Vasoconstrictor. Readily absorbed by g.i.t., and blood levels persist 6–12 hr. Partially demethylated and oxidized and excreted as 1-methyluric acid. |
| cryst. as sodium salt | Sodium salt, readily soluble in water | Inhibits cell wall synthesis. Action similar to penicillins causing lysis of growing bacterial cells by inhibiting polymerization of UDP-muramic acid peptides; approx. 0.1% activity of benzylpenicillin against *S. aureus*. Induces penicillinase in *S. aureus* and *B. cereus* but resistant to penicillinase action. Attacked by cephalosporinase and by acetylesterase, both found in many bacteria. Low antibacterial activity increased by chemical replacement of aminoadipic sidechain. |
| wh. cryst.; M.p. 93–4 | s. EtOH, acet.; sl. s. $H_2O$; i. pet. eth. | Inhibits fatty acid synthetase (rat liver at 4–20 µg/ml, *E. coli* at 4–8 µg/ml). Inhibits HMG-CoA synthetase and prevents sterol synthesis. Antifungal, antibacterial; *B. subtilis* growth inhibited at 20 µg/ml, reversed by palmitic acid. Inhibition of peptidase reported. Review, *Bacteriol. Rev.* **40**, 681 (1976). Stable in neutral and acidic solns. |
| cryst.; M.p. 95, B.p. 247 | s. EtOH, benz., eth., ethylene glycol monomethyl ether; i. $H_2O$ | Enzyme inhibitor at $10^{-3}$–$10^{-4}$ M. Lachrymatory. |
| wh. leaflets; M.p. 179 | s. EtOH; sl. s. $H_2O$ | Inhibits L-glutamic dehydrogenase: mechanism mixed comp.-non-comp. |
|  | v.s. $H_2O$ | Enzyme inhibitor at $10^{-5}$ M. Titration of –SH groups in proteins, *JBC* **203**, 563 (1953). *Class characteristics* of organic mercurials: Reaction RSH + R'HgX → R–S–HgR' + HX. Generally fairly high specificity at low concentration, reversed by thiols (e.g. mercaptoethanol); may react with other protein groups at high concentration. Have high affinity for –SH and react rapidly, useful for quantitative determination of –SH. *Note*: Inorganic $Hg^{2+}$ salts (and those of other heavy metals) have also been used as –SH enzyme inhibitors and for –SH analysis. Anion constitution of medium may affect reactivity and specificity; the reactive species may be derivatives formed with buffer anions. Review: *Metabolic Inhibitors*, vol. 2, pp. 119–44 (1963). |

| Name | Synonyms | Formula | M. wt. |
|------|----------|---------|--------|
| Cycloserine | Oxamycin; D-4-amino-3-isoxazolidone | | 102.1 |
| 4-Deoxypyridoxine | 2,4-Dimethyl-3-hydroxy-5-hydroxymethylpyridine | | 153.2 |
| Desferrioxamine B | Deferoxamine | | 560.7 |
| Desthiobiotin | | | 214.3 |
| Diethyldithiocarbamic acid, Na salt | DIECA | | 171.3 |
| Diethylpyrocarbonate | DEP; diethyl dicarbonate; ethoxyformic acid anhydride | | 162.2 |
| Diisopropylphosphofluoridate | Diisopropylfluorophosphonate; DFP | | 184.2 |
| Dimethylethanolamine | Dimethyl-2-hydroxyethylamine; $N,N$-Dimethyl-2-aminoethanol | | 89.1 |
| $m$-Dimethylaminophenylmethylcarbamate · HCl | | | 230.7 |

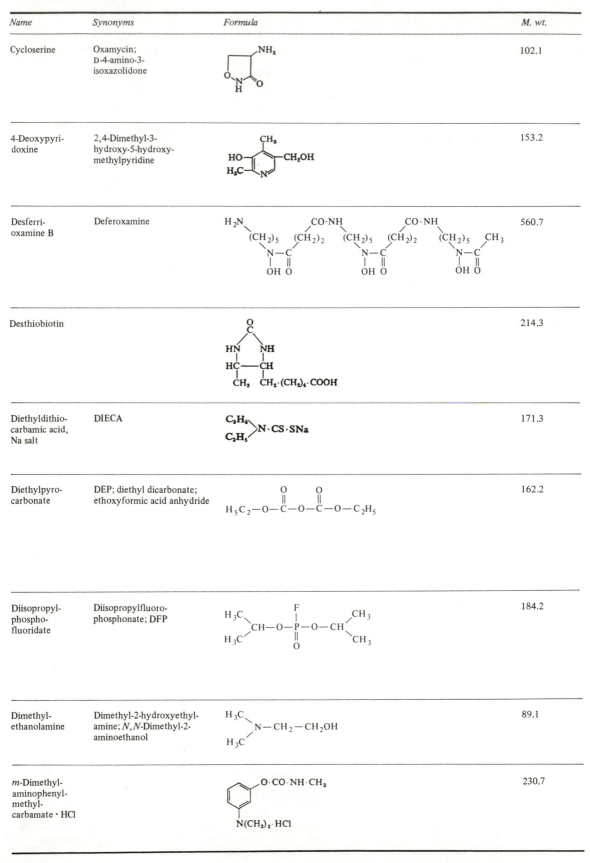

| Physical properties | Solubility | General remarks |
|---|---|---|
| cryst.; decomp. 155—6 | s. $H_2O$; sl. s. MeOH, propylene glycol | Inhibits cell wall synthesis in both gram + ve and gram − ve organisms. Prevents bacterial growth and causes lysis by blocking conversion of L-alanine to D-alanine required for formation of D-alanyl-D-alanine; also inhibits D-alanine:D-alanine ligase. Inhibition reversed competitively by D-alanine. Forms salts with acids and bases. Neutral or acid solutions are unstable. Aq. soln. buffered to pH 10 with $Na_2CO_3$ can be stored for a week at $+4\,°C$. |
| wh. cryst. | s. $H_2O$; sl. s. EtOH | An anti-pyridoxin in chickens. Inhibits the growth of most bacteria which require pyridoxin. In bacterial cells is phosphorylated to an inhibitor of amino acid decarboxylases. |
| | | Used as inhibitor of ferrochelatase; chelates iron extremely tightly (binding constant for $Fe^{3+}$ of order of $10^{30}$). Produced by microorganisms as iron transport molecule. Inhibits haem biosynthesis at approx. $500\,\mu g/ml$. A family of related structures known, *Science* **156**, 1443 (1967). Desferrioxamine mesylate (methanesulphonate), M. wt. 656.8, decomposes when exposed to air; more stable in desiccator at $4\,°C$. Solns. freshly prepared for use, *JBC* **250**, 9215 (1975). |
| wh. needles; M.p. DL- 165 | s. $H_2O$ | Competes with biotin utilization of *L. casei* but stimulates growth of *Saccharomyces cerevisiae* in a biotin-deficient medium. Only D-isomer active. |
| | s. $H_2O$; sl. s. EtOH | Irreversible inhibition of Cu enzymes at $10^{-3}$ M. Inhibits diamine oxidase, *BJ* **59**, 609 (1955). May also react with Zn, Fe, and other metallo-enzymes. Unstable in acid solutions. *See also* data in Chelating Agents. |
| oily liq.; B.p. 74—6 at 7 mm Hg; fruity odour | 0.6 d. $H_2O$; v.s. EtOH, organic solvents | Destroys enzymes by ethoxyformylation of proteins. Has been used to inhibit nucleases during RNA extraction but known to destroy biological activity of mRNA (reacts with single-stranded RNA). Often used to destroy trace nuclease contamination in reagents before use − 0.1% renders solns. nuclease free, *Biochem.* **10**, 3014 (1972); left overnight DEP decomposes into $CO_2$ and EtOH; pH may fall. Toxicity low but caution in handling recommended because of potential mutagenic effects. Comprehensive review on DEP, *PNARMB* **16**, 189 (1976). See also p. 388. |
| col. liq; B.p. 183 | s. organic solvents; $1.54^{25}\,H_2O$ | Highly toxic nerve gas to be handled with extreme precautions; absorbed via skin; decontaminate glassware in 1M-NaOH in 50% EtOH. Inhibits serine esterases by covalent attachment to active site serine. Pseudocholinesterase inhibitor at $10^{-7}-10^{-9}$ M, chymotrypsin and trypsin at $10^{-3}-10^{-5}$ M (less hazardous PMSF, TLCK, and TPCK (q.v.) may be preferred as inhibitors for latter two enzymes). DFP usually stored as stock solns. in dry *i*-PrOH (stable at $-10\,°C$ for months). Aq. solns. unstable. |
| liq.; $pK_a$ 9.24; $d_4^{20}$ 0.887; B.p. 135 | $\infty\,H_2O$, EtOH, eth. | Analogue of choline, incorporated into cellular phospholipids, *PNAS* **71**, 4072 (1974). Inhibitor of ethanolamine phosphokinase, *BBA* **276**, 143 (1972). |
| wh. prisms; M.p. 170 | s. EtOH, acet. | Inhibits liver esterase at $10^{-6}$ M. |

## 13F  Other enzyme inhibitors

| Name | Synonyms | Formula | M. wt. |
|---|---|---|---|
| α,α-Dimethyl-choline chloride | | 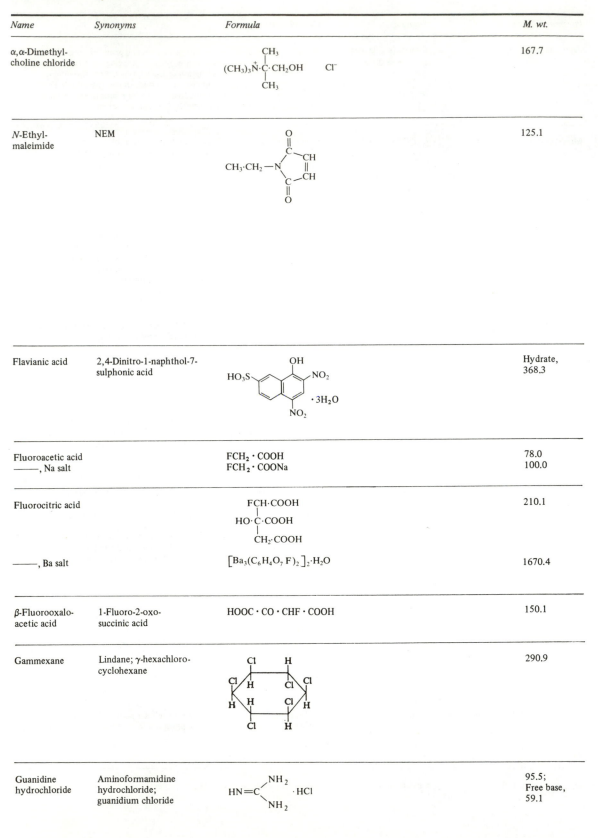 | 167.7 |
| N-Ethyl-maleimide | NEM | | 125.1 |
| Flavianic acid | 2,4-Dinitro-1-naphthol-7-sulphonic acid | | Hydrate, 368.3 |
| Fluoroacetic acid | | $FCH_2 \cdot COOH$ | 78.0 |
| ———, Na salt | | $FCH_2 \cdot COONa$ | 100.0 |
| Fluorocitric acid | | $FCH \cdot COOH$ $HO \cdot C \cdot COOH$ $CH_2 \cdot COOH$ | 210.1 |
| ———, Ba salt | | $[Ba_3(C_6H_4O_7 F)_2]_2 \cdot H_2O$ | 1670.4 |
| β-Fluorooxalo-acetic acid | 1-Fluoro-2-oxo-succinic acid | $HOOC \cdot CO \cdot CHF \cdot COOH$ | 150.1 |
| Gammexane | Lindane; γ-hexachloro-cyclohexane | | 290.9 |
| Guanidine hydrochloride | Aminoformamidine hydrochloride; guanidium chloride | | 95.5; Free base, 59.1 |

| Physical properties | Solubility | General remarks |
|---|---|---|
| cryst. | s. EtOH; i. eth. | Antimetabolite of choline in rats. |
| col. cryst.; sublimes 44 | v.s. $H_2O$. Stable at pH 5 (22 hr). Slow hydrolysis to N-ethylmaleamate at pH 7 – rate increased at higher pH values. Use fresh solutions. | *Class characteristics* of maleimide alkylating reagents: Reaction |

$$R{-}SH + R'{-}N\underset{\overset{\displaystyle\|}{C}-CH}{\overset{\overset{\displaystyle O}{\|}}{C}-CH} \longrightarrow R'{-}N\underset{\overset{\displaystyle\|}{C}-CH_2}{\overset{\overset{\displaystyle O}{\|}}{C}-\overset{H}{\underset{\phantom{x}}{C}}-S-R}$$

essentially irreversible, fairly specific for –SH at low concentration, rapid reaction. Usually only most reactive –SH groups of proteins react. Forms acid-resistant adduct. Abs. max. at 305 nm disappears on reaction with –SH, used for quantitative –SH group determination, *Meth. Enzymol.* **25**, 453 (1972). Commercial preps. may contain impurities troublesome in –SH determination. Synthesis may be desirable, *PNAS* **54**, 891 (1965). Reaction between NEM and glutathione complete within 1 min at R.T. and pH 7. Reaction rate decreases at lower pH values. Reaction product of NEM + RSH gives intense, unstable red colour in alkali: used for detection on chromatograms. Slow reaction of NEM with peptide-$NH_2$, imidazoles. Used frequently as inhibitor of transport and enzymic processes. Lachrymator when liquid.

| Physical properties | Solubility | General remarks |
|---|---|---|
| yel. needles; M.p. 100 | s. $H_2O$, EtOH | Inhibits phosphate-activated glutaminase at $10^{-3}$ M; non-comp. with glutamine. |
| wh. cryst.; M.p. 33; $pK_a$ 2.66 col. cryst. | s. $H_2O$, EtOH | Forms fluorocitrate (q.v.) *in vivo* through action of acetyl-CoA synthetase and citrate synthase. |
| anhyd., col. needles; hydrated, col. cryst.; both v. deliq. | s. $H_2O$, EtOH, eth. | Inhibits aconitase at $10^{-5}$ M. Difference between natural and synthetic compounds probably due to presence of different stereoisomers. Biologically-active isomer is (−)-*erythro*-fluorocitrate. 10–100 nM irreversibly inhibits citrate influx in isolated mitochondria from rat brain. Effect on citrate transport related more directly to toxic effect than inhibition of aconitase, *Mol. Pharmacol.* **14**, 172 (1978). Site of inhibition: a citryl-glutathione-thioester forming enzyme system, *PNAS* **74**, 4942 (1977). |
| cryst.; M.p. 86 | s. $H_2O$ | Comp. inhibits malate dehydrogenase at $10^{-3}$ M. Crystalline acid decomposes on standing. |
| cryst.; M.p. 113 | v.s. acet.; sl. s. EtOH; i. $H_2O$ | Probably an antimetabolite of inositol in *Neurospora* and in plants. Powerful insecticide. Early commercial samples were mixtures of isomers–now 99% γ-isomer. |
| deliq. cryst.; $pK_a$ 13.6 | v. s. $H_2O$, EtOH; i. eth. Soln. of free base alk., absorbs $CO_2$ from air; soln. of hydrochloride neutral. | Used at 6M to destroy RNase in RNA extraction; reported to give less degradation than by phenol (q.v.). Extraction procedure, *Meth. Enzymol.* **12B**, 120 (1968). Strong hydrogen bonding agent. General protein denaturant and solubilizing agent for large complexes whose structure depends on hydrogen bonds. |

## 13F Other enzyme inhibitors

| Name | Synonyms | Formula | M. wt. |
|------|----------|---------|--------|
| δ-Guanidino-valeric acid | | $\underset{NH_2}{\overset{NH}{>}}$CH·NH·CH$_2$·CH$_2$·CH$_2$·CH$_2$·COOH | 160.2 |
| Hydroxylamine | | NH$_2$OH | 33.0; Hydrochloride, 69.5 |
| p-Hydroxymercuri-benzoic acid, Na salt | | NaOOC—⟨benzene ring⟩—HgOH | 360.7 |
| Imidazole | Glyoxaline; 1,3-diazole; iminazole | ⟨imidazole ring⟩ | 68.1 |
| Iodoacetamide | | ICH$_2$·CO·NH$_2$ | 185.0 |
| Iodoacetic acid ———, Na salt | | ICH$_2$·COOH ICH$_2$·COONa | 186.0 208.0 |
| Iproniazid | Isonicotinic acid 2-iso-propylhydrazine; Marsilid | ⟨pyridine ring⟩CO·NH·NH·CH(CH$_3$)$_2$ | 179.2 |
| Isoniazid | Isonicotinic acid hydrazide | ⟨pyridine ring⟩CO·NH·NH$_2$ | 137.1 |
| Isopropyl-hydrazine | | $\underset{CH_3}{\overset{CH_3}{>}}$CH·NH—NH$_2$ | 74.1 |
| Levamisole hydrochloride | L-(−)-2,3,5,6-tetrahydro-6-phenylimidazo{2,1-b}thiazole; tetramisol | ⟨phenyl-imidazothiazole ring⟩ . HCl | 240.8 |
| Levulinic acid | Laevulinic acid; 4-oxopentanoic acid | CH$_3$·CO·CH$_2$·CH$_2$·COOH | 116.1 |

| Physical properties | Solubility | General remarks |
|---|---|---|
| cryst.; M.p. 265 | s. $H_2O$, EtOH | Comp. inhibits carboxypeptidase B at $10^{-3}$ M. Similar action by δ-amino-valeric acid and ε-aminocaproic acid which also inhibits plasmin. |
| wh. needles or col. liq.; M.p. 33 | s. $H_2O$, EtOH | Inhibits amino acid decarboxylases at $10^{-5}$ M. Also γ-aminobutyrate-α-oxo-glutarate transaminase and serine and threonine dehydratases. Inhibits glucose oxidase by unknown mechanism. Similar inhibition by most carbonyl reagents which combine with pyridoxal phosphate. |
| amorph. wh. powder or cryst. | s. $H_2O$, alkali; i. acid. Dissolve in small amount of 0.2M-NaOH, dilute and carefully neutralize to pH 8. | This compound is often referred to as p-chloromercuribenzoate in the literature. p-Chloromercuribenzoic acid converts to p-hydroxymercuribenzoate under conditions in which sodium salt is prepared. Enzyme inhibitor at $10^{-5}$ M. Titration of —SH groups in proteins. Reaction rates maximal at pH 4.5—5.0, though pHs near neutral may also be used. In some cases inhibition reversed by ethylenediaminetetra-acetate. Pptd. by phosphate at pH 7. Solubility increased in presence of pyrophosphate, glycylglycine, Tris. Increase in u.v. absorption at 250—5 nm on formation of mercaptide used in —SH analysis, *JACS* **76**, 4331 (1954); *Meth. Enzymol.* **25**, 449 (1972). |
| prisms from benz.; M.p. 90—1; $pK_a$ 7.1 | s. $H_2O$, EtOH, eth., $CHCl_3$, pyr.; sl. s. benz.; v. sp. s. pet. eth. | Inhibits low $K_m$ cAMP phosphodiesterase and stimulates high $K_m$ cAMP phosphodiesterase at 10—40 mM in some cases, *Diabetes*, **17**, 308 (1968); *Adv. Cyclic Nucleotide Res.* **7**, 249 (1976). Good buffer in range 6.2—7.8. |
| M.p. 95 | s. $H_2O$ | Enzyme inhibitor at $10^{-3}$ M. See iodoacetic acid. |
| col. cryst.; M.p. 82—3; $pK_a$ 3.13 | Free acid, s. $H_2O$, EtOH; sl. s. eth. Salt, s. $H_2O$ | *Class characteristics* of halogenated alkylating agents: Reaction R—SH + R'X → R—S—R' + HX, essentially irreversible; *not highly specific*. Review of carboxymethylation procedures, *Meth. Enzymol.* **25**, 424 (1972). Reacts also with —$NH_2$ and phenolic —OH and with methionine, lysine and histidine (pH dependent) (more slowly than with —SH). Increased rate of reaction at high pH values (pH 9) indicates that reaction is probably with RS⁻. Enzyme inhibitor at $10^{-3}$ M. Triosephosphate dehydrogenase is the 'classic' sensitive enzyme. Slow decomp. in solution; store away from light. |
| needles; M.p. 113 | s. $H_2O$, EtOH | Antitubercular activity probably not related to anti-pyridoxine activity. Used as a 'psychic energiser' in depressed states. Inhibits amino acid decarboxylation *in vivo* and *in vitro*, and also amine oxidases. |
| wh. cryst.; M.p. 170—3 | v.s. $H_2O$; sl. s. EtOH, $CHCl_3$ | An antagonist of pyridoxin in some bacteria but not in mycobacteria as the effect in latter not reversed by pyridoxin. Causes peripheral neuritis in man, reversed by pyridoxin. Antibacterial action probably due to chelation of metals. |
| col. liq. | s. $H_2O$, EtOH | Inhibits diamine oxidase at $10^{-9}$ M; no inhibition of monoamine oxidase. |
| M.p. 226—9 (230—3); $[\alpha]^{21}$ −127.3 (c = 0.9 in $H_2O$) | s. $H_2O$, MeOH; sp. s. EtOH | Alkaline phosphatase inhibitor at $10^{-5}$ M of enzyme from various mammalian tissues, except intestine, *BBA* **289**, 158 (1972). Antihelminthic. $LD_{50}$ in mice, rats: 22, 24 mg/kg i.v; 84, 130 mg/kg s.c.; 210, 480 mg/kg orally. |
| plates or leaflets; M.p. 33—5; protect from light | s. $H_2O$, EtOH, eth.; i. aliphatic hydro-carbons | Inhibits δ-aminolaevulinic acid dehydratase. Inhibitor of chlorophyll synthesis, *BBRC* **49**, 364 (1972). Readily formed when many carbohydrates are heated in acid solution. |

## 13F Other enzyme inhibitors

| Name | Synonyms | Formula | M. wt. |
|---|---|---|---|
| MERCAP | 2-Mercaptobenzothiazole | 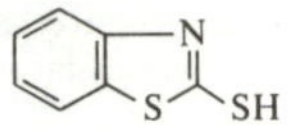 | 167.3 |
| MIX | 1-Methyl-3-isobutylxanthine | 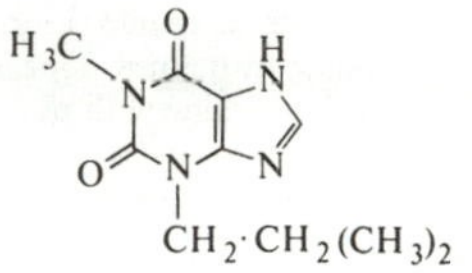 | 223.3 |
| Neostigmine bromide | Prostigmine | 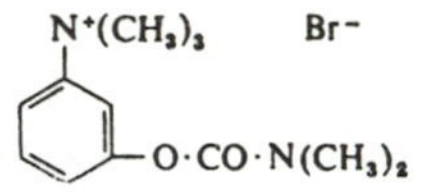 | 303.2 |
| Oxamic acid | | $\begin{matrix} COOH \\ | \\ CONH_2 \end{matrix}$ | 89.1 |
| Oxythiamine chloride hydro-chloride | | 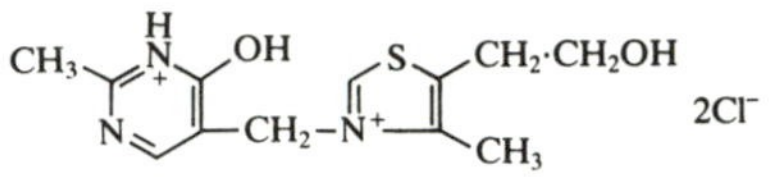 | 338.3 |
| Parapyruvate | $\gamma$-Methyl-$\gamma$-hydroxy-$\alpha$-ketoglutaric acid | $\begin{matrix} CH_3 \\ | \\ HOOC \cdot C \cdot CH_2 \cdot CO \cdot COOH \\ | \\ OH \end{matrix}$ | 176.1 |
| Penicillin | | All penicillins have the $\beta$-lactam-thiazolidine structure shown below:<br><br>Penicillin G, benzylpenicillin R = PhCH$_2$—<br><br>——, Na salt | 334.4 (free acid)<br><br>356.4 |
| 2-Phenylcyclo-propylamine hydrochloride | SKF trans-385 | 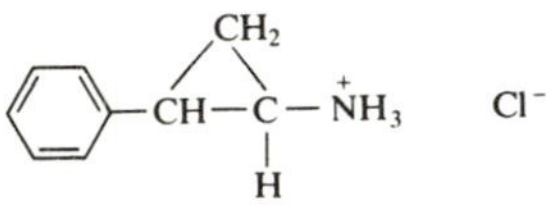 | 169.7 |
| Phenylmethane-sulphonyl fluoride | PMSF; $\alpha$-toluenesulphonyl fluoride | 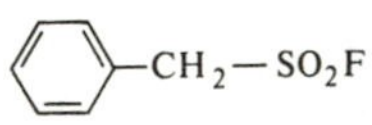 | 174.2 |
| Phenylpanto-thenone | | | 279.3 |

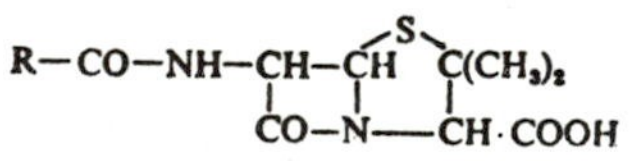

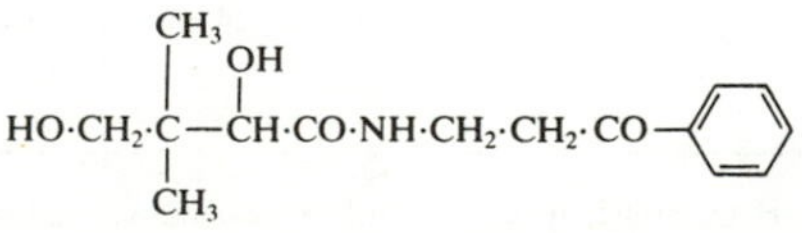

| Physical properties | Solubility | General remarks |
|---|---|---|
| pale yel. monoclinic needles; M.p. 180–2 | i. $H_2O$; $2^{25}$ EtOH; $1^{25}$ eth.; $10^{25}$ acet.; s. alk. and alk. carbonates | Inhibits polyphenoloxidase (at $10^{-7} - 2 \times 10^{-5}$ M) by Cu-chelating activity, *Science* **157**, 200 (1967). Since it is also an —SH compd., used to replace EDTA or EGTA plus cysteine or mercaptoethanol in isolating mitochondria, *Meth. Enzymol.* **31**, 592 (1974). |
| M.p. 200–1 | | Inhibitor of cAMP phosphodiesterase. Lipolytic activity seen at conc. producing <20% inhibition of phosphodiesterase; MIX 19× more active than theophylline (0.05 mM), *Mol. Pharmacol.* **6**, 597 (1970); *Adv. Cyclic Nucleotide Res.* **7**, 225 (1976). |
| wh. cryst. powder; M.p. 168 d. | v.s. cold $H_2O$; s. EtOH | Brain, red blood cell and plasma cholinesterase inhibitor at $10^{-7}-10^{-8}$ M. Protect solutions from light. |
| col. cryst.; M.p. 210 | s. $H_2O$; v. sl. s. EtOH | Inhibits heart lactic dehydrogenase at $10^{-5}$ M by competing with pyruvate, *JBC* **234**, 1143 (1959). Has been used to inhibit glycolysis in neoplastic cells. |
| wh. needles; M.p. 195 d. | s. MeOH; i. eth. | Thiamine antagonist in chicken and mouse, effects reversed by thiamine. Unlike pyrithiamine is phosphorylated *in vivo* to an inhibitor of carboxylase. |
| | s. $H_2O$ | Specifically inhibits at $10^{-3}$ M the oxidation of α-oxoglutarate in tissue preps. Parapyruvate exists in equilibrium with the corresponding lactone, the latter amounting to 25% at equilibrium. |
| Free acid, amorph. wh. powder / Sodium salt, cryst. from MeOH-ethyl acetate | Free acid, s. MeOH, EtOH, eth., acet., ethyl acetate; sp. s. $H_2O$; i. pet. eth. / Sodium salt, v.s. $H_2O$; sl. s. EtOH; pract. i. acet., eth., $CHCl_3$, ethyl acetate | Blocks cell wall formation in growing cells resulting in accumulation of uracil nucleotides of muramic acid peptides and in the formation of protoplasts preceding lysis. Covalently links to proteins in membrane. Probably critical action is to block final transpeptidation reaction in the transfer of the muramic acid peptide from its UDP carrier to polymerized position in the cell wall. Resistant strains of susceptible organisms occur which produce inducible penicillinase. The free acid retains its activity when dry but is rapidly inactivated by small amounts of water. |
| col. needles | s. EtOH; i. eth. | Inhibits amine oxidase, essentially irreversibly, at $10^{-7}$ M. Both *cis-* and *trans-*isomers active. Neither has significant effect on diamine oxidase. |
| cryst.; M.p. 91–2 | sl. s. $H_2O$ | Specific chymotrypsin and trypsin inhibitor; sulphonylates protein exclusively at active site histidine. Aq. solns. hydrolyse 50% in 100 min at 25 °C, pH 7. Stock solns. in 2-PrOH (7 mg/ml) used. |
| wh. cryst.; M.p. 126 | v.s. EtOH; s. $H_2O$ | Powerful antagonist of pantothenic acid in many microorganisms, irrespective of dietary requirement for this factor. Effects reversed by pantothenic acid only in those species with dietary requirement. Formation of CoA inhibited by this analogue and by the even more effective tolylpantothenone. |

| Name | Synonyms | Formula | M. wt. |
|---|---|---|---|
| Phenyl-β-D-thiogalactoside | | 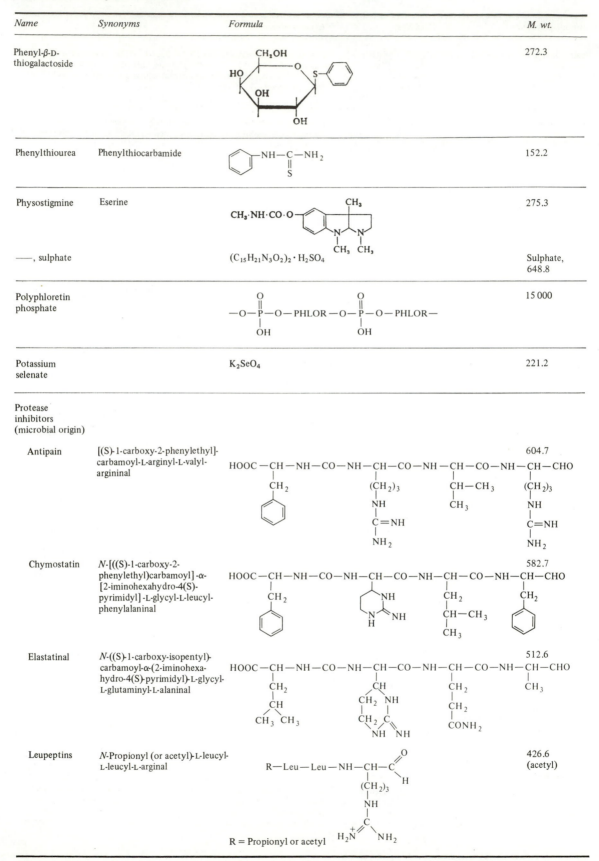 | 272.3 |
| Phenylthiourea | Phenylthiocarbamide | | 152.2 |
| Physostigmine | Eserine | | 275.3 |
| ——, sulphate | | $(C_{15}H_{21}N_3O_2)_2 \cdot H_2SO_4$ | Sulphate, 648.8 |
| Polyphloretin phosphate | | | 15 000 |
| Potassium selenate | | $K_2SeO_4$ | 221.2 |
| Protease inhibitors (microbial origin) | | | |
|   Antipain | [(S)-1-carboxy-2-phenylethyl]-carbamoyl-L-arginyl-L-valyl-argininal | | 604.7 |
|   Chymostatin | N-[((S)-1-carboxy-2-phenylethyl)carbamoyl]-α-[2-iminohexahydro-4(S)-pyrimidyl]-L-glycyl-L-leucyl-phenylalaninal | | 582.7 |
|   Elastatinal | N-((S)-1-carboxy-isopentyl)-carbamoyl-α-(2-iminohexa-hydro-4(S)-pyrimidyl)-L-glycyl-L-glutaminyl-L-alaninal | | 512.6 |
|   Leupeptins | N-Propionyl (or acetyl)-L-leucyl-L-leucyl-L-arginal | R = Propionyl or acetyl | 426.6 (acetyl) |

| Physical properties | Solubility | General remarks |
|---|---|---|
| M.p. 112 | s. $H_2O$ | Comp. inhibits $\beta$-galactosidase at $10^{-3}$ M. Is not an inducer of $\beta$-galactosidase in *E. coli*. |
| M.p. 154 | 0.25 $H_2O$; s. EtOH | Inhibits tyrosinase, *Meth. Enzymol.* **17A**, 620 (1970); bitter or tasteless depending on heredity. $LD_{50}$ orally in rats, rabbits: 3, 40 mg/kg. |
| col. cryst. prisms (unstable form); M.p. 105 (86); $pK_a$ 6.12, 12.24 | s. EtOH, $CHCl_3$, eth.; sl. s. $H_2O$ | Serum and muscle cholinesterase inhibitor at $10^{-5}-10^{-8}$ M. Must be kept in the dark. |
| M.p. 145 | v. s. $H_2O$; s. EtOH | |
| light green or brown powder | s. $H_2O$ | Inhibits alkaline phosphatase at 0.025 $\mu$g/ml and hyaluronidase at 0.1 $\mu$g/ml. Other polyphosphates act similarly. |
| col. rh. cryst. | s. $H_2O$ | Inhibits ATP-sulphurylase and many reactions involving sulphate. |
| | | A series of relatively specific protease inhibitors have been isolated from culture filtrates. Review: *Cold Spring Harbour Symposium* (1976) on *Proteases*, p. 429. |
| Di-HCl: M.p. 170–7 | Di-HCl: s. $H_2O$, MeOH, DMSO; sl. s. EtOH; i. eth., $CHCl_3$ | Action resembles leupeptin (q.v.) but inhibits plasmin less and cathepsin A more than leupeptin; 50% inhibition levels ($\mu$g/ml) papain 0.16, trypsin 0.26, cathepsin A 1.19, B 0.59, D 125, plasmin $>$93, chymotrypsin, pepsin $>$250, *J. Antibiotics* **25**, 263, 267 (1972) |
| wh. cryst.; M.p. 205–7 d. | s. acetic acid, DMSO; sl. s. $H_2O$, EtOH; i. eth. | Inhibits chymotrypsin strongly, papain and cathepsins weakly, inactive on trypsin. 50% inhibition levels ($\mu$g/ml) chymotrypsin 0.15, papain 7.5, cathepsin A 62.5, B 2.6, D 49.0, plasmin, trypsin $>$250, *J. Antibiotics* **23**, 425 (1970); **26**, 625 (1973). Leucine in structure may be replaced by isoleucine or valine. |
| $pK_a$ 3.7, $>$11 | s. $H_2O$, DMSO; sl. s. EtOH, acet.; i. eth. | Strong inhibitor of elastase; 50% inhibition at 0.29 $\mu$g/ml; $>$250 $\mu$g/ml for other proteases, *J. Antibiotics* **26**, 787 (1973); **28**, 337 (1975). Unstable in alkaline soln. |
| | HCl: s. $H_2O$, EtOH, DMSO; i. acet. | Leupeptin has propionyl and acetyl derivatives in 3:1 ratio. Strongly inhibits plasmin, trypsin, papain, and cathepsin B. 50% inhibition levels ($\mu$g/ml) 8, 2, 0.5, and 0.44 resp. Chymotrypsin, pepsin, cathepsins A and D insensitive. 50% inhibition levels ($\mu$g/ml) $>$500, $>$500, 1680, 109 resp., *J. Antibiotics* **22**, 283, 558 (1969); **25**, 515 (1972). |

| Name | Synonyms | Formula | M. wt. |
|---|---|---|---|
| Pepstatin A | | R—L-Val—L-Val—AHMHA—L-Ala—AHMHA<br><br>R=Isovaleric acid<br>AHMHA=4-Amino-3-hydroxy-6-methylheptanoic acid | 685.9 |
| Phosphor-amidon | *N*-(α-L-rhamnopyranosyloxy-hydroxyphosphinyl)-L-leucyl-L-tryptohan | | 543.6 |
| 6-Pteridyl-aldehyde | 2-Amino-4-hydroxy-6-formylpteridine | | 191.2 |
| Pyrazole | 1,2-Diazole | | 68.1 |
| Pyridine-3-sulphonic acid | | | 159.2 |
| Pyrithiamine bromide hydro-bromide | Neopyrithiamine | | 420.2 |
| Pyrogallol | Pyrogallic acid | | 126.1 |
| Riboflavin 5-sulphate | | | 456.4 |
| Saccharo-lactone | D-Glucaro-1,4-lactone | | 192.1 |

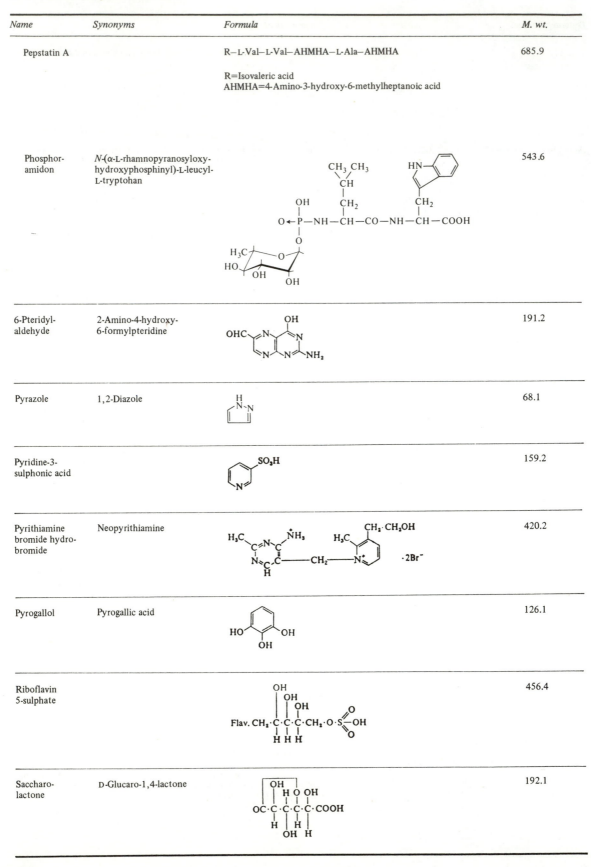

| Physical properties | Solubility | General remarks |
|---|---|---|
| col. needles; M.p. 228–9 | s. MeOH, EtOH, DMSO; sl. s. $H_2O$, eth. | Inhibits acid proteases strongly. First pepstatin isolated; 50% inhibition levels pepsin $1.5 \times 10^{-8}$ M, cathepsin D $1.5 \times 10^{-8}$ M, trypsin, plasmin, chymotrypsin, elastase, thermolysin $>3.6 \times 10^{-4}$ M. Also inhibits renin ($6.0 \times 10^{-6}$ M). Precise 50% inhibition concentration varies somewhat with substrate. Other pepstatins isolated differing in R-group or amino acids; antirenin activity increases as R-group increases in hydrophobicity. *J. Antibiotics* **23**, 259, 263 (1970); **24**, 687 (1971); **25**, 689 (1972). |
| | Na salt: s. $H_2O$, DMSO; sl. s. EtOH; i. eth. | Inhibits thermolysin strongly, collagenase weakly (50% inhibition at 0.4, 33 µg/ml resp.), inactive on trypsin, chymotrypsin, papain, and pepsin (50% inhibition at $>250$ µg/ml), *J. Antibiotics* **26**, 621 (1973); *Tetrahedron Letts.* **1**, 97 (1972). |
| yel. powder | | Inhibits milk xanthine oxidase at $10^{-9}$ M. |
| needles or prisms from pet. eth.; M.p. 70 | s. $H_2O$, EtOH, eth., benz. | Inhibitor of alcohol dehydrogenase, *Alcoholism: Clin. and Exper. Res.* **1**, 7 (1977). 4-Methyl derivative is more effective. |
| needles or plates; M.p. 357 d. | v.s. $H_2O$; sl. s. EtOH | Nicotinamide antagonist in some microorganisms and in nicotinic acid-deficient dogs. Forms an inhibitory analogue of NAD *in vivo*. |
| hygr. needles; M.p. 220 | s. $H_2O$, EtOH, $CHCl_3$ | Competitive antagonist of thiamine in microorganisms and in higher animals. Effects produced differ from those caused by oxythiamine. Inhibits enzyme forming co-carboxylase but may have other effects. |
| wh. cryst.; darken in air and light; M.p. 131 | s. $H_2O$, EtOH, eth. | Comp. inhibits catechol *O*-methyl transferase at $10^{-5}$ M. Potentiates action of adrenaline and noradrenaline *in vivo*. |
| yel. cryst. | s. $H_2O$ | Inhibits amino acid oxidase at $10^{-5}$ M by competing for riboflavin moiety of FAD. Does not prevent FMN combining with 'old yellow enzyme', *Nature, Lond.* **180**, 922 (1957). |
| col. cryst.; M.p. Hydrate, 90 | s. $H_2O$, acet. | Comp. inhibits β-glucuronidase at $10^{-5}$ M. The lactone is formed to about 30% on boiling a solution of potassium hydrogen saccharate for 30 min. It is unstable at a pH greater than 6. |

## 13F Other enzyme inhibitors

| Name | Synonyms | Formula | M. wt. |
|------|----------|---------|--------|
| Sinefungin | | | 367.3 |
| Sodium fluoride | | NaF | 42.0 |
| Sodium sulphite | | $Na_2SO_3 \cdot 7H_2O$ | 252.2 |
| SKF 525-A | 2-Diethylamino-ethyl-2-diphenyl-propylacetate | | 353.5 |
| Sulphadiazine | $N^1$-2-Pyrimidyl-sulphanilamide | | 250.3 |
| Sulphaguanidine | $N^1$-Guanylsulphanilamide | | 214.3 |
| Sulphamethazine | $N^1$-(4,6-Dimethyl-2-pyrimidyl)sulphanilamide | | 278.3 |
| Sulphanilamide | $p$-Aminobenzene-sulphonamide | | 172.2 |
| Sulphapyridine | $N^1$-2-Pyridylsulphanilamide | | 249.3 |
| Sulphathiazole | $N^1$-2-Thiazolylsulphanilamide | | 255.3 |
| Suramin | Hexasodium $sym.$-bis-($m$-aminobenzoyl-$m$-amino-$p$-methylbenzoyl-1-naphthyl-amino-4,6,8-trisulphonate)-carbamide; Antrypol; Bayer 205; Germanin; Fourneau 309 | | 1429.2 |

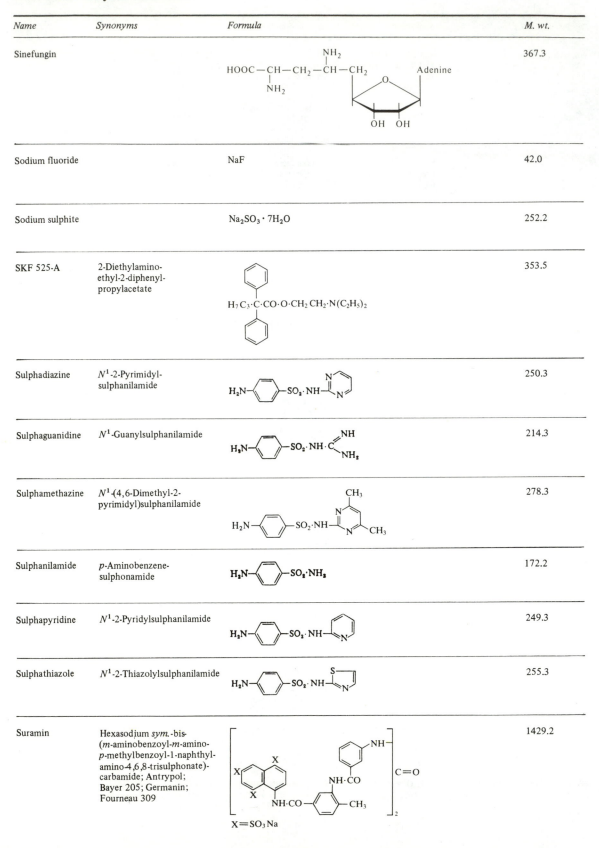

| Physical properties | Solubility | General remarks |
|---|---|---|
| | | Methyl transferase inhibitor. Structurally resembles $S$-adenosylhomocysteine; inhibits mRNA-(guanine-7)methyl transferase in Newcastle disease virions and mRNA-nucleoside-$2'$-$O$-methyl transferase of vaccinia virions ($K_i$:12.0, 40 nM resp.). Prevents formation of m$^7$GpppN at $5'$-terminus of mRNA molecules and inhibits viral multiplication, $JBC$ **253**, 4075 (1978). In L-cells, vaccinia growth inhibited 62% at 10 $\mu$M. $S$-Adenosylhomocysteine also inhibits but less effectively (ref. above). |
| wh. cubic cryst.; p$K_a$ 3.2 (free acid) | s. $H_2O$ | Inhibits many $Mg^{2+}$-requiring enzymes such as enolase and acid phosphatase. Activates adenylate cyclase by modification of $Mg^{2+}$ requirement, $PNAS$ **74**, 92 (1977), $Adv.\ Cyclic\ Nucleotide\ Res.$ **3**, 23 (1973). |
| efflor. col. monocl. cryst. | s. $H_2O$; sl. s. EtOH | Inhibits sulphatases at $10^{-4}$ M or less. General reagent for cleaving protein disulphide bonds, $Chem.\ Rev.$ **59**, 583 (1959). |
| | | Inhibits hepatic drug metabolism by cytochrome $P_{450}$ system. Potentiates the action of many drugs (e.g. barbiturates) $in\ vivo$. |
| wh. cryst.; M.p. 252 | s. dil. acid and alkali; sl. s. $H_2O$, EtOH Na salt: s. $H_2O$ | E. H. Northey, $The\ sulphonamides\ and\ allied\ compounds$, Am. Chem. Soc. Monograph Series (1948). All sulphonamides are antagonists of $p$-aminobenzoic acid, preventing the formation of folic acid. |
| needles; M.p. 190–3 | s. hot $H_2O$, dil. acid; sl. s. $H_2O$, EtOH | |
| wh. cryst.; M.p. 176 | s. dil. alkali; sl. s. $H_2O$ Na salt: v. s. $H_2O$ | |
| wh. cryst.; M.p. 165–7 | s. dil. acid and alkali; sl. s. $H_2O$, EtOH | Inhibits carbonic anhydrase at $10^{-6}$ M. |
| wh. cryst.; M.p. 191–3 | s. dil. acid and alkali; v. sl. s. $H_2O$ Na salt: s. $H_2O$ | |
| wh. cryst.; M.p. 200–3 | s. dil. acid Na salt: s. $H_2O$ | |
| wh. or creamy wh. powder | freely s. $H_2O$; sp. s. 95% EtOH; i. benz., eth., $CHCl_3$ | Inhibits trypsin, fumarase, hyaluronidase, urease, hexokinase, succinic dehydrogenase, choline dehydrogenase, ribonuclease, $\beta$-galactosidase, and lysozyme. Active against these enzymes at concentrations within the range $10^{-4}$–$10^{-5}$ M ($BJ$ **47**, 158 (1950)). Unstable in solution. Has been used in a rapid method for determination of the isoelectric point of certain sensitive enzymes, the method being particularly useful in early stages of enzyme purification ($BJ$ **50**, 421 (1952)). |

## 13F  Other enzyme inhibitors

| Name | Synonyms | Formula | M. wt. |
|------|----------|---------|--------|
| L(+)-Tartaric acid | *d*-Tartaric acid; D(+)-tartaric acid (See *JBC* **207**, 275 (1954)) | 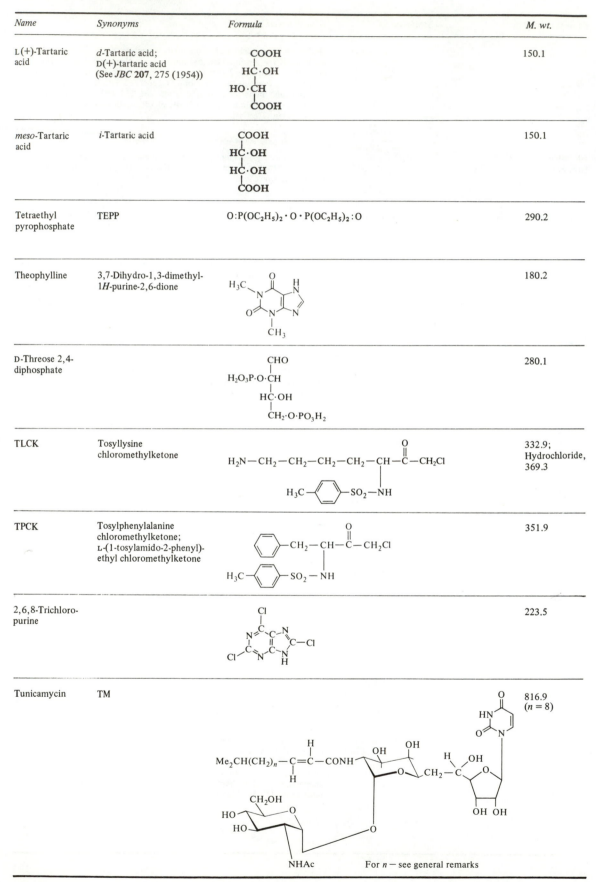 | 150.1 |
| *meso*-Tartaric acid | *i*-Tartaric acid | | 150.1 |
| Tetraethyl pyrophosphate | TEPP | $O:P(OC_2H_5)_2 \cdot O \cdot P(OC_2H_5)_2:O$ | 290.2 |
| Theophylline | 3,7-Dihydro-1,3-dimethyl-1*H*-purine-2,6-dione | | 180.2 |
| D-Threose 2,4-diphosphate | | | 280.1 |
| TLCK | Tosyllysine chloromethylketone | | 332.9; Hydrochloride, 369.3 |
| TPCK | Tosylphenylalanine chloromethylketone; L-(1-tosylamido-2-phenyl)-ethyl chloromethylketone | | 351.9 |
| 2,6,8-Trichloro-purine | | | 223.5 |
| Tunicamycin | TM | | 816.9 ($n = 8$) |

For *n* — see general remarks

| Physical properties | Solubility | General remarks |
|---|---|---|
| col. monocl. cryst.; M.p. 170 | s. $H_2O$, EtOH; i. benz. | Inhibits acid phosphatase (liver, kidney, and prostate) at $10^{-3}$ M. D(−)-isomer inactive. Erythrocyte or plasma enzyme not inhibited—basis of clinical differentiation. |
| col. plates; M.p. 140 | s. $H_2O$, EtOH | Inhibits fumarase at $10^{-5}$ M. |
| col. hygr. oil | s. EtOH, $H_2O$. Soln. hydrolyses to EtOH and $H_3PO_4$ | Brain and plasma cholinesterase inhibitor at $10^{-8}$–$10^{-9}$ M. Plant acetylesterase inhibitor at $10^{-6}$ M. No effect on trypsin; reacts v. slowly with chymotrypsin; compare DFP. |
| Monohydrate; thin monoclinic crystals from $H_2O$; M.p. 270–4 | 0.9 $H_2O$; 1.25 EtOH; s. hot $H_2O$, alk. hydroxides, dil. acids; sp. s. eth. | Inhibits cAMP phosphodiesterase competitively, $K_i = 1 \times 10^{-4}$ M in purified beef heart enzyme, *JBC* **237**, 1244 (1962). 10 mM gives 100% inhibition. Caffeine less potent. *Adv. Cyclic Nucleotide Res.* **3**, 65 (1973); **7**, 225 (1976); **8**, 119 (1977) for other inhibitors. Used as diuretic, cardiac stimulant, smooth muscle relaxant. $LD_{50}$ orally in mice: 540 mg/kg. |
| | s. $H_2O$ | Non-comp. inhibition of glyceraldehyde-3-phosphate dehydrogenase. Inhibitor not isolated but prepared by oxidation of corresponding arabitol phosphate. |
| | sl. s. $H_2O$ | Inactivates trypsin but not chymotrypsin [cf. reverse with TPCK (q.v.)]; reacts stoichiometrically with active centre. Fresh solns. used. |
| M.p. 102–3 | s. MeOH | Specific inhibitor of chymotrypsin but not trypsin [cf. reverse with TLCK (q.v.)]. Alkylates active centre histidine; preparation of enzyme derivative in 3–5% MeOH or 10% MeOH–10% DMSO, *Meth. Enzymol.* **25B**, 655 (1972). Stock solns. in MeOH. |
| platelets of pentahydrate; M.p. Hydrate, 187 | sl. s. $H_2O$; v. sl. s. EtOH, acet. | Inhibits uricase at $10^{-6}$ M. Other tri-substituted purines act similarly. |
| $\lambda_{max}$ 205, 260 nm $A_{1\,cm}^{1\%}$ 230, 110 (MeOH) | s. MeOH, $H_2O$ at alkaline pH; sl. s. EtOH; i. acet. | Inhibitor of bacterial and eukaryote *N*-acetylglucosamine transferases; prevents formation of *N*-acetylglucosamine lipid intermediates and prevents glycosylation of newly synthesized glycoproteins in eukaryote and bacterial cells. Inhibits replication of VSV in mammalian cells: 99% at 0.5 $\mu$g/ml, *J. Virol.* **21**, 375 (1977). Review, *PNARMB* **22**, 193 (1979). Unstable in acids, stable alkaline pH. Four different homologues exist in which $n = 8$, 9, 10, and 11. Mechanism of action, *Biochem.* **18**, 2186 (1979). |

# 14 Pharmacologically active compounds

**Fluorescence data**

A = wavelength of maximum activation (nm); F = wavelength of maximum fluorescence (nm).

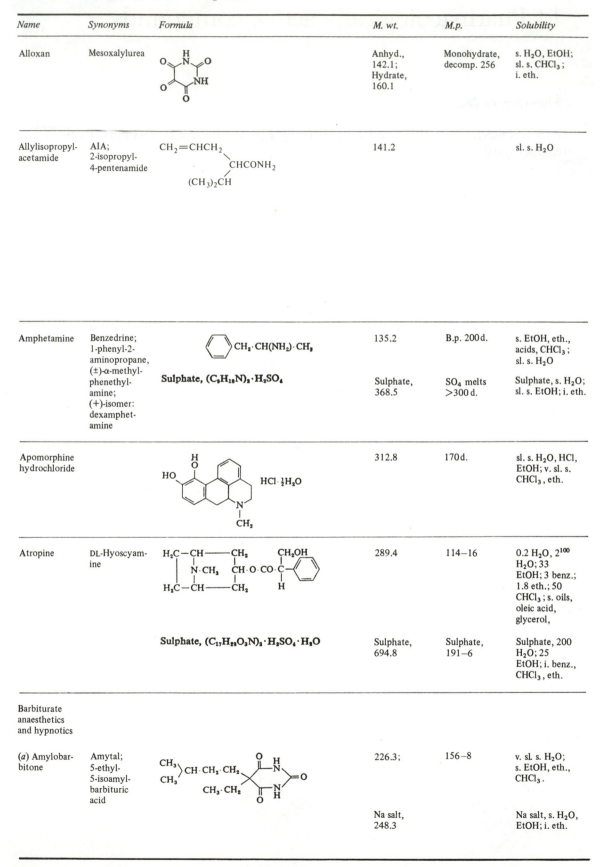

| Name | Synonyms | Formula | M. wt. | M.p. | Solubility |
|---|---|---|---|---|---|
| Alloxan | Mesoxalylurea | | Anhyd., 142.1; Hydrate, 160.1 | Monohydrate, decomp. 256 | s. $H_2O$, EtOH; sl. s. $CHCl_3$; i. eth. |
| Allylisopropyl-acetamide | AIA; 2-isopropyl-4-pentenamide | $CH_2=CHCH_2$ ... $CHCONH_2$ ... $(CH_3)_2CH$ | 141.2 | | sl. s. $H_2O$ |
| Amphetamine | Benzedrine; 1-phenyl-2-aminopropane, (±)-α-methyl-phenethyl-amine; (+)-isomer: dexamphet-amine | $CH_2 \cdot CH(NH_2) \cdot CH_3$ <br><br> Sulphate, $(C_9H_{13}N)_2 \cdot H_2SO_4$ | 135.2 <br><br> Sulphate, 368.5 | B.p. 200d. <br><br> $SO_4$ melts >300 d. | s. EtOH, eth., acids, $CHCl_3$; sl. s. $H_2O$ <br><br> Sulphate, s. $H_2O$; sl. s. EtOH; i. eth. |
| Apomorphine hydrochloride | | $HCl \cdot \frac{1}{2}H_2O$ | 312.8 | 170d. | sl. s. $H_2O$, HCl, EtOH; v. sl. s. $CHCl_3$, eth. |
| Atropine | DL-Hyoscyam-ine | $H_2C$—CH——$CH_2$ ... $N \cdot CH_3$ $CH \cdot O \cdot CO \cdot C$ ... $H_2C$—CH——$CH_2$ ... $CH_2OH$ ... H <br><br> Sulphate, $(C_{17}H_{23}O_3N)_2 \cdot H_2SO_4 \cdot H_2O$ | 289.4 <br><br><br> Sulphate, 694.8 | 114–16 <br><br><br> Sulphate, 191–6 | 0.2 $H_2O$, $2^{100}$ $H_2O$; 33 EtOH; 3 benz.; 1.8 eth.; 50 $CHCl_3$; s. oils, oleic acid, glycerol, <br><br> Sulphate, 200 $H_2O$; 25 EtOH; i. benz., $CHCl_3$, eth. |
| Barbiturate anaesthetics and hypnotics | | | | | |
| (a) Amylobar-bitone | Amytal; 5-ethyl-5-isoamyl-barbituric acid | $CH_3$ $\rangle$CH·CH_2·CH_2$ ... $CH_3$ ... $CH_3 \cdot CH_2$ | 226.3; <br><br><br> Na salt, 248.3 | 156–8 | v. sl. s. $H_2O$; s. EtOH, eth., $CHCl_3$. <br><br> Na salt, s. $H_2O$, EtOH; i. eth. |

| Action | Route | Absorption and fate | General remarks |
|---|---|---|---|
| Cytotoxic, diabetogenic. At $10^{-3}$ M inhibits skeletal muscle hexokinase; inhibition reversed by cysteine. Succinic dehydrogenase also inhibited | i.v., oral | Absorbed orally, parenterally. Rapidly destroyed. Part reduced to alloxantin | Monohydrate, col. rh. prisms efflor.; anhyd., yel. powder. Cellular mechanism unknown. Action very rapid. Prevented by SH compounds, nicotinic acid. Diabetogenic dosage: Dogs, 50—70 mg/kg i.v. Rabbits, 200 mg/kg i.v. Rats, 50 mg/kg i.v. Reversibly nephrotoxic above diabetogenic dosage. Fluorescent product with $o$-phenylene diamine. |
| Porphyrinogenic agent; causes rapid induction of hepatic δ-aminolaevulinic acid synthase and excretion of δ-aminolaevulinic acid and porphobilinogen. Also induces in isolated hepatocytes and cultured chick embryo liver cells, *JBC* **249**, 851 (1974). Causes destruction of haem prosthetic group of liver microsomal cytochrome $P_{450}$ with formation of green pigment, *BBRC* **83**, 132 (1978). | s.c. (15 mg/100 g body weight in rats). oral (40 mg/100 g body weight in rats) | | |
| Central stimulant, peripheral sympathomimetic | oral, i.v. | Absorbed g.i.t. Part deaminated, part excreted unchanged | Dextrorotatory form has twice the potency of racemate. Stronger inhibitor of amine oxidase than ephedrine. Used in barbiturate intoxication. |
| Centrally acting emetic. C.n.s. depressant | s.c., oral, i.v., i.m. | Absorbed all routes | Cryst.; decomposes in light and air. Emetic dose in the dog 2—10 mg. |
| Antagonist of muscarinic actions of acetylcholine. Central excitant and depressant | i.m., oral, topical | Rapidly absorbed by g.i.t., from mucosal surfaces and to some extent from intact skin. Disappears quickly from the blood. The tissues, especially liver, hydrolyse it to tropine and tropic acid. In man about 10% excreted in urine. Species differences in occurrence of atropinase. Blackbird and most strains of rabbit are resistant. | Col. microcryst. Reduces salivary and gastric secretions. Pupil of the eye dilated and accommodation paralysed. Sweat glands inhibited. Tolerance soon develops in man. Unstable to autoclaving. |
| | | After absorption barbiturates distributed throughout the tissues | Readily cross placental barrier. |
| Hypnotic of intermediate duration | oral | Degraded by the liver | Fluor., A 265 nm F 410 nm (pH 14). |

# 14 Pharmacologically active compounds

| Name | Synonyms | Formula | M. wt. | M.p. | Solubility |
|------|----------|---------|--------|------|------------|
| (b) Barbitone | Barbital; veronal; 5,5-diethyl-barbituric acid; 5,5-diethyl-malonylurea. Na salt; barbitone soluble | | 184.2 <br><br><br><br><br> Na salt, 206.2 | 189–92 | 0.84 $H_2O$; s. EtOH, eth., $CHCl_3$, acet. <br><br><br><br> Na salt, s. $H_2O$ |
| (c) Pentobarbitone sodium | Nembutal; sodium 5-ethyl-5-(1-methylbutyl)-barbiturate | | 248.3 | 128.5–130 (free acid) | s. $H_2O$, EtOH; i. eth. |
| (d) Thiopentone sodium | Pentothal sodium | | 264.3 | | s. $H_2O$, EtOH; i. eth., benz. |
| Chlorpromazine | 10-($\gamma$-Dimethyl-aminopropyl)-2-chloro-phenothiazine HCl; thorazine; largactil | | 355.3 | 179–80 | s. $H_2O$, $CHCl_3$, EtOH, MeOH |
| Dicoumarol | Bishydroxy-coumarin; 3,3'-methylene-bis(4-hydroxy-coumarin) | | 336.3 | 287–93 | sl. s. $CHCl_3$; sp. s. $H_2O$, EtOH; s. aq. alkalis, organic bases |
| Dihydro-$\beta$-erythroidine | | | 275.3 <br><br><br> HBr, 356.3 | 85–86 d.; <br><br><br> HBr salt, 242 d. | Base, s. $CHCl_3$, EtOH. <br><br><br> HBr, s. $H_2O$, EtOH |
| Diphenhydramine | Benadryl HCl; 2-(benzhydryl-oxy)-N,N-di-methylethyl-amine hydro-chloride | | 291.8 | 161–2 | s. $H_2O$, EtOH, $CHCl_3$; sp. s. eth., benz. |
| Ephedrine | l-Ephedrine; $\alpha$-(1-methyl-aminoethyl)-benzyl alcohol; l-1-phenyl-2-methylamino-propanol | | 165.2 <br><br><br><br> HCl, 201.7 | 38 <br><br><br><br> HCl, 216–20 | s. $H_2O$, EtOH, $CHCl_3$, eth., oils. <br><br><br> HCl and sulphate, s. $H_2O$, EtOH; i. eth. |

| Action | Route | Absorption and fate | General remarks |
|---|---|---|---|
| Hypnotic, sedative (long lasting) | oral | Readily absorbed. Not bound to plasma proteins, excreted mainly by the kidney | Onset of effect is slow. Often used as sodium salt. Phenobarbitone is also long lasting. |
| Hypnotic of short duration used as surgical anaesthetic in animals (dose 35–40 mg/kg i.p.) | oral, i.v., i.p. | 50% bound to plasma proteins. Degraded by the liver. | Wh. cryst. powder or granules. Fluor., A 265 nm F 440 nm (pH 13–14). |
| Very short acting general anaesthetic | i.v. | 75–80% bound to plasma proteins. Rapidly taken up by body fat, degraded by the liver | Yel.-wh. hygr. powder. Alliaceous odour. Solns. are unstable. Immediate onset of anaesthesia. Fluor., A 315 nm F 513 nm (pH 13–14). |
| Central depressant, adrenolytic, antifibrillatory, antiedemic, hypothermic, antipyretic, antiemetic, local anaesthetic | oral, i.m. | Readily absorbed g.i.t. Highest blood level 3 hr. Distribution or metabolism unknown. Little urinary excretion (7–8% rabbits). Metabolized to the sulphoxide | Whitish grey powder sensitive to light. Enhances analgesic and hypnotic drugs and disrupts conditioned reflexes. A 5% aq. soln. stable at least 1 day and has pH 4.9. Fluor., A 350 nm F 480 nm (pH 11). Used as a calmodulin inhibitor, see p. 304. |
| Blood anticoagulant. Uncouples phosphorylation associated with oxidation of butyrate by liver mitochondria. At $10^{-5}$ M inhibits $NADH_2$ oxidase activity of heart muscle preps. | oral | Absorbed (variably) from g.i.t. Transformed slowly into intermediates. Bound to plasma proteins (especially albumin) up to 99% at dosage levels. Little urinary excretion | Wh. hexag. prisms. Acts by competitive interference with hepatic utilization of vitamin K in prothrombin synthesis. Other hepatic functions unaffected. Vitamin K does not affect disappearance rate from plasma. Latent period 24–96 hr (man). |
| Neuromuscular and ganglionic blocking agent. Inhibits cholinergic synaptic transmission to Renshaw cells | oral | | Longer acting than β-erythroidine and six times as active. |
| Antihistaminic | oral | Readily absorbed. Peak tissue concentration in 60 min. Concentration: lungs > spleen > kidney > liver > brain > muscle > skin. Excreted kidney, some unchanged, rest as unidentified degradation products, in 20–24 hr | Protective against death from anaphylactic shock, in dogs and guinea-pigs. |
| Sympathomimetic. Competitive inhibitor of choline dehydrogenase | oral, s.c. | Readily absorbed g.i.t. Over 50% eliminated by kidney in 12 hr. Unchanged in man. Dog excretes it mostly as norephedrine | Waxy crystal decomposing in light; HCl wh. needles. Predominant alkaloid of *Ephedra* spp. Aq. soln. stable to light, air, and heat. |

| Name | Synonyms | Formula | M. wt. | M.p. | Solubility |
|------|----------|---------|--------|------|------------|
| Heparin (Na salt) | | Heteropolysaccharide with repeating 4-$O$-($\alpha$-D-glucuronido)-D-glucosamine-$N$-sulphate units linked by $\alpha$-(1 → 4) hexosaminidic bonds and bearing between one and two $O$-sulphate groups per disaccharide | approx. 16 000– 17 000 | | s. $H_2O$; v. sp. s. EtOH, eth., $CHCl_3$ |
| Insulin | | A protein containing 51 amino-acid residues. For complete structure see BJ **60**, 541 (1955) | 5734 | | s. $H_2O$ |
| Isoproterenol | Isoprenaline; $N$-isopropyl-noradrenaline | HO—⟨ring⟩—CH(OH)CH$_2$NHCH(CH$_3$)$_2$ (with OH groups) | 211.2 | dl 155.5  <br> dl HCl, 170–1 | s. EtOH  <br> HCl, s. $H_2O$; sl. s. EtOH; i. $CHCl_3$, eth., benz. |
| Mechloreth-amine hydro-chloride | Mustargen; methyl-bis-($\beta$-chloro-ethyl)-amine hydrochloride | $CH_3 \cdot N \begin{cases} CH_2 \cdot CH_2Cl \\ CH_2 \cdot CH_2Cl \end{cases} \cdot HCl$ | 192.5 | 109–10 | v.s. $H_2O$; s. EtOH |
| Methonium compounds (a) Hexa-methonium | Hexamethyl-ene-bis(tri-methyl-ammonium); hexameton chloride. Bromide: Vegalysen | $(CH_3)_3\overset{+}{N}$—$[CH_2]_6$—$\overset{+}{N}(CH_3)_3$  <br> $Cl^-$  $Cl^-$ | Chloride, 273.3 | 289–92 d. | s. $H_2O$, EtOH; i. eth., $CHCl_3$ |
| (b) Deca-methonium | Decamethyl-ene-bis(tri-methyl-ammonium). Bromide: Syncurine | $(CH_3)_3\overset{+}{N}$—$[CH_2]_{10}$—$\overset{+}{N}(CH_3)_3$  <br> $Br^-$  $Br^-$ | Bromide, 418.4 | 255–67 d. | s. $H_2O$, EtOH; sl. s. $CHCl_3$; i. eth. |
| (c) Suxame-thonium bromide | Succinyl choline; bis(2-dimethyl-aminoethyl)-succinate bis-(metho-bromide); Brevidil M. | $Br^-$ $(CH_3)_3\overset{+}{N} \cdot CH_2 \cdot CH_2 \cdot O \cdot \overset{O}{\underset{}{C}} \cdot CH_2$  <br> $Br^-$ $(CH_3)_3\overset{+}{N} \cdot CH_2 \cdot CH_2 \cdot O \cdot \underset{O}{C} \cdot CH_2$ | Bromide, 450.2; Chloride, (dihydrate) 397.3 | 225  <br> 156–63 (dihydrate) | s. $H_2O$; sl. s. EtOH; i. eth. |
| Metrazol | Pentyl-enetetrazol; leptazol; cardiazol | ⟨ring structure⟩ | 138.2 | 57–60 | v.s. $H_2O$, EtOH, s. $CHCl_3$, $CCl_4$, eth. |

| Action | Route | Absorption and fate | General remarks |
|---|---|---|---|
| Anticoagulant | i.v., i.m., s.c. | Destroyed in g.i.t. After i.v. injection, disappears rapidly from plasma | Wh. amorph. powder; isolated as Na salt. May be sterilized by autoclaving, 110 °C, 30 min. $\alpha$- and $\beta$-forms known. Has chylocytic properties $[\alpha]_D + 65$ (in $H_2O$). Inhibits RNAase. Inhibits casein kinase II, $I_{50}$ 21 mg/ml, *Curr. Top. Cell. Regul.* **21**, 101 (1982). |
| Produces hypoglycaemia | i.m., i.v., s.c. | Rapidly absorbed from injection site, disappears from circulation, and is bound by tissues. Believed to be destroyed by insulinase present in muscle, liver, kidney; none excreted. | Zn insulin cryst. = 22 units/mg. Rapidly destroyed by proteolytic enzymes of g.i.t. Impure samples usually contaminated with glucagon, which mobilizes hepatic glycogen and increases blood sugar level. |
| $\beta$-Adrenergic activator, sympathomimetic, bronchodilator | oral (slowly absorbed) iv., inhalation | i.v. half-life in minutes, excreted in urine unchanged or conjugated, also some 3-methoxyisoprenaline and its conjugate formed and excreted by same route | Decomposes in neutral or alkaline solution; $pK_a$ 8.64. *L*-form of hydrochloride $[\alpha]_D^{19} - 50$. $\beta$-Receptor activation, *Ann. Rev. Biochem.* **52**, 159 (1983); *Adv. Cyc. Nuc. Res.* **14**, 51 (1981). |
| Cytotoxic, mitotic arrest, mutagenic | i.v. | Absorbed from g.i.t. and parenteral sites (local reaction). Active form is extremely short-lived. None excreted | Local vesicant. Mean lethal dose may produce delayed death in laboratory animals. In neutral or alkaline soln. rapid cyclization to highly reactive quaternary ammonium compound occurs. |
| Ganglionic blocking agent | oral, s.c., i.m., i.v. | Poorly absorbed g.i.t.; distributed extracellular fluids; excreted unchanged in urine | pH of 10% aq. soln. 5.5—6.5. Can be autoclaved. |
| Neuromuscular blocking agent | i.v. | Similar to hexamethonium | Aqueous soln. stable. Produces block by depolarization; does not pass placental barrier. |
| Short-acting neuromuscular blocking agent | i.v. | Rapid enzymic hydrolysis by non-specific plasma choline esterase; 5—15% excreted in urine | Solutions slightly acidic, not stable. |
| Central nervous system stimulant | i.v., oral | Rapidly absorbed, 75% excreted unchanged in urine. Metabolite temporarily stored in the liver | Wh. cryst. Will protect against toxic doses of central depressants. No direct effect on the heart. |

| Name | Synonyms | Formula | M. wt. | M.p. | Solubility |
|------|----------|---------|--------|------|------------|
| Morphine | | Hydrochloride, $C_{17}H_{19}NO_3 \cdot HCl \cdot 3H_2O$<br><br>Sulphate, $(C_{17}H_{19}NO_2)_2 \cdot H_2SO_4 \cdot 5H_2O$ | Hydrate, 303.3; Anhyd., 285.3<br><br>HCl (tri-hydrate), 375.8<br><br>Sulphate (penta-hydrate), 758.8 | Anhyd., 254d.<br><br>HCl, 250d.<br><br>$SO_4$, decomp. 250 | s. alkalis; sl. s. EtOH, MeOH; sp. s. $H_2O$, eth., $CHCl_3$<br><br>HCl and sulphate, s. $H_2O$; sl. s. EtOH; i. eth., $CHCl_3$ |
| Nicotine | | Hydrochloride, $C_{10}H_{14}N_2 \cdot 2HCl$ | 162.2<br><br>Di-HCl, 235.2 | B.p. 247 | Base and hydro-chloride, s. $H_2O$, EtOH, MeOH, $CHCl_3$ |
| Phenoxy-benzamine | Dibenzyline; dibenyline; N-(2-chloro-ethyl)-N-(1-methyl-2 phenoxy-ethyl)-benzyl-amine | | 303.8 | 38–40; Hydro-chloride, 137.5–40 | s. benz. HCl, s. EtOH, propylene glycol, $CHCl_3$; sp. s. $H_2O$ |
| Phentolamine | Regitine | | 281.4<br><br>HCl, 317.9 | 174–5<br><br>HCl, 239 | HCl, sl. s. $H_2O$ and EtOH; i. acet., Et. acetate |
| Picrotoxin | Cocculin | Picrotoxinin + Picrotin | Picrotoxinin, 292.3; Pircrotin, 310.3 | 203 | 0.3 $H_2O$; 8.3 EtOH; v.s. alkalis; sl. sl. $CHCl_3$, eth. |
| Pilocarpine | | | 208.3 | 34 | s. $H_2O$, EtOH, $CHCl_3$; sp. s. eth., benz.; i. pet. eth. |
| Probenecid | Benemid; p-(dipropyl-sulphamyl)-benzoic acid | | 285.4 | 198–200 | i. $H_2O$; s. $CHCl_3$, alkalis |

| Action | Route | Absorption and fate | General remarks |
|---|---|---|---|
| On c.n.s., narcotic and anal-gesic, respiratory depressant | oral, i.v. | Readily absorbed g.i.t. The majority is excreted, mainly as an unknown conjugated form in the urine | Loses $H_2O$ of cryst. at 110 °C. $[\alpha]_D^{20}$ −133 to −135 (c = 1 in EtOH). HCl, $[\alpha]_D^{20}$ −97 to −99 (c = 2 in $H_2O$). $SO_4$, $[\alpha]_D^{25}$ −107 to −109 (c = 2 in $H_2O$). Addiction and tolerance develop. Central excitation sometimes observed. Diacetylmorphine = heroin; morphine methyl ether = codeine. Morphine can be converted to a fluorescent derivative by treatment with conc. $H_2SO_4$ and then make alkaline with $NH_4OH$. Fluoresence in isobutanol, A 365 nm F 420 nm. |
| Cholinomimetic at ganglia and neuromuscular junction, central stimulant | | Absorbed rapidly from g.i.t., mucous membranes, and skin. Mainly metabolized in liver, kidney, and lungs but 10–20% excreted unchanged in man | Col. oil with burning taste; Di-HCl, hygr. cryst. Tolerance develops. Nor-nicotine is demethylated nicotine. |
| Adrenergic blocking agent | i.v., oral | 20–30% absorbed g.i.t.; maximum effect 1 h after i.v. injection. 50% excreted in urine and bile within 12 h | Does not block inhibitory adrenergic response. I.v. must be given slowly. Store in concentrated solution at pH 2.5–3. |
| α-Adrenergic blocker; vasodilator | oral; i.v. (4 times more active) | 5% of oral dose and 10% of i.v. dose excreted in urine in man | Aqueous solutions decompose especially if iron salts present. |
| C.n.s. stimulant and con-vulsant | i.v. | Absorbed all channels; leaves blood rapidly. Distri-bution unknown. Only pres-ent in urine if large amounts ingested | Shiny rh. leaflets. Bitter principle of *Anamirta cocculus*. Equimolecular compound of picrotin and picrotoxinin. Antidote to barbiturates. Protect from light. |
| Parasympathomimetic (selective action on tissue innervated by post-ganglionic cholinergic nerves) | oral, s.c. | After absorption most ex-creted in conjugated form | Oil. HCl. hygr. cryst. Nitrate generally used. Resembles muscarine and arecoline. Atropine antagonist. Stimulant to gastric secretion, miotic, diaphoretic. |
| Inhibitor of renal tubular transport | oral | Absorbed rapidly by g.i.t. Portion bound plasma pro-teins. Urinary excretion (free form) low. Slow con-jugation with glucuronic acid | Decreases elimination of organic acids (e.g. *p*-amino-salicylic acid, *p*-aminobenzoic acid). Inhibits glycine conjugation by preventing benzoyl-CoA formation. |

# 14 Pharmacologically active compounds

| Name | Synonyms | Formula | M. wt. | M.p. | Solubility |
|---|---|---|---|---|---|
| Procaine | Ethocaine; diethylamino-ethyl-*p*-amino-benzoate | $(C_2H_5)_2N \cdot CH_2 \cdot CH_2 \cdot O \cdot C$ (phenyl) $NH_2$, C=O | 236.3; HCl, 272.8 | Anhyd., 61; HCl, 154–6 | s. $H_2O$, EtOH; sl. s. $CHCl_3$, eth. HCl, s. $H_2O$; 12.5 95% EtOH; sl. s. $CHCl_3$; i. eth. |
| Propranolol | Inderal; propanolol | $OCH_2CHCH_2NHCH(CH_3)_2$, OH | 259.3 HCl, 295.8 | (±) 96 (+) or (−)73 HCl, (±) 163–4 (+) or (−) 192 | sl. s. cyclohexane; s. EtOH HCl, s. $H_2O$; EtOH; i. eth., benz., Et acetate |
| Propylthio-uracil | 6-Propyl-2-thiouracil | $C_2H_5 \cdot CH_2$ (thiouracil ring) | 170.2 | 219 | sl. s. $H_2O$, EtOH, $CHCl_3$, eth.; i. benz. |
| Prosta-glandins | | | | | |
| $E_1$ | 11α-15(S)-Dihydroxy-9-oxo-13-*trans*-prostenoic acid; $PGE_1$ | | 354.5 | 115–17 | v. sl. s. $H_2O$; s. MeOH, EtOH, ethyl-acetate, $CHCl_3$ |
| $E_2$ | 11α-15(S)-Dihydroxy-9-oxo-5-*cis*,13-*trans*-prosta-dienoic acid; $PGE_2$ | | 352.5 | 68–9 | |
| $A_1$ | 15(S)-Hydroxy-9-oxo-10,13-*trans*-prosta-dienoic acid; $PGA_1$ | | 336.5 | 42–4 | |
| $A_2$ | 15(S)-Hydroxy-9-oxo-5-*cis*, 10,13-*trans*-prostatrienoic acid; $PGA_2$ | | 334.5 | | |
| $F_{1α}$ | 9α,11α, 15(S)-Trihydroxy-5-*cis*-13-*trans*-prostenoic acid; $PGF_{1α}$ | | 356.5 | 102–3 | |

| Action | Route | Absorption and fate | General remarks |
|---|---|---|---|
| Local anaesthetic | infiltration | Readily absorbed after parenteral administration. Hydrolysed to PABA and diethylaminoethanol by choline esterase | Used as hydrochloride (needles). Procaine-sulphonamide antagonism exists (interferes with sulphonamide estimation). 0.2–2.0% for nerve block. Soln. unstable and slowly oxidized especially in the presence of heavy metals and alkali. Fluor., A 275 nm F 345 nm (pH 11). Calmodulin antagonist, PNAS **78**, 795 (1981). |
| $\beta$-Adrenergic blocker; abolishes oubain-induced arrhythmias | oral, i.v. | Peak plasma concentrations in 1–2 h. Decomposition products largely excreted in the urine within 24 h | The (−) isomer is much more active at blocking $\beta$-adrenergic stimulation. Neutral or alkaline solutions in $H_2O$ decompose with discolouration. More stable at pH 3. |
| Goitrogenic | oral | Readily absorbed g.i.t. 60% destroyed, 40% excreted in 24 hr | Wh. cryst. with bitter taste. Interferes with synthesis of thyroxine, triiodothyronine. Thyroid hyperplasia occurs in response to thyrotrophic hormone secretion. Less toxic than thiouracil. |
| Complex effects on reproductive, respiratory, g.i.t. and cardiovascular systems and mobilize free fatty acids from adipose tissues. Antagonists of hypotensive and diuretic action of angiotensin. | i.v. (can cause effect on blood vessels) | Can be absorbed from g.i.t. but the motility and secretion of the latter can be affected. Rapidly catabolized especially in the lungs. | Optical rotations measured in tetrahydrofuran $PGE_1 [\alpha]_{578}$ −61.6 (c = 0.56) $PGE_2 [\alpha]_D^{26}$ −61 (c = 1) $PGF_{2\alpha} [\alpha]_D^{25}$ +23.5 (c = 1) Generally unstable in aqueous solutions which are acid or alkaline. Maximum stability of $PGE_1$ and $PGE_2$ between pH 6–7. $PGF_{1\alpha}$ and $PGF_{2\alpha}$ stable at pH 5–11 at room temperature, but decompose under more acid conditions. Reviews, *J. Pharmaceutical Sciences* **61**, 1861 (1972) *Prog. Chem. Fats and other Lipids*, **9**, 233 (1968). *Meth. Enzymol.* **86** (1982). *Prostaglandins* (ed. J. B. Lee). Elsevier, New York (1982). |

| Name | Synonyms | Formula | M. wt. | M.p. | Solubility |
|------|----------|---------|--------|------|------------|
| Prosta-glandins (cont.) | | | | | |
| $F_{2\alpha}$ | $9\alpha,11\alpha,15(S)$-Trihydroxy-5-*cis*,13-*trans*-prostadienoic acid; $PGF_{2\alpha}$ | | 354.5 | 25–35 | |
| Reserpine | 3,4,5,Tri-methoxyben-zoyl methyl reserpate; Serpasil | | 608.9 | 264–5 d. | s. $CHCl_3$, benz., gl. acetic; sp. s. $H_2O$. HCl, s. $H_2O$. $H_2SO_4$, s. $H_2O$ |
| Strychnine | | $C_{21}H_{22}N_2O_2$ | 334.4 | 268 d. | s. $CHCl_3$; sl. s. benz., EtOH; sp. s. $H_2O$, eth. |
| | | Hydrochloride, $C_{21}H_{22}N_2O_2 \cdot HCl \cdot 2H_2O$ | HCl, 406.9 | | Hydrochloride and sulphate, s. $H_2O$; sl. s. $CHCl_3$, EtOH; i. eth. |
| | | Sulphate, $(C_{21}H_{22}N_2O_2)_2 \cdot H_2SO_4 \cdot 5H_2O$ | Sulphate, 857.0 | Anhyd. $SO_4$, 200 d. | |
| Tetraethyl-ammonium chloride | TEA chloride; etamon chloride | $(C_2H_5)_4N^+Cl^-$ | 165.7 (anhyd.) | Tetra-hydrate, 37.5 | v.s. $H_2O$, EtOH, $CHCl_3$, acet. |
| Tubo-curarine chloride | *d*-Tubo-curarine chloride | $2Cl^-$  $5H_2O$ | Anhyd., 695.7 Hydrate, 785.8 | Anhyd., de-comp. 274–5; Hydrate, 268–9 d. | s. alkalis; sp. s. $H_2O$, EtOH, MeOH; i. $CHCl_3$, acet. pyr. |
| Urethane | Ethyl carbamate | $NH_2 \cdot CO \cdot OC_2H_5$ | 89.1 | 50 | v.s. $H_2O$, EtOH, $CHCl_3$, eth.; s. vegetable oils, glycerol |

| Action | Route | Absorption and fate | General remarks |
|---|---|---|---|
| Hypotensive tranquilizer. Sedative | oral, s.c. | Absorbed g.i.t. Trimethoxy-benzoic acid excreted in urine of mice. Up to 15% unchanged in faeces | Long prisms. $pK_a$ 6.6. Releases catechol amines and 5-HT from stores in tissues. Fluor., A 300 nm F 375 nm (pH 1). Thought to interact with 4-aminobutyrate receptor sites on postsynaptic membranes, thus preventing access of the inhibitory transmitter, glycine. |
| Blocks postsynaptic inhibition. Convulsant | oral, i.m. | Readily absorbed by g.i.t. and from injection sites. Rapidly enters tissues especially c.n.s. Mainly destroyed by liver but some excreted unchanged | Col. rh. cryst. with very bitter taste; HCl and $SO_4$, efflor. cryst. |
| Ganglionic blocking agent. Sympathetic and parasympathetic ganglionic transmission blocked. Raises excitation threshold for acetylcholine. | i.m. | Poor absorption g.i.t. Rapid, quantitative excretion by kidney (glomerular and tubular) | Deliq. cryst,; prisms $+ 4H_2O$. |
| Autonomic blocking agent. Action brief. | i.v. (i.m.) | Distributed throughout body tissues; not bound to plasma proteins. About 30% excreted in urine (man) | Hex. and pent. platelets (from water). Quaternary base isolated from *Chondrodendron tomentosum*. In presence of moisture anhyd. form is rapidly converted to pentahydrate. |
| Cytotoxic, mitotic inhibitor; weak hypnotic | oral, i.p. | Absorbed rapidly g.i.t., greater part rapidly metabolized | Wh. prisms or needles with salty taste. Mechanism of cytotoxic effect undetermined. Less potent than nitrogen mustards. Used as an anaesthetic for small animals (1.2–1.5 g/kg i.p.) and fish (1:40 000 in $H_2O$). |

# 15 Artificial and natural substrates

## A. ELECTRON DONORS, CARRIERS AND ACCEPTORS

### General references

D. S. Bendall, Electron and Proton Transfer in Chloroplasts, Ch. 2 *in International Review of Biochemistry*, vol. 13, *Plant Biochemistry II*, ed. D. H. Northcote, University Park Press, Baltimore (1977), p. 41.

W. M. Clark, *Oxidation-reduction Potentials of Organic Systems*, Baillère, Tindall and Cox, London (1960).

G. Hauska, Artificial Acceptors and Donors, Ch. II. 15 in *The Encyclopedia of Plant Physiology* (N.S) vol. 5, *Photosynthesis I*, eds. A. Trebst and M. Avron, Springer-Verlag, Berlin (1977), p. 253.

A. Trebst, Measurement of Hill Reactions and Photoreduction, Ch. 14 in *Meth. Enzymol.* **24**, *Photosynthesis and Nitrogen Fixation, Part B.* ed. A. San Pietro, Academic Press, New York (1972), p. 146.

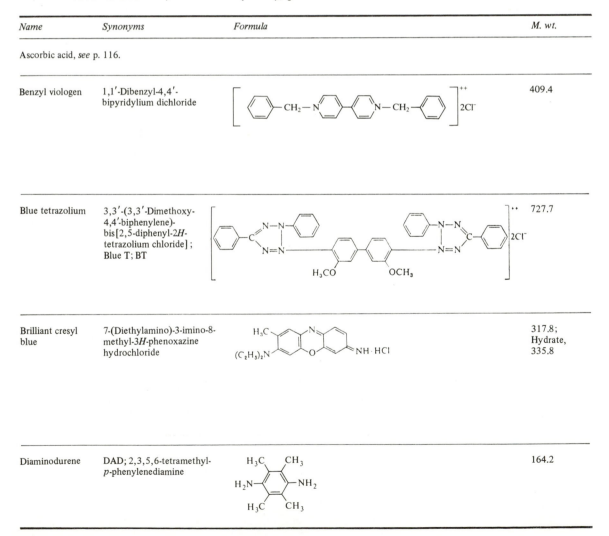

| *Name* | *Synonyms* | *Formula* | *M. wt.* |
|---|---|---|---|
| Ascorbic acid, *see* p. 116. | | | |
| Benzyl viologen | 1,1'-Dibenzyl-4,4'-bipyridylium dichloride | | 409.4 |
| Blue tetrazolium | 3,3'-(3,3'-Dimethoxy-4,4'-biphenylene)-bis[2,5-diphenyl-2*H*-tetrazolium chloride]; Blue T; BT | | 727.7 |
| Brilliant cresyl blue | 7-(Diethylamino)-3-imino-8-methyl-3*H*-phenoxazine hydrochloride | | 317.8; Hydrate, 335.8 |
| Diaminodurene | DAD; 2,3,5,6-tetramethyl-*p*-phenylenediamine | | 164.2 |

| Physical properties | Solubility | General remarks |
|---|---|---|
| col. cryst; $E_0'$ $-0.359$ V (30 °C; independent of pH) | s. $H_2O$, MeOH; i. acet. | Low potential electron acceptor and carrier. Oxidized form colourless to pale yellow, reduced form blue to violet. Reduced compd. v. readily oxidized by $O_2$; benzyl viologen used either anaerobically or as carrier to $O_2$ or non-autoxidizable acceptors. Reduced compd. used as an electron donor. Reduced by dithionite, borohydride. Stable reduced compd. at neutral pH formed by addition of one electron. *Reduced compd.*: $\lambda_{max}$ 555 nm at room temp. At higher temp. 555 nm peak diminishes and peak at 598 nm appears. At 80 °C only 598 nm peak is visible. |
| yel. needles; M.p. 245–7d | sl. s. $H_2O$; v.s. MeOH, EtOH, $CHCl_3$; i. acet., eth., Et acetate | Electron acceptor. Oxidized form colourless; reduced form (bis-formazan) blue to black. Reduced by flavoprotein enzymes, rate increased by intermediate electron carriers such as phenazine methosulphate. Hydrogen acceptor in Hill reaction. Used in estimation and detection of reducing steroids on chromatograms, especially adrenocortical steroids with α-ketol group. Not appreciably photolabile. |
| *Reduced compd.*: blue black needles; M.p. 244 | *Reduced compd.*: i. $H_2O$; s. most organic solvents | *Reduced compd.*: $\lambda_{max}$ about 520 nm (in EtOH), varies widely in other solvents. Not oxidized by $O_2$. |
| green needles $+ 1$ $H_2O$ from dil. EtOH; $E_0'$ $+0.047$ V (pH 7, 30 °C) | s. $H_2O$, EtOH, acet., gl. acetic; i. eth., benz. | Electron acceptor. Oxidized form blue, reduced form colourless. Reduced by flavoprotein enzymes, but not by soluble succinic dehydrogenase. Unstable in aq. soln., esp. alkaline solns., or as solid in presence of $H_2O$. Spectrum depends upon conc.; at 40 mg/l $\lambda_{max}$ 625 nm, at 1 g/l $\lambda_{max}$ 575 nm. Reduced by dithionite. Recryst. from pet. eth. Commercial product is now usually diethylamino compd., but may also be, esp. in older literature, dimethylamino compd. which has similar properties. *Reduced compd.*: reoxidized by air at pH 7 and above, but *not* below pH 6.4. Reoxidized by ferricyanide at all pHs. |
| $E_0'$ $+0.3$ V (pH 6.2); $pK_a$ 4.3; M.p. 153 | s. EtOH | Electron donor for PS I, best available for whole chloroplasts, *Meth. Enzymol.* **24**, 162 (1972). |

| Name | Synonyms | Formula | M. wt. |
|------|----------|---------|--------|
| 2,6-Dichloro-phenol-indophenol, Na salt | 2,6-Dichloroindo-phenol; N-(p-hydroxy-phenyl)-2,6-dichloro-p-benzoquinoneimine; DCPIP; DPIP | 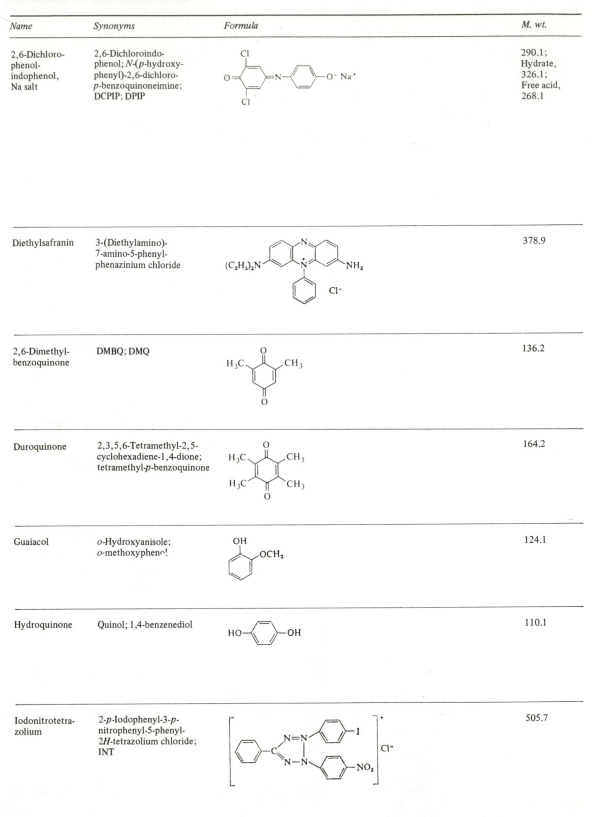 | 290.1; Hydrate, 326.1; Free acid, 268.1 |
| Diethylsafranin | 3-(Diethylamino)-7-amino-5-phenyl-phenazinium chloride | | 378.9 |
| 2,6-Dimethyl-benzoquinone | DMBQ; DMQ | | 136.2 |
| Duroquinone | 2,3,5,6-Tetramethyl-2,5-cyclohexadiene-1,4-dione; tetramethyl-p-benzoquinone | | 164.2 |
| Guaiacol | o-Hydroxyanisole; o-methoxyphenol | | 124.1 |
| Hydroquinone | Quinol; 1,4-benzenediol | | 110.1 |
| Iodonitrotetra-zolium | 2-p-Iodophenyl-3-p-nitrophenyl-5-phenyl-2H-tetrazolium chloride; INT | | 505.7 |

| Physical properties | Solubility | General remarks |
|---|---|---|
| dark green powder $+ 2H_2O$; hydration somewhat variable; $E_0' + 0.217$ V (pH 7, 30 °C); Oxidized $pK_a$ 5.9; Reduced $pK_a$ 7.0, 10.1; $\lambda_{max}$ approx. 600 nm ($\epsilon_{600}$ 22 000 (pH 7)) *BBA* **86**, 194 (1964). | s. $H_2O$; v.s. EtOH | Electron acceptor for PSII. Oxidized form blue at neutral pH, pink in acid, reduced form colourless. Reduced by flavoprotein enzymes; used in their assay, often with phenazine methosulphate as intermediate electron carrier. Addition of phenazine methosulphate allows coupling to nicotinamide nucleotide-linked dehydrogenases. Reduced compd. only v. slowly oxidized by $O_2$, so exclusion of air *not* necessary. Volumetric reagent, e.g. for ascorbic acid. Solid stable for years in air if kept dark, decomp. by heat and light. Aq. solns. decomp. slowly at neutral pH, rapidly below pH 3 or if strongly alkaline, and must be standardized daily for volumetric use. Reduced by ascorbic acid, dithionite, borohydride, reduced phenazine methosulphate, reduced ubiquinones, reduced vitamin K. Commercial preparations often impure. Purify by repeated transfer of acid form into ether, and alkaline form into carbonate/bicarbonate mixture. Salt out from carbonate/bicarbonate with NaCl. |
| $E_0' - 0.251$ V (pH 7); $\lambda_{max}$ 555 nm ($\epsilon$ approx. 49 000). | s. $H_2O$ | Reduced compd. used as hydrogen donor in fumarate reductase — *Meth. Biochem. Anal.* **4**, 307 (1957) — and similar reactions. Oxidized form red, reduced form colourless. Reduced form v. readily oxidized by $O_2$, generally prepared *in situ* by action of dithionite on oxidized form. Unstable esp. to acid and to air; prepare fresh daily. Generally impure because starting material, Janus Green B, is impure. |
| yel. cryst.; $E_0' + 0.18$ V (pH 7, 25 °C) | s. EtOH | Electron acceptor for photosystem II. 2,5-Dimethylbenzoquinone has been used similarly. |
| yel. cryst.; M.p. 110–2; $E_0' + 0.05$ V (pH 7, 25 °C) | s. EtOH | Electron acceptor for mitochondria and chloroplasts. Reduction to durohydroquinone, *FEBS Lett.* **96**, 252 (1978). |
| wh. or sl. yel. cryst. mass or col. to yel. liq.; M.p. 28; B.p. 204–6 | 1.5 $H_2O$; ∞ EtOH, $CHCl_3$, eth., gl. acetic | Hydrogen donor in assay of peroxidase, *Meth. Biochem. Anal.* **1**, 357 (1954). On oxidation forms tetraguaiacol which has $\lambda_{max}$ at 470 nm. Colour fades rapidly. Protect from light. |
| col. hexagonal prisms; dimorphous; stable form from $H_2O$; M.p. 170–1; B.p. 286–7; $pK_a$ 9.85, 11.4; $E_0' + 0.285$ V (pH 7, 25 °C) | 7 $H_2O$; s. EtOH, eth., acet.; sl. s. benz. | Electron donor. Reduces cytochrome c. Antioxidant. Keep well closed and protected from light. Soln. oxidizes in air, v. rapidly in presence of alkali. |
| buff or cream powder; M.p. 245d *Reduced compd.*: red-purple needles; M.p. 185–6 | $0.5^{25}$ $H_2O$ *Reduced compd.*: i. $H_2O$; s. most organic solvents | Electron acceptor. Oxidized form colourless, reduced form reddish purple. Readily reduced by flavoprotein enzymes; rate may be increased by intermediate electron carriers such as phenazine methosulphate. Used in assay of dehydrogenases by non-enzymic coupling to NADH or NADPH with phenazine methosulphate, *JBC* **235**, 499 (1960); *Analyt. Biochem.* **1**, 317 (1960). Much less photolabile than triphenyltetrazolium. Soln. stable at 5 °C for months. Reduced by reducing sugars, ascorbic acid, $NH_2OH$ in alkaline soln., by reduced phenazine methosulphate, reduced ubiquinones, reduced vitamin K at neutral pH. *Reduced compd.* (formazan): $\lambda_{max}$ about 500 nm (varies slightly with solvent). Not oxidized by $O_2$. |

| Name | Synonyms | Formula | M. wt. |
|------|----------|---------|--------|
| Menadione | Vitamin K₃; menaphthone; 2-methyl-1,4-naphthoquinone; menaquinone | | 172.2 |
| Methylene blue | Methylthionine chloride; 3,7-bis(dimethylamino)-phenazathionium chloride | | 319.9 (anhyd.) |
| Methyl viologen | 1,1′-Dimethyl-4,4′-bipyridylium dichloride; Paraquat | | 257.2; + 3H₂O, 311.3 |
| Neotetrazolium | 3,3′-(4,4′-Biphenylene)-bis[2,5-diphenyl-2H-tetrazolium chloride]; NeoT; NT | | 667.6 |
| Nitroblue tetrazolium | 3,3′-(3,3′-Dimethoxy-4,4′-biphenylene)-bis[2-(p-nitrophenyl)-5-phenyl-2H-tetrazolium chloride]; NitroBT | | 817.7 |

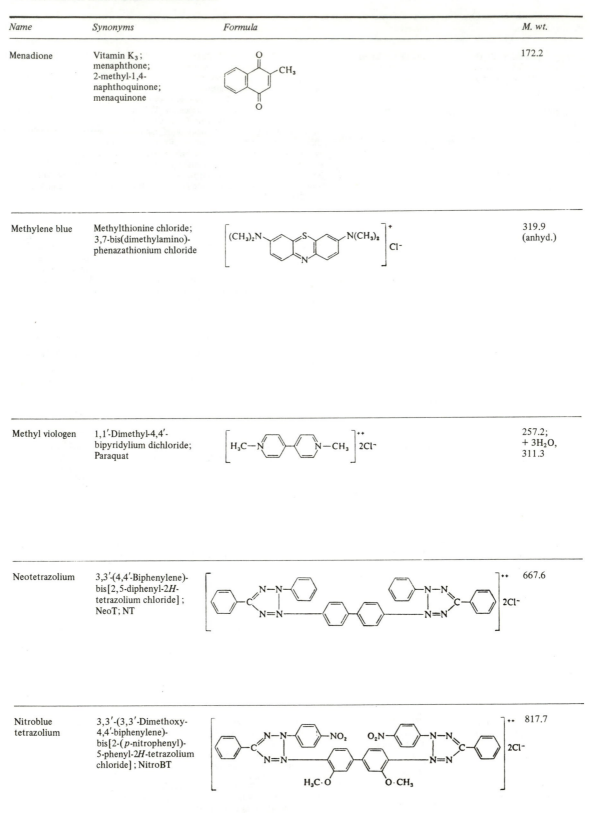

| Physical properties | Solubility | General remarks |
|---|---|---|
| bright yel. needles; M.p. 105–7; $E_0'$ 0 V (pH 7, 25 °C) | 1.7 EtOH; 10 benz.; s. eth., CHCl$_3$, CCl$_4$; i. H$_2$O | Electron carrier. Reduced by flavoprotein enzymes. Oxidation-reduction may be followed at 262 nm. Frequently used as an electron carrier to O$_2$ or non-autoxidizable acceptors such as indophenols or tetrazolium salts. Effect of pH on redox potential, *FEBS Lett.* **105**, 189 (1979). Cofactor of cyclic photophosphorylation. Stable in air but decomp. by sunlight. Solns. stable at 120°C but destroyed by reducing agents or alkalis. In hexane, $\lambda_{max}$ 244, 253, 264, 328 nm $\epsilon$ 19 800, 19 700, 16 800, 3100. In aq. buffer pH 6.24, $\lambda_{max}$ 250, 263–4, 340 nm. *Reduced compd.* (menadiol): greyish-wh. powder, M.p. 160–7, PREP. *JBC* **133**, 391 (1940), $\lambda_{max}$ 241, 330 nm (in aq. buffer pH 6.24), p$K_a$ 9.5, 11.0 (approx.). Readily oxidized by air at neutral or alkaline pH, very slowly oxidized at pH 6.3 and below. |
| dark green cryst. + 3–5 H$_2$O; $E_0'$ + 0.011 V (pH 7, 30 °C) | 4.3 H$_2$O; 1.5 EtOH; sl. s. CHCl$_3$; i. eth. *Reduced compd.*: v. sl. s. H$_2$O | Electron acceptor. Oxidized form blue; reduced form colourless. Reduced by flavoprotein enzymes, but not by soluble succinic dehydrogenase; rate often increased by intermediate electron carriers such as phenazine methosulphate. Reduced compd. readily reoxidized in air, so methylene blue is either used anaerobically or as carrier to O$_2$. Oxidizes on standing as solid and esp. in soln. to give demethylated forms. Loses H$_2$O of cryst. only with partial decomp. Spectrum depends upon concentration; at $10^{-5}$ M $\lambda_{max}$ 665 nm. Above $10^{-4}$ M main peak between 610 and 570 nm tending to lower wavelengths at higher concs. Peak at 665 nm falls and virtually disappears at $10^{-3}$ M. See *JACS* **77**, 4197 (1955). Reduced by dithionite, reduced flavins, reduced phenazine methosulphate, reduced quinones. Possesses vitamin E activity. *Reduced compd.*: Tends to stick to glass surfaces. Reoxidized by O$_2$ or anaerobically by light; oxidation rate increases with pH. Stable under N$_2$ in dark. |
| col. needles + 3H$_2$O, lose H$_2$O at 50 °C; $E_0'$ − 0.446 V (30 °C, independent of pH) | s. H$_2$O, MeOH; i. acet. | V. low potential electron acceptor. Oxidized form colourless, reduced form blue to violet. Reduced compd. v. readily oxidized by O$_2$, so methyl viologen is used anaerobically or as carrier to O$_2$ or non-autoxidizable acceptor. Reduced compd. used as electron donor, e.g. in hydrogenase reaction. Reduced by dithionite, borohydride. Stable reduced form at neutral pH formed by addition of one electron. The 1,1′-dimethyl-4,4′-bipyridylium ion, usually as the dimethosulphate, is a herbicide, 'Paraquat'. Estimation, *Nature, Lond.* **199**, 1011 (1963). *Reduced compd.*: $\lambda_{max}$ 601 nm, shoulder at 570 nm. |
| col. needles; M.p. 230d *Reduced compd.*: dark violet needles; M.p. 219–20 d. | s. H$_2$O; 5 MeOH *Reduced compd.*: i. H$_2$O; s. most organic solvents | Electron acceptor. Oxidized form pale yellow, reduced form (bis-formazan) magenta. Reduced by flavoprotein enzymes, rate increased by intermediate electron carriers such as phenazine methosulphate. Use in assay of succinoxidase, *BJ* **73**, 314 (1959). Not sensitive to sunlight, no decomp. of soln. in 4 hr in direct sunlight. Reduced by reducing sugars, ascorbic acid, NH$_2$OH at alkaline pH, by reduced phenazine methosulphate, reduced ubiquinones, reduced vitamin K$_3$ at neutral pH. *Reduced compd.*: $\lambda_{max}$ about 520 nm (varies widely with solvent). Not oxidized by O$_2$. |
| cryst. containing solvent; trihydrate, M.p. 156 d; anhydrous chloride hydroxide, M.p. 134 *Reduced compd.*: black cryst.; M.p. 270–2d. | s. H$_2$O *Reduced compd.*: i. H$_2$O; s. most organic solvents | Electron acceptor. Oxidized form colourless; reduced form (bis-formazan) blue to black. Rapidly reduced by flavoprotein enzymes, rate increased by electron carriers such as phenazine methosulphate. Most commonly used tetrazolium salt for histochemical detection of dehydrogenases, see Burstone, *Enzyme Histochemistry*, Academic Press (1962). Used, with phenazine methosulphate, in detection of dehydrogenases on electrophoretograms, *Meth. Enzymol.* **6**, 958 (1963). Not appreciably photolabile. *Reduced compd.* (bis-formazan): has v. marked affinity for protein, e.g. *not* extracted into Et acetate from aq. suspension containing gelatin. $\lambda_{max}$ approx. 550 nm (varies widely with solvent). |

## 15 Artificial and natural substrates

| Name | Synonyms | Formula | M. wt. |
|---|---|---|---|
| Phenazine methosulphate | *N*-Methyl-phenazinium methylsulphate; PMS | (structure) $CH_3SO_4^-$ | 306.3 |
| *p*-Phenylene diamine | 1,4-Diaminobenzene | $H_2N$—(benzene ring)—$NH_2$ | 108.1; 2 HCl, 181.1 |
| Plastoquinone, *see* p. 132 | | | |
| Potassium ferricyanide | | $K_3[Fe(CN)_6]$ | 329.3 |
| Pyocyanine | | (structure) | 210.2; Hydrate, 228.3 |
| Pyrogallol | 1,2,3-Trihydroxy-benzene | (structure) OH, OH, OH | 126.1 |
| Sodium boro-hydride | | $NaBH_4$ | 37.8 |

| Physical properties | Solubility | General remarks |
|---|---|---|
| yel. to brown parallelepipeds from EtOH; M.p. 167; $E_0' + 0.080$ V (pH 7, 30 °C) *Reduced compd.*: M.p. 164 | 10 $H_2O$ *Reduced compd.*: v. sl. s. $H_2O$ | Electron acceptor and electron carrier. Oxidized form yellow, reduced form colourless, green semiquinone sometimes observed. Rapidly reduced by flavoprotein enzymes, incl. succinic dehydrogenase — *Meth. Biochem. Anal.* **4**, 307 (1957). Reduced compd. v. readily oxidized by $O_2$, so PMS normally used in assays as electron carrier between enzymes and $O_2$, cytochrome c, or less readily autoxidizable electron acceptors e.g. indophenols or tetrazolium salts. $H_2O_2$ formed on autoxidation of $PMSH_2$ and since PMS completely inhibits catalase, other provision to remove $H_2O_2$, e.g. $CN^-$ or 8-hydroxyquinoline, may be necessary. PMS reduced non-enzymically by NADH and NADPH; used to couple dehydrogenases to other electron acceptors, e.g. indophenols, tetrazolium salts. Electron carrier in cyclic photophosphorylation and stimulates Hill reaction. Reduced compd. used as an electron donor, e.g. to reduce cytochrome c or in photosynthetic expts. For use in enzymic reactions best to use enzymically reduced material (tissue prep. + NADH). Solid stable years in dark. Prepare solns. in $H_2O$ *not* neutral buffers; such solns. keep frozen and in dark for several months. Unstable to light, forming pyocyanine and other products; in sunlight decomp. in 5–10 min, but takes hours in diffuse light. Stabilized by polyvalent cations. Reduced by dithionite, borohydride, NADH, NADPH, ascorbic acid, reduced ubiquinones, reduced vitamin K. Reacts with –SH compds., incl. –SH enzymes. $\lambda_{max}$ 387 nm ($\epsilon$ 26 300) (pH 2–8); $\Delta\epsilon$ (ox-red) 25 000. *Reduced compd.*: Solid stored 2–3 weeks in air at −20 °C, but in soln. and at working temp. v. rapidly oxidized by $O_2$. Rapidly reduces cytochrome c, indophenol dyes, tetrazolium salts, and many other electron acceptors, *Meth. Enzymol.* **24**, 162 (1972). |
| wh. cryst., darken on exposure to air; M.p. 145–7; B.p. 267; $pK_a$ 2.67, 6.16 | 1 $H_2O$; s. hot $H_2O$, EtOH, $CHCl_3$, eth. | Electron donor. Reduces cytochrome c, *Meth. Enzymol.* **24**, 161 (1972). Store in dark and well closed. |
| monocl. red cryst.; decomp. on heating; $E_0' + 0.42$ V (pH >3.5, 25 °C) | 48.8$^{25}$ $H_2O$; sl. s. MeOH, EtOH, acet. | Electron acceptor for PS II and mild oxidizing agent. Reduction may be followed by decrease in absorbance at 420 nm ($\epsilon$ 1020). Reduced at several sites in electron transport chain. Oxidizes reduced cytochrome c. Redox potential under various conditions, *BBA* **292**, 509 (1973). Aq. soln. decomp. slowly on standing, protect from light. Oxidizes –SH groups to –S–S–. |
| dark blue needles + 1 $H_2O$ from $H_2O$; loses $H_2O$ *in vacuo* over $P_2O_5$ at 50 °C; M.p. 133; $E_0' - 0.034$ V (pH 7, 30 °C) | v.s. $CHCl_3$; s. hot $H_2O$, hot EtOH, acet., gl. acetic, pyr., phenol, Et acetate; sl. s. cold $H_2O$, benz., i. eth., pet. eth., $CCl_4$ | Electron acceptor and carrier. PREP. *Org. Synth.* **Coll. 3**, 753 (1955); *JCS* **1937**, 1704. Oxidized form blue, reduced form colourless. Very effective cofactor of cyclic photophosphorylation, *Pl. Physiol.* **34**, 240 (1959). Reduced pyocyanine used as an electron donor in fumarate reductase; best prepared enzymically with tissue prep. + NADH, *JBC* **229**, 755 (1957). Solid stable weeks in dry and dark, decomp. on long storage. Reduced by dithionite, borohydride, and in alkaline soln. by glucose. Formed by cultures of *Pseudomonas aeruginosa*. $\lambda_{max}$ 239, 312, 379, 690 nm (pH 7–8) $\epsilon_{700}$ 3400 (pH 7). *Reduced compd.*: V. rapidly oxidized by $O_2$. |
| wh. cryst.; M.p. 133; B.p. 309; $pK_a$ 9.0 | 62.5$^{25}$ $H_2O$; 78$^{25}$ EtOH; 64$^{25}$ eth.; sl. s. benz., $CHCl_3$, $CS_2$ | Hydrogen donor in peroxidase assay, *Meth. Biochem. Anal.* **1**, 357 (1954). On oxidation forms purpurogallin, which has $\lambda_{max}$ at 430 nm ($\epsilon$ 2470). Oxygen absorber in strongly alkaline solution. Poisonous. Keep well closed and protected from light. Aq. soln. oxidizes in air, rapidly when alkaline. Strong reducing agent. |
| cubic cryst.; decomp. >300 | 10 isopropylamine; 3 pyr.; 1 morpholine; 0.8 dimethyl cellosolve; s. $H_2O$; sl. s. tetrahydrofuran | Powerful reducing agent, reduces many physiological and artificial electron carriers. Reduces pyridoxal phosphate Schiff's bases to stable –$CH_2$–NH– links. Solid stable if dry, decomp. in moist air. Reacts slowly with water at room temp., less rapidly if NaOH is added. |

| Name | Synonyms | Formula | M. wt. |
|---|---|---|---|
| Sodium dithionite | Sodium hydrosulphite; sodium sulphoxylate | $Na_2S_2O_4 \cdot 2H_2O$ | 210.2; Anhydrous, 174.1 |
| $N,N,N',N'$-Tetramethyl-*p*-phenylene diamine | TMPD | 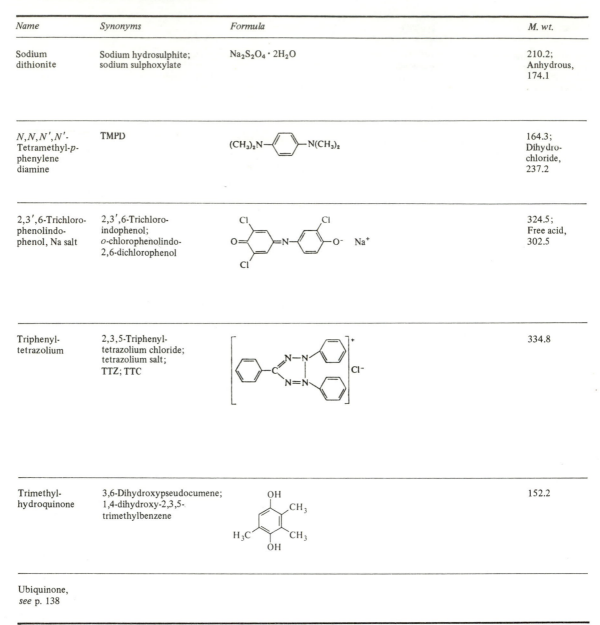 | 164.3; Dihydrochloride, 237.2 |
| 2,3′,6-Trichlorophenolindophenol, Na salt | 2,3′,6-Trichloroindophenol; *o*-chlorophenolindo-2,6-dichlorophenol | | 324.5; Free acid, 302.5 |
| Triphenyltetrazolium | 2,3,5-Triphenyltetrazolium chloride; tetrazolium salt; TTZ; TTC | | 334.8 |
| Trimethylhydroquinone | 3,6-Dihydroxypseudocumene; 1,4-dihydroxy-2,3,5-trimethylbenzene | | 152.2 |

Ubiquinone,
*see* p. 138

| Physical properties | Solubility | General remarks |
|---|---|---|
| monocl. cryst. or yel. powder; decomp. 52; $pK_a$ 2.4, 6.4; $\lambda_{max}$ 314 nm $\epsilon$ 8000. For redox potentials, *see EJB* **85**, 535 (1978). | $25.4^{20}$ $H_2O$; s. alkalis, dil. acids; sp. s. EtOH | Powerful reducing agent, used to reduce many physiological and artificial electron carriers including NAD, NADP, flavins and cytochromes. Oxidizes in air, readily when damp or in soln., but dry solid only v. slowly. Solutions should normally be prepared in buffer, pH $>7.5$ preferably. Generates $SO_2$ in solution. |
| leaflets from aq. EtOH or ligroin; M.p. 51; B.p. 260; $E_0'$ + 0.26 V (pH 7) | v.s. EtOH, eth., $CHCl_3$, benz.; s. ligroin; sp. s. $H_2O$ | Electron donor. Reduces cytochrome c; generally used in catalytic amounts with ascorbate as bulk electron donor. Keep solid protected from light. Soln. unstable. Oxidized form (Wurster's blue) is a stable free radical $\lambda_{max}$ 560 nm $\epsilon$ 12 100, 606 nm $\epsilon$ 11 600. PREP. *JACS* **65**, 1747 (1948). Dihydrochloride, cryst., M.p. 222–4; solubility 10 $H_2O$. |
| green cryst. + up to 17% $H_2O$; $E_0'$ + 0.219 V (pH 7, 30 °C) | s. $H_2O$; v.s. EtOH | Electron acceptor. In neutral soln., oxidized form blue, reduced form colourless. Reduced by flavoprotein enzymes. Used as acceptor in Hill reaction. Reduced compd. used as electron donor, e.g. in nitrate reductase. Oxidation by $O_2$ occurs v. slowly. Solid stable in air if kept dark, decomp. slowly in light. Aq. solns. decomp. on standing, esp. at acid pH. Reduced by ascorbic acid, dithionite, reduced phenazine methosulphate. $\lambda_{max}$ approx. 645 nm $\epsilon$ 27 000 (pH 7.3). *Reduced compd.*: Stable several days under $H_2$ at R.T. |
| solvated needles, lose solvent on heating; M.p. 243 d.; $E_0'$ − 0.080 V (pH 7) *Reduced compd.*: red leaflets; M.p. 173.5 | 25 $H_2O$; s. MeOH, EtOH; sl. s. acet., $CHCl_3$; i. eth. *Reduced compd.*: i. $H_2O$; s. most organic solvents | Electron acceptor. Oxidized form colourless to pale yellow, reduced form red. Slowly reduced by flavoprotein enzymes, rate increased by intermediate electron carriers such as phenazine methosulphate or pyocyanine. For testing seed viability, *Science* **113**, 751 (1951). Indicator of bacterial growth in bioautography, *Appl. Microbiol.* **2**, 29 (1954). Least toxic to bacteria of tetrazolium salts. Review of uses, *Tetrazolium Salts*, B.D.H. Ltd., Poole, England. Turns yellow on exposure to light. Decomp. by visible or u.v. light. Nonenzymic reduction by reducing sugars, ascorbic acid, $NH_2OH$ requires alkaline pH. *Reduced compd.* (formazan): $\lambda_{max}$ about 490 nm (varies slightly with solvent). Not oxidized by $O_2$. |
| $E_0'$ + 0.115 V (pH 7, 25 °C); M.p. 169–72 | 10 MeOH | Electron donor. Mid-point oxidation-reduction potentials of the trimethylbenzoquinone system as a function of pH given in *International Review of Biochemistry* **13**, p. 66, but note the semiquinone potentials should be 30 mV nearer each other than shown. |

# B. SUBSTRATES FOR PEPTIDASES

## Assay of peptidases

Methods of assay of peptidases, using natural and artificial substrates, are described in *Meth. Biochem. Anal.* **2**, 215 (1955); **4**, 171 (1957); *Meth. Enzymol.* **2**, 3–114 (1955); Bergmeyer, *Methods of Enzymatic Analysis*, pp. 800–36, Academic Press (1963).

| Name | Synonyms | Formula | M. wt. |
|---|---|---|---|
| *N*-Acetyl-L-tyrosine ethyl ester | ATEE | HO—⟨C₆H₄⟩—$CH_2 \cdot CH \cdot CO \cdot O \cdot C_2H_5$, $NH \cdot CO \cdot CH_3$ | 251.3; Hydrate, 269.3 |
| α-*N*-Benzoyl-L-arginin-amide hydrochloride | BAA | $H_2N—C—NH \cdot (CH_2)_3 \cdot CH \cdot CO \cdot NH_2$, NH, $NH \cdot CO \cdot C_6H_5$  ·HCl | 313.8; Hydrate, 331.8; Free base, 277.3 |
| α-*N*-Benzoyl-L-arginine ethyl ester hydrochloride | BAEE | $H_2N \cdot C \cdot NH \cdot (CH_2)_3 \cdot CH \cdot CO \cdot O \cdot C_2H_5$, NH, $NH \cdot CO \cdot C_6H_5$  ·HCl | 342.8; Free base, 306.4 |
| *N*-Benzoyl-L-tyrosine ethyl ester | BTEE | HO—⟨C₆H₄⟩—$CH_2 \cdot CH \cdot CO \cdot O \cdot C_2H_5$, $NH \cdot CO \cdot C_6H_5$ | 313.4 |
| Glycylglycine | Diglycine | $H_2N \cdot CH_2 \cdot CO \cdot NH \cdot CH_2 \cdot COOH$ | 132.1 |
| Glycylglycyl-glycine | Diglycylglycine; triglycine | $H_2N \cdot CH_2 \cdot CO$  $NH \cdot CH_2 \cdot COOH$, $NH \cdot CH_2 \cdot CO$ | 189.2 |
| Glycyl-L-phenylalanin-amide acetate | | $H_2N \cdot CH_2 \cdot CO \cdot NH \cdot CH \cdot CO \cdot NH_2$, $CH_2$, ⟨C₆H₅⟩ · $CH_3 \cdot COOH$ | 281.3; Free base, 221.3 |
| Glycyl-L-proline | | $H_2C—CH_2$, $H_2C$  $CH \cdot COOH$, N, $H_2N \cdot CH_2 \cdot CO$ | 172.2; Hydrate, 181.2 |

| Physical properties | Solubility | General remarks |
|---|---|---|
| pale cream powder $+ 1 H_2O$; M.p. 87–88; $[\alpha]_D^{20} + 24$ (c = 1 in EtOH) | v. sl. s. $H_2O$; s. hot $H_2O$ | Substrate for assay of chymotrypsin. Hydrolysis followed by decrease in absorbance at 237 nm (pH 7), *BBA* **16**, 570 (1955), or by appearance of carboxyl gps., *Meth. Biochem. Anal.* **2**, 215 (1955), **4**, 171 (1957). Super-saturated solns. (0.01 M–0.02 M), stable for 6–12 hours, prepared by dissolving at 85 °C and rapid cooling to room temp. (25 °C). Stronger solns. must be maintained at elevated temp. |
| cryst. $+ 1 H_2O$; sinters 120–3, loses $H_2O$ 135–40, decomp. $> 260$; $[\alpha]_D^{25} - 17.2$ (in $H_2O$) | s. $H_2O$ | Substrate for assay of trypsin, papain, cathepsin B, ficin, bromelin. Hydrolysis followed by release of carboxyl gps. or of ammonia, *Meth. Biochem. Anal.* **2**, 215 (1955); *Biochem. Preps.* **6**, 61 (1958). Soln. keeps for months at 5 °C with thymol as preservative. |
| hygr. cryst.; M.p. 129.5–131; $[\alpha]_D^{22} - 17.5$ (c = 2 in $H_2O$) | s. $H_2O$ | Substrate for assay of trypsin, papain, ficin. Hydrolysis followed by increase in absorbance at 253 nm (pH 8), *BBA* **16**, 570 (1955), or by release of carboxyl groups, *Meth. Biochem. Anal.* **2**, 215 (1955), **4**, 171 (1957). Hydrolyses slowly in soln., 4% in 24 hr at 4 °C and pH 8. |
| cryst.; M.p. 122–3; $[\alpha]_D^{20} - 23.7$ (c = 3.7 in EtOH) | v. sl. s. $H_2O$; s. aq. MeOH, EtOH | Substrate for assay of chymotrypsin, completely resistant to trypsin. Hydrolysis followed by increase in absorbance at 256 nm, *Can. J. Biochem. Physiol.* **37**, 1393 (1959), or by release of carboxyl gps., *Meth. Biochem. Anal.* **2**, 215 (1955), **4**, 171 (1957). |
| col. plates; M.p. 215–20d. ($> 250$d.); $pK_a$ 3.14, 8.25 | $13.4^{25}$ $H_2O$, v.s. hot $H_2O$; v. sl. s. EtOH; i. eth. | Substrate for the assay of glycylglycine dipeptidase, see *Meth. Enzymol.* **2**, 107 (1955), *Meth. Biochem. Anal.* **2**, 215 (1955). Used as a buffer. Hydrochloride, needles $+ 1H_2O$. |
| monocl. cryst. from $H_2O$; M.p. 244–6d; $pK_a$ 3.23, 8.09 | $6.2^{25}$ $H_2O$, v.s. hot $H_2O$; i. EtOH, eth. | Substrate for the assay of aminotripeptidase, see *Meth. Enzymol.* **2**, 83 (1955), *Meth. Biochem. Anal.* **2**, 215 (1955). |
| cryst.; $[\alpha]_D^{26} + 28.8$ (c = 5 in $H_2O$) | s. $H_2O$ | Substrate for assay of cathepsin C, also hydrolysed by chymotrypsin. Hydrolysis followed by release of $NH_3$ or of carboxyl groups, *Meth. Biochem. Anal.* **2**, 215 (1955), or by transfer to hydroxylamine, *Meth. Enzymol.* **2**, 64 (1957). |
| hygr. prisms $+ \frac{1}{2}H_2O$; M.p. 185; $pK_a$ 2.81, 8.65; $[\alpha]_D^{24} - 115.2$ (c = 1 in $H_2O$) | v.s. $H_2O$; sl. s. EtOH | Soln. keeps only a few days at 5 °C due to diketopiperazine formation. Substrate for the assay of prolidase (imidodipeptidase), see *Meth. Enzymol.* **2**, 100 (1955), *Meth. Biochem. Anal.* **2**, 215 (1955). |

| Name | Synonyms | Formula | M. wt. |
|------|----------|---------|--------|
| Glycyl-L-tyrosinamide acetate | | | 297.3; Free base, 237.3 |
| Hide powder blue | | | |
| Hippuryl-L-arginine | Benzoylglycyl-L-arginine | | 335.4 |
| Hippuryl-L-phenylalanine | Benzoylglycyl-L-phenylalanine | | 326.4 |
| L-Leucinamide hydrochloride | | $(CH_3)_2CH \cdot CH_2 \cdot CH(NH_2) \cdot CO \cdot NH_2 \cdot HCl$ | 166.7; Free base, 130.2 |
| L-Leucylglycine | | | 188.2 |
| L-Prolylglycine | | | 172.2; Hydrate, 190.2 |
| $\alpha$-N-Toluene-p-sulphonyl-L-arginine methyl ester hydrochloride | p-Tosyl-L-arginine methyl ester hydrochloride; TAME | | 378.9; Free base, 342.4 |
| L-Tyrosine ethyl ester hydrochloride | | $HO-\langle\rangle-CH_2 \cdot CH(NH_2) \cdot CO \cdot OC_2H_5 \cdot HCl$ | 245.7; Free base, 209.2 |

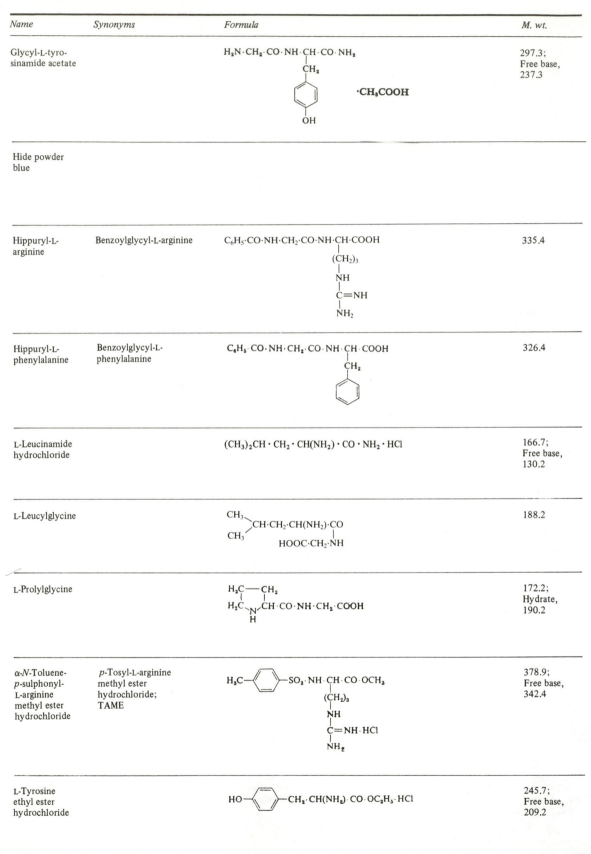

| Physical properties | Solubility | General remarks |
|---|---|---|
| cryst.; $[\alpha]_D^{22} + 28.0$ (c = 10 in $H_2O$) | s. $H_2O$ | Substrate for assay of cathepsin C, also hydrolysed by chymotrypsin. Hydrolysis followed by release of $NH_3$ or of carboxyl groups, *Meth. Biochem. Anal.* **2**, 215 (1955), or by transfer to hydroxylamine, *Meth. Enzymol.* **2**, 64 (1957). Slow spontaneous hydrolysis occurs at pHs above 7.8, even at 4 °C. Negligible over 2–3 hour period but significant after a few days storage. |
| | i. $H_2O$ | An insoluble substrate derived from hide powder labelled covalently with Remazolbrilliant Blue. Measure dye released by proteases at 595 nm. Not affected by presence of albumin. For comparison with Azacoll (a dyed denatured collagen prep.; dye released assayed at 580 nm), see *Clin. Chim. Acta* **21**, 197 (1968). |
| M.p. 182–6; $[\alpha]_D^{20} - 2.8$ (c = 2 in MeOH) | s. $H_2O$, MeOH | Substrate for assay of carboxypeptidase B. Hydrolysis followed by increase in absorbance at 254 nm, *JBC* **235**, 2272 (1960), or by release of amino N, *Meth. Biochem. Anal.* **2**, 215 (1955). |
| $[\alpha]_D^{25} + 39$ (c = 5 in 95% EtOH) | | Substrate for assay of carboxypeptidase A. Hydrolysis followed by increase in absorbance at 254 nm, *JBC* **238**, 3884 (1963), or by release of amino N, *Meth. Biochem. Anal.* **2**, 215 (1955). |
| long needles from MeOH-eth.; M.p. 246–8d.; $[\alpha]_D^{25} + 10.0$ (c = 1 in $H_2O$) | s. $H_2O$, MeOH | Substrate for assay of leucine aminopeptidase. Hydrolysis followed by release of $NH_3$ or of carboxyl groups, *Biochem. Preps.* **6**, 35 (1958); *Meth. Biochem. Anal.* **2**, 215 (1955). Soln. keeps several weeks at pH 8.5 and 5 °C with thymol added as preservative. |
| needles from EtOH/$H_2O$; M.p. 245 d.; $pK_a$ 3.25, 8.28; $[\alpha]_D^{21} + 89.8$ (c = 2.4 in $H_2O$) | s. $H_2O$ | Substrate for the assay of peptidases, especially leucine aminopeptidase, see *Meth. Biochem. Anal.* **2**, 215 (1955); *Meth. Enzymol.* **2**, 88 (1955). |
| rods or needles + $1H_2O$, sl. hygr.; M.p. 236 d.; $pK_a$ (at I = 0.16) 3.19, 8.97; $[\alpha]_D^{20} - 22.5$ (c = 0.1–2 anhyd. in $H_2O$) | s. $H_2O$ | Substrate for assay of iminodipeptidase (prolinase), see *Meth. Biochem. Anal.* **2**, 215 (1955), *Meth. Enzymol.* **2**, 97 (1955). Soln. keeps only a few days at 5 °C due to diketopiperazine formation. |
| M.p. 147.5–148; $[\alpha]_D^{18} - 14.4$ (c = 4 in $H_2O$) | s. $H_2O$ | Substrate for assay of trypsin, not attacked by chymotrypsin. Also hydrolysed by papain, plasmin, and thrombin. Hydrolysis followed by release of carboxyl groups, *Meth. Biochem. Anal.* **2**, 215 (1955), **4**, 171 (1957). Hydrolyses slowly above pH 9. |
| M.p. 166–8; $[\alpha]_D^{20} - 6.8$ (c = 2 in $H_2O$) | v. sl. s. $H_2O$; s. aq. MeOH | Substrate for assay of chymotrypsin, not hydrolysed by trypsin. Hydrolysis followed by decrease in absorbance at 233.5 nm (pH 6.5), *BBA* **16**, 570 (1955), or by release of carboxyl groups, *Meth. Biochem. Anal.* **2**, 215 (1955), **4**, 171 (1957). Hydrolyses slowly in soln., 4% in 24 hr at 4 °C and pH 7. Free ester, prisms, M.p. 108–9, $[\alpha]_D^{20} + 20.4$ (c = 4.85 in EtOH). |

# C. SUBSTRATES AND INDUCERS FOR GLYCOSIDASES

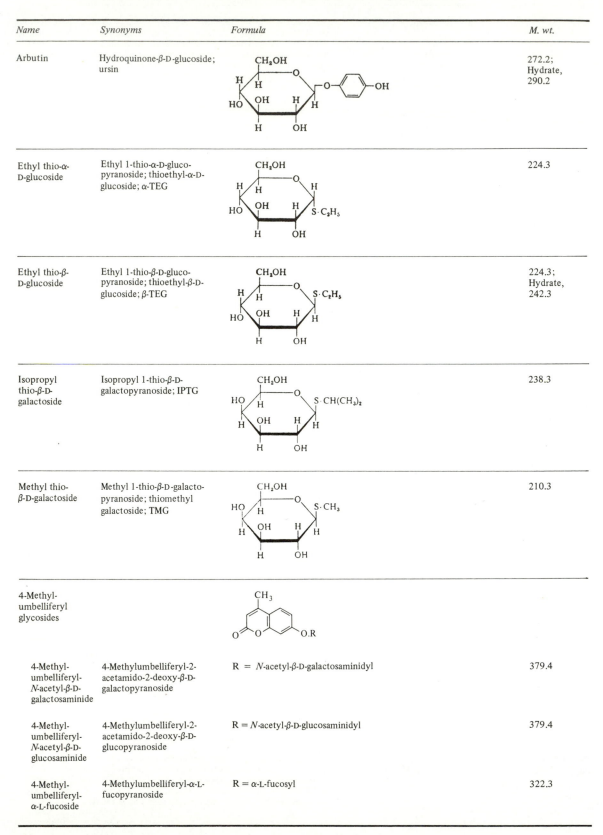

| Name | Synonyms | Formula | M. wt. |
|---|---|---|---|
| Arbutin | Hydroquinone-β-D-glucoside; ursin | | 272.2; Hydrate, 290.2 |
| Ethyl thio-α-D-glucoside | Ethyl 1-thio-α-D-gluco-pyranoside; thioethyl-α-D-glucoside; α-TEG | | 224.3 |
| Ethyl thio-β-D-glucoside | Ethyl 1-thio-β-D-gluco-pyranoside; thioethyl-β-D-glucoside; β-TEG | | 224.3; Hydrate, 242.3 |
| Isopropyl thio-β-D-galactoside | Isopropyl 1-thio-β-D-galactopyranoside; IPTG | | 238.3 |
| Methyl thio-β-D-galactoside | Methyl 1-thio-β-D-galacto-pyranoside; thiomethyl galactoside; TMG | | 210.3 |
| 4-Methyl-umbelliferyl glycosides | | | |
| 4-Methyl-umbelliferyl-N-acetyl-β-D-galactosaminide | 4-Methylumbelliferyl-2-acetamido-2-deoxy-β-D-galactopyranoside | R = N-acetyl-β-D-galactosaminidyl | 379.4 |
| 4-Methyl-umbelliferyl-N-acetyl-β-D-glucosaminide | 4-Methylumbelliferyl-2-acetamido-2-deoxy-β-D-glucopyranoside | R = N-acetyl-β-D-glucosaminidyl | 379.4 |
| 4-Methyl-umbelliferyl-α-L-fucoside | 4-Methylumbelliferyl-α-L-fucopyranoside | R = α-L-fucosyl | 322.3 |

| Physical properties | Solubility | General remarks |
|---|---|---|
| long needles +1H$_2$O; M.p. 200; $[\alpha]_D^{20} - 64$ (c = 3 in H$_2$O) | s. H$_2$O, EtOH, eth. | Non-reducing sugar. Colour with FeCl$_3$-blue. Substrate for $\beta$-glucosidase. |
| needles; M.p. 117; $[\alpha]_D^{20} + 261.5$ (c = 2 in H$_2$O) | s. H$_2$O | Inducer of $\alpha$-glucosidase; *not* hydrolysed by this enzyme. |
| cryst. + 1 H$_2$O, M.p. 42–44; Anhyd., M.p. 99.5; $[\alpha]_D - 55$ (c = 4 anhyd. in H$_2$O) | s. H$_2$O, EtOH; sl. s. acet.; v. sl. s. eth. | Inducer of $\beta$-glucosidase (cellobiase), *not* hydrolysed by this enzyme, *BBA* **36**, 47 (1959). Loses H$_2$O of cryst. *in vacuo* at 65 °C. |
| col. needles; M.p. 109.5–110.5; $[\alpha]_D^{22} - 31.4$ (in H$_2$O) | v.s. H$_2$O, MeOH, EtOH; sl. s. acet., CHCl$_3$; i. eth. | Inducer of $\beta$-galactosidase and $\beta$-galactoside permease; *not* hydrolysed by $\beta$-galactosidase, *BBA* **31**, 525 (1959). Substrate for thiogalactoside trans-acetylase, *JBC* **237**, 253 (1962). |
| col. needles; M.p. 174–5; $[\alpha]_D^{20} + 10.7$ (in H$_2$O) | s. H$_2$O, MeOH; i. eth., CHCl$_3$ | Inducer of $\beta$-galactosidase and $\beta$-galactoside permease; *not* hydrolysed by $\beta$-galactosidase, *BBA* **31**, 525 (1959). |
| | | Fluorimetric assay of glycosidases, *Meth. Biochem. Anal.* **17**, 256 (1969). These substrates show relatively little fluorescence but on hydrolysis yield 4-methylumbelliferone which fluoresces intensely in alkaline soln. At pH 10.3, excitation max. is at 364 nm, fluorescence max. at 448 nm. Substrates stable at −20 °C, stored dry and protected from light. |
| | | Substrate for assay of *N*-acetyl-$\beta$-D-galactosaminidase. |
| | | Substrate for assay of *N*-acetyl-$\beta$-D-glucosaminidase. |
| | | Substrate for assay of $\alpha$-L-fucosidase. |

## 15  Artificial and natural substrates

| Name | Synonyms | Formula | M. wt. |
|---|---|---|---|
| 4-Methyl-umbelliferyl-α-D-galactoside | 4-Methylumbelliferyl-α-D-galactopyranoside | R = α-D-galactosyl | 338.3 |
| 4-Methyl-umbelliferyl-α-D-glucoside | 4-Methylumbelliferyl-α-D-glucopyranoside | R = α-D-glucosyl | 338.3 |
| 4-Methyl-umbelliferyl-β-D-glucoside | 4-Methylumbelliferyl-β-D-glucopyranoside | R = β-D-glucosyl | 338.3 |
| 4-Methyl-umbelliferyl-β-D-glucuronide | | R = β-D-glucuronidyl | 352.3; Trihydrate, 406.3 |
| 4-Methyl-umbelliferyl-α-D-mannoside | 4-Methylumbelliferyl-α-D-mannopyranoside | R = α-D-mannosyl | 338.3 |
| 4-Methyl-umbelliferyl-β-D-xyloside | 4-Methylumbelliferyl-β-D-xylopyranoside | R = β-D-xylosyl | 308.3 |
| o-Nitrophenyl β-D-galactoside | o-Nitrophenyl β-D-galactopyranoside; Niphegal; ONPG | | 301.3 |
| o-Nitrophenyl β-D-glucoside | o-Nitrophenyl β-D-glucopyranoside | | 301.3 |
| p-Nitrophenyl N-acetyl-β-D-glucosaminide | p-Nitrophenyl 2-acetamido-2-deoxy-β-D-glucopyranoside | | 342.3 |
| p-Nitrophenyl β-D-galactoside | p-Nitrophenyl β-D-galactopyranoside | | 301.3 |

| Physical properties | Solubility | General remarks |
|---|---|---|
| | | Substrate for assay of α-D-galactosidase. Enzyme deficient in Fabry's disease. |
| | | Substrate for assay of α-D-glucosidase. |
| M.p. 212–14;<br>$[\alpha] - 94.5$<br>(c = 1 in $H_2O$) | | Substrate for assay of β-D-glucosidase. Enzyme deficient in Gaucher's disease. |
| | | Substrate for assay of β-D-glucuronidase. |
| | | Substrate for assay of α-D-mannosidase. |
| $[\alpha] - 30.2$ (c = 0.3 in $H_2O$) | | Substrate for β-D-xylosidase. |
| needles; M.p. 193–4; $[\alpha]_D^{20} - 66$<br>(c = 1 in $H_2O$) | s. $H_2O$, MeOH | Substrate for the assay of β-galactosidase (lactase). Hydrolysis followed by release of o-nitrophenol which is yellow in alkaline soln. ($\lambda_{max}$ 420 nm $\epsilon$ 21 300 at pH 10.2), *Adv. Carbohydr. Chem.* **16**, 239 (1961); *Meth. Enzymol.* **1**, 241 (1957). |
| needles + $H_2O$ from $H_2O$.<br>Hydrate, M.p. 130–1, Anhyd.,<br>M.p. 168–70; $[\alpha]_D^{18.5} - 140.4$<br>(c = 2.14 anhyd. in $H_2O$) | s. $H_2O$ | Substrate for β-glucosidase, hydrolysed by emulsin enzyme, *BJ* **57**, 1 (1954), but not by that from *Stachybotrys atra*, *Aust. J. Biol. Sci.* **8**, 541 (1955). Hydrolysis followed by release of o-nitrophenol which is yellow in alkaline soln. ($\lambda_{max}$ 420 nm $\epsilon$ 21 300 at pH 10.2). Loses $H_2O$ of cryst. *in vacuo* over $P_2O_5$ at 110 °C. |
| M.p. 210–12; $[\alpha]_D^{20} - 15$ (c = 0.5 in $H_2O$);<br>$\lambda_{max}$ 300 nm $\epsilon$ 10 800 (in 0.1M-NaOH). | $0.78^{20}$ $H_2O$ | Substrate for assay of N-acetyl-β-D-glucosaminidase. Hydrolysis followed by release of p-nitrophenol which is yellow in alkaline soln. ($\lambda_{max}$ 400 nm $\epsilon$ 18 300 at pH 10.2), *BJ* **78**, 106 (1961). Sensitive to daylight or u.v. but not tungsten light in strongly alkaline soln. but stable at pH 9.2 or below. |
| cryst.; M.p. 185–90d; $[\alpha]_D^{21} - 84$<br>(c = 0.3 in $H_2O$) | s. $H_2O$, MeOH | Substrate for assay of β-galactosidase (lactase). Hydrolysis followed by release of p-nitrophenol which is yellow in alkaline soln. ($\lambda_{max}$ 400 nm $\epsilon$ 18 300 at pH 10.2), *BJ* **83**, 331 (1962). |

## 15 Artificial and natural substrates

| Name | Synonyms | Formula | M. wt. |
|---|---|---|---|
| *p*-Nitrophenyl α-D-glucoside | *p*-Nitrophenyl α-D-glucopyranoside | | 301.3 |
| *p*-Nitrophenyl β-D-glucoside | *p*-Nitrophenyl β-D-glucopyranoside | | 301.3 |
| Phenolphthalein β-D-glucuronide | Phenolphthalein β-D-glucopyranosiduronic acid | | 494.5 |
| Salicin | Saligenin β-D-glucopyranoside | | 286.2 |

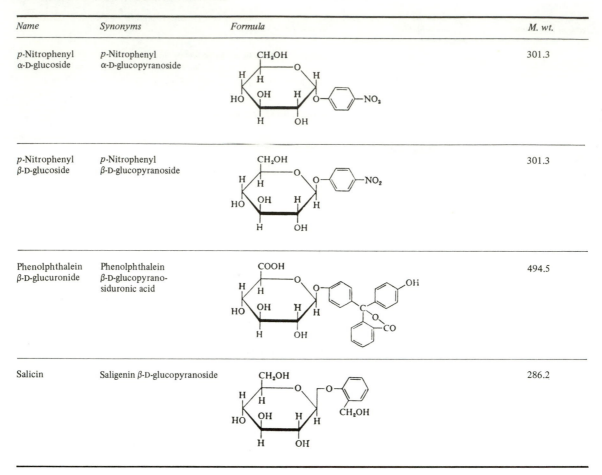

| Physical properties | Solubility | General remarks |
|---|---|---|
| prisms; M.p. 216–17; $[\alpha]_D^{17} + 215$ (c = 1 in $H_2O$) | s. $H_2O$ | Substrate for the assay of α-glucosidases (maltase and isomaltase). Hydrolysis followed by release of p-nitrophenol which is yellow in alkaline soln. ($\lambda_{max}$ 400 nm $\epsilon$ 18 300 at pH 10.2), *BBA* **30**, 28 (1958). |
| col. needles from $H_2O$; dry *in vacuo* at 90 °C; Anhyd., M.p. 164–5; $[\alpha]_D^{20} - 108$ (c = 1 anhyd. in $H_2O$) | s. $H_2O$ | Substrate for assay of β-glucosidase (cellobiase). Hydrolysis followed by release of p-nitrophenol which is yellow in alkaline soln. ($\lambda_{max}$ 400 nm $\epsilon$ 18 300 at pH 10.2), *BZ* **337**, 146 (1963); *JBC* **233**, 1113 (1958). |
|  | s. $H_2O$ | Substrate for the assay of β-glucuronidase. Hydrolysis followed by formation of phenolphthalein which is red in alkaline soln., max. colour development at pH 10.3–11.2 ($\lambda_{max}$ approx. 550 nm $\epsilon$ 26 600), *Adv. Carbohydr. Chem.* **14**, 381 (1959); *Meth. Enzymol.* **1**, 262 (1957); *Meth. Biochem. Anal.* **15**, 77 (1967). Soln. stable at 0 °C for months. $\lambda_{max}$ 420 nm $\epsilon$ 130 (pH 10). |
| needles or prisms; M.p. 201; $[\alpha]_D^{20} - 62$ (c = 5 in $H_2O$) | s. $H_2O$, NaOH soln., gl. acetic, pyridine; v. sl. s. EtOH; i. $CHCl_3$, eth. | Substrate for β-glucosidase. Non-reducing sugar. Colour with conc. $H_2SO_4$ – purple. |

## D. SUBSTRATES FOR PHOSPHATASES

For naturally occurring phosphate esters, *see* Phosphate esters, pp. 55–73.

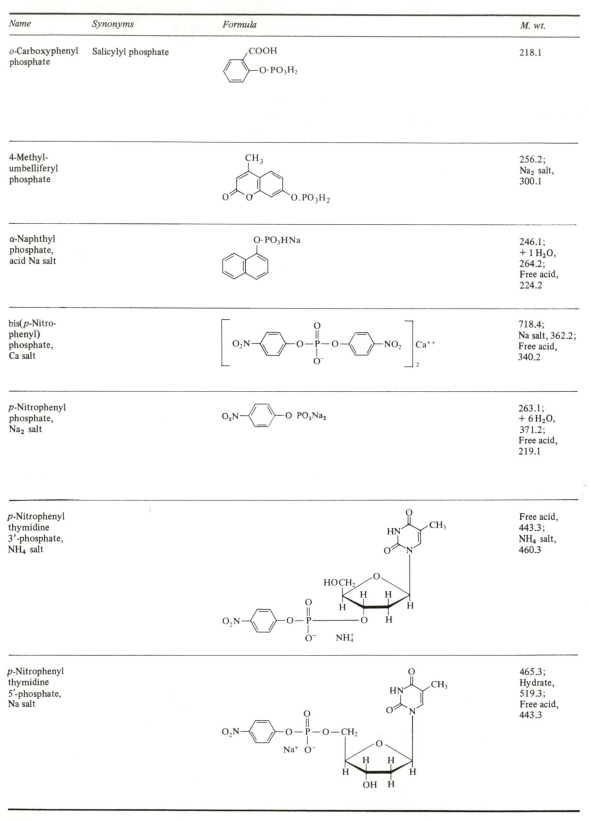

| Name | Synonyms | Formula | M. wt. |
|------|----------|---------|--------|
| *o*-Carboxyphenyl phosphate | Salicylyl phosphate | | 218.1 |
| 4-Methyl-umbelliferyl phosphate | | | 256.2; Na$_2$ salt, 300.1 |
| α-Naphthyl phosphate, acid Na salt | | | 246.1; + 1 H$_2$O, 264.2; Free acid, 224.2 |
| bis(*p*-Nitrophenyl) phosphate, Ca salt | | | 718.4; Na salt, 362.2; Free acid, 340.2 |
| *p*-Nitrophenyl phosphate, Na$_2$ salt | | | 263.1; + 6 H$_2$O, 371.2; Free acid, 219.1 |
| *p*-Nitrophenyl thymidine 3′-phosphate, NH$_4$ salt | | | Free acid, 443.3; NH$_4$ salt, 460.3 |
| *p*-Nitrophenyl thymidine 5′-phosphate, Na salt | | | 465.3; Hydrate, 519.3; Free acid, 443.3 |

| Physical properties | Solubility | General remarks |
|---|---|---|
| non-hygr. needles; M.p. 154–5; p$K_a$ 0.95, 3.5, 6.11 | v.s. $H_2O$, EtOH, dioxan; i. pet. eth., toluene | Phosphomonoesterase substrate, *ABB* **51**, 139 (1954). Hydrolysis followed by increase in absorbance at 310 nm due to release of salicylic acid. $\lambda_{max}$ for salicylic acid is at 295–300 nm, use of 310 nm avoids slight absorbance due to the phosphate and to protein. Advantage that salicylic acid absorbs over whole pH range, $\epsilon_{310}$ 1900 above pH 5, at lower pH $\epsilon_{310}$ rises to 3200 at pH 1. Non-enzymic hydrolysis occurs at max. rate at pH 5.2, slowly at room temp., complete in 1 hr at 80–90 °C. Stable in soln. above pH 8, almost completely stable below pH 2. |
| | | Substrate for alkaline phosphatase. At pH 10.3, 4-methylumbelliferone formed is intensely fluorescent, excitation max. at 364 nm, fluorescence max. at 448 nm. At pH 5 the fluorescence is less intense but still easily measureable, excitation max. then shifted to 330 nm, *Meth. Biochem. Anal.* **17**, 254 (1969). Bis(4-methylumbelliferyl) phosphate used for detection of phosphodiesterase in membranes, *BBA* **465**, 667 (1977). |
| wh. cryst. | s. $H_2O$ | Substrate for phosphomonoesterases, especially prostatic enzyme, *Am. J. Clin. Path.* **32**, 88 (1959). Hydrolysis releases α-naphthol which is estimated colorimetrically after coupling with a diazonium salt, e.g. tetrazotized *o*-dianisidine, or by fluorimetry, *BJ* **76**, 32P (1960). Useful for detection of phosphatases on electrophoretograms. Stable in soln. above pH 8, but slow hydrolysis occurs below pH 6. Free acid, wh. cryst., M.p. 155–6, p$K_a$ 0.97, 5.85. |
| | s. $H_2O$ | Substrate for phosphodiesterases, *JBC* **198**, 293 (1952). Hydrolysis releases *p*-nitrophenol which is yellow in alkaline soln. ($\lambda_{max}$ 400 nm $\epsilon$ 18 300 at pH 9–10). Early methods used 440 nm but 400 nm preferable. Store in cold, dry and dark. Soln. keeps weeks in cold if sl. acid but deteriorates rapidly if alkaline. Virtually no absorbance at 400 nm in alkali. Na salt, wh. cryst. powder, M.p. 174–6. |
| light yel. cryst.; hydration variable; $\lambda_{max}$ 290 nm (pH 2.3) 310 nm (pH 9.2) $\epsilon$ 9500 (all pHs). Free acid, p$K_{a2}$ 5.70. | s. $H_2O$ | Substrate for phosphomonoesterases, *BBA* **258**, 178 (1972); *Meth. Enzymol.* **4**, 371 (1957); gives higher rates than glycerol phosphate, phenyl phosphate, or phenolphthalein phosphate. Hydrolysis releases *p*-nitrophenol which is yellow in alkaline soln. ($\lambda_{max}$ 400 nm $\epsilon$ 18 300 at pH 9–10). *p*-Nitrophenyl phosphate has slight absorbance at 400 nm so 405–20 nm sometimes used. Store solid in cold and dark. Soln. decomposes slowly; store in cold and dark and renew every few weeks. Completely hydrolysed by M-HCl in 3 hr at 100 °C. |
| anhyd. cryst.; $\lambda_{max}$ 270.5 nm $\epsilon$ 15 400. | s. $H_2O$ | Substrate for spleen phosphodiesterase and enzymes of similar specificity, *Meth. Enzymol.* **6**, 245 (1963). Not hydrolysed by venom enzyme. Hydrolysis releases *p*-nitrophenol which is yellow in alkaline soln. ($\lambda_{max}$ 400 nm $\epsilon$ 18 300 at pH 9–10). |
| cryst. +3$H_2O$; loses $H_2O$ at 100 °C under reduced pressure; $\lambda_{max}$ 270 nm $\epsilon$ 16 250 (pH 2). | s. $H_2O$, MeOH; i. eth. | Substrate for venom phosphodiesterase and enzymes of similar specificity, *Meth. Enzymol.* **6**, 237 (1963). Gives rate many times higher than bis(*p*-nitrophenyl) phosphate. Not hydrolysed by spleen enzyme. Hydrolysis releases *p*-nitrophenol which is yellow in alkaline soln. ($\lambda_{max}$ 400 nm $\epsilon$ 18 300 at pH 9–10). |

## 15 Artificial and natural substrates

| Name | Synonyms | Formula | M. wt. |
|---|---|---|---|
| Phenolphthalein phosphate, Na$_4$ salt | Phenolphthalein diphosphate | 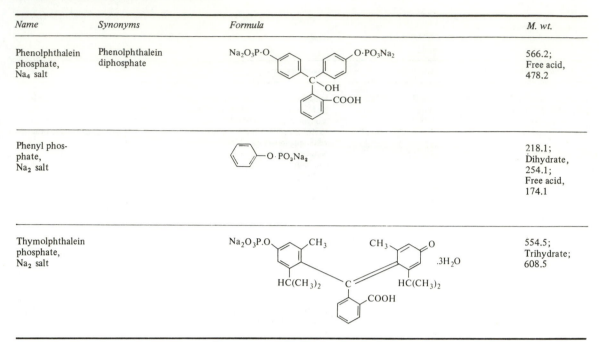 | 566.2; Free acid, 478.2 |
| Phenyl phosphate, Na$_2$ salt | | | 218.1; Dihydrate, 254.1; Free acid, 174.1 |
| Thymolphthalein phosphate, Na$_2$ salt | | | 554.5; Trihydrate; 608.5 |

| Physical properties | Solubility | General remarks |
|---|---|---|
| amorphous | s. $H_2O$ | Substrate for phosphomonoesterases, *Enzymologia* **31**, 309 (1966); *Clin. Chem.* **13**, 941 (1967); *J. Assoc. Off. Anal. Chem.* **64**, 196 (1981). Hydrolysis releases phenolphthalein which is red ($\lambda_{max}$ approx. 550 nm) in alkaline soln., max. colour at pH 10.3–11.4. Stable if stored cold, dry and dark. No absorbance at 550 nm in alkaline soln. |
| wh. cryst.<br>Free acid, M.p. 94, p$K_{a2}$ 5.73. | s. $H_2O$, MeOH, eth. | Substrate for phosphomonoesterases, *Meth. Biochem. Anal.* **4**, 257 (1957); Bergmeyer, *Methods of Enzymatic Analysis*, p. 785, Academic Press (1963), *J. Assoc. Off. Anal. Chem.* **64**, 196 (1981). Hydrolysis releases phenol which may be estimated colorimetrically or by increase in absorbance at 287 nm in alkaline soln., *BBA* **52**, 36 (1961). Keep cold, dry and dark. Solns. deteriorate slowly; store in cold and prepare fresh every 1–2 weeks. |
|  |  | Substrate for alkaline phosphatase. Hydrolysis releases thymolphthalein, measured at pH 10, $\lambda_{max}$ approx. 600 nm, *Clin. Chem.* **17**, 1093 (1971). |

## E. SUBSTRATES FOR ESTERASES AND LIPASES

Any ester is a potential esterase substrate. Hydrolysis may be followed by measurement of acid released, by titration, e.g. in a pH stat (*Meth. Biochem. Anal.* **4**, 171, 1957), or by measurement of unhydrolysed ester by the hydroxamic acid method, *JBC* **180**, 249 (1949).

| Name | Synonyms | Formula | M. wt. |
|------|----------|---------|--------|
| Acylsalicylic acids | 2-Acyloxybenzoic acids | COOH / $-O \cdot CO \cdot R$ | 120.1 + M. wt. of *acid* OR 165.1 + R; Acetyl, 180.2 |
| Fluorescein diacetate | | $CH_3-CO-O-$ ... $-O-CO-CH_3$ $\cdot CO$ | 416.4 |
| 4-Methyl-umbelliferyl esters | | $CH_3$ / $O$ ... $O \cdot R$ | |
| ——, acetate | | $R = -CO \cdot CH_3$ | 218.2 |
| ——, butyrate | | $R = -CO \cdot (CH_2)_2 \cdot CH_3$ | 246.3 |
| ——, elaidate (*trans*) | | $R = -CO \cdot (CH_2)_7 \cdot CH = CH \cdot (CH_2)_7 \cdot CH_3$ | 440.5 |
| ——, heptanoate | | $R = -CO \cdot (CH_2)_5 \cdot CH_3$ | 288.4 |
| ——, nonanoate | | $R = -CO \cdot (CH_2)_7 \cdot CH_3$ | 316.4 |
| ——, oleate (*cis*) | | $R = -CO \cdot (CH_2)_7 \cdot CH = CH \cdot (CH_2)_7 \cdot CH_3$ | 440.5 |
| ——, palmitate | | $R = -CO \cdot (CH_2)_{14} \cdot CH_3$ | 414.6 |
| ——, propionate | | $R = -CO \cdot CH_2 \cdot CH_3$ | 232.2 |
| β-Naphthyl esters | 2-Naphthyl esters | $O \cdot CO \cdot R$ | 126.2 + M. wt. of *acid* OR 171.2 + R; Acetate, 186.2; Laurate, 326.5 |
| *p*-Nitrophenyl esters | | $O_2N-$ ... $-O \cdot CO \cdot R$ | 121.1 + M. wt. of *acid* OR 166.1 + R; Acetate, 181.2 |
| Phenyl esters | | $-O \cdot CO \cdot R$ | 76.1 + M. wt. of *acid* OR 121.1 + R; Acetate, 136.2 |

| Physical properties | Solubility | General remarks |
|---|---|---|
| Acetyl, needles, M.p. 135; Higher homologues, cryst. solids | sl. s. H₂O, decreasing with increasing chain length of acid; s. alkali; s. organic solvents | Substrates for assay of esterases. Hydrolysis releases salicylic acid which has $\lambda_{max}$ 290–300 nm, not found in its esters, *JBC* **199**, 357 (1952). Keep solns. in cold and prepare fresh daily. |
| needles from EtOH; M.p. 200 | | Fluorogenic substrate for assay of esterases, *Meth. Biochem. Anal.* **17**, 251 (1969). Use as an indicator of cell viability, *PNAS* **55**, 134 (1966); *Stain Tech.* **47**, 189 (1972). |
| | s. H₂O | Fluorogenic substrates for the assay of esterases and lipases, *Anal. Biochem.* **21**, 279 (1967). |

| | | *Enzymes assayed:* |
|---|---|---|
| | | Esterases |
| M.p. 91 | | Esterases |
| | | Lipases |
| M.p. 41–2 | | Esterases |
| M.p. 47–9 | | Esterases; lipases |
| M.p. 38–40 | | Lipases |
| M.p. 70–2 | | Lipases |
| | | Esterases |

| Physical properties | Solubility | General remarks |
|---|---|---|
| wh. solids; Acetate, M.p. 70; Laurate, M.p. 58–60; Stearate, M.p. 73–75 | sl. s. H₂O, decreasing with increasing chain length of acid; s. EtOH, acet., eth., CHCl₃ | β-Naphthyl acetate used as substrate for assay of esterases, *J. Clin. Invest.* **29**, 31 (1950); β-naphthyl laurate for assay of lipase, *JBC* **181**, 343 (1949), Bergmeyer, *Methods of Enzymatic Analysis*, p. 776, Academic Press (1963). Hydrolysis releases β-naphthol which may be estimated colorimetrically by coupling with a diazotized amine. Stock solns. in acet. keep at 4 °C for at least 14 days. Dilute with water or buffer, to form soln. or emulsion depending on chain length of acid, immediately before use. |
| Acetate, pyramidal cryst., M.p. 81; Propionate, wh. needles, M.p. 62–63; *n*-Butyrate, liq. | Acetate, 0.06²⁵ H₂O; 0.03²⁵ 0.025 M-NaHCO₃–CO₂ buffer pH 7.5; s. organic solvents | Substrates for assay of esterases. Hydrolysis followed by release of acid (see above) or of *p*-nitrophenol which is yellow in alk. soln., $\lambda_{max}$ 400 nm $\epsilon$ 18 300, *JBC* **170**, 467 (1947). Also hydrolysed, particularly acetate, by chymotrypsin and trypsin, *BJ* **50**, 672 (1952), **56**, 288 (1954). Slow spontaneous hydrolysis occurs at neutral pH, for which correction must be made. Store solid in dark. To prepare soln. or emulsion, dissolve in MeOH and dilute with water or buffer. |
| Acetate, liq., d¹⁵₁₅ 1.081, B.p. 195.7; Propionate, prisms, M.p. 20, B.p. 211; Higher homologues, liq. or low melting cryst. solids | Acetate, sl. s. H₂O Higher homologues, i. H₂O; s. EtOH, eth., acet., CHCl₃ | Substrates for assay of esterases. Hydrolysis releases phenol which may be estimated colorimetrically, *BJ* **57**, 692 (1954). Commercial samples often contain some free phenol, purification, *BJ* **57**, 692 (1954). |

# 15 Artificial and natural substrates

| Name | Synonyms | Formula | M. wt. |
|------|----------|---------|--------|
| Triacetin | Glyceryl triacetate; acetin | $CH_2 \cdot O \cdot CO \cdot CH_3$<br>$\mid$<br>$CH \cdot O \cdot CO \cdot CH_3$<br>$\mid$<br>$CH_2 \cdot O \cdot CO \cdot CH_3$ | 218.2 |
| Tributyrin | Glyceryl tributyrate; butyrin | $CH_2 \cdot O \cdot CO \cdot CH_2 \cdot CH_2 \cdot CH_3$<br>$\mid$<br>$CH \cdot O \cdot CO \cdot CH_2 \cdot CH_2 \cdot CH_3$<br>$\mid$<br>$CH_2 \cdot O \cdot CO \cdot CH_2 \cdot CH_2 \cdot CH_2$ | 302.4 |

| Physical properties | Solubility | General remarks |
|---|---|---|
| cryst., M.p. 3.2; col. liq., $d_4^{25}$ 1.156; B.p. 258–60 | 0.685 $H_2O$; s. EtOH, eth., benz., $CHCl_3$ | Substrate for assay of esterases. Hydrolysis followed by release of acid, see above. |
| col. liq., bitter taste, $d^{20}$ 1.032; B.p. 305–10 | i. $H_2O$; s. EtOH, eth., acet. | Substrate for assay of esterases and lipase, *J. Lab. Clin. Med.* **33**, 1047 (1948). Hydrolysis followed by release of acid, see above. |

# 16 Biochemical reagents

## A PROTECTIVE AGENTS

This table includes compounds used primarily to protect enzymes against inactivation, caused by oxidation of −SH groups or by traces of heavy metals, or by toxic endogenous tissue components (e.g. phenols, quinones, fatty acids). Reagents used to protect against endogenous enzyme attack (RNAase and protease) are to be found in Section 13F, Other enzyme inhibitors (pp. 316–335).

# 16 A Biochemical reagents – protective agents

| Name | Synonyms | Formula | M. wt. |
|------|----------|---------|--------|
| Bovine serum albumin | BSA | | 67 000 |
| Cysteine, cysteamine, glutathione, *see* pp. 12 and 16 | | | |
| 2,3-Dimercapto-propan-1-ol | British anti-Lewisite; BAL; dimercaprol; 1,2-dithioglycerol | $CH_2SH$<br>$\|$<br>$CHSH$<br>$\|$<br>$CH_2OH$ | 124.2 |
| 1,4-Dithioerythritol | DTE; *erythro*-2,3 dihydroxy-1,4-dithiol-butane | $\begin{array}{cc} H & H \\ \| & \| \\ HSCH_2-C-C-CH_2SH \\ \| & \| \\ OH & OH \end{array}$ | 154.3 |
| 1,4-Dithiothreitol | DTT; Cleland's reagent; *threo*-2,3-dihydroxy-1,4-dithiolbutane | $\begin{array}{cc} H & OH \\ \| & \| \\ HSCH_2-C-C-CH_2SH \\ \| & \| \\ OH & H \end{array}$ | 154.3 |
| Mercap; *see* Other enzyme inhibitors, p. 326 | | | |
| 2-Mercapto-ethanol | Monothioethylene glycol | $HS \cdot CH_2 \cdot CH_2 \cdot OH$ | 78.1 |
| Polyethylene glycol | PEG; α-hydro-ω-hydroxypoly (oxy-1,2-ethanediyl); Carbowax. | Liquid or solid polymers of the general formula: $H(OCH_2CH_2)_nOH$, where $n$ is $\geqslant 4$.<br>e.g. PEG 400, average $n = 8.2-9.1$<br>PEG 4000, average $n = 68-84$ | 340–420<br>3500–4500 |
| Polyvinylpyrro-lidone, soluble | PVP; 1-ethenyl-2-pyrrolidinone polymers; Plasdone; Povidone | $\left[\begin{array}{c} H_2C\!-\!\!-\!\!-CH_2 \\ \| \quad\quad \| \\ H_2C_{\diagdown N}C\!\!=\!\!O \\ \| \\ -CH-CH_2- \end{array}\right]_n$ | Average M.wt. ranges available from 10 000–360 000 |

| Physical properties | Solubility | General remarks |
| --- | --- | --- |
| pI 4.7 | s. $H_2O$ | Used at 0.1–1.0% in isolation of mitochondria and chloroplasts as a phenol and quinone absorbent or to bind free fatty acids and inhibit further lipolytic activity, *Meth. Enzymol.* **31**, 306, 524, 531, 536, 603 (1974). 6.5% needed to maintain rod-like mitochondria from potato, *Tissue Cell* **1**, 575 (1969). |
| | | Frequently used to protect enzymes against inactivation caused by oxidation of –SH groups |
| viscous col. to yel. liq.; pungent odour; $d^{20}$ 1.2463; B.p. 86–90[1] | $6.8^{20}$ $H_2O$ (slow decomp.); s. EtOH, eth., vegetable oils | Protects many enzymes from inactivation (used at about $10^{-3}$ M), since an excess of dimercaptopropanol maintains protein –SH groups in reduced state and it is a strong chelating agent for heavy metals. Combines with trivalent As compds. Reverses inhibition, esp. of pyruvic and $\alpha$-ketoglutaric oxidases, by trivalent arsenicals and will cause reversal in many cases of inhibition by heavy metal reagents. Conversely, inactivates many enzymes and other proteins containing disulphide links or heavy metal prosthetic groups, e.g. catalase, peroxidase, carbonic anhydrase. Used medicinally, sometimes as less toxic glucoside, as antidote in arsenical and heavy metal poisoning. Pure liq. stable if kept $O_2$-free in sealed containers, oxidizes slowly in air. Aq. soln. oxidizes to disulphide in air, rate negligible at pH 5 but rapid in alkaline soln. |
| M.p. 82–84; pK 9.0, 9.9 | | Preferred agent for reducing –S–S– to –SH; low redox potential (−0.33 V, pH 7) ensures most thiols reduced; reaction yields intramolecular disulphide ensuring reductions proceed to completion. Disulphide reduction complete in minutes at pH 8. Specific and sensitive assay for disulphide groups based on determination of resulting monothiols with DTNB in presence of arsenite, *JBC* **243**, 716 (1968). DTT solns. oxidize relatively |
| cryst; M.p. 43; sl. hygr.; pK 8.3, 9.5 | s. $H_2O$, MeOH, EtOH, acet., $CHCl_3$ | slowly in air. Erythroisomer (DTE) appears identical in properties but DTT more easily prepared and commonly used [*Biochem.* **3**, 480 (1964)]. DTE slightly better in disulphide assay because of faster reaction rate of its arsenite complex with DTNB. |
| liq.; characteristic odour; B.p. $157d.^{748}$, $68^{20}$, $53.5^{10}$; $d^{25}$ 1.1196 | $\infty$ $H_2O$, EtOH, eth., benz. | Protects many enzymes from inactivation (generally used at about 0.01 M), since an excess of mercaptoethanol maintains protein –SH groups in reduced state. Also forms mercaptides with heavy metals. In some cases inhibition rather than activation is observed. Used to maintain readily oxidized substances particularly thiols, such as CoASH, and tetrahydrofolic acid in reduced state (concs. 0.01 M–1.0 M). Pure liq. decomp. only slowly in air, 8% in 6 months. Aq. solns. readily oxidized in air to disulphide, esp. at alkaline pH. Decomp. by mineral acids esp. HCl. |
| PEG 400: visc., sl. hygr. liq.; M.p. 1–5 PEG 4000: white powder; M.p. 59–61 | s. $H_2O$, aromatic hydrocarbons; sl.s. aliphatic hydrocarbons | Effective macromolecules (8% Carbowax 20 000) for keeping mitochondria rod-like during isolation, *Meth. Enzymol.* **31**, 599 (1974). PEG 4000 or 20 000 (1%) used in enzyme preparation when polyphenols are troublesome. Weaker phenol absorbent than PVP or BSA but solubility in acetone is a useful property, *Meth. Enzymol.* **13**, 577, 562 (1969). PEG 300–PEG 6000 (at 50–55%, w/w) induce cell hybridization, *Meth. Cell Biol.* **15**, 325 (1977). Used as a plasmolyticum. *Planta* **71**, 81 (1966); *New Phytol.* **69**, 501 (1970). Dialysis [*Science* **133**, 1486 (1981)] or passing through ion exchange resins may be necessary, *Plant Physiol.* **61**, 708 (1978). Possible complications, *see Ann. Rev. Plant Physiol.* **24**, 538, 541 (1973). Solvent action on some plastics. Low toxicity: $LD_{50}$ orally in rats: *ca* 40–60 g/kg. PEGs do not hydrolyse or deteriorate on storage; will not support mould growth. For use of PEG as fusogen to obtain hybridomas for monoclonal antibody production, *see Meth. Enzymol.* **92**, 10 (1983). |
| | s. $H_2O$ (giving a colloidal solution), EtOH, $CHCl_3$; i. eth | Used in isolating plant mitochondria and ribosomes (essential to use pharmaceutical grades) and as a phenol or quinone absorbent, *Meth. Enzymol.* **31**, 534 (1974). |

## 16 A Biochemical reagents — protective agents

| Name | Synonyms | Formula | M. wt. |
|---|---|---|---|
| Polyvinylpyrrolidone, insoluble | Polyclar AT | Cross-linked PVP | |
| Thioglycollic acid | Mercaptoacetic acid | $HS \cdot CH_2 \cdot COOH$ | 92.1 |
| ———, Na salt | | $HS \cdot CH_2 \cdot COONa$ | 114.1 |

| Physical properties | Solubility | General remarks |
|---|---|---|
| | i. $H_2O$ | Used in isolating soluble enzymes from plant material, *Meth. Enzymol.* **31**, 534 (1974). May be purified by boiling 10 min in 10% HCl and then washing in glass-distilled water until free of $Cl^-$. Final $Cl^-$ removed more easily by neutralizing with KOH and continuing washing. |
| liq.; strong unpleasant odour; $d^{20}$ 1.325; M.p. — 16.5; B.p. 108[15]; $pK_a$ 3.68, 10.7 | $\infty$ $H_2O$, EtOH, eth., $CHCl_3$, benz., most organic solvents | Protects many enzymes against inactivation (usually at $10^{-3}$ M to $10^{-2}$ M); an excess of thioglycollate maintains protein —SH groups in reduced state and it forms mercaptides with heavy metals. Frequently used in bacteriological media to maintain reducing conditions. Readily oxidized by air, esp. at alkaline pHs. |
| hygr. cryst. | v.s. $H_2O$; sl. s. EtOH | |

## B. REAGENTS FOR PROTEIN MODIFICATION

The allocation of compounds between this Section and Section 13, Antimetabolites, Antibacterial Agents and Enzyme Inhibitors is necessarily arbitrary. In particular, compounds used to modify thiol (—SH) groups are included in Section 13F, Other Enzyme Inhibitors. In cases of doubt, the **Index** should be consulted to locate a particular compound.

### References

*General*

G. E. Means and R. E. Feeney, *Chemical modification of proteins,* Holden-Day (1971).
*Meth. Enzymol.* **4**, 247 (1957); **11**, 481–711 (1967); **25**, 387–671 (1972); **47**, 407–498 (1977).

| Name | Synonyms | Formula | M. wt. |
|---|---|---|---|
| Acetic anhydride | Ethanoic anhydride | $CH_3-C(=O)-O-$ ; $CH_3-C(=O)-O$ (acetic anhydride structure) | 102.1 |
| *N*-Acetylimidazole | 1-Acetylimidazole | imidazole $-N-CO\cdot CH_3$ | 110.1 |
| Bis-imidates | Bis-imidoesters | $R'-O-\underset{\underset{NH}{\|}}{C}-R-\underset{\underset{NH}{\|}}{C}-O-R'$ | |
| Dimethyl adipimidate | DMA | $H_3C-O-\underset{\underset{NH}{\|}}{C}-(CH_2)_4-\underset{\underset{NH}{\|}}{C}-O-CH_3$ | 172.2; Di-HCl, 245.2 |
| Dimethyl 3,3'-dithiobispropionimidate | DTBP | $H_3C-O-\underset{\underset{NH}{\|}}{C}-(CH_2)_2-S-S-(CH_2)_2-\underset{\underset{NH}{\|}}{C}-O-CH_3$ | 236.4; Di-HCl, 309.3 |
| Dimethyl malonimidate | | $H_3C-O-\underset{\underset{NH}{\|}}{C}-CH_2-\underset{\underset{NH}{\|}}{C}-O-CH_3$ | 130.2; Di-HCl, 203.1 |
| Dimethyl suberimidate | DMS | $H_3C-O-\underset{\underset{NH}{\|}}{C}-(CH_2)_6-\underset{\underset{NH}{\|}}{C}-O-CH_3$ | 200.3; Di-HCl, 273.2 |

A. N. Glazer, in *The proteins,* eds. H. Neurath and R. L. Hill, vol. II, pp. 1–103, 3rd edition, Academic Press (1976).

A. N. Glazer, R. J. DeLange, and D. S. Sigman, *Chemical modification of proteins,* in *Laboratory techniques in biochemistry and molecular biology,* eds. T. S. Work and E. Work, vol. 4, part I, North Holland-Elsevier (1975).

*Bifunctional cross-linking reagents*

*Meth. Enzymol.* **25**, 623 (1972).
*Ann. Rev. Biochem.* **46**, 523 (1977).
*BBA* **559**, 39 (1979).

## Definition

'Acid hydrolysis' in this Section refers to the procedure used for the acid hydrolysis of proteins to yield free amino acids, viz. 6M-HCl at 110 °C *in vacuo* for 24 hr.

| Physical properties | Solubility | General remarks |
|---|---|---|
| pungent, irritant liq.; readily combustible; M.p. −73; B.p. 139 | Slowly s. $H_2O$ forming acetic acid; ∞ EtOH forming ester; s. $CHCl_3$, benz. | Reagent of choice for acetylating protein amino groups, *Meth. Enzymol.* **25**, 494 (1972). At neutral or mildly alkaline pH (7–9.5), reacts with unprotonated α- and ε-$NH_2$ groups rendering them electrically neutral. Tyrosine −OH also readily acetylated, but acetyl groups removed under moderately alkaline conditions or by M-$NH_2OH$ at pH 7–9, 0 °C, 2 hr. Serine −OH, threonine −OH and −SH also acetylated; acetyl groups removed by $NH_2OH$ at alkaline pH. Half-life of acetic anhydride in $H_2O$, 50 min at 0 °C, 4.5 min at 25 °C. |
| hygr. solid; M.p. 101.5–102.5 | s. $H_2O$, benz. | Acetylates tyrosine −OH at pH 7.5 or below; reagent and *O*-acetyltyrosine unstable at more alkaline pH. May also react slowly with −$NH_2$, but at pH 7.5 more selective for tyrosine −OH than acetic anhydride. Acetyl groups removed from tyrosine −OH (but not −$NH_2$) by M-$NH_2OH$ at pH 7–9, *Meth. Enzymol.* **25**, 500 (1972). Acetylation of tyrosine quantitated by decrease in tyrosine absorbance at 278 nm, $\Delta\epsilon_{278}$ 1160. Reagent stable as solid if dry, and for 1 month in soln. in dry benz. Hydrolysed in aqueous soln., most stable at pH 7.5. |
| | | Bifunctional cross-linking reagents; see reviews listed above. Highly specific for −$NH_2$ groups, reacting over the pH range 7–10 yielding amidine derivs. (−R−C−NH−Protein). The amidine group retains the +ve charge of the ‖ NH amino group with a higher $pK_a$ value than the −$NH_3^+$ group. Amidine derivs. are stable in mildly acid and neutral solns., but break down in alk. solns. Bis-imidates are unstable in aq. soln., with half-life of several min to 40 min depending on pH. |
| Di-HCl: hygr. solid, M.p. 223 | Di-HCl, s. $H_2O$ | Approx. max. link distance, 0.9 nm. |
| | Di-HCl, s. $H_2O$ | −S−S− bond can be cleaved with 10mM-mercaptoethanol; useful in detection of cross-linked components in two-dimensional SDS-gel electrophoresis. Related reagents have linker containing glycol, cleavable by periodate, see reviews above. |
| | Di-HCl, s. $H_2O$ | Approx. max. link distance, 0.5 nm. |
| Di-HCl: hygr. solid., M.p. 213–14 | Di-HCl, s. $H_2O$ | Approx. max. link distance 1.1 nm. |

## 16B Reagents for protein modification

| Name | Synonyms | Formula | M. wt. |
|------|----------|---------|--------|
| *N*-Bromo-succinimide | NBS | | 178.0 |
| 2,3-Butanedione | Diacetyl; dimethyl diketone; dimethyl glyoxal; 2,3-dioxobutane | $CH_3 \cdot CO \cdot CO \cdot CH_3$ | 86.1 |
| Carbodiimides | | | |
| 1-Benzyl-3-(3-dimethylamino-propyl)carbodi-imide hydro-chloride | BDC | | 253.9 |
| 1-Cyclohexyl-3-(2-morpholinyl-4-ethyl)car-bodiimide methyl *p*-toluenesul-phonate | CMC | | 423.6 |
| 1-Ethyl-3-(3-dimethylamino-propyl)carbodi-imide hydro-chloride | EDC | $CH_3 \cdot CH_2 \cdot N=C=N \cdot CH_2 \cdot CH_2 \cdot CH_2 \cdot N(CH_3)_2 \cdot HCl$ | 191.8 |
| Citraconic anhydride | 2-Methylmaleic anhydride | | 112.1 |
| Cyanogen bromide | CNBr | | 105.9 |
| 1,2-Cyclo-hexanedione | Dihydrocatechol; 1,2-dioxocyclo-hexane | | 112.1 |

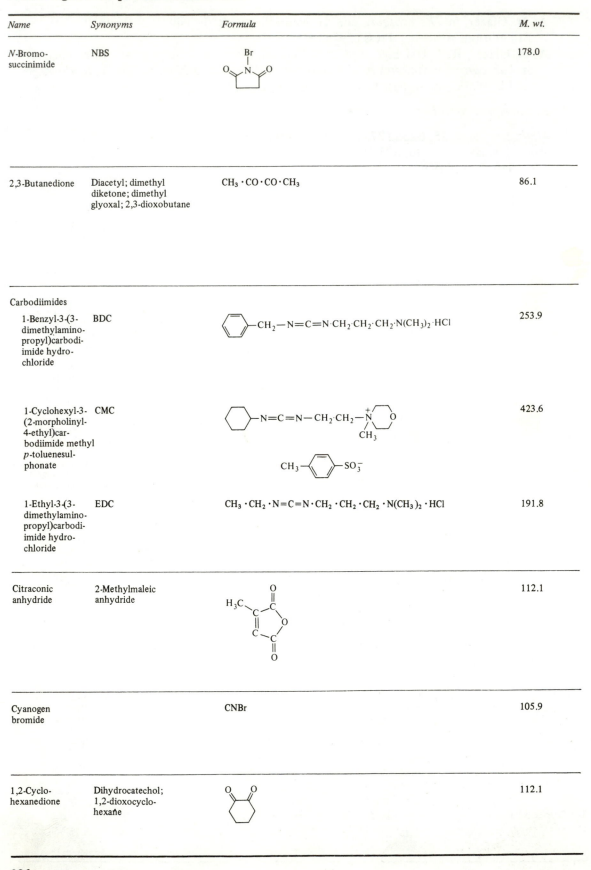

| Physical properties | Solubility | General remarks |
|---|---|---|
| cryst.; M.p. 173–5 d. | s. $H_2O$, acet., gl. acetic | At pH 3–4, in acetate or formate buffers, the indole group of tryptophan is oxidized, and peptide bonds on carboxyl side of tryptophan residues are cleaved. NBS is a strong oxidizing agent; it rapidly oxidizes —SH groups and reacts more slowly with tyrosine, histidine, and methionine. At higher pHs (e.g. 7) little or no peptide bond cleavage occurs, and in absence of —SH groups NBS is relatively specific for tryptophan. Reaction with tryptophan is accompanied by a decrease in absorbance at 280 nm and an increase at 261 nm, $\Delta\epsilon_{261}$ 10 300. Reviews, *Meth. Enzymol.* **11**, 283, 498, 506 (1967), **78**, 452, 456 (1978); *Adv. Protein Chem.* **24**, 97 (1970). |
| yellowish-green liq.; quinone odour; b.p. 88. Trimer: col. needles; M.p. 112.5–14 | s. $H_2O$; $\infty$ EtOH, eth. Trimer: s. $H_2O$ | Modifies arginine residues under mild conditions, pH 7.5–8; use of borate buffers increases rate of reaction. Acid hydrolysis causes partial regeneration of arginine; treatment with M-HCl prior to acid hydrolysis prevents this regeneration and allows quantitation of extent of modification by amino acid analysis. Under neutral and slightly alkaline conditions, 2,3-butanedione readily forms trimer, which is cryst. and stable at room temp. if dry. Trimer also used as a modifying reagent for arginine at similar pHs, also reacts slowly with —NH₂ groups, *Meth. Enzymol.* **25**, 566 (1972). |
| | s. $H_2O$ | Water-soluble carbodiimides are used to modify —COOH. Reaction is usually performed at pH 4.5–5 in presence of an amine, commonly glycine methyl ester. The —COOH group is converted to an amide of the added amine, the reaction being promoted by the carbodiimide. Carbodiimides react at similar rates with —SH groups and more slowly with tyrosine —OH. Tyrosine derivs. decompose on treatment with 1M-NH₂OH at pH 7, but —SH derivs. are more stable. CMC reacts with the active-centre serine residue of serine proteases. |
| solid; M.p. 113–15 | s. $H_2O$ | |
| M.p. 113–15 | s. $H_2O$ | |
| liq.; M.p. 7–8; B.p. 213; $d_4^{20}$ 1.245 | s. $H_2O$ decomp.; v.s. EtOH; s. acet. | Used for reversible blocking of protein —NH₂ groups, reacting at pH 8–9, *Meth. Enzymol.* **25**, 546 (1972). Citraconyl blocking groups are stable for many hours at neutral or mildly alkaline pH, but removed by acid conditions, e.g. pH 4.2 at 40 °C for 3 hr (lysozyme), pH 2 at room temp. for 6 hr (aldolase). Two isomeric citraconyl half-amides can be formed in the blocking reaction, but they have similar stabilities. Also reacts with —SH forming stable derivs. and with serine and threonine —OH forming derivs. decomposed by alk. NH₂OH. |
| volatile cryst.; M.p. 52; B.p. 61–2 | v.s. $H_2O$, EtOH, eth. | Selectively cleaves peptide bonds on carboxyl side of methionine residues at room temp. under strongly acid conditions, see *JBC* **242**, 5434 (1967) for conditions. Methionine residue is converted into homoserine lactone residue. Solid cyanogen bromide is volatile at room temp.; vapour extremely toxic (similar to HCN); unstable in alkali; impure solids may be explosive. |
| cryst.; M.p. 35–8; B.p. 193–5 | s. $H_2O$ | Selectively modifies arginine residues in borate buffers, pH 8–9, at 25–40 °C, *JBC* **250**, 557 (1975). Earlier procedures used more alkaline conditions (0.2M-NaOH, *JBC* **242**, 1036 (1967); pH 11–12, *Biochem.* **7**, 2886 (1968)) and tend to cause denaturation. Under some conditions may also react with —NH₂ groups, forming yellow colour with $\lambda_{max}$ approx. 440 nm. |

| Name | Synonyms | Formula | M. wt. |
|---|---|---|---|
| Dansyl chloride | 5-Dimethylamino-naphthalene-1-sulphonyl chloride | | 269.8 |
| Diazonium-benzene sulphonic acid | DABS | | 184.2 |
| Diazonium-1$H$-tetrazole | DHT | | 97.1 |
| Diethyl pyro-carbonate | Ethoxyformic anhydride; diethyloxydiformate; diethyl dicarbonate; DEP | | 162.1 |
| 2,4-Dinitro-fluorobenzene | 1-Fluoro-2,4-dinitro-benzene; DNFB | | 186.1 |
| 5,5′-Dithiobis-(2-nitrobenzoic acid) | DTNB; Ellman's reagent | | 396.4 |
| Dithiobis-(succinimidyl-propionate) | DSP | | 404.4 |

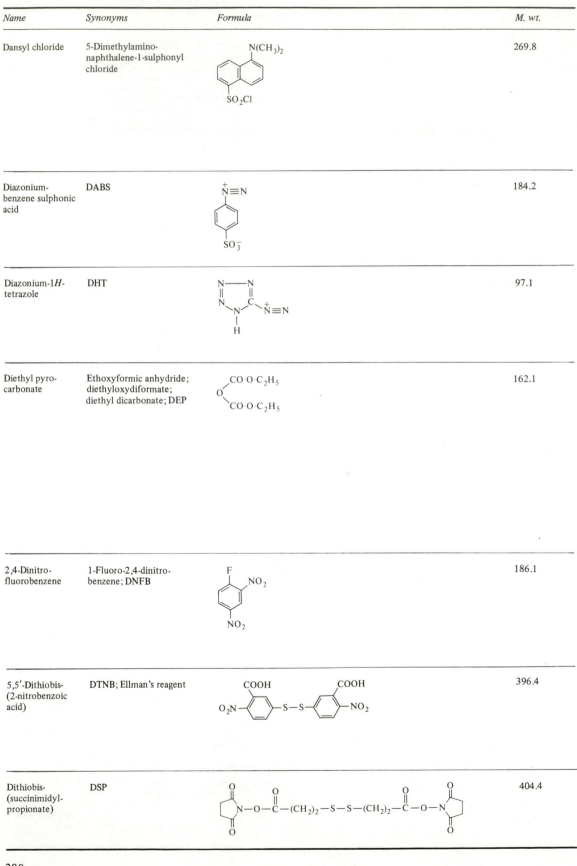

| Physical properties | Solubility | General remarks |
|---|---|---|
| yel. or orange cryst.; M.p. 74–6 | i. $H_2O$; s. acet., pyr., benz., dioxan | Reacts with $-NH_2$ groups to attach a fluorescent dimethylaminonaph-thalenesulphonyl (DNS or dansyl) group. Used for amino end-group analysis and sequence analysis of proteins on an ultramicro scale, *BJ* **89**, 379 (1963), *Meth. Enzymol.* **25**, 121, 333 (1972). Reaction usually performed at pH 8.5–9; under these conditions dansyl chloride also reacts with $-SH$, tyrosine $-OH$, lysine $\epsilon$-$NH_2$ and histidine imidazole; thiol and imidazole derivs. unstable in acid reforming amino acid. DNS-amino acid compounds (except DNS-proline and DNS-serine) are stable to acid hydrolysis. Dansyl chloride slowly decomp. by $H_2O$. Solid stable over $CaCl_2$ for months. Conjugates, absorbance max. 340 nm, fluorescence max. 525 nm. |
| | sl. s. $H_2O$, EtOH; s. dil. HCl, dil. NaOH | Non-penetrating, water-soluble membrane probe, covalently attaches to $-NH_2$, $-SH$, imidazole and tyrosine $-OH$ groups of proteins. Soln. of diazonium salt prepared when required from sulphanilic acid and $HNO_2$, *J. Membrane Biol.* **8**, 163 (1972); soln. can be stored frozen. Cryst. DABS readily explodes with friction, on impact or on heating and should be kept moist. |
| | s. $H_2O$ | Reacts with histidine and tyrosine forming both mono- and di-substituted derivs. Reaction can be quantitated spectrophotometrically, *Meth. Enzymol.* **25**, 521 (1972). May also react with $-NH_2$ groups. Reagent is prepared as dilute soln. when required from 5-amino-1*H*-tetrazole. Reagent is VIOLENTLY EXPLOSIVE in dry state and in solns. stronger than 0.2 M; solns. should not be allowed to dry on glassware, etc. |
| liq., $d_4^{20}$ 1.12; B.p. 155 | 0.6 $H_2O$ with decomp.; v.s. EtOH, eth. | Reacts with histidine residues, usually at pH 6–8, to form *N*-carbethoxy-histidine, absorption max. 230–50 nm, $\Delta\epsilon_{230}$ 3000, $\Delta\epsilon_{240}$ 3200. *N*-Carbeth-oxyimidazole fairly stable at neutral pH, half-life at 25 °C and pH 7 is 55 hr, rapidly deacylated at neutral pH by $NH_2OH$, not stable to acid hydrolysis, histidine being regenerated. Possibility of cleavage of imidazole ring rendering modification of histidine irreversible, *FEBS Lett.* **72**, 155 (1976). Reasonably selective reagent for histidine but may react with tyrosine $-OH$, causing fall in absorbance at 278 nm ($\Delta\epsilon_{278}$ 1310) and in 230–50 nm region; reaction with tyrosine reversed by $NH_2OH$. May also react slowly with $-SH$ and $-NH_2$, not reversed by $NH_2OH$. Review, *Meth. Enzymol.* **47**, 431 (1977). Diethyl pyrocarbonate hydrolyses in aq. soln., half-life in phosphate buffer at 25 °C, 24 min at pH 6, 9 min at pH 7; hydrolysis accelerated by Tris, half-life in Tris buffer at 25 °C, 1.25 min at pH 7.5, 0.37 min at pH 8.2. Solns. made up immediately before use in anhyd. EtOH or anhyd. acetonitrile. Irritant. See also p. 320. |
| oily liq. or cryst; M.p. 26; B.p. $130^1$ | s. benz., eth., organic solvents; $0.16^{15}$ $H_2O$ | Reacts with $-NH_2$, $-SH$, tyrosine $-OH$ and imidazole groups under mildly alkaline conditions forming dinitrophenyl (DNP) derivs. DNP-compounds have $\lambda_{max}$ approx. 365 nm, decompose in the light. Imidazole deriv. unstable to acid hydrolysis. Use in identification of amino terminal amino acids, *Meth. Enzymol.* **4**, 221 (1957), as a reagent for protein modification, *Meth. Enzymol.* **11**, 548 (1967). 2,4-Dinitrofluorobenzene is a vesicant, avoid skin contact. $\lambda_{max}$ 360 nm, $\epsilon$ 14 800 (0.01 M-NaOH), darkens on standing esp. in light. |
| yel. powder; M.p. 243–5d. | s. $H_2O$ (pH 8) | Reacts with $-SH$ groups under mild alkaline conditions (pH 7–8) to form the thionitrobenzoate-protein mixed disulphide and stoichiometric amounts of thionitrobenzoate dianion, which has intense yellow colour, $\Delta\epsilon_{412}$ 13 600 (pH 7–8), see also *Anal. Biochem.* **94**, 75 (1979). May be used both for quantitative estimation of $-SH$ groups in proteins and other compounds (e.g. CoA-SH) and for modification of protein $-SH$ groups. Review, *Meth. Enzymol.* **25**, 457 (1972). |
| | | Bifunctional cross-linking reagent (see refs. above) reacting primarily with $-NH_2$ groups forming amide bonds. Also reacts with $-SH$ and imidazole groups. The $-S-S-$ bond may be cleaved by $-SH$ compds., e.g. mercapto-ethanol, allowing separation of cross-linked sub-units. |

| Name | Synonyms | Formula | M. wt. |
|------|----------|---------|--------|
| Ethyl acetimidate hydrochloride | | $CH_3 \cdot C \cdot O \cdot CH_2 \cdot CH_3$ <br> $\parallel$ <br> $NH \cdot HCl$ | Hydro-chloride, 123.7; Free base, 87.2 |
| Ethylenimine | Azacyclopropane | $CH_2 \!-\! CH_2$ <br> $\diagdown N \diagup$ <br> $H$ | 43.1 |
| Fluorescein isothiocyanate | FITC | 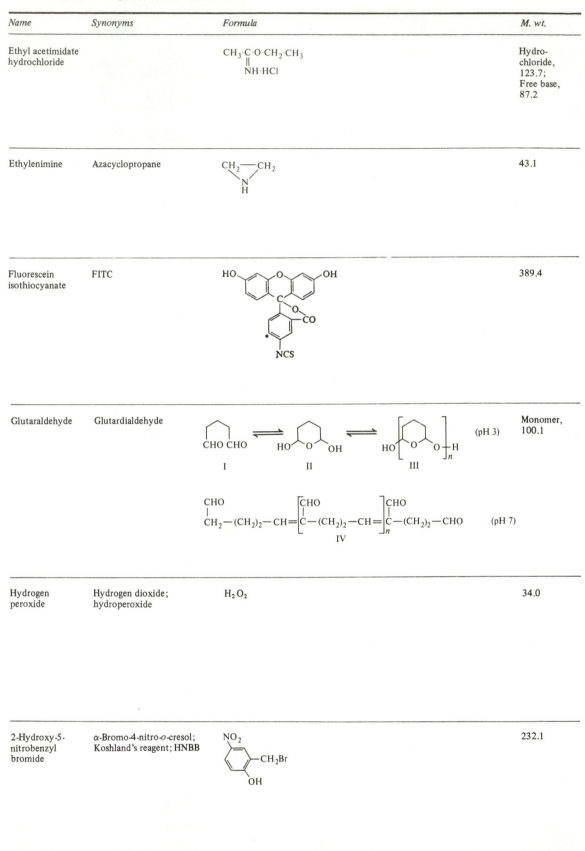 | 389.4 |
| Glutaraldehyde | Glutardialdehyde | | Monomer, 100.1 |
| Hydrogen peroxide | Hydrogen dioxide; hydroperoxide | $H_2O_2$ | 34.0 |
| 2-Hydroxy-5-nitrobenzyl bromide | α-Bromo-4-nitro-o-cresol; Koshland's reagent; HNBB | | 232.1 |

| Physical properties | Solubility | General remarks |
|---|---|---|
| HCl: cryst.; M.p. 112–14 | s. H$_2$O | Reacts with $\alpha$- and $\epsilon$-NH$_2$ groups at pH 7–10 forming amidines. Amidine derivs. retain +ve charge of original amino group, p$K_a$ of amidine somewhat higher than that of —NH$_3^+$. $\epsilon$-Amidine groups are partially converted back into $\epsilon$-NH$_2$ during acid hydrolysis. Ethyl acetimidate is slowly hydrolysed in aq. soln. to acetamide and ethanol. Between pH 7 and 11, rate of hydrolysis is slow compared to rate of reaction with amines. |
| liq., ammoniacal smell; B.p. 55–6 | $\infty$ H$_2$O; s. EtOH | Handle with extreme care in a hood — toxic, irritant, carcinogenic, strongly alkaline. Polymerizes, fairly stable over NaOH pellets. Reacts with cysteine —SH groups at slightly alkaline pH, forming H$_2$N-CH$_2$-S— and introducing a new trypsin-sensitive site into protein chain. For conditions of reaction, see *JBC* **241**, 3457 (1966). May react with methionine residues at low pH. |
| bright yel. powder | s. H$_2$O, acet. | Used, frequently adsorbed on Celite, to add a fluoresecent group to proteins, e.g. for fluorescent antibody tracing, R.C. Nairn (ed.) *Fluorescent protein tracing,* 3rd ed., Livingstone (1969); *Nature* **193**, 167 (1962), and in immunological research, *J. Neurochem.* **31**, 1375 (1978). Decomp. in H$_2$O, solid stable at least one year at room temp. Two isomers known; one (FITC II) is as shown, FITC I has isothiocyanate group in position marked with asterisk. Absorption max. of conjugates 495 nm, fluorescence max. of conjugates *ca.* 520 nm. Prep. of fluorescein-labelled proteins, see, for example, *Meth. Enzymol.* **26**, 38 (1972), **81**, 70 (1982), **93**, 151 (1983). |
| | s. H$_2$O | Bifunctional cross-linking reagent, reacting with —NH$_2$ groups to form Schiff's bases. Commercial 25% aq. solns. of glutaraldehyde at approx. pH 3 contain 3% glutaraldehyde (I), the hemiacetal (II), and polymers of the latter (III). Schiff's bases formed by I at pH 3 are unstable to acid hydrolysis. At neutral or slightly alkaline pHs, where reagent is commonly used for protein modification, glutaraldehyde forms polymers (IV), the value of *n* increasing with pH until pptn. occurs. At pH 7 or above, IV forms acid-stable Schiff's bases involving the conjugated, internal aldehyde groups; Schiff's bases formed by terminal —CHO groups in IV are not stable to acid hydrolysis. Because of variability of *n*, cross-linking distance cannot be specified. Review, *Ann. Rev. Biochem.* **46**, 523 (1977). Used as a fixative in electron microscopy. |
| col. liq.; M.p. − 1.7; B.p. 152 | $\infty$ H$_2$O; s. EtOH, eth. | Oxidizes methionine residues to methionine sulphoxide. Oxidation of cysteine —SH also occurs at neutral and alkaline pHs. At acid pH, oxidation of methionine is much more rapid than that of cysteine, so that at pH 2.5 H$_2$O$_2$ is a reasonably specific reagent for methionine residues. Methionine sulphoxide decomposes to methionine in about 85% yield on acid hydrolysis, but is not destroyed by alkaline hydrolysis and can also be estimated by indirect methods, see *Meth. Enzymol.* **11**, 487 (1967). Methionine sulphoxide can be reduced to methionine by treatment with thiols. Review, *Meth. Enzymol.* **11**, 485 (1967); **25**, 393 (1972). |
| leaflets or needles; M.p. 147–9 | s. EtOH, eth., acet., dioxan; sl.s. benz., H$_2$O decomp. | Reacts rapidly under mild conditions with the indole ring of tryptophan; reaction is normally carried out in pH range 2.5–5. Reacts more slowly with —SH, and under strongly alk. conditions with tyrosine —OH. In absence of —SH and at acid pH, reagent is specific for tryptophan. Extent of reaction with tryptophan may be quantitated at 410 nm after removal of hydrolysed reagent and raising pH to > 10, $\Delta\epsilon_{410}$ 18 450 (in 2M-NaOH), *Meth. Enzymol.* **25**, 468 (1972). Reagent hydrolyses very rapidly in aq. soln., half-life less than 1 min, and is made up immediately before use in acet. or dioxan. |

| Name | Synonyms | Formula | M. wt. |
|------|----------|---------|--------|
| Iodination reagents | | | |
| *p*-Iodophenyl-sulphonyl chloride | Pipsyl chloride | I—⟨benzene ring⟩—SO$_2$Cl | 302.5 |
| Lissamine Rhodamine B | RB 200; Sulphorhodamine B | (C$_2$H$_5$)$_2$N— [xanthene ring system] —N$^+$(C$_2$H$_5$)$_2$ ; SO$_3^-$ ; SO$_3$Na | 580.7 |
| Methyl 3-(4-azidophenyl-dithio)propion-imidate | MADP | N≡N$^+$—⟨benzene ring⟩—S—S—CH$_2$—CH$_2$—C—O—CH$_3$  (C has =NH) | 280.4 |
| Maleic anhydride | *cis*-Butenedioic anhydride; 2,5-furandione | [maleic anhydride ring: HC=CH with two C=O groups bridged by O] | 98.1 |
| Methyl acetimidate | | CH$_3$—C—O—CH$_3$  (C has =NH) | 73.1 |

| Physical properties | Solubility | General remarks |
|---|---|---|
| | | Iodination of proteins may be used to modify tyrosine residues and to incorporate a radioactive [131]I or [125]I label into a protein. Tyrosine and, more slowly, histidine residues are modified to mono- and di-substituted derivs. Monoiodo- and diiodo-tyrosine may be distinguished spectrophotometrically, *JBC* **237**, 2778 (1962). Iodo derivs. of histidine break down during acid hydrolysis. —SH groups are oxidized under mild conditions, and under harsh conditions tryptophan and methionine may also be modified, *JBC* **238**, 1343 (1963). A wide variety of conditions and reagents have been used for protein iodination, including potassium triiodide (see e.g. *Biochem.* **5**, 3770 (1966), *JBC*, **243**, 720 (1968)), iodine monochloride (*Meth. Enzymol.* **25**, 438 (1972)), I⁻ + chloramine T (*BJ* **89**, 114 (1963)), I⁻ + lactoperoxidase + $H_2O_2$, which avoids protein denaturation and provides a non-penetrating agent for surface labelling of membrane proteins (*BBRC* **40**, 284 (1970)); lactoperoxidase linked to agarose permits easy removal of the enzyme (*Biochem.* **13**, 1014 (1974)). Micro-scale iodination prior to electrophoresis, *Anal. Biochem.* **95**, 568 (1979). To label compounds that lack tyrosine or are labile under the conditions encountered in the chloramine T and lactoperoxidase methods, use the Bolton—Hunter reagent (iodinated *N*-succinimidyl 3-(4-hydroxyphenyl)propionate), which reacts with lysine residues under mild conditions, *Meth. Enzymol.* **70A**, 221 (1980). |
| col. cryst.; M.p. 86; sublimes 150³ | s. organic solvents | Reacts with —NH₂ and tyrosine —OH groups forming stable *p*-iodophenyl-sulphonyl (pipsyl) derivs. Use in sequence determination, *Meth. Enzymol.* **4**, 238 (1957). Radioactive substance, especially [131]I, tends to become coloured over long periods, but is satisfactory for use. Non-radioactive reagent is stable. |
| red powder | s. H₂O; sl. s. EtOH | Used as acid chloride, frequently adsorbed on Celite, to add a fluorescent group to proteins, e.g. for fluorescent antibody tracing, R.C. Nairn (ed.), *Fluorescent protein tracing*, 3rd ed., Livingtone (1969), *Nature, Lond.* **193**, 167 (1962). Absorption max. of conjugates 575 nm., fluorescence max. of conjugates 595 nm. Acid chloride is slowly hydrolysed by H₂O. |
| | | Photosensitive heterobifunctional cross-linking reagent. Imido ester group reacts conventionally with —NH₂ groups (see entries for methyl acetimidate and bisimidates). Azide group is relatively unreactive until activated by light of ~ 350 nm to form highly reactive nitrene group, which forms a variety of cross-linked products. The half-life of the nitrene groups is $10^{-2}$–$10^{-4}$ s, which minimizes cross-linking of proteins brought together by random collision. The —S—S— bridge can be cleaved with thiol compounds, e.g. mercaptoethanol. |
| cryst.; M.p. 52.8; B.p. 202 | s. acet., CHCl₃, Et acetate; sl. s. benz.; sl. s. EtOH forming ester; s. H₂O decomp. | Reacts with α- and ε-NH₂ groups under mildly alkaline conditions (pH 8.5–9.0) forming a monoamide, *BJ* **112**, 679 (1969). Product is stable at neutral and alkaline pH, but hydrolyses regenerating original amine at acid pH; half-life of ε-maleyllysine at pH 3.5 and 37 °C is ~ 11 hr (more stable than ε-citraconyllysine). Extent of maleylation may be quantitated by increase in absorbance below 280 nm, $\Delta\epsilon_{250}$ 3360 at pH 8, *Biochem.* **7**, 1941 (1968). Maleylation replaces the +ve charge on —NH₃⁺ by a —ve charge on the free —COO⁻ of the maleyl group, which tends to cause disaggregation of oligomeric proteins into subunits and prevents trypsin cleavage at modified lysine residues. Also reacts with —SH groups forming stable derivs. (cf. *N*-ethylmaleimide), and slowly with tyrosine —OH (deriv. alkali-labile), serine and threonine —OH (reversed by NH₂OH at pH 9). Review, *Meth. Enzymol.* **25**, 191 (1972). |
| | s. H₂O | Reacts with α- and ε-NH₂ groups at pH 7–10 forming amidines. Amidine derivs. retain +ve charge of original amino group, p$K_a$ of amidine somewhat higher than that of —NH₃⁺. ε-Amidine groups are partially converted back into ε-NH₂ during acid hydrolysis. Methyl acetimidate is slowly hydrolysed in aq. soln. to acetamide and methanol. Between pH 7 and 11, rate of hydrolysis is slow compared to rate of reaction with amines. |

## 16B  Reagents for protein modification

| Name | Synonyms | Formula | M. wt. |
|------|----------|---------|--------|
| *O*-Methylisourea | 2-Methylpseudourea | $$\begin{array}{c} NH \\ \| \\ C-O-CH_3 \\ \| \\ NH_2 \end{array}$$ | 74.1; Hydrogen sulphate, 172.2 |
| Nitrous acid | | $HNO_2$ | 47.2 |
| Performic acid | Peroxyformic acid; permethanoic acid; formyl hydroperoxide | $H \cdot COOOH$ | 62.0 |
| Phenylglyoxal | Benzoylformaldehyde | | 134.1; Hydrate, 152.1 |
| Phenyl isothiocyanate | PITC | | 135.2 |

### Photo-oxidation dyes

| Name | Synonyms | Formula | M. wt. |
|------|----------|---------|--------|
| Methylene Blue | Methylthionine chloride; tetramethylthionine chloride | | Anhyd., 319.9 |
| Rose Bengal | 4,5,6,7-Tetrachloro 2′,4′,5′,7′-tetraiodofluorescein | | Unionised, acid, 973.6; Na$_2$ salt, 1017.6; K$_2$ salt, 1049.8 |

| Physical properties | Solubility | General remarks |
|---|---|---|
| cryst.; M.p. 44.5. Hydrogen sulphate: M.p. 118–20 | v.s. $H_2O$, EtOH | Reacts with $\epsilon$-$NH_2$ groups converting lysine to homoarginine and thus retaining the +ve charge on the residue. $\alpha$-$NH_2$ groups react much more slowly or not at all. Reaction is usually performed at pH 10–11, using 0.2–1M reagent for several days. Homoarginine is stable to acid hydrolysis, so that the degree of modification may be estimated by amino acid analysis; homoarginine emerges shortly after arginine. Review, *Meth. Enzymol.* **11**, 584, 589 (1967). A similar reagent is 1-guanyl-3,5-dimethylpyrazole, which reacts under somewhat milder conditions, pH $\sim$ 9.5, but also reacts with $\alpha$-$NH_2$ groups (*Meth. Enzymol.* **25**, 558 (1972)). *O*-Methylisourea should be stored at $-30\,^{\circ}$C in sealed, evacuated ampoules; it is slowly hydrolysed in aq. soln., 41% in 24 hr at room temp. |
| known only in soln.; pale blue | | Nitrous acid is generated in soln. from $NaNO_2$ and acid, e.g. acetic acid pH 4.35. Converts $-NH_2$ groups to $-OH$ with quantitative evolution of $N_2$. $\alpha$-$NH_2$ groups react more rapidly than $\epsilon$-$NH_2$. Also reacts with the indole ring of tryptophan, the ring of tyrosine, $-SH$ groups and possibly methionine side chains. |
| col. liq. | $\infty$ $H_2O$, EtOH, eth.; s. $CHCl_3$, benz. | Chief use is for the quantitative estimation of cysteine and cystine residues, both of which are oxidised to cysteic acid. Performic acid also oxidizes methionine to methionine sulphone and tryptophan to formylkynurenine and other products. Tyrosine, serine, and threonine may also be oxidized, but much more slowly and usually only under harsh conditions. Conditions for the complete oxidation of cysteine, cystine, and methionine residues vary with different proteins, side reactions being minimized at low temp., *JBC* **219**, 611 (1956), *Meth. Enzymol.* **11**, 59 (1967). Cysteic acid and methionine sulphone are stable to acid hydrolysis and may be estimated by amino acid analysis. Performic acid is generated *in situ* by mixing $H_2O_2$ and formic acid; it can be explosive especially in the presence of other substances. |
| yel. liq.; B.p. 120$^{50}$ Hydrate: needles $+1H_2O$; M.p. 91 | s. $H_2O$ | Reacts with guanidino group of arginine residues at pHs close to neutral, yielding derivs. containing two phenylglyoxal moieties per guanidino group, *JBC* **243**, 6171 (1968). Derivs. are stable in mildly acid conditions (pH < 4), but decompose slowly at neutral and alkaline pHs regenerating most of the original guanidino groups. Phenylglyoxal also reacts, under these conditions, with $\alpha$-$NH_2$ groups forming $\alpha$-oxo acid residues; $\epsilon$-$NH_2$ groups may react on extensive treatment with phenylglyoxal. |
| col. liq., $d_4^{25}$ 1.1288; M.p. $-21$; B.p. 221$^{760}$, 95$^{12}$ | i. $H_2O$; s. EtOH, eth. | Combines with $-NH_2$ groups to form phenylthiocarbamyl (PTC) derivs. In the Edman degradation used for protein sequence determination, the $\alpha$-PTC-deriv. of the amino terminal amino acid residue is cleaved from the polypeptide and cyclizes to form the phenylthiohydantoin (PTH) derived from that amino acid. |
| dark green cryst. containing up to 5$H_2O$ | s. $H_2O$, EtOH, $CHCl_3$; i. eth. | Cysteine, histidine, methionine, tryptophan, and tyrosine residues in proteins can be oxidized in the presence of a photo-active dye by irradiation with visible light, *ABB* **110**, 57 (1965), *Meth. Enzymol.* **11**, 490 (1967), **25**, 401 (1972). Many different dyes have been used, most commonly methylene blue, rose bengal, eosin Y, fluorescein, crystal violet and riboflavin. It is frequently found that photo-oxidation of a particular protein results in modification of only one or two types of residue, *EJB* **26**, 125 (1972), *BBRC* **65**, 652 (1975), so that the technique has been widely used to investigate the active sites of enzymes, e.g. *PNAS* **57**, 107 (1967), *J. Biochem., Tokyo* **69**, 363 (1971), *Biochem.* **10**, 2143 (1971), *BBA* **295**, 543 (1973). The pathway of oxidation varies according to the conditions and the dye used (*Science* **162**, 963 (1968)) leading to a variety of oxidation products, *ABB* **33**, 90 (1951), *Meth. Enzymol.* **11**, 490 (1967), *Biochem.* **8**, 5149 (1969), *Ann. N.Y. Acad. Sci.* **171**, 149 (1970), *Aust. J. Chem.* **24**, 1285 (1971). |
| bright bluish pink cryst. | s. $H_2O$ | |

## 16B  Reagents for protein modification

| Name | Synonyms | Formula | M. wt. |
|------|----------|---------|--------|
| Potassium cyanate | | KNCO (K salt)<br>H—N=C=O (free acid) | 81.1;<br>Free acid, 43.0 |
| Sodium borohydride | Sodium tetrahydroborate | NaBH₄ | 37.8 |
| Succinic anhydride | Butanedioic anhydride;<br>2,5-dioxotetrahydrofuran | 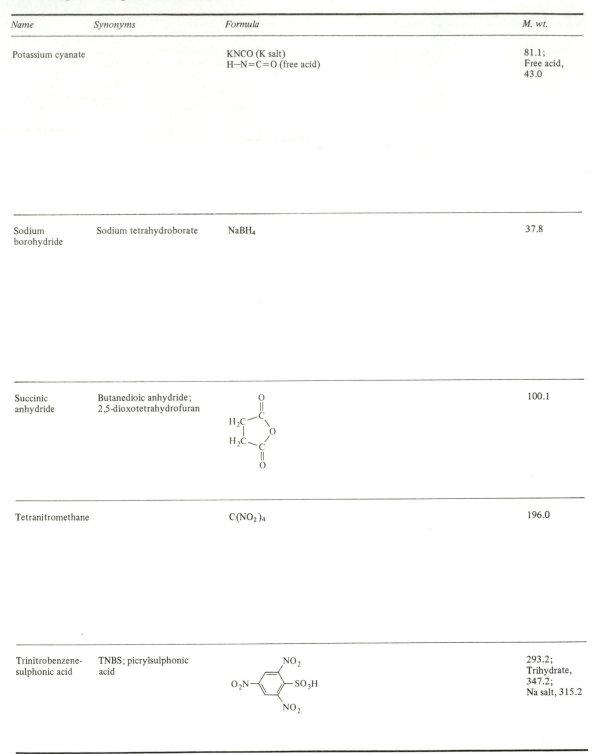 | 100.1 |
| Tetranitromethane | | $C(NO_2)_4$ | 196.0 |
| Trinitrobenzene-sulphonic acid | TNBS; picrylsulphonic acid | | 293.2;<br>Trihydrate, 347.2;<br>Na salt, 315.2 |

| Physical properties | Solubility | General remarks |
|---|---|---|
| K salt: col. cryst. <br> Free acid: liq.; <br> M.p. − 86; B.p. 23.5 | K salt: s. $H_2O$; <br> v. sl. s. EtOH <br> Free acid: <br> s. $H_2O$, eth., benz., <br> toluene | Reacts with −$NH_2$ (at pH 5 and above), −SH, imidazole, tyrosine −OH, and −COOH groups forming carbamyl derivs. ($-\overset{\text{O}}{\underset{\|}{\text{C}}}-NH_2$). Derivs. of −SH, imidazole and tyrosine −OH are labile at alkaline pH (though −SH and tyrosine −OH derivs. are stable below pH 5), and reaction with −COOH occurs only at acid pH, e.g. pH 5.3, so that at pH 8 only −$NH_2$ groups form a stable reaction product with cyanate. At pH 7 and below, α-$NH_2$ groups react at 100 × the rate of ε-$NH_2$ groups. Review, *Meth. Enzymol.* **11**, 590 (1967). Cyanate solns. tend to polymerize on standing forming cyanuric acid and cyamelide, and also decompose in $H_2O$ to $CO_2$ and $NH_3$. Dilute solns. of free acid in eth., benz., or toluene are stable for several weeks, solns. in $H_2O$ at 0 °C are stable for several hours. Rapid heating of HNCO may result in explosion. |
| hygr. cryst. forming a dihydrate; <br> M.p. 36−7 (dihydrate), > 300 d. <br> (anhyd.) | s. $H_2O$, MeOH, liq. <br> $NH_3$; sl.s. EtOH, <br> tetrahydrofuran | Used in reductive alkylation of α- and ε-$NH_2$ groups. Schiff's base formed between −$NH_2$ group and oxo compound, e.g. formaldehyde, pyridoxal phosphate, is reduced by $NaBH_4$. Reaction in presence of small molar excess of HCHO proceeds efficiently at pH 9 and 0−4 °C yielding ε-*N,N*-dimethyl-lysine residues (stable to acid hydrolysis) as principal product, *Biochem.* **7**, 2192 (1968), *Meth. Enzymol.* **47**, 469 (1977). Reaction involving pyridoxal phosphate can be used to identify −$NH_2$ groups at active sites of pyridoxal phosphate enzymes or generally to introduce a fluorescent group into a protein, particularly those with phosphate binding sites. Also reduces −S−S− groups (*JBC* **244**, 6289 (1969)) and many natural and artificial electron acceptors. Solid $NaBH_4$ stable if dry, decomp. in moist air. Aq. solns. stable for several days in presence of 0.2% NaOH, rapidly decomp. below pH 7 forming borate and hydrogen. |
| wh. cryst; M.p. 120 | s. $CHCl_3$, EtOH <br> forming ester; sl.s. $H_2O$ <br> decomp., eth. | Reacts preferentially with −$NH_2$ groups at pH 7−9, converting +ve charge on amino group to a −ve charge, *Biochem.* **8**, 2890 (1969). Introduction of −ve charges tends to dissociate proteins into sub-units (cf. maleic anhydride). Succinyl half-amide derivs. are more stable than maleyl derivs. but hydrolysed by 6M-HCl at 100 °C. Modification may also occur of tyrosine −OH (*O*-succinyltyrosine unstable above pH 5), of serine and threonine −OH (reversed by $NH_2OH$, *JBC* **242**, 2739 (1967)), and possibly of −SH. Succinic anhydride in $H_2O$ at 25 °C has half-life of 4.3 min. |
| pale yel. liq.; M.p. 13.8; B.p. 126; <br> $d_4^{25}$ 1.6229 | i. $H_2O$; s. EtOH, eth. | Modifies tyrosine residues forming 3-nitrotyrosine; reaction usually carried out at pH 8, no reaction at pH 6, *Meth. Enzymol.* **25**, 515 (1972). Nitro-tyrosine may be quantitated by absorbance, $\lambda_{max}$ 428 nm ε 4200 (pH 9.0), $\lambda_{max}$ 360 nm ε 2790 (in acid soln.), isosbestic point 381 nm ε 2200 (prior removal of nitroformate ion, which is formed in the reaction and absorbs strongly at 350 nm, is necessary); nitrotyrosine is stable to acid hydrolysis and may be estimated by amino acid analysis, *BBRC* **27**, 20 (1967). Treatment with tetranitromethane can give rise to cross-linking, normally oxidizes −SH groups, and may also modify methionine and tryptophan residues. Reagent is a skin and lung irritant and is explosive in presence of impurities. |
| Trihydrate: wh. flaky cryst. | s. $H_2O$, benz. | Reacts with α- and ε-$NH_2$ groups at mildly alkaline pH, usually 9.5, forming trinitrophenyl deriv. Also reacts with −SH groups, but not with arginine, imidazole, tyrosine, serine, or threonine. Extent of reaction may be estimated by the absorbance of the TNP-amino acids at 335−345 nm at acid pH, *Anal. Biochem.* **14**, 328 (1966), or by absorbance of the TNP-amino acid-sulphite complexes at 420 nm, *Meth. Enzymol.* **25**, 464 (1972), or by amino acid analysis after acid hydrolysis. |

# 17 Stability constants of metal complexes

The general order of complexing ability of metal ions can be expressed as: alkali metals ($Na^+$, $K^+$, etc.) < alkaline earths ($Mg^{2+}$, $Ca^{2+}$, etc.) < transition metals.

Alkali and alkaline earth metals combine most strongly with oxyanions, the transition metals with N and to a lesser extent with S, metals such as Zn and Hg combine most strongly with S. For the divalent ions of the transition metals the complexing ability usually follows the Irving-Williams series, viz. Mn < Fe < Co < Ni < Cu > Zn.

## Stability constants

For the reaction between metal (M) and ligand (L), $M + L \rightleftharpoons ML$, the stability constant is defined by $K_1 = [ML]/[M][L]$.

The metal may combine with more than one molecule of ligand, e.g.

$$\text{for } ML + L \rightleftharpoons ML_2, K_2 = [ML_2]/[ML][L], \text{etc.}$$

Experimentally, where more than one complex is formed, the *cumulative stability constants* are determined. These are defined by

$$\beta_2 = K_1 K_2$$

$$\beta_n = K_1 K_2 \ldots K_n$$

Other stability constants which may occur are $K_{MHL}^M = [MHL]/[M][HL]$ for the reaction $M + HL \rightleftharpoons MHL$, and $K_{M_2L}^M = [M_2L]/[M][ML]$ for the reaction $M + ML \rightleftharpoons M_2L$.

Constants are taken mainly from references 1–3. For methods of determination of stability constants, see Rossotti and Rossotti (ref. 4). As far as possible, all results are quoted at 25–30°C, at ionic strengths ranging within 0.01 to 0.5, and the $pK_a$ values were obtained under the same conditions. The effects of these variables is not negligible (ref. 4) so that these are not 'thermodynamic' constants. Many gaps in the Tables reflect the present lack of quantitative data.

## Use of tables

### (a) Conversion of absolute to 'apparent' constants

Unless indicated otherwise, the stability constants are expressed as absolute values, i.e. independent of pH. In practice, it is more usual to require the 'apparent' value at a particular pH. An apparent stability constant considers all forms of complexing species, whereas an absolute constant considers only the most anionic,

i.e. $$K_{app} = [ML]/[M]([L]_T - [ML]) = [ML]/[M][L]_{T'}$$

where $[L]_{T'}$ is the sum of all the individual uncomplexed forms of the ligand present in a solution.

To a first approximation, where the $pK_a$ of the ligand is more than one unit above the pH under consideration, the log of the absolute stability constant is reduced by $\log \alpha$, the difference between the $pK_a$ and the pH, to give the log of the apparent stability constant, e.g. for $\alpha$-alanine; $pK_{a2} = 9.9$

At pH 7.0, $$\log \alpha = pK_a - pH = 9.9 - 7.0 = 2.9$$

$$\log K_1 (\text{app}) (Cu^{2+}) = 8.5 - 2.9 = 5.6.$$

To convert cumulative constants to apparent values:

$$\log \beta_2 \, (\text{app}) = \log \beta_2 - 2\log \alpha$$

$$\log \beta_3 \, (\text{app}) = \log \beta_3 - 3\log \alpha, \text{ etc.}$$

This approach is illustrated in Table A where the results for EDTA include the apparent stability constants at pH 7.0 and pH 8.0.

For a ligand, L, with $n$ $pK_a$ values, $\alpha$ is given by

$$\alpha = [H^+]^n/K_{a1}K_{a2}\ldots K_{an} + [H^+]^{n-1}/K_{a1}K_{a2}\ldots K_{an-1} + \ldots + [H^+]/K_{a1} + 1.$$

Thus EDTA has 4 $pK_a$ values and, at pH 7.0, $\alpha = 2.08 \times 10^3$, so that $\log \alpha = 3.3$. For Mg-EDTA at pH 7.0: $\log K_1 \, (\text{app}) = 8.7 - 3.3 = 5.4$. The apparent stability constants will be indistiguishable from the absolute stability constants at pH values two or more units above the $pK_a$ value.

*(b) Calculation of free metal and ligand concentrations*

(i) When the ligand is present in excess, and only 1:1 complexes are formed:

$$[\text{ML}] \simeq [\text{M}]_T$$

$$[\text{L}]_{T'} \simeq [\text{L}]_T - [\text{M}]_T = [\text{L}],$$

and the free metal ion concentration is

$$[\text{M}] = [\text{M}_T]\alpha/K_1([\text{L}]_T - [\text{M}]_T).$$

(ii) When the metal ion is present in excess,

$$[\text{ML}] \approx [\text{L}]_T$$

$$[\text{M}] \simeq [\text{M}]_T - [\text{L}]_T$$

and the free ligand concentration is

$$[\text{L}] = [\text{L}]_T/K_1([\text{M}]_T - [\text{L}]_T).$$

These equations enable the concentrations of the species M, L, and ML, and hence

# A  Table of chelating agents

| Name | Synonym | Formula | M. wt. | $pK_a$ |
|---|---|---|---|---|
| Ammonium *N*-nitrosophenyl-hydroxylamine | Cupferron | $C_6H_5 \cdot N(NO) \cdot ONH_4$ | 155.1 | 4.2 |
| Ammonium purpurate | Murexide | $\cdot NH_4^+$ | 284.2; Hydrate, 302.2 | 9.2 10.5 |
| α-Benzoin oxime | Cupron | $C_6H_5 \cdot CHOH \cdot C(:NOH) \cdot C_6H_5$ | 227.3 | |

the composition of metal ion and ligand buffers (ref. 5) to be calculated under a given set of conditions. Computer programs are available for more complicated systems, involving ML, $ML_2$, $ML_3$, etc., or mixed complexes. (See, for example, ref. 5 for a fuller discussion of metal-ion buffers and the concept of p$M$.)

Complex formation modifies the oxidation–reduction potential of metal ion pairs, the shift in potential depending on the difference in the stability constants of the metal complexes in the two valence states concerned. For a quantitative treatment see ref. 6.

A notable omission from the present Tables are the macrocyclic ligands such as the crown ethers which form lipid-soluble metal complexes in which the metal is 'hidden' from the solvent. In spite of their important biological applications there is currently little quantitative information about their stability constants. (See ref. 7 for further discussion.)

## References

1. *Stability constants of metal-ion complexes* (1964). Compiled by L. G. Sillén and A. E. Martell. Special Publication No. 17, The Chemical Society, London.
2. *Stability constants of metal-ion complexes. Supplement No. 1* (1971). Compiled by L. G. Sillén and A. E. Martell. Special Publication No. 25, The Chemical Society, London.
3. *Stability constants of metal-ion complexes: organic ligands* (1979). Compiled by D. D. Perrin. Pergamon Press, Oxford.
4. F. J. C. Rossotti and H. Rossotti. *The determination of stability constants*, McGraw-Hill, New York (1961).
5. D. D. Perrin and B. Dempsey, *Buffers for pH and metal-ion control*, Chapman and Hall, London (1974).
6. D. D. Perrin, *Organic complexing reagents*, Robert E. Krieger Publ. Co., Huntington, New York (1978).
7. C. J. Pederson and H. K. Frensdorff, *Angew. Chem. (Internat. Edn.)* **11**, 16 (1972).
8. W. J. O'Sullivan & G. W. Smithers, Stability constants for biologically important metal-ligand complexes. *Meth. Enzymol.* **63**, 294 (1979).

| Main form of ligand at pH 7.0 | Type of stability constant | Log stability constant | | | | | | | | General remarks |
|---|---|---|---|---|---|---|---|---|---|---|
| | | Mg | Ca | Mn | Fe | Co | Ni | Cu | Zn | |
| $L^-$ | | | | | | | | | | Sol. in $H_2O$ and EtOH. Metal complexes insol. in $H_2O$, sol. in $CCl_4$, used in solvent extraction separations. Reagent and complexes generally unstable. |
| $H_2L^-$ | $K_1$ $K_{MH_2L}^M$ | 2.2 | 5 2.7 | | | 2.5 | | 3.5 | 3.1 | Sol. in $H_2O$. Forms sol. coloured complexes with divalent metals. Used particularly for analysis of $Ca^{2+}$ concns., also for $Cu^{2+}$, $Ni^{2+}$, $Co^{2+}$. Other complexes too unstable for analytical purposes. |
| | | | | | | | | | | Slightly sol in $H_2O$, complexes insol. in $H_2O$. Used for estimation of Mo(VI). |

| Name | Synonym | Formula | M. wt. | $pK_a$ |
|---|---|---|---|---|
| $N,N$-Bis-(hydroxyethyl)-glycine | Bicine | $(HO \cdot CH_2 \cdot CH_2)_2 N \cdot CH_2 \cdot COOH$ | 163.2 | 1.7<br>8.1 |
| 2,3-Butane-dione dioxime | Dimethylglyoxime | $CH_3 \cdot C(:NOH) \cdot C(:NOH) \cdot CH_3$ | 116.1 | 12.8 |
| *trans*-1,2-Diaminocyclo-hexanetetra-acetic acid | CDTA | | 346.3;<br>+ $H_2O$<br>364.3 | 2.4<br>3.5<br>6.1<br>12.4 |
| Diethylene-triaminopenta-acetic acid | DTPA | | 393.4 | 1.8<br>2.6<br>4.4<br>8.8<br>10.4 |
| 4,5-Dihydroxy-benzene-1,3-disulphonic acid | Catechol-3,5-disulphonic acid; tiron | | 270.2;<br>$Na_2$ salt,<br>314.2 | 7.7<br>12.6 |
| 2,3-Dimercapto-1-propanol | BAL; dimercaprol | $CH_2.OH$<br>$HC.SH$<br>$CH_2.SH$ | 124.2 | 8.7 |
| Diphenylthio-carbazone | Dithizone | $C_6H_5 \cdot N{:}N \cdot CS \cdot NH \cdot NH \cdot C_6H_5$ | 256.3 | 4.5 |
| 2,2'-Dipyridyl | $\alpha,\alpha'$-Bipyridyl | | 156.2 | 4.4 |
| 3,6-Disulpho-1,8-dihydroxy-naphthalene | Chromotropic acid | | Hydrate,<br>356.2 (2$H_2O$)<br>$Na_2$ salt<br>+ 2$H_2O$<br>400.3 | 5.4 |

| Main form of ligand at pH 7.0 | Type of stability constant | Log stability constant | | | | | | | | General remarks |
|---|---|---|---|---|---|---|---|---|---|---|
| | | Mg | Ca | Mn | Fe | Co | Ni | Cu | Zn | |
| L⁻ | $K_1$ | | 2.8 | 3.1 | 4.3 | 5.3 | 6.4 | 8.1 | 5.4 | |
| | $\beta_2$ | | | 5.4 | 7.3 | 8.8 | 10.8 | 13.3 | 8.6 | |
| HL | $K_1$ | | | | | 8.4 | | 9.1 | | Insol. in $H_2O$; sol. in EtOH. Forms sol. complexes with $Co^{2+}$, $Cu^{2+}$, $Fe^{2+}$, insol. complexes with $Ni^{2+}$. Used for quantitative estimation of $Ni^{2+}$. |
| | $\beta_2$ | | | | | 17.0 | 17.0 | 18.5 | | |
| HL³⁻ | $K_1$ | 11.0 | 13.2 | 17.4 | 28.1 (Feᴵᴵᴵ) | 19.6 | 19.4 | 22.0 | 19.3 | Used in preventing pptn. of Mn in 3M-alkali during the estimation of org. compds. in alk. soln. |
| H₂L³⁻ | $K_1$ | 9.3 | 10.6 | 15.1 | 28.6 (Feᴵᴵᴵ) | 19.0 | 20.2 | 21.1 | 18.7 | |
| H₂L²⁻ | $K_1$ | 6.9 | 5.8 | 8.6 | | 9.5 | 10.0 | 14.5 | 10.4 | Log $K_{app}(Ca^{2+}) = 1.8$ at pH 7.2. Log $\beta_2$ ($Zn^{2+}$) = 18.6. Used in colorimetric estimation of $Fe^{3+}$ |
| | $\beta$ | | | | 47.7 | | | 25.5 | | |
| | $K_{MHL}^{M}$ | 2.0 | 2.2 | | 20.8 (Feᴵᴵᴵ) | 3.1 | 3.0 | 5.5 | 3.3 | |
| H₂L | $K_1$ | | | 5.2 | | | | | 13.5 | Insol. in $H_2O$. General chelator of heavy metals. Used in therapeutic treatment of Pb, As, Hg poisoning. |
| | $\beta_2$ | | | 10.4 | 15.8 | | 23.0 | | 23.0 | |
| L⁻ | | | | | | | | | | Dithizone and its complexes insol. in $H_2O$; sol. in org. solvents. Used in extraction of heavy metal contaminants from aq. soln. Complexes highly coloured and used for analytical determination of many metals, e.g. Zn, *ABB* **46**, 345 (1953); *JBC* **237**, 1129 (1962); *Anal. Chim. Acta* **110**, 21 (1979). |
| L | $K_1$ | 0.5 | | 2.5 | 4.3 | 5.6 | 7.1 | 8.5 | 5.4 | |
| | $\beta_2$ | | | 4.6 | 7.9 | 11.2 | 13.9 | 14.0 | 9.8 | |
| | $\beta_3$ | | | 6.3 | 17.3 | 16.0 | 20.1 | 17.9 | 13.5 | |
| HL³⁻ | $K_1$ | | | | | | | 13.4 | | Sol. in $H_2O$. Complexes (sol. in $H_2O$ and usually coloured) with heavy metals, also Al, Be. |

| Name | Synonym | Formula | M. wt. | $pK_a$ |
|---|---|---|---|---|
| Dithiooxamide | Rubeanic acid | HN=C——C=NH<br>    SH    SH | 120.2 | 10.6 |
| Eriochrome Black T | 1-(1-Hydroxy-2-napththylazo)-2-hydroxy-5-nitro-naphthalene-4-sulphonic acid | *(structure)* | 439.4;<br>Na salt,<br>461.4 | 6.3<br>11.6 |
| Ethylene-diamine | 1,2-Diaminoethane | $NH_2 \cdot CH_2 \cdot CH_2 \cdot NH_2$ | 60.1 | 7.2<br>9.9 |
| Ethylene-diaminetetra-acetic acid | EDTA; versene; sequestrol | HOOC CH$_2$⟍    ⟋CH$_2$COOH<br>      N·CH$_2$·CH$_2$N<br>HOOC CH$_2$⟋    ⟍CH$_2$COOH | 292.2 | 2.0<br>2.7<br>6.2<br>10.3 |
| ——, Na$_2$ salt | | $C_{10}H_{14}O_8N_2Na_2 \cdot 2H_2O$ | 372.3 | |
| (Ethylene-dioxy)diethyl-enedinitrilo-tetraacetic acid | EGTA | HOOC—CH$_2$⟍                    ⟋CH$_2$·COOH<br>      N·CH$_2$·CH$_2$·O·CH$_2$·CH$_2$·O·CH$_2$·CH$_2$·N<br>HOOC—CH$_2$⟋                    ⟍CH$_2$·COOH | 380.4 | <2<br>2.7<br>8.8<br>9.5 |
| o-Hydroxybenz-aldehyde oxime | Salicylaldoxime | *(structure)* CH:NOH / OH | 137.1 | 8.9<br>11.1 |
| N-(2′-Hydroxy-ethyl)iminodi-acetic acid | HIMDA | $HO \cdot CH_2 \cdot CH_2 \cdot N \cdot (CH_2COOH)_2$ | 177.2 | 2.2<br>8.7 |
| 8-Hydroxy-quinoline | Oxine, quinolinol | *(structure)* N / OH | 145.2 | 5.1<br>9.9 |
| 8-Hydroxy-quinoline-5-sulphonic acid | Sulphoxine | *(structure)* SO$_3$H / N / OH | 225.2 | 1.3<br>4.1<br>8.7 |
| 4-Methyl-1,2-dimercapto-benzene | Dithiol, toluene-3,4-dithiol | *(structure)* SH SH / CH$_3$ | 156.3 | |

| Main form of ligand at pH 7.0 | Type of stability constant | Log stability constant | | | | | | | | General remarks |
|---|---|---|---|---|---|---|---|---|---|---|
| | | Mg | Ca | Mn | Fe | Co | Ni | Cu | Zn | |
| $H_2L$ | | | | | | | | | | Sol. in aq. EtOH. Forms coloured complexes with transition and heavy metals. Used in localization of Cu (green ppt.) on chromatograms and in histochemical preparations. Other complexes sol. in $H_2O$, except Co and Ni complexes (sol. in acid solns). |
| $HL^{2-}$ | $K_1$ | 7.0 | 5.5 | | | 20.0 | | 21.4 | 12.3 | Sol. in $H_2O$. Forms coloured complexes with many divalent metal ions. Used particularly for analytical determination of Mg. |
| $H_2L^{2+}$ | $K_1$ | 0.4 | | 2.7 | 4.3 | 5.9 | 7.6 | 10.7 | 6.0 | |
| | $\beta_2$ | | | 4.8 | 7.5 | 10.7 | 14.0 | 20.0 | 11.0 | |
| | $\beta_3$ | | | 5.7 | 9.5 | 13.8 | 18.5 | | 13.0 | |
| $HL^{3-}$ | $K_1$ | 8.7 | 10.6 | 14.0 | 14.2 | 16.0 | 18.6 | 18.8 | 16.4 | Log $K_1(Na^+) = 1.7$. Used as a metal buffer and in metal titrations. Used to eliminate inhibition of enzyme-catalysed reactions due to traces of heavy metals. See *BJ* **79**, 584 (1961); *BBA* **64**, 83 (1962); **77**, 142 (1963). Poor complexing ability with $Ag^+$. |
| | $K_1$ (app) at pH 7 | 5.4 | 7.3 | 10.7 | 10.9 | 12.7 | 15.3 | 15.5 | 13.1 | |
| | $K_1$ (app) at pH 8 | 6.4 | 8.3 | 11.7 | 11.9 | 13.7 | 16.3 | 16.5 | 14.1 | |
| $H_2L^{2-}$ | $K_1$ | 5.2 | 11.0 | 12.1 | 11.8 | 12.3 | 11.8 | 17.7 | 12.9 | Used to chelate $Ca^{2+}$ in the presence of $Mg^{2+}$, *Helv. chim. Acta* **47**, 1801 (1964). |
| | $K^M_{MHL}$ | 3.4 | 5.3 | 7.0 | 6.4 | 8.0 | 8.3 | 12.6 | 8.4 | |
| $H_2L$ | $K^M_{MHL}$ | 0.6 | 0.9 | | | 8.1 | 3.8 | 4.2 | | Slightly sol. in $H_2O$. Complexes heavy metals; yellow-green ppt. with Cu. |
| $HL^-$ | $K_1$ | 3.5 | 4.7 | 5.6 | 6.8 | 8.1 | 9.4 | 11.9 | 8.4 | Log $K_1(Fe^{III}) = 11.6$ |
| | $\beta_2$ | | | 9.4 | | 12.4 | 14.5 | 16.0 | 12.3 | |
| $HL$ | $K_1$ | 4.7 | 3.3 | 6.8 | 8.0 | 9.1 | 9.9 | 12.2 | 8.5 | Slightly sol. in $H_2O$. Mg and Ca complexes sparingly sol., others insol. |
| | $\beta_2$ | | | 12.6 | 15.0 | 17.2 | 18.7 | 23.4 | 17.6 | |
| $HL^-$ | $K_1$ | 4.8 | 3.5 | 6.9 | 8.4 | 8.8 | 9.8 | 12.5 | 8.7 | Higher solubilities of ligand and complexes than for oxine. |
| | $\beta_2$ | 8.4 | | | 15.1 | 15.9 | 18.5 | 23.1 | 16.2 | |
| $H_2L$ | | | | | | | | | | Slightly sol. in aq. alkali; sol. in org. solvents. Forms slightly soluble coloured complexes with heavy metals. |

| Name | Synonym | Formula | M. wt. | $pK_a$ |
|---|---|---|---|---|
| Nitrilotriacetic acid | NTA | $N(CH_2COOH)_3$ | 191.1; Na$_3$ salt + 1 H$_2$O 275.1 | 1.9 2.5 9.8 |
| 5-Nitro-1,10-phenanthroline | | | 225.2 | 3.2 |
| 1,10-Phenanthroline | o-Phenanthroline | | Hydrate, 198.2 (H$_2$O) | 5.0 |
| Potassium ethyl xanthate | Potassium xanthogenate | $C_2H_5O \cdot CS \cdot SK$ | 160.3 | |
| Salicylic acid | o-Hydroxybenzoic acid | | 138.1 | 2.9 13.1 |
| Sodium diethyldithio-carbamate | Cupral | $(C_2H_5)_2N \cdot CS \cdot SNa$ | Hydrate, 225.3 (3 H$_2$O) | |
| 2-Thenoyl-2-furoylmethane | | | 220.3 | 12.3 |
| Thenoyl-trifluoro-acetone | 4,4,4-Trifluoro-1-(2-thienyl)-1,3-butanedione | | 222.2 | 6.2 |
| Thiourea | Thiocarbamide | $NH_2 \cdot CS \cdot NH_2$ | 76.1 | |
| Triethylene-tetramine | Trien | $H_2N \cdot CH_2 \cdot CH_2 \cdot NH \cdot CH_2 \cdot CH_2 \cdot NH \cdot CH_2 \cdot CH_2 \cdot NH_2$ | 146.2; 2 HCl, 219.2 | 3.3 6.6 9.1 9.8 |

| Main form of ligand at pH 7.0 | Type of stability constant | Log stability constant | | | | | | | | General remarks |
|---|---|---|---|---|---|---|---|---|---|---|
| | | Mg | Ca | Mn | Fe | Co | Ni | Cu | Zn | |
| $HL^{2-}$ | $K_1$ | 5.5 | 6.5 | 7.4 | 15.9 (Fe$^{III}$) | 10.8 | 11.5 | 13.1 | 10.4 | |
| L | $K_1$<br>$\beta_3$ | 3.5 | | | 5.1<br>18.0 | 6.3<br>16.6 | 7.0<br>20.4 | 8.0<br>17.7 | 5.5 | Other substituted 1,10-phenanthrolines (e.g. 5-Br, 5-Me) have similar chelating ability. 2-Substituted compounds have weaker chelating ability. |
| L | $K_1$<br>$\beta_2$<br>$\beta_3$ | 1.5 | 0.5 | 3.9<br>7.0<br>10.0 | 5.8<br>11.2<br>16.5 | 7.3<br>14.0<br>20.0 | 8.6<br>16.7<br>24.0 | 6.3<br>12.5<br>18.0 | 6.4<br>12.1<br>17.0 | Used in removal of Zn from Zn-metalloenzymes (*JBC* **235**, 64 (1960)). Also for spectrophotometric determination of Fe$^{2+}$. |
| $L^-$ | | | | | | | | | | Soluble in H$_2$O but solns. unstable. Forms coloured complexes (insol. in H$_2$O) with heavy metals. Used in analysis of Mo. |
| $HL^-$ | $K_1$ | | 0.5 | 5.9 | 6.6 | 6.7 | 7.0 | 10.6 | | Slightly sol. in water. Forms strong complexes with Cu, Al, Fe$^{3+}$. Used to remove Be (log $K_1 = 4.3$) in Be poisoning. |
| L | $\beta_2$ | | | | | | 12.5 | | 11.5 | Sol. in H$_2$O but solns. unstable. Metal complexes insol. in H$_2$O. Used in immiscible solvents to extract heavy metals; also for colorimetric determinations of Cu, Ni, and Co. |
| HL | | | | | | | | | | Insol. in H$_2$O; sol. in org. solvents. Complexes (insol. in H$_2$O) with heavy metals. |
| $L^-$ | | | | | | | | | | Slightly sol. in H$_2$O; sol. in C$_6$H$_6$. Complexes (usually insol. in H$_2$O, sol. in benz.) with heavy metals. Used in solvent extraction procedures. |
| L | | | | | | | | | | Sol. in H$_2$O. Forms sol. complexes with heavy metals. Used esp. as a masking agent for Cu$^{2+}$. Fairly strong reducing agent. |
| $H_2L^{2+}$ | $K_1$<br>$K_{MHL}^M$ | | | 4.9 | 7.8 | | 14.0<br>8.9 | 20.4<br>14.0 | 12.1<br>7.3 | |

# B Metal binding properties of compounds used in biochemistry

| Name | $pK_a$ | Principal form of ligand at pH 7.0 | Type of constant | Log stability constant | | | | | | | |
|---|---|---|---|---|---|---|---|---|---|---|---|
| | | | | Mg | Ca | Mn | Fe | Co | Ni | Cu | Zn |
| **Anions*** | | | | | | | | | | | |
| Cyanide, $CN^-$ | 9.4 | HL | $\beta_4$ | | | | | | 12 | 25 | 16.9 |
| | | | $\beta_6$ | | | | 35 | 19 | | | |
| Phosphate, $PO_4^{3-}$ | 2.1 7.2 12.0 | $H_2L^-$ | $K_{MHL}^M$ | 2.5 | 2.2 | 2.6 | | 2.2 | 2.1 | 3.2 | 2.4 |
| Pyrophosphate, $P_2O_7^{4-}$ | 0.9 2.0 6.0 9.1 | $HL^{3-}$ | $K_1$ | 4.7 | 5.0 | | | 7.4 | 5.8 | 6.7 | |
| | | | $\beta_2$ | | | | | | 7.3 | 9.0 | 6.5 |
| Thiocyanate, $SCN^-$ | | $L^-$ | $K_1$ | | | | 1.0 | 1.2 | | | 1.6 |
| | | | $\beta_3$ | | | | | | 1.8 | 5.2 | |
| Thiosulphate, $S_2O_3^{2-}$ | | $L^{2-}$ | $K_1$ | 1.8 | 2.0 | 2.0 | 2.2 | 2.1 | 2.1 | | 2.4 |
| | | | $\beta_2$ | | | | | | | 12.3 | |
| Triphosphate, $P_3O_{10}^{5-}$ | 5.4 7.9 | $HL^{4-}$ | $K_1$ | 5.8 | 5.0 | 7.2 | | 8.1 | 7.9 | 9.8 | 7.6 |
| | | | $K_{MHL}^M$ | 3.7 | 3.1 | 3.8 | | | | | 3.9 |
| Sulphate, $SO_4^{2-}$ | 2.0 | $L^{2-}$ | $K_1$ | 2.4 | 2.3 | 2.3 | 2.3 | 2.5 | 2.4 | 2.2 | 2.3 |
| **Amino acids and related compounds** | | | | | | | | | | | |
| $\alpha$-Alanine | 2.34 9.87 | HL | $K_1$ | 2.0 | 1.2 | 3.1 | | 4.4 | 5.5 | 8.2 | 4.6 |
| | | | $\beta_2$ | | | 6.1 | 7.3 | 7.9 | 10.0 | 15.0 | 8.6 |
| $\beta$-Alanine | 3.56 10.22 | HL | $K_1$ | | | 2.1 | | 3.6 | 4.7 | 7.1 | 4.1 |
| | | | $\beta_2$ | | | | 4.0 | 6.1 | 8.1 | 12.6 | 7.2 |

*Other anions:* $AsO_4^{3-}$ and $CO_3^{2-}$ generally form insoluble salts with divalent metals; $Cl^-$, possible very weak complexes with Mn, Fe, Cu; $F^-$, weak complexes with Mg, Ni, Co, Zn but usually gives insoluble salts, strong complexes with tri- and tetravalent cations; $NO_3^-$, possible weak complexes with Co, Cu.

*Hydrolysis of metal ions:*
In aqueous solutions, divalent metal ions undergo hydrolysis according to the equation $M_{aq}^{2+} \rightleftharpoons MOH^+ + H^+$, with a subsequent step $MOH^+ \rightleftharpoons M(OH)_2 + H^+$, leading to precipitation of insoluble hydroxide. The $pK_a$ value for the formation of $MOH^+$ is the pH at which $M_{aq}^{2+}$ and $MOH^+$ are present in equal concentrations. Some useful $pK_a$ values are: Mg, 11.4; Ca, 12.6; Mn, 10.6; Fe(II), 6.7; Fe(III), 2.5; Co, 8.9; Ni, 9.9; Cu, 8.0; Zn, 9.0. For further values, see *Dissociation constants of inorganic acids and bases* (1969), D.D. Perrin, Butterworths, London. Onset of precipitation occurs about 2–3 pH units below the $pK_a$ value.

| Name | $pK_a$ | Principal form of ligand at pH 7.0 | Type of constant | Log stability constant | | | | | | | |
|------|--------|------|------|------|------|------|------|------|------|------|------|
| | | | | Mg | Ca | Mn | Fe | Co | Ni | Cu | Zn |
| α-Aminobutyric acid | 2.23<br>9.63 | HL | $K_1$<br>$\beta_2$ | | | | 3.4 | 4.3<br>7.6 | 5.5<br>9.8 | 8.2<br>14.7 | 4.5<br>8.7 |
| Arginine | 2.17<br>9.36<br>(12.48) | $H_2L^+$ | $K_1$<br>$\beta_2$<br>$\beta_3$ | 1.3 | 2.2 | 2.6 | 3.2 | 4.0<br>7.2<br>9.2 | 5.2<br>9.5 | 7.9<br>14.6 | 4.1<br>8.1 |
| Asparagine | 2.16<br>8.75 | HL | $K_1$<br>$\beta_2$<br>$\beta_3$ | 4.0 | | 4.5 | 6.5 | 4.6<br>8.3<br>10.0 | 10.6 | 7.9<br>14.4 | 8.7 |
| Aspartic acid | 1.94<br>3.70<br>9.62 | $HL^-$ | $K_1$<br>$\beta_2$ | 2.4 | 1.6 | 3.7 | 8.5 | 5.9<br>10.2 | 6.7<br>12.0 | 8.6<br>15.4 | 5.8<br>10.2 |
| Cysteine | 1.96<br>8.48<br>10.55 | $H_2L$ | $K_1$<br>$\beta_2$ | <4 | | 4.6 | 6.2<br>11.8 | 9.3<br>16.9 | 9.8<br>20.2 | | 9.2<br>18.2 |
| Glutamic acid | 2.30<br>4.28<br>9.67 | $HL^-$ | $K_1$<br>$\beta_2$ | 1.9 | 1.4 | 3.3 | 4.6 | 4.5<br>8.1 | 5.9<br>10.3 | 7.9<br>14.6 | 5.5<br>9.5 |
| Glycine | 2.43<br>9.63 | HL | $K_1$<br>$\beta_2$<br>$\beta_3$ | 1.3 | 1.4 | 2.9<br>5.5 | 4.1<br>7.7 | 4.6<br>8.5<br>10.8 | 5.7<br>10.5 | 8.1<br>15.2 | 5.0<br>9.2 |
| Glycylglycine | 2.91<br>8.22 | HL | $K_1$<br>$\beta_2$ | 1.1 | 1.2 | 2.2 | | 2.9<br>5.2 | 4.1<br>7.2 | 5.6<br>11.0 | 3.5<br>6.4 |
| Histamine | 6.10<br>9.8 | $HL^+$ | $K_1$<br>$\beta_2$<br>$\beta_3$ | | | 3.0 | | 5.2<br>8.7<br>10.0 | 6.8<br>11.7<br>14.9 | 9.6<br>16.2 | 5.7<br>8.7 |
| Histidine | 1.82<br>6.05<br>9.17 | HL | $K_1$<br>$\beta_2$ | | | 3.4<br>5.8 | 9.3 | 6.8<br>13.9 | 8.9<br>15.9 | 10.2<br>18.3 | 6.7<br>11.8 |
| Imidazole | 7.1 | $HL^+$ | $K_1$<br>$\beta_2$<br>$\beta_3$<br>$\beta_4$ | | 0.1 | 1.6<br>2.9 | 3.3<br>6.4 | 2.4<br>4.4<br>6.0<br>7.2 | 2.9<br>5.4<br>7.3<br>8.7 | 4.2<br>7.7<br>10.1<br>12.5 | 2.0<br>4.2<br>6.6<br>9.5 |
| Leucine | 2.36<br>9.60 | HL | $K_1$<br>$\beta_2$ | | | 2.8<br>5.5 | 3.4 | 4.6<br>8.3 | 5.6<br>10.2 | 7.9<br>14.3 | 4.9<br>8.9 |
| Lysine | 2.18<br>9.18<br>10.72 | $H_2L^+$ | $K_1$<br>$\beta_2$ | | | 2 | 4.5 | 3.6<br>6.8 | 5.5<br>8.8 | 7.6<br>13.7 | 7.6 |
| Methionine | 2.20<br>9.10 | HL | $K_1$<br>$\beta_2$ | | | 2.8<br>4.8 | 6.7 | 4.4<br>7.9 | 5.2<br>9.8 | 8.0<br>14.8 | 4.4<br>8.5 |

# 17B  Metal binding properties of compounds used in biochemistry

| Name | $pK_a$ | Principal form of ligand at pH 7.0 | Type of constant | Mg | Ca | Mn | Fe | Co | Ni | Cu | Zn |
|---|---|---|---|---|---|---|---|---|---|---|---|
| Norleucine | 2.25 | HL | $K_1$ | | | | | | 5.4 | | |
| | 9.70 | | $\beta_2$ | 4 | | 5 | 8.6 | 9.4 | 9.9 | 15.4 | 10.4 |
| Ornithine | 1.96 | $H_2L^+$ | $K_1$ | | | 2 | 5.0 | 4.0 | 4.9 | 6.9 | 4.1 |
| | 8.65 | | $\beta_2$ | | | | | 6.9 | 8.5 | 12.5 | 7.3 |
| | 10.7 | | | | | | | | | | |
| Phenylalanine | 1.85 | HL | $K_1$ | | | 2.4 | 3.7 | 4.1 | 5.6 | 8.3 | 4.4 |
| | 9.13 | | $\beta_2$ | | | | 6.3 | 7.9 | 10.2 | 14.7 | 8.4 |
| Proline | 1.93 | HL | $K_1$ | | | 2.8 | | 5.0 | 6.2 | 8.9 | 5.1 |
| | 10.68 | | $\beta_2$ | 4 | | 5.5 | 8.3 | 9.3 | 11.3 | 16.8 | 9.7 |
| Serine | 2.15 | HL | $K_1$ | | 1.4 | 3.9 | | 4.5 | 5.4 | 7.9 | 4.7 |
| | 9.60 | | $\beta_2$ | | | 6.3 | 7.0 | 8.0 | 9.8 | 14.5 | 8.7 |
| Tryptophan | 2.38 | HL | $K_1$ | | | 2.9 | 2.9 | 4.6 | 5.7 | 8.3 | 5.2 |
| | 9.39 | | $\beta_2$ | 4 | | 5 | 7.6 | 8.5 | 10.2 | 15.9 | 9.3 |
| Tyrosine | 2.20 | $H_2L$ | $K^M_{MHL}$ | 2 | 1.5 | 2.4 | | 4.0 | 5.1 | 7.9 | 4.2 |
| | 9.19 | | $K^M_{M(HL)_2}$ | | | | 7.1 | 7.8 | 9.6 | 14.8 | 8.3 |
| | 10.4 | | | | | | | | | | |
| Valine | 2.3 | HL | $K_1$ | | | 2.8 | | 4.6 | 5.3 | 8.1 | 5.0 |
| | 9.7 | | $\beta_2$ | | | 5.6 | 6.8 | 8.4 | | | |

**Zwitterionic buffers**

| Name | $pK_a$ | Principal form of ligand at pH 7.0 | Type of constant | Mg | Ca | Mn | Fe | Co | Ni | Cu | Zn |
|---|---|---|---|---|---|---|---|---|---|---|---|
| $N$-(2-Acetamido)-2-aminoethane-sulphonic acid (ACES)* | 6.88 | $L^-$ | $K_1$ | | 0.4 | 0.4 | | | | | 4.6 |
| $N$-(2-Acetamido)-iminodiacetic acid (ADA)* | 6.52 | $L^{2-}$ | $K_1$ | | 2.5 | 4.0 | 4.9 | | | | 9.7 |
| 2-($N$-Morpholino)-ethanesulphonic acid (MES)* | 6.15 | $L^-$ | $K_1$ | | 0.8 | 0.7 | 0.7 | | | | |
| $N$-Tris(hydroxy-methyl)methyl-glycine (Tricine)* | 8.15 | HL | $K_1$ | | 1.2 | 2.4 | 2.7 | | | | 7.3 |
| Tris(hydroxy-methyl)methyl-amine (Tris) | 8.09 | $HL^+$ | $K_1$ | | | | | | | 2.6 | 4.0 |
| | | | $\beta_2$ | | | | | | | 4.5 | 7.6 |
| | | | $\beta_3$ | | | | | | | | 11.0 |

*A 'Good' buffer: see ADA, HEPES, MES, etc., *Biochemistry* **5**, 467 (1966). Binding of Mg, Ca, and Mn by PIPES, cholamine chloride, BES, TES, and HEPES is negligible, as also is binding of Cu by HEPES, cholamine chloride, and PIPES. Log $K_1$ for Cu with BES is 3.5, with TES it is 3.2.

| Name | $pK_a$ | Principal form of ligand at pH 7.0 | Type of constant | Log stability constant | | | | | | | |
|------|--------|-----------------------------------|------------------|-----|-----|-----|-----|-----|-----|-----|-----|
| | | | | Mg | Ca | Mn | Fe | Co | Ni | Cu | Zn |
| **Carboxylic acids** | | | | | | | | | | | |
| Acetic acid | 4.64 | $L^-$ | $K_1$ | 0.5 | 0.5 | 1.2 | 1.4 | 1.5 | 0.7 | 1.6 | 1.3 |
| | | | $\beta_2$ | | | | | 1.9 | 1.3 | 2.7 | 2.1 |
| Citric acid | 3.1 | $L^{3-}$ | $K_1$ | 3.6 | 3.6 | 3.7 | 4.4 | 5.0 | 5.4 | 5.9 | 5.0 |
| | 4.7 | | $K^M_{MHL}$ | 1.8 | 2.1 | 2.1 | 2.7 | 3.0 | 3.3 | 3.4 | 3.0 |
| | 6.4 | | $K^M_{MH_2L}$ | | 1.2 | | | | 1.3 | 1.8 | 2.3 | 1.3 |
| Formic acid | 3.77 | $L^-$ | $K_1$ | 1.4 | 1.4 | 0.8 | | | | 2.0 | |
| Fumaric acid | 3.02 | $L^{2-}$ | $K_1$ | | 2.0 | 1.0 | | | | 2.5 | |
| | 4.39 | | | | | | | | | | |
| Gluconic acid | 3.56 | $L^-$ | $K_1$ | 0.7 | 1.2 | | | | | 1.8 | 1.7 |
| Lactic acid | 3.77 | $L^-$ | $K_1$ | 0.9 | 1.1 | 0.9 | | 1.4 | 1.6 | 2.6 | 1.6 |
| | | | $\beta_2$ | 1.3 | 1.2 | 1.4 | | 2.3 | 2.7 | 3.9 | 2.8 |
| Maleic acid | 1.92 | $L^{2-}$ | $K_1$ | | 2.4 | 1.7 | | | 2.0 | 3.9 | 2.0 |
| | 6.22 | | | | | | | | | | |
| Malic acid | 3.23 | $L^{2-}$ | $K_1$ | 1.6 | 1.9 | 2.2 | | 2.0 | | 3.4 | 2.8 |
| | 4.77 | | $K^M_{MHL}$ | 1.7 | 2.0 | | | 2.9 | 3.2 | 3.4 | 2.9 |
| Malonic acid | 2.62 | $L^{2-}$ | $K_1$ | 2.1 | 1.5 | 3.3 | | 3.0 | 3.3 | 5.0 | 3.0 |
| | 5.30 | | $\beta_2$ | | | | 2.2 | 4.4 | 4.9 | 7.7 | 4.5 |
| Oxalic acid | 1.14 | $L^{2-}$ | $K_1$ | 2.6 | 3 | 3.9 | 4.7 | 4.7 | 5.3 | 4.4 | 4.9 |
| | 3.85 | | $\beta_2$ | 4.4 | | 5.3 | 9.2 | 6.7 | 12.9 | 8.5 | 7.4 |
| | | | $\beta_3$ | | | | 14.4 | | 14.0 | | 8.2 |
| Propionic acid | 4.7 | $L^-$ | $K_1$ | 0.5 | 0.5 | | | 0.8 | | 2.2 | 1.0 |
| Pyruvic acid | 2.5 | $L^-$ | $K_1$ | | 0.8 | 1.3 | | | 1.2 | 2.2 | 1.3 |
| Succinic acid | 3.90 | $L^{2-}$ | $K_1$ | 1.2 | 1.2 | | | 1.7 | | 2.9 | 1.8 |
| | 5.19 | | $K^M_{MHL}$ | | 0.5 | | | 1.0 | | 1.7 | 1.0 |
| Tartaric acid | 2.88 | $L^{2-}$ | $K_1$ | 1.4 | 1.8 | | 2.2 | 2.4 | 3.1 | 3.4 | 2.7 |
| | 3.94 | | $\beta_2$ | | | | 5.0 | | 5.4 | 5.8 | |
| | | | ($\log K_1$ 5.7, $\log \beta_2$ 10.5 for $Fe^{III}$) | | | | | | | | |
| **Miscellaneous compounds of biological interest** | | | | | | | | | | | |
| Adenine | 4.18 | HL | $K_1$ | 3.1 | 3.0 | 3.4 | | 8.1 | 8.3 | 8.5 | 8.2 |
| | 9.7 | | $\beta_2$ | | | | | | | 13.5 | |

411

# 17B  Metal binding properties of compounds used in biochemistry

| Name | $pK_a$ | Principal form of ligand at pH 7.0 | Type of constant | Log stability constant | | | | | | | |
|---|---|---|---|---|---|---|---|---|---|---|---|
| | | | | Mg | Ca | Mn | Fe | Co | Ni | Cu | Zn |
| Aureomycin | 3.3 7.44 9.27 | $H_2L$ | $K_1$ $\beta_2$ | | | 4.3 | 5.7 10.4 | 4.8 | | 7.6 12.6 | 4.5 |
| Flavine adenine dinucleotide (FAD) | | | $K_{app}$, pH 8.2 | 2.0 | 2.0 | 2.4 | | 2.4 | | | |
| Flavine mono-nucleotide (FMN) | | | $K_{app}$, pH 8.2 | 2.1 | 2.1 | 2.2 | | 2.4 | | | |
| Guanosine | 2.2 9.3 | HL | $K_1$ $K^M_{MHL}$ | | | | 4.8 | 3.2 | 3.8 | 6.0 2.2 | 4.6 |
| Glucose 1-phosphate | 1.11 6.13 | $HL^{2-}$ | $K_1$ | | 2.5 | 2.3 | | | | | |
| Glucose 6-phosphate | 0.94 6.11 | $HL^{2-}$ | $K_1$ | | | 2.3 | | | | | |
| Hypoxanthine | 1.98 8.94 12.1 | HL | $K_1$ $K^M_{MHL}$ | 6.7 | 6.5 | 6.9 2.4 | 3.9 | 7.1 3.8 | 7.2 4.7 | 7.5 1.9 | 7.1 |
| Inosine | 1.2 8.8 | HL | $K_1$ | | | | 3.0 | 2.6 | 3.3 | 5.0 | |
| Phosphoarginine | <2 2.0 4.5 9.6 11.2 | $HL^{3-}$ | $K^M_{MHL}$ | 2.0 | | | | | | | |
| Phosphocreatine | 2 2.7 4.5 | $HL^{3-}$ | $K^M_{MHL}$ | 1.6 | 1.3 | 2.0 | | | | | |
| Phosphoenol-pyruvic acid | | | $K_1$ | 2.3 | | 2.7 | | 3.5 | 2.3 | | 3.0 |
| 2-Phosphoglyceric acid | | | $K_1$ | 2.4 | | 3.1 | | 3.0 | 2.9 | | 3.4 |
| Pteroylglutamic acid (folic acid) | 8.26 | $HL^{2-}$ | $\beta_2$ | | | 6 | 7.9 | 8.1 | 9.0 | 7.8 | 7.5 |
| Pyridine | 5.45 | L | $K_1$ $\beta_2$ | | | 0.1 | 0.7 1.0 | 1.1 1.8 | 1.9 3.1 | 2.5 4.4 | 1.4 1.1 |
| Pyridoxamine | 3.37 8.0 10.1 | $H_2L^{2+}$ | $K_1$ $\beta_2$ | | | 3.6 | | 5.1 9.6 | 6.0 10.9 | 10.2 16.0 | 5.7 |

| Name | $pK_a$ | Principal form of ligand at pH 7.0 | Type of constant | Log stability constant | | | | | | | | |
|------|--------|-----------------------------------|------------------|------|------|------|------|------|------|------|------|
| | | | | Mg | Ca | Mn | Fe | Co | Ni | Cu | Zn |
| Riboflavin | 3.6 | HL | $K_1$ | | | 3.7 | 7.1 | 4.1 | 4.2 | 6.5 | 4.2 |
| | 9.5 | | $K_{MHL}^M$ | | | 3.2 | | | 3.5 | 3.5 | 3.7 | 3.7 |
| Terramycin | 3.10 | $H_2L$ | $K_1$ | 3.8 | | 4.3 | 5.6 | 5.1 | 5.8 | 7.2 | 4.6 |
| | 7.26 | | $\beta_2$ | | | 8.0 | 10.4 | | 10.6 | 12.2 | |
| | 9.1 | | | | | | | | | | |
| Xanthosine | 2.5 | $L^-$ | $K_1$ | | | | 2 | 2.8 | 3.0 | 3.4 | 2.4 |
| | 5.67 | | | | | | | | | | |

## C  Metal nucleotide complexes

Detailed information is presented for the alkali metals and for $Mg^{2+}$, $Ca^{2+}$, and $Mn^{2+}$ complexes with ADP and ATP. There is considerable variation in the values available from the literature (see *The enzymes*, vol. 2, p. 3, Academic Press, New York (1960)) and this Table is based largely on the results of Burton (*BJ* **71**, 388 (1959)) and O'Sullivan and Perrin (*BBA* **52**, 612 (1961); *Biochemistry* **3**, 18 (1964)). (Cf. *The enzymes*, vol. 6, p. 515, Academic Press, New York (1962)). Where values are 'apparent' stability constants the pH is reported. The $pK_a$ values of ATP (6.53 and 4.06) and ADP (6.44 and 3.93, all values at $25^{\circ}$C and 0.1 M-$KNO_3$) indicate that the ligands are fully ionized at pH 8.

### Other metal nucleotide complexes

In general the substitution of a deoxyribose sugar for ribose or changing the identity of the purine or pyrimidine base would only slightly alter the magnitude of the stability constants (*The enzymes*, vol. 2, p. 3, Academic Press, New York (1960); *Biochemistry* **3**, 18 (1964); *Acta Chem. Scand.*, **12**, 528 (1958)). Thus these figures are a fairly reliable guide for complexes formed by other nucleotides with $Mg^{2+}$ and $Ca^{2+}$ and possibly $Mn^{2+}$.

Values for complexes with other metals have been reported (expressed as log $K$): $CoATP^{2-}$, 4.62; $CoADP^-$, 3.68 (*Acta Chem. Scand.* **12**, 528 (1958)); $SrATP^{2-}$, 3.03; $SrADP^-$, 2.50 (*JACS* **78**, 2376 (1956)); $CoATP^{2-}$, 4.71; $NiATP^{2-}$, 4.54; $ZnATP^{2-}$, 4.80; $CuATP^{2-}$, 5.77 (*Helv. Chim. Acta* **44**, 935 (1961)).

Estimates for metal complexes with DNA and RNA have also been reported (expressed as log $K$): MgDNA, 2.10; CaDNA, 2.10; MnDNA, 2.44; MgRNA, 2.32; CaRNA, 2.32 (*ABB* **72**, 66 (1957)). Measurements at $\mu = 0.15$, pH 7.2 (0.11 M-Na barbital).

| Complex | Conditions | log K | References |
|---------|-----------|-------|-----------|
| $MgADP^-$ | 0.085 M-tributylethylammonium bromide + 0.05 M-triethanolamine, pH 7.9, 25°C | 3.34 | *BJ* **71**, 388 (1959) |
| | 0.1 M-*N*-ethylmorpholine, pH 8.0, 30°C | 3.60 | *Biochemistry* **3**, 18 (1964) |
| | 0.1 M-tetrabutylammonium bromide, 25°C ($K_{MHL}^M = 1.82$) | 3.44 | *JACS* **88**, 2631 (1966) |
| | 0.1 M-$KNO_3$, 25°C ($K_{MHL}^M = 1.64$) | 3.17 | *JACS* **89**, 5585 (1967) |

## 17C Metal nucleotide complexes

| Complex | Conditions | log K | References |
|---|---|---|---|
| CaADP$^-$ | 0.085 M-tributylethylammonium bromide + 0.05 M-triethanolamine, pH 7.9, 25°C | 2.89 | *BJ* **71**, 388 (1959) |
| | 0.1 M-$N$-ethylmorpholine, pH 8.0, 30°C | 3.34 | *Biochemistry* **3**, 18 (1964) |
| | 0.1 M-KNO$_3$, 25°C ($K_{MHL}^M$ = 1.60) | 2.86 | *JACS* **89**, 5585 (1967) |
| NaADP$^{2-}$ | 0.2 M-tetraethylammonium bromide, 25°C | 0.65 | *The enzymes*, vol. 6, p. 515, Academic Press, New York (1962); *JBC* **208**, 615 (1954). |
| KADP$^{2-}$ | 0.2 M-tetraethylammonium bromide, 25°C | 0.68 | *The enzymes*, vol. 6, p. 515, Academic Press, New York (1962); *JBC* **208**, 615 (1954). |
| MnADP$^-$ | 0.1 M-tetramethylammonium chloride + 0.05 M-tris, pH 7.5 | 4.00 | *Nature, Lond.* **193**, 1037 (1962) |
| | 0.1 M-$N$-ethylmorpholine, pH 8.0, 30°C | 4.40 | *Biochemistry* **3**, 18 (1964) |
| | 0.05 M-KNO$_3$ + 0.05 M-tris, pH 7.05, 38°C | 3.89 | *ABB* **92**, 94 (1961) |
| | 0.1 M-KNO$_3$, 25°C ($K_{MHL}^M$ = 1.89) | 4.16 | *JACS* **89**, 5585 (1967) |
| ZnADP$^-$ | 0.1 M-KCl, 25°C ($K_{MHL}^M$ = 2.34) | 4.13 | *Z. physiol. Chem.* **313**, 212 (1958) |
| | 0.1 M-KNO$_3$, 25°C ($K_{MHL}^M$ = 2.04) | 4.28 | *JACS* **89**, 5585 (1967) |
| MgATP$^{2-}$ | 0.11 M-tributylethylammonium ion, 25°C, pH 8.4 | 4.58 | *BJ* **71**, 388 (1959) |
| | 0.1 M-tris, 30°C, pH 8.0 | 4.30 | *BBA* **52**, 612 (1961) |
| | 0.1 M-triethanolamine buffer, 30°C, pH 8.0 | 4.80 | *Biochemistry* **3**, 18 (1964) |
| | 0.1 M-tetrabutylammonium bromide, 25°C ($K_{MHL}^M$ = 2.9) | 4.63 | *JACS* **88**, 2631 (1966) |
| | 0.1 M-KNO$_3$, 25°C ($K_{MHL}^M$ = 2.29) | 4.22 | *JACS* **88**, 668 (1966) |
| CaATP$^{2-}$ | 0.1 M-tributylethylammonium ion, 25°C, pH 8.0 | 4.45 | *BJ* **71**, 388 (1959) |
| | 0.1 M-$N$-ethylmorpholine, 30°C, pH 8.0 | 4.40 | *Biochemistry* **3**, 18 (1964) |
| | 0.165 M-Na$^+$, pH 7.4, 37°C | 3.82 | *Biochemistry* **3**, 18 (1964), corrected according to *BJ* **71**, 388 (1959) |
| | 0.1 M-KNO$_3$, 25°C ($K_{MHL}^M$ = 2.13) | 3.97 | *JACS* **88**, 668 (1966) |
| NaATP$^{3-}$ | 0.1 M-$N$-ethylmorpholine, 30°C, pH 8.0 | 1.18 | *Biochemistry* **3**, 18 (1964) |
| | 0.2 M-tetramethylammonium ion, 25°C | 1.0 | *The enzymes*, vol. 6, p. 515, Academic Press, New York, (1962); *JBC* **208**, 615 (1954) |
| KATP$^{3-}$ | 0.1 M-$N$-ethylmorpholine, 30°C, pH 8.0 | 1.15 | *Biochemistry* **3**, 18 (1964) |
| | 0.2 M-tetramethylammonium ion, 25°C | 1.0 | *The enzymes*, vol. 6, p. 515, Academic Press, New York, (1962); *JBC* **208**, 615 (1954) |
| MnATP$^{2-}$ | 0.1 M-tetraethylammonium chloride + 0.05 M-tris, pH 8.0 | 4.88 | *Nature, Lond.* **193**, 1037 (1962) |
| | 0.05 M-$N$-ethylmorpholine, 25°C, pH 7.5 | 5.0 | *JBC*, **241**, 3104 (1966) |
| | 0.1 M-tetramethylammonium bromide, 30°C ($K_{MHL}^M$ = 2.62) | 5.19 | *BBA* **127**, 35 (1966) |
| | 0.1 M-KNO$_3$, 25°C ($K_{MHL}^M$ = 2.39) | 4.78 | *JACS* **88**, 668 (1966) |
| ZnATP$^{2-}$ | 0.1 M-tetramethylammonium bromide, 30°C ($K_{MHL}^M$ = 2.91) | 5.52 | *BBA* **127**, 35 (1966) |
| | 0.1 M-KNO$_3$, 25°C ($K_{MHL}^M$ = 2.67) | 4.85 | *JACS* **88**, 668 (1966) |
| | 0.1 M-NaClO$_4$, 25°C | 5.21 | *BBA* **148**, 655 (1967) |

## Stability constants of some Mg-Nucleotide complexes

| Ligand | $pK_a$ | Type of constant | Log stability constant (Mg) | General remarks |
|--------|--------|------------------|-----------------------------|-----------------|
| AMP | 3.80<br>6.23 | $K_1$ | 1.8 | Also log $K_1$ = 1.8 (Ca); 2.4 (Mn); 2.5 (Co); 2.6 (Ni); 3.2 (Cu); 2.7 (Zn) |
| CMP | 4.35<br>6.35 | $K_1$ | 1.8 | Also log $K_1$ = 1.9 (Ni); 2.5 (Zn) |
| CDP | 4.56<br>6.38 | $K_1$<br>$K_{MHL}^M$ | 3.2<br>1.6 | Also log $K_1$ = 3.5 (Ni); log $K_{MHL}^M$ = 1.9 (Ni) |
| CTP | | $K_1$ | 2.0 | |
| IDP | | $K_1$<br>$K_{MHL}^M$ | 2.4<br>3.8 | |
| ITP | 6.9 | $K_1$<br>$K_{MHL}^M$ | 3.3<br>2.4 | Also log $K_1$ = 3.4 (Ca); 4.5 (Mn); 5.0 (Co); 5.1 (Ni); 5.8 (Cu); 4.6 (Zn) |
| GDP | | $K_1$ | 3.4 | |
| GMP | 6.5 | $K_1$ | 1.8 | |
| UMP | | $K_1$ | 1.7 | |
| UDP | | $K_1$ | 3.5 | |

# 18 pH, buffers, and physiological media

---

# THE STANDARDIZATION AND MEASUREMENT OF pH

## DISSOCIATION CONSTANTS OF ACIDS AND BASES

For an acid dissociating thus:

$$HA \rightleftharpoons H^+ + A^-$$

the thermodynamic dissociation constant, $K_a$, is defined by the equation

$$K_a = \frac{a_{H^+} \times a_{A^-}}{a_{HA}}$$

$$= \frac{c_{H^+} \times c_{A^-}}{c_{HA}} \times \frac{f_{H^+} \times f_{A^-}}{f_{HA}}$$

and

$$pK_a = -\log_{10} K_a$$

where $a$ = activity, $c$ = concentration, and $f$ = activity coefficient,
in each case of the molecular or ionic species indicated by the subscript.

For a base dissociating thus:

$$BH^+ \rightleftharpoons B + H^+,$$

$$K_a = \frac{a_{H^+} \times a_B}{a_{BH^+}}.$$

If the activity coefficients are neglected, the classical or stoichiometric dissociation constant, $K_c$ (but frequently denoted by $K_a$ in biochemical literature), is obtained:

$$K_c = \frac{c_{H^+} \times c_{A^-}}{c_{HA}} = \frac{[H^+][A^-]}{[HA]},$$

where square brackets denote the concentration of the species indicated within the brackets.

In biochemical literature a clear distinction is not always made between values of the thermodynamic dissociation constant, which may be obtained by extrapolation of determined values of $K_c$ to zero ionic strength ($I = 0$), and 'practical' values of the dissociation constant obtained at finite ionic strengths. Where 'practical' values are quoted, the conditions of measurement, particularly the ionic

418

strength, should be given. Note that 'practical' values may differ appreciably (in some cases by as much as 3-fold, i.e. 0.5 p$K$ unit) from the thermodynamic dissociation constants.

## NOTES ON pH MEASUREMENT

These notes apply to pH determination using the usual commercial pH assemblies with glass electrodes.

*Calibration. At least two standard buffer solutions should be used to calibrate the* pH *assembly.*

*Temperature.* The standard solutions used to calibrate the pH assembly and the unknowns must all be at the same temperature. This requirement is not dispensed with by the use of the 'temperature' compensator control of the pH meter which usually only compensates for the 'slope factor' (pH–e.m.f. relationship) and sometimes also for the zero shift.

## NOTES ON THE PROPERTIES OF BUFFER SOLUTIONS

*Buffer capacity (buffer value).* In the tables of buffers the van Slyke buffer value, $\beta = db/d$pH, is given where possible; $db$ is an increment of a strong base, in equivalents, added to 1 litre of buffer solution. An increment of strong acid, equivalent in effect to a negative increment, $-db$, of strong base produces a decrease in pH. Therefore $db/d$pH is always positive.

Where the buffer value is not available in the tables it can be determined experimentally but can also be calculated from theoretical considerations. For a weak acid system,

$$\beta = \frac{db}{d\text{pH}} \approx 2.303 \left( \frac{cKc_{\text{H}}}{(K + c_{\text{H}})^2} + c_{\text{H}} + c_{\text{OH}} \right),$$

where $c$ is the *total* molar concentration of weak acid HA and its salt MA; $K$ is the dissociation constant of HA, $c_{\text{H}}$ and $c_{\text{OH}}$ are the concentrations of $H_3O^+$ and $OH^-$ respectively.

Between pH 3 and 11 the buffer value is determined almost wholly by the first term within the brackets. The maximum buffer effect for a given value of $c$ is found when $c_{\text{H}} = K$ (pH $\approx$ p$K$), i.e. when there are present equivalent amounts of HA and MA. The actual buffer value, $\beta_{\text{max}}$, is then given by:

$$\beta_{\text{max}} = \frac{2.303}{4} c$$

(interionic effects impose a practical upper limit for $\beta$ of approx. 0.2).

If the ratio of HA to MA is increased or decreased tenfold, i.e. 10:1 or 1:10, the pH $\approx$ p$K + 1$ and p$K - 1$ respectively. The buffer capacity is then only about one-third of the maximum value. If the pH lies within the range of p$K - 1$ and p$K + 1$ the buffer capacity is appreciable, but outside this range it falls off to such an extent as to be of little value. **Therefore a given system only has useful buffer action in a range of one pH unit on either side of the p$K$ of the weak acid.**

The same equation applies to systems consisting of a weak base (B) and its conjugate acid (BH$^+$) using $K_{bh}$, the dissociation constant of BH$^+$ (where p$K_{bh}$ = p$K_w$ − p$K_b$).

While aqueous solutions of strong acids and bases are not normally classified as buffer solutions they do display 'buffer capacity' at pH values below about 2.4 and above pH 11.6 ($db/d$pH $\approx 2.303(c_{\text{H}} + c_{\text{OH}})$).

*Dilution value.* The dilution values ($\Delta$pH$_{1/2}$) given in the tables refer to the change of pH suffered by a solution of initial concentration $c_i$, upon dilution with an equal volume of pure water.

## 18 pH, buffers, and physiological media

$$\Delta pH_{1/2} = (pH)_{c_i/2} - (pH)_{c_i}.$$

It is positive when the pH increases with dilution and negative when it decreases.

*Dilution values* $(\Delta pH_{1/2})$ *for equimolal amine buffer solutions between* pH 4.5 *and* 9.5 *in* pH *units*

(Bates, *Ann. N.Y. Acad. Sci.* **92**, 341 (1961))

| $m$ (molality) | $\Delta pH_{1/2}$ | $m$ | $\Delta pH_{1/2}$ |
|---|---|---|---|
| 0.0025 | $-0.007$ | 0.025 | $-0.019$ |
| 0.005 | $-0.010$ | 0.05 | $-0.023$ |
| 0.01 | $-0.013$ | 0.1 | $-0.028$ |
| 0.02 | $-0.017$ | | |

*Salt effects.* The effect on the pH of adding neutral salt to a buffer solution is readily predicted in a qualitative manner from a consideration of the buffer equilibria.

Some indication of the magnitude of the effects to be expected is given in the following tables.

*Salt effect caused by addition of neutral salt* (0.1 M) *to typical buffers*

(From Bates (1973) *Determination of pH: theory and practice*, 2nd edn. Wiley, New York.)

| Solution | $\Delta pH$ |
|---|---|
| 0.005M-HCl | $+0.10$ |
| 0.005M-NaOH | $-0.10$ |
| 0.005M-$CH_3COOH$ | 0 |
| 0.005M-$NH_3$ | 0 |
| 0.005M-$CH_3COOH$ $-$ 0.005M-$CH_3COONa$ | $-0.10$ |
| 0.005M-$NH_3$ $-$ 0.005M-$NH_4Cl$ | $+0.10$ |

*Salt effects on three standard buffers*

(From Bates (1973) *Determination of pH: theory and practice*, 2nd edn. Wiley, New York.)

| Buffer solution | $\Delta pH$ 0.02M *added salt* | $\Delta pH$ 0.05M *added salt* |
|---|---|---|
| 0.05M-KH phthalate (added KCl) | $-0.019$ | $-0.044$ |
| 0.025M-$KH_2PO_4$ $-$ 0.025M-$Na_2HPO_4$ (added NaCl) | $-0.022$ | $-0.051$ |
| 0.01M-$Na_2B_4O_7$ (added NaCl) | $-0.014$ | $-0.035$ |

*Approximate salt effects (in pH units) for amine buffer solutions at 25°C*

(Bates, *Ann. N.Y. Acad. Sci.* **92**, 341 (1961))

| $m$ (molality) | Salt effect for $\Delta I$ equal to[†] | | | |
|---|---|---|---|---|
| | 0.01 | 0.02 | 0.05 | 0.1 |
| 0.01 | + 0.016 | + 0.027 | + 0.049 | + 0.070 |
| 0.02 | + 0.011 | + 0.020 | + 0.039 | + 0.058 |
| 0.05 | + 0.006 | + 0.012 | + 0.024 | + 0.039 |
| 0.1 | + 0.003 | + 0.007 | + 0.015 | + 0.025 |

† Molality of added salt, $m_s$, is given by $m_s = \Delta I$ (uni-univalent salts such as NaCl, $KNO_3$), $m_s = \frac{1}{3}\Delta I$ (ternary salts such as $Na_2SO_4$ or $Ba(NO_3)_2$).

*Temperature effects.* The effect of temperature on the pH of the buffer solutions is given in the tables where possible. There is a considerable variation in the magnitude of $d\text{pH}/dt$ for the different buffers.

*Metal ion effects.* Bjerrum first noted a correlation between the affinity for hydrogen ions of a *closely related* series of ligands and their affinity for a given metal ion. *Thus all buffers are potential ligands for forming metal complexes.*

Caution must be exercised in the use of buffers in the investigation of metal complexes. Some workers consider the interaction of certain nitrogen base buffers, e.g. *N*-ethylmorpholine, triethanolamine, and collidine with alkali and alkaline earth metal ions is negligible and may be small with transition metal ions. However, such buffers should not be used in a particular instance without prior investigation.

# REVISED N.B.S. STANDARD BUFFER SOLUTIONS FOR pH MEASUREMENTS FROM 0°C TO 95°C

(Bates, *J. Res. Natn. Bur. Stand.* **66A**, 179 (1962))

## PRIMARY STANDARDS

Composition and properties of the five primary standard buffers at 25°C (see notes on preparation, below).

| | Buffer solution | | | | |
|---|---|---|---|---|---|
| | Tartrate | Phthalate | Phosphate D | Phosphate E | Borate |
| Buffer substance | $KHC_4H_4O_6$ | $KHC_8H_4O_4$ | $KH_2PO_4 +$ $Na_2HPO_4$ | $KH_2PO_4 +$ $Na_2HPO_4$ | $Na_2B_4O_7 \cdot$ $10H_2O$ |
| g/l soln. at 25 °C | Saturated at 25 °C | 10.12 | [b]3.39 [c]3.53 | [b]1.179 [c]4.30 | 3.80 |
| Molality ($m$) | 0.0341 | 0.05 | [a]0.025 | [b]0.008695 [c]0.03043 | 0.01 |
| Molarity (M) | 0.034 | 0.04958 | [a]0.02490 | [b]0.008665 [c]0.03032 | 0.009971 |
| Density (g/ml) | 1.0036 | 1.0017 | 1.0028 | 1.0020 | 0.9996 |
| pH at 25 °C | 3.557 | 4.008 | 6.865 | 7.413 | 9.180 |
| Dilution value, $\Delta\text{pH}_{1/2}$ | + 0.049 | + 0.052 | + 0.080 | [d]+ 0.07 | + 0.01 |
| Buffer value, $\beta$, equiv./pH | 0.027 | 0.016 | 0.029 | 0.016 | 0.020 |
| Temp. coeff., $d\text{pH}(S)/dt$, units/°C | − 0.0014 | + 0.0012 | − 0.0028 | − 0.0028 | − 0.0082 |

[a] Concentration of each phosphate salt.　　[b] $KH_2PO_4$.　　[c] $Na_2HPO_4$.
[d] Calculated value.

# 18 pH, buffers, and physiological media

Recommended standard values of pH(S) for primary standard buffers (estimated limits of accuracy ± 0.005 over the temperature range 0–60 °C and ± 0.008 from 60–90 °C).

| Temp. (°C) | Buffer pH | | | | |
|---|---|---|---|---|---|
| | Tartrate | Phthalate | Phosphate D | Phosphate E | Borate |
| 0 | | 4.003 | 6.984 | 7.534 | 9.464 |
| 5 | | 3.999 | 6.951 | 7.500 | 9.395 |
| 10 | | 3.998 | 6.923 | 7.472 | 9.332 |
| 15 | | 3.999 | 6.900 | 7.448 | 9.276 |
| 20 | | 4.002 | 6.881 | 7.429 | 9.225 |
| 25 | 3.557 | 4.008 | 6.865 | 7.413 | 9.180 |
| 30 | 3.552 | 4.015 | 6.853 | 7.400 | 9.139 |
| 35 | 3.549 | 4.024 | 6.844 | 7.389 | 9.102 |
| 38 | 3.548 | 4.030 | 6.840 | 7.384 | 9.081 |
| 40 | 3.547 | 4.035 | 6.838 | 7.380 | 9.068 |
| 45 | 3.547 | 4.047 | 6.834 | 7.373 | 9.038 |
| 50 | 3.549 | 4.060 | 6.833 | 7.367 | 9.011 |
| 55 | 3.554 | 4.075 | 6.834 | | 8.985 |
| 60 | 3.560 | 4.091 | 6.836 | | 8.962 |
| 70 | 3.580 | 4.126 | 6.845 | | 8.921 |
| 80 | 3.609 | 4.164 | 6.859 | | 8.885 |
| 90 | 3.650 | 4.205 | 6.877 | | 8.850 |
| 95 | 3.674 | 4.227 | 6.886 | | 8.833 |

## Notes on the preparation of the above standard buffers solutions

The compositions of the above solutions to which pH(S) values have been assigned by the N.B.S., using the Bates–Guggenheim convention, are **on the molal scale**. Errors in pH(S) resulting from the use of an $x$ molar solution in place of an $x$ molal solution are small for the dilute solutions presented, but if third decimal accuracy is required the compositions of the solutions must be adjusted more carefully. Consequently the density of the standard solutions is listed above, together with the corresponding molarity to enable the solutions to be prepared precisely by volume methods.

The buffer solutions should be stored in bottles of borosilicate glass (e.g. Pyrex) or of polyethylene (pure). The tartrate solution is subject to mould growth accompanied by an increase in the pH value; it must therefore be freshly made every few days or a few crystals of thymol added as a preservative. Mould may appear slowly in the phthalate buffer and sediment may appear in the phosphate buffers. It is recommended that these buffers be remade every month.

Of the buffer salts only $Na_2HPO_4$ is appreciably hygroscopic. The tartrate, phthalate, and phosphates may be dried at 110 °C for 1–2 hr before use. Potassium tetroxalate dihydrate should not be dried at temperatures above 60 °C, nor should borax be heated above normal room temperature. Good quality distilled water should be used to prepare the buffer solutions (specific conductance should be less than $2 \times 10^{-6}$ ohm$^{-1}$ cm$^{-1}$ at 25 °C).

## SECONDARY STANDARDS
Composition and properties of the two secondary standard buffers at 25 °C

|  | Buffer solution | |
|---|---|---|
|  | Tetroxalate | Calcium hydroxide |
| Buffer substance | $KH_3(C_2O_4)_2 \cdot 2H_2O$ | $Ca(OH)_2$ |
| g/l of soln. at 25 °C | 12.61 | Saturated at 25 °C |
| Molality ($m$) | 0.05 | 0.0203 |
| Molarity (M) | 0.04962 | 0.02025 |
| Density (g/ml) | 1.0032 | 0.9991 |
| pH at 25 °C | 1.679 | 12.454 |
| Dilution value, $\Delta pH_{1/2}$ | + 0.186 | − 0.28 |
| Buffer value, $\beta$, equiv./pH | 0.070 | 0.09 |
| Temp. coeff., $d$pH(S)/$dt$, units/°C | + 0.001 | − 0.033 |

Recommended standard values of pH(S) for the secondary buffer standards.

| Temp. (°C) | Buffer pH | |
|---|---|---|
|  | Tetroxalate | Calcium hydroxide |
| 0 | 1.666 | 13.423 |
| 5 | 1.668 | 13.207 |
| 10 | 1.670 | 13.003 |
| 15 | 1.672 | 12.810 |
| 20 | 1.675 | 12.627 |
| 25 | 1.679 | 12.454 |
| 30 | 1.683 | 12.289 |
| 35 | 1.688 | 12.133 |
| 38 | 1.691 | 12.043 |
| 40 | 1.694 | 11.984 |
| 45 | 1.700 | 11.841 |
| 50 | 1.707 | 11.705 |
| 55 | 1.715 | 11.574 |
| 60 | 1.723 | 11.449 |
| 70 | 1.743 | |
| 80 | 1.766 | |
| 90 | 1.792 | |
| 95 | 1.806 | |

*Note.* See above for remarks on drying potassium tetroxalate dihydrate.

## APPROXIMATE p$K_a$ VALUES OF SUBSTANCES USEFUL FOR BUFFER SYSTEMS

| p$K_a$ at 25 °C | Compound | $\Delta$ pH/$\Delta t$ (pH *units per* °C) |
|---|---|---|
| 1.27 | $k_1$ Oxalic acid | |
| 1.97 | $k_1$ Maleic acid | |
| 2.15 | $k_1$ Phosphoric acid | |
| 2.35 | $k_1$ Glycine† | |
| 2.95 | $k_1$ Phthalic acid† | |
| 3.02 | $k_1$ Fumaric acid | |
| 3.04 | $k_1$ Tartaric acid | |
| 3.13 | $k_1$ Citric acid† | |
| 3.14 | $k_1$ Glycylglycine | |

† A table of buffer composition is given for these compounds in the next section.

| p$K_a$ *at* 25 °C | | *Compound* | ΔpH/Δ*t* (pH *units per* °C) |
|---|---|---|---|
| 3.17 | | Furoic acid | |
| 3.71 | $k_1$ | β,β′-Dimethylglutaric acid† | |
| 3.75 | | Formic acid | |
| 4.04 | | Barbituric acid | |
| 4.20 | | Benzoic acid | |
| 4.21 | $k_1$ | Succinic acid† | |
| 4.27 | $k_2$ | Oxalic acid | |
| 4.37 | $k_2$ | Tartaric acid | |
| 4.38 | $k_2$ | Fumaric acid | |
| 4.76 | | Acetic acid† | 0.000 |
| 4.76 | $k_2$ | Citric acid† | |
| 5.05 | $k_2$ | Malic acid | |
| 5.41 | $k_2$ | Phthalic acid† | |
| 5.64 | $k_2$ | Succinic acid† | |
| 6.04 | $k_2$ | Histidine | |
| 6.09 | | MES {2-(*N*-Morpholino)ethanesulphonic acid}† | −0.011 |
| 6.12 | $k_3$ | Pyrophosphoric acid | |
| 6.24 | $k_2$ | Maleic acid† | |
| 6.27 | | Cacodylic acid† | |
| 6.34 | $k_2$ | β,β′-Dimethylglutaric acid† | |
| 6.35 | $k_1$ | Carbonic acid† | |
| 6.39 | | 5(4)-Hydroxymethylimidazole | |
| 6.40 | $k_3$ | Citric acid | |
| 6.57 | | ADA {*N*-(2-Acetamido)iminodiacetic acid} | −0.011 |
| 6.65 | $k_2$ | Glycerol 2-phosphoric acid | |
| 6.76 | | PIPES {Piperazine-*NN*′-bis-(2-ethanesulphonic acid)} | −0.0085 |
| 6.82 | $k_2$ | Phosphoric acid† | −0.003 |
| 6.85 | $k_1$ | Ethylenediamine | −0.027 |
| 6.95 | | Imidazole† | |
| 6.98 | $k_2$ | Arsenic acid | |
| 7.07 | | BES {*N,N*-(Bis-2-hydroxyethyl)-2-aminoethanesulphonic acid} | −0.016 |
| 7.15 | | MOPS {3-(*N*-Morpholino)-propanesulphonic acid} | −0.011 |
| 7.40 | | TES {*N*-((Trishydroxymethyl)methyl)-2-aminoethanesulphonic acid} | −0.020 |
| 7.43 | | 2,4,6-Collidine† | |
| 7.47 | | HEPES {*N*-2-Hydroxyethylpiperazine-*N*′-2-ethanesulphonic acid}† | −0.015 |
| 7.52 | | 5(4)-Methylimidazole | |
| 7.67 | | *N*-Ethylmorpholine† | |
| 7.76 | | Triethanolamine | −0.020 |
| 7.95 | | EPPS {*N*-2-Hydroxyethylpiperazine-*N*′-3-propanesulphonic acid}† | −0.011 |
| 7.98 | | Diethylbarbituric acid† | −0.014 |
| 8.05 | | TRICINE {*N*-((Trishydroxymethyl)-methyl)glycine}† | −0.021 |
| 8.08 | | Tris(hydroxymethyl)aminomethane† | −0.028 |
| 8.25 | | Glycylglycine | −0.026 |
| 8.26 | | BICINE {*N,N*-(Bis-2-hydroxyethyl)-glycine}† | −0.018 |
| 8.36 | | 2,5(4)-Dimethylimidazole | |
| 8.79 | | 2-Amino-2-methyl-1,3-propanediol† | −0.029 |
| 8.80 | | 2-Amino-2-ethyl-1,3-propanediol | |
| 8.88 | | Diethanolamine | −0.025 |

† A table of buffer composition is given for these compounds in the next section.

| $pK_a$ at 25 °C | Compound | $\Delta pH/\Delta t$ (pH *units per* °C) |
|---|---|---|
| 8.95 | $k_4$ Pyrophosphoric acid | |
| 9.11 | 4-Aminopyridine | −0.028 |
| 9.21 | Serine | −0.025 |
| 9.24 | Boric acid† | |
| 9.25 | Ammonia | −0.031 |
| 9.50 | Ethanolamine | −0.030 |
| 9.50 | CHES {2-(Cyclohexylamino)-ethanesulphonic acid} | −0.011 |
| 9.54 | Ephedrine | |
| 9.66 | Hydroxyproline | |
| 9.69 | 2-Amino-2-methyl-1-propanol | −0.032 |
| 9.74 | Leucine | |
| 9.78 | Glycine† | −0.026 |
| 9.80 | Trimethylamine | |
| 9.87 | α-Alanine | −0.027 |
| 9.93 | $k_2$ Ethylenediamine | −0.029 |
| 10.00 | Aspartic acid | |
| 10.24 | β-Alanine | −0.028 |
| 10.33 | $k_2$ Carbonic acid† | −0.009 |
| 10.56 | γ-Aminobutyric acid | −0.030 |
| 10.57 | *n*-Propylamine | |
| 10.62 | Methylamine | |
| 10.63 | Ethylamine | |
| 10.64 | *n*-Butylamine | |
| 10.72 | Triethylamine | |
| 10.77 | Dimethylamine | |
| 10.93 | $k_2$ Hexamethylenediamine | −0.034 |
| 10.93 | Diethylamine | |
| 11.12 | Piperidine | −0.031 |
| 12.38 | $k_3$ Phosphoric acid† | . |

† A table of buffer composition is given for these compounds in the next section.

p$K$ values for many other compounds are given in the main tables of biochemical compounds.

*Preparation of buffers.* Buffers may be prepared from these or other suitable compounds by the addition of acid or alkali as appropriate. The amount of acid or alkali required can be calculated from the Henderson–Hasselbalch equation

$$pH = pK + \log_{10} \frac{[\text{salt}]}{[\text{acid}]} .‡$$

The table below gives [salt]/[acid] ratios corresponding to pH values between p$K$ − 1 and p$K$ + 1, which represents the useful buffering range of a buffer system.

| pH | [salt]/[acid] ‡ | pH | [salt]/[acid] ‡ |
|---|---|---|---|
| p$K$ − 1.0 | 0.10 | p$K$ + 0.1 | 1.26 |
| − 0.9 | 0.13 | + 0.2 | 1.58 |
| − 0.8 | 0.16 | + 0.3 | 2.00 |
| − 0.7 | 0.20 | + 0.4 | 2.51 |
| − 0.6 | 0.25 | + 0.5 | 3.16 |
| − 0.5 | 0.32 | + 0.6 | 3.98 |
| − 0.4 | 0.40 | + 0.7 | 5.01 |
| − 0.3 | 0.50 | + 0.8 | 6.31 |
| − 0.2 | 0.63 | + 0.9 | 7.94 |
| − 0.1 | 0.79 | + 1.0 | 10.0 |
| p$K$ | 1.0 | | |

‡ [base]/[salt] ratio for cation buffers.

## BUFFER SOLUTIONS FOR pH 1–13

Data are given in this section for buffer solutions which have wide application in biochemistry. Their concentration and ionic strength can be altered readily to make them more suitable for specific purposes. In general the pH values of these solutions have not been determined with high precision, and are given to the first decimal place. In other cases, marked with an asterisk, the pH values have been accurately determined and are given to two decimal places.

*Clark and Lubs solutions,* pH 1.0–2.2*

(Bower and Bates, *J. Res. Natn. Bur. Stand.* **55**, 197 (1955))

25 ml 0.2M-KCl (14.919 g/l), $x$ ml 0.2M-HCl; diluted to 100 ml with $H_2O$.

| pH, 25 °C | $x$ | Buffer value ($\beta$) |
|---|---|---|
| 1.00 | 67.0 | 0.31 |
| 1.10 | 52.8 | 0.24 |
| 1.20 | 42.5 | 0.19 |
| 1.30 | 33.6 | 0.16 |
| 1.40 | 26.6 | 0.13 |
| 1.50 | 20.7 | 0.10 |
| 1.60 | 16.2 | 0.077 |
| 1.70 | 13.0 | 0.060 |
| 1.80 | 10.2 | 0.049 |
| 1.90 | 8.1 | 0.037 |
| 2.00 | 6.5 | 0.030 |
| 2.10 | 5.1 | 0.026 |
| 2.20 | 3.9 | 0.022 |

*Glycine–HCl buffer solutions,* pH 2.2–3.6 at 25 °C

(Sørensen, *BZ* **21**, 131 (1909); Gomori, *Meth. Enzymol.* **1**, 141 (1955))

Glycine, $C_2H_5NO_2$, M. wt. 75.07
25 ml 0.2M-glycine (15.01 g/l), $x$ ml 0.2M-HCl; diluted to 100 ml with $H_2O$.

| pH, 25 °C | $x$ ml 0.2M-HCl |
|---|---|
| 2.2 | 22.0 |
| 2.4 | 16.2 |
| 2.6 | 12.1 |
| 2.8 | 8.4 |
| 3.0 | 5.7 |
| 3.2 | 4.1 |
| 3.4 | 3.2 |
| 3.6 | 2.5 |

*Clark and Lubs solutions,* pH 2.2–4.0* (*J. Res. natn. Bur. Stand.* **55**, 197 (1955))
50 ml 0.1M-KH phthalate (20.42 g/l), *x* ml 0.1M-HCl; diluted to 100 ml with $H_2O$.

| pH, 25 °C | x | Buffer value ($\beta$) |
|---|---|---|
| 2.20 | 49.5 | |
| 2.30 | 45.8 | 0.036 |
| 2.40 | 42.2 | 0.035 |
| 2.50 | 38.8 | 0.034 |
| 2.60 | 35.4 | 0.033 |
| 2.70 | 32.1 | 0.032 |
| 2.80 | 28.9 | 0.032 |
| 2.90 | 25.7 | 0.033 |
| 3.00 | 22.3 | 0.034 |
| 3.10 | 18.8 | 0.033 |
| 3.20 | 15.7 | 0.030 |
| 3.30 | 12.9 | 0.026 |
| 3.40 | 10.4 | 0.023 |
| 3.50 | 8.2 | 0.020 |
| 3.60 | 6.3 | 0.018 |
| 3.70 | 4.5 | 0.017 |
| 3.80 | 2.9 | 0.015 |
| 3.90 | 1.4 | 0.014 |
| 4.00 | 0.1 | 0.014 |

*Citric acid*–$Na_2HPO_4$ (*McIlvaine*) *buffer solutions,* pH *approx.* 2.6–7.6

(McIlvaine, *JBC* **49**, 183 (1921))

Citric acid monohydrate, $C_6H_8O_7 \cdot H_2O$, M. wt. 210.14; 0.1M-solution contains 21.01 g/l. $Na_2HPO_4$, M. wt. 141.98; 0.2M-solution contains 28.40 g/l, or $Na_2HPO_4 \cdot 2H_2O$, M. wt. 178.05; 0.2M-solution contains 35.61 g/l. *x* ml 0.1M-citric acid and *y* ml 0.2M-$Na_2HPO_4$ mixed.

| pH | x ml 0.1M-citric acid | y ml 0.2M-$Na_2HPO_4$ |
|---|---|---|
| 2.6 | 89.10 | 10.90 |
| 2.8 | 84.15 | 15.85 |
| 3.0 | 79.45 | 20.55 |
| 3.2 | 75.30 | 24.70 |
| 3.4 | 71.50 | 28.50 |
| 3.6 | 67.80 | 32.20 |
| 3.8 | 64.50 | 35.50 |
| 4.0 | 61.45 | 38.55 |
| 4.2 | 58.60 | 41.40 |
| 4.4 | 55.90 | 44.10 |
| 4.6 | 53.25 | 46.75 |
| 4.8 | 50.70 | 49.30 |
| 5.0 | 48.50 | 51.50 |
| 5.2 | 46.40 | 53.60 |
| 5.4 | 44.25 | 55.75 |
| 5.6 | 42.00 | 58.00 |
| 5.8 | 39.55 | 60.45 |
| 6.0 | 36.85 | 63.15 |
| 6.2 | 33.90 | 66.10 |
| 6.4 | 30.75 | 69.25 |
| 6.6 | 27.25 | 72.75 |
| 6.8 | 22.75 | 77.25 |
| 7.0 | 17.65 | 82.35 |
| 7.2 | 13.05 | 86.95 |
| 7.4 | 9.15 | 90.85 |
| 7.6 | 6.35 | 93.65 |

## 18 pH, buffers, and physiological media

*Citric acid–sodium citrate buffer solutions,* pH 3.0–6.2

(N. Hemington and R. M. C. Dawson, unpublished data)

Citric acid monohydrate, $C_6H_8O_7 \cdot H_2O$, M. wt. 210.14; 0.1M-solution contains 21.01 g/l. Trisodium citrate dihydrate, $C_6H_5O_7Na_3 \cdot 2H_2O$, M. wt. 294.12; 0.1M-solution contains 29.41 g/l.

$x$ ml 0.1M-citric acid and $y$ ml 0.1M-trisodium citrate mixed.

| pH | $x$ ml 0.1M-*citric acid* | $y$ ml 0.1M-*trisodium citrate* |
|---|---|---|
| 3.0 | 82.0 | 18.0 |
| 3.2 | 77.5 | 22.5 |
| 3.4 | 73.0 | 27.0 |
| 3.6 | 68.5 | 31.5 |
| 3.8 | 63.5 | 36.5 |
| 4.0 | 59.0 | 41.0 |
| 4.2 | 54.0 | 46.0 |
| 4.4 | 49.5 | 50.5 |
| 4.6 | 44.5 | 55.5 |
| 4.8 | 40.0 | 60.0 |
| 5.0 | 35.0 | 65.0 |
| 5.2 | 30.5 | 69.5 |
| 5.4 | 25.5 | 74.5 |
| 5.6 | 21.0 | 79.0 |
| 5.8 | 16.0 | 84.0 |
| 6.0 | 11.5 | 88.5 |
| 6.2 | 8.0 | 92.0 |

*β,β′-Dimethylglutaric acid*–NaOH *buffer solutions,* pH 3.2–7.6 *at* 21 °C

This buffer was outlined by Stafford, Watson, and Rand, *BBA* **18**, 318 (1955), for use in enzyme studies where low u.v. absorption of the buffer was required. No details of mixtures were given. The following approximate pH data were kindly supplied by R. Hems.

β,β′-Dimethylglutaric acid, $C_7H_{12}O_4$, M. wt. 160.2.
50 ml 0.1M-β,β′-dimethylglutaric acid (16.02 g/l), $x$ ml 0.2M-NaOH; diluted to 100 ml with $H_2O$.

| pH, 21 °C | $x$ ml 0.2M-NaOH |
|---|---|
| 3.2 | 4.15 |
| 3.4 | 7.35 |
| 3.6 | 11.0 |
| 3.8 | 13.7 |
| 4.0 | 16.65 |
| 4.2 | 18.4 |
| 4.4 | 19.9 |
| 4.6 | 20.85 |
| 4.8 | 21.95 |
| 5.0 | 23.1 |
| 5.2 | 24.5 |
| 5.4 | 26.0 |
| 5.6 | 27.9 |
| 5.8 | 29.85 |
| 6.0 | 32.5 |
| 6.2 | 35.25 |
| 6.4 | 37.75 |
| 6.6 | 42.35 |
| 6.8 | 44.0 |
| 7.0 | 45.2 |
| 7.2 | 46.05 |
| 7.4 | 46.6 |
| 7.6 | 47.0 |

*Sodium acetate—acetic acid buffer solutions,* pH 3.7—5.6

Sodium acetate trihydrate, $CH_3COONa \cdot 3H_2O$, M. wt. 136.09; 0.2M-solution contains 27.22 g/l.
$x$ ml 0.2M-NaOAc and $y$ ml 0.2M-HOAc mixed.

| pH, 18 °C | $x$ ml 0.2M-NaOAc | $y$ ml 0.2M-HOAc |
|---|---|---|
| 3.7 | 10.0 | 90.0 |
| 3.8 | 12.0 | 88.0 |
| 4.0 | 18.0 | 82.0 |
| 4.2 | 26.5 | 73.5 |
| 4.4 | 37.0 | 63.0 |
| 4.6 | 49.0 | 51.0 |
| 4.8 | 59.0 | 41.0 |
| 5.0 | 70.0 | 30.0 |
| 5.2 | 79.0 | 21.0 |
| 5.4 | 86.0 | 14.0 |
| 5.6 | 91.0 | 9.0 |

*Succinic acid—NaOH buffer solutions,* pH 3.8—6.0 *at* 25 °C

(Gomori, *Meth. Enzymol.* **1**, 141 (1955))

Succinic acid, $C_4H_6O_4$, M. wt. 118.09.
25 ml 0.2M-succinic acid (23.62 g/l), $x$ ml 0.2M-NaOH; diluted to 100 ml with $H_2O$.

| pH, 25 °C | $x$ ml 0.2M-NaOH |
|---|---|
| 3.8 | 7.5 |
| 4.0 | 10.0 |
| 4.2 | 13.3 |
| 4.4 | 16.7 |
| 4.6 | 20.0 |
| 4.8 | 23.5 |
| 5.0 | 26.7 |
| 5.2 | 30.3 |
| 5.4 | 34.2 |
| 5.6 | 37.5 |
| 5.8 | 40.7 |
| 6.0 | 43.5 |

## 18  pH, buffers, and physiological media

*Clark and Lubs solutions,* pH 4.1–5.9*

(Bower and Bates, *J. Res. Natn. Bur. Stand.* **55**, 197 (1955))

50 ml 0.1M-KH phthalate (20.42 g/l), $x$ ml 0.1M-NaOH; diluted to 100 ml with $H_2O$.

| pH, 25 °C | $x$ | Buffer value $(\beta)$ |
|---|---|---|
| 4.10 | 1.3 | 0.016 |
| 4.20 | 3.0 | 0.017 |
| 4.30 | 4.7 | 0.018 |
| 4.40 | 6.6 | 0.020 |
| 4.50 | 8.7 | 0.022 |
| 4.60 | 11.1 | 0.025 |
| 4.70 | 13.6 | 0.027 |
| 4.80 | 16.5 | 0.029 |
| 4.90 | 19.4 | 0.030 |
| 5.00 | 22.6 | 0.031 |
| 5.10 | 25.5 | 0.031 |
| 5.20 | 28.8 | 0.030 |
| 5.30 | 31.6 | 0.026 |
| 5.40 | 34.1 | 0.025 |
| 5.50 | 36.6 | 0.023 |
| 5.60 | 38.8 | 0.020 |
| 5.70 | 40.6 | 0.017 |
| 5.80 | 42.3 | 0.015 |
| 5.90 | 43.7 | 0.013 |

*Sodium cacodylate–HCl buffer solutions,* pH 5.0–7.4 at 15 °C

(Plumel, *Bull. Soc. Chim. Biol.* **30**, 129 (1948))

Sodium cacodylate trihydrate, $Na(CH_3)_2AsO_2 \cdot 3H_2O$, M. wt. 214.02.
50 ml 0.1M-$Na(CH_3)_2AsO_2 \cdot 3H_2O$ (21.40 g/l), $x$ ml 0.1M-HCl; diluted to 100 ml with $H_2O$.

| pH, 15 °C | $x$ ml 0.1M-HCl |
|---|---|
| 5.0 | 46.75 |
| 5.2 | 45.05 |
| 5.4 | 42.6 |
| 5.6 | 39.2 |
| 5.8 | 34.8 |
| 6.0 | 29.55 |
| 6.2 | 23.85 |
| 6.4 | 18.75 |
| 6.6 | 13.3 |
| 6.8 | 9.3 |
| 7.0 | 6.3 |
| 7.2 | 4.15 |
| 7.4 | 2.7 |

*Sodium hydrogen maleate*–NaOH *buffer solutions,* pH 5.2–6.8 *at* 25 °C

(Temple, *JACS* **51**, 1754 (1929))

Sodium hydrogen maleate, $NaHC_4H_2O_4 \cdot 3H_2O$, M. wt. 192.11.
0.2M-solution is prepared by dissolving in $H_2O$, 23.2 g maleic acid and mixing with
200 ml 1M-NaOH and diluting to 1 litre with $H_2O$.
25 ml 0.2M-NaH maleate, $x$ ml 0.1M-NaOH; diluted to 100 ml with $H_2O$.

| pH, 25 °C | $x$ ml 0.1M-NaOH |
|---|---|
| 5.2 | 7.2 |
| 5.4 | 10.5 |
| 5.6 | 15.3 |
| 5.8 | 20.8 |
| 6.0 | 26.9 |
| 6.2 | 33.0 |
| 6.4 | 38.0 |
| 6.6 | 41.6 |
| 6.8 | 44.4 |

*Tris(hydroxymethyl)aminomethane*–*maleate buffer solutions,* pH 5.4–8.4

(Gomori, *PSEBM* **68**, 354 (1948); *Meth. Enzymol.* **1**, 138 (1955))

25 ml 0.2M-tris-maleate (24.2 g tris + 23.2 g maleic acid/l) + $x$ ml 0.2M-NaOH
diluted to 100 ml

$dpH/dt \simeq -0.0067$ units/degree rise

| pH, 23 °C | $x$ ml 0.2M-NaOH |
|---|---|
| 5.4 | 5.40 |
| 5.6 | 7.75 |
| 5.8 | 10.25 |
| 6.0 | 13.00 |
| 6.2 | 15.75 |
| 6.4 | 18.50 |
| 6.6 | 21.25 |
| 6.8 | 22.50 |
| 7.0 | 24.00 |
| 7.2 | 25.50 |
| 7.4 | 27.00 |
| 7.6 | 29.00 |
| 7.8 | 31.75 |
| 8.0 | 34.50 |
| 8.2 | 37.50 |
| 8.4 | 40.50 |

*2-(N-Morpholino)ethanesulphonic acid*(MES)–NaOH *buffer solutions,* pH 5.4–6.8

25 ml 0.1M-MES (19.523 g/l) + $x$ ml 0.1M-NaOH diluted to 50 ml with $H_2O$

| pH | $x$ ml 0.1M-NaOH | |
|---|---|---|
| | 21 °C | 37 °C |
| 5.4 | – | 4.4 |
| 5.6 | 4.6 | 5.7 |
| 5.8 | 6.2 | 7.3 |
| 6.0 | 8.0 | 9.4 |
| 6.2 | 10.3 | 12.0 |
| 6.4 | 12.9 | 14.9 |
| 6.6 | 15.3 | 16.9 |
| 6.8 | 17.4 | – |

$Na_2HPO_4-NaH_2PO_4$ *buffer solutions,* pH 5.8–8.0 *at* 25 °C

(Gomori, after Sørensen, *Meth. Enzymol.* **1**, 143 (1955))

$Na_2HPO_4 \cdot 2H_2O$, M. wt. 178.05; 0.2M-solution contains 35.61 g/l.
$Na_2HPO_4 \cdot 12H_2O$, M. wt. 358.22; 0.2M-solution contains 71.64 g/l.
$NaH_2PO_4 \cdot H_2O$, M. wt. 138.01; 0.2M-solution contains 27.6 g/l.
$NaH_2PO_4 \cdot 2H_2O$, M. wt. 156.03; 0.2M-solution contains 31.21 g/l.
$x$ ml 0.2M-$Na_2HPO_4$, $y$ ml 0.2M-$NaH_2PO_4$; diluted to 100 ml with $H_2O$.

| pH, 25 °C | $x$ ml 0.2M-$Na_2HPO_4$ | $y$ ml 0.2M-$NaH_2PO_4$ |
|---|---|---|
| 5.8 | 4.0 | 46.0 |
| 6.0 | 6.15 | 43.85 |
| 6.2 | 9.25 | 40.75 |
| 6.4 | 13.25 | 36.75 |
| 6.6 | 18.75 | 31.25 |
| 6.8 | 24.5 | 25.5 |
| 7.0 | 30.5 | 19.5 |
| 7.2 | 36.0 | 14.0 |
| 7.4 | 40.5 | 9.5 |
| 7.6 | 43.5 | 6.5 |
| 7.8 | 45.75 | 4.25 |
| 8.0 | 47.35 | 2.65 |

*Clark and Lubs solutions,* pH 5.8–8.0*

(Bower and Bates, *J. Res. Natn. Bur. Stand.* **55**, 197 (1955))

50 ml 0.1M-$KH_2PO_4$ (13.60 g/l), $x$ ml 0.1M-NaOH; diluted to 100 ml with $H_2O$.

| pH, 25 °C | $x$ | Buffer value $(\beta)$ |
|---|---|---|
| 5.80 | 3.6 | |
| 5.90 | 4.6 | 0.010 |
| 6.00 | 5.6 | 0.011 |
| 6.10 | 6.8 | 0.012 |
| 6.20 | 8.1 | 0.015 |
| 6.30 | 9.7 | 0.017 |
| 6.40 | 11.6 | 0.021 |
| 6.50 | 13.9 | 0.024 |
| 6.60 | 16.4 | 0.027 |
| 6.70 | 19.3 | 0.030 |
| 6.80 | 22.4 | 0.033 |
| 6.90 | 25.9 | 0.033 |
| 7.00 | 29.1 | 0.031 |
| 7.10 | 32.1 | 0.028 |
| 7.20 | 34.7 | 0.025 |
| 7.30 | 37.0 | 0.022 |
| 7.40 | 39.1 | 0.020 |
| 7.50 | 40.9 | 0.016 |
| 7.60 | 42.4 | 0.013 |
| 7.70 | 43.5 | 0.011 |
| 7.80 | 44.5 | 0.009 |
| 7.90 | 45.3 | 0.008 |
| 8.00 | 46.1 | |

*Sodium bicarbonate*–5% $CO_2$ *buffer solutions,* pH 6.0–8.0 *at* 37 °C

Calculated from the Henderson–Hasselbalch equation

$$pH = pK' + \log \frac{[HCO_3^-]}{[CO_2]}.$$

Concentrations of bicarbonate are approximately correct when atmospheric pressure varies between 725 and 760 mm Hg. Temperature: for temperatures below 37 °C (down to 20 °C) the bicarbonate concentration given in the tables should be decreased by approximately 1.88% per degree to give the required pH.

| pH, 37 °C | Conc. of $NaHCO_3$ (*M. wt.* 84.02) in equilibrium with gas phase containing 5% $CO_2$ |
|---|---|
| 6.0 | $5.86 \times 10^{-4}$ M |
| 6.2 | $9.29 \times 10^{-4}$ M |
| 6.4 | $1.47 \times 10^{-3}$ M |
| 6.6 | $2.33 \times 10^{-3}$ M |
| 6.8 | $3.70 \times 10^{-3}$ M |
| 7.0 | $5.86 \times 10^{-3}$ M |
| 7.2 | $9.29 \times 10^{-3}$ M |
| 7.4 | $1.47 \times 10^{-2}$ M |
| 7.6 | $2.33 \times 10^{-2}$ M |
| 7.8 | $3.70 \times 10^{-2}$ M |
| 8.0 | $5.86 \times 10^{-2}$ M |

*Imidazole (glyoxaline)*–HCl *buffer solutions,* pH 6.2–7.8 *at* 25 °C

(Mertz and Owen, *PSEBM* **43**, 204 (1940))

Imidazole, $C_3H_4N_2$, M. wt. 68.08.
25 ml 0.2M-imidazole (13.62 g/l), $x$ ml 0.2M-HCl, diluted to 100 ml with $H_2O$.

| pH, 25 °C | $x$ ml 0.2M-HCl |
|---|---|
| 6.2 | 21.45 |
| 6.4 | 19.9 |
| 6.6 | 17.75 |
| 6.8 | 15.2 |
| 7.0 | 12.15 |
| 7.2 | 9.3 |
| 7.4 | 6.8 |
| 7.6 | 4.65 |
| 7.8 | 3.0 |

## 18  pH, buffers, and physiological media

*2,4,6-Trimethylpyridine (2,4,6-collidine)*–HCl *buffer solutions,* pH 6.4–8.3

(Gomori, *PSEBM* **62**, 33 (1946))

2,4,6-Trimethylpyridine, $C_8H_{11}N$, M.wt. 121.18.
25 ml 0.2M-2,4,6-trimethylpyridine (24.24 g/l), $x$ ml 0.2M-HCl; diluted to 100 ml with $H_2O$.

| pH | | |
|---|---|---|
| 23 °C | 37 °C | $x$ ml 0.2M-HCl |
| 6.4 | 6.4 | 22.5 |
| 6.6 | 6.5 | 21.25 |
| 6.8 | 6.7 | 20.0 |
| 6.9 | 6.8 | 18.75 |
| 7.0 | 6.9 | 17.5 |
| 7.1 | 7.0 | 16.25 |
| 7.2 | 7.1 | 15.0 |
| 7.3 | 7.2 | 13.75 |
| 7.4 | 7.3 | 12.5 |
| 7.5 | 7.4 | 11.25 |
| 7.6 | 7.5 | 10.0 |
| 7.7 | 7.6 | 8.75 |
| 7.8 | 7.7 | 7.5 |
| 7.9 | 7.8 | 6.25 |
| 8.0 | 7.9 | 5.0 |
| 8.2 | 8.1 | 3.75 |
| 8.3 | 8.3 | 2.5 |

*Morpholinopropanesulphonic acid (MOPS)* – KOH *buffer solutions,* pH 6.6–7.8 *at* 22 °C

25 ml 0.1M-MOPS (20.93 g/l) + $x$ ml 0.1M-KOH diluted to 50 ml with $H_2O$

| | $x$ ml 0.1M-KOH | |
|---|---|---|
| pH | 22 °C | 37 °C |
| 6.4 | – | 5.8 |
| 6.6 | 4.8 | 7.8 |
| 6.8 | 6.7 | 10.1 |
| 7.0 | 8.7 | 13.0 |
| 7.2 | 11.5 | 16.4 |
| 7.4 | 15.0 | 19.3 |
| 7.6 | 18.0 | 21.8 |
| 7.8 | 20.6 | – |

*Sodium 5,5-diethylbarbiturate (veronal sodium; barbitone sodium)–HCl buffer solutions,* pH 6.8–9.6 *at* 18 °C

(Britton and Robinson, *JCS* **1931**, 1456)

Sodium 5,5-diethylbarbiturate, $C_8H_{11}N_2O_3Na$, M.wt. 206.18; 0.04M-solution contains 8.25 g/l.
$x$ ml 0.04M-sodium diethylbarbiturate and $y$ ml 0.2M-HCl mixed.

| pH, 18 °C | $x$ ml 0.04M-*sodium diethylbarbiturate* | $y$ ml 0.2M-HCl |
|---|---|---|
| 6.8 | 100 | 18.4 |
| 7.0 | 100 | 17.8 |
| 7.2 | 100 | 16.7 |
| 7.4 | 100 | 15.3 |
| 7.6 | 100 | 13.4 |
| 7.8 | 100 | 11.47 |
| 8.0 | 100 | 9.39 |
| 8.2 | 100 | 7.21 |
| 8.4 | 100 | 5.21 |
| 8.6 | 100 | 3.82 |
| 8.8 | 100 | 2.52 |
| 9.0 | 100 | 1.65 |
| 9.2 | 100 | 1.13 |
| 9.4 | 100 | 0.70 |
| 9.6 | 100 | 0.35 |

*N-Ethylmorpholine–HCl buffer solutions,* pH 7.0–8.2 *at* 20 °C

(Prof. A. Albert, private communication)

*N*-Ethylmorpholine, $C_6H_{13}NO$, M. wt. 115.17.
*N*-Ethylmorpholine should be dried and freshly distilled (B.p. 138–9 °C, 763 mm).
50 ml 0.2M-*N*-ethylmorpholine (23.03 g/l), $x$ ml 1M-HCl; diluted to 100 ml with $H_2O$.

| pH, 20 °C | $x$ ml 1M-HCl |
|---|---|
| 7.0 | 8.0 |
| 7.2 | 7.1 |
| 7.4 | 6.1 |
| 7.6 | 5.0 |
| 7.8 | 4.0 |
| 8.0 | 2.9 |
| 8.2 | 2.0 |

*Tris(hydroxymethyl)aminomethane buffer solutions,* pH 7.1–8.9 *at* 25 °C*

(Bates and Bower, *Analyt. Chem.* **28**, 1322 (1956))

$C_4H_{11}NO_3$, M. wt. 121.14.
50 ml 0.1 M-Tris† (12.114 g/l), $x$ ml 0.1 M-HCl; diluted to 100 ml with $H_2O$.

$$I = 0.001x.$$

$$d\text{pH}/dt \approx -0.028 \text{ pH units/deg.}$$

† Tris solutions absorb $CO_2$ from the air (see Bates and Hetzer, *Analyt. Chem.* **33**, 1285 (1960)).

| pH, 25 °C | $x$ | Buffer value ($\beta$) | $\Delta\text{pH}_{1/2}$ ‡ |
|---|---|---|---|
| 7.10 | 45.7 | 0.010 | |
| 7.20 | 44.7 | 0.012 | |
| 7.30 | 43.4 | 0.013 | |
| 7.40 | 42.0 | 0.015 | |
| 7.50 | 40.3 | 0.017 | −0.02 |
| 7.60 | 38.5 | 0.018 | |
| 7.70 | 36.6 | 0.020 | |
| 7.80 | 34.5 | 0.023 | |
| 7.90 | 32.0 | 0.027 | |
| 8.00 | 29.2 | 0.029 | −0.02 |
| 8.10 | 26.2 | 0.031 | |
| 8.20 | 22.9 | 0.031 | |
| 8.30 | 19.9 | 0.029 | −0.01 |
| 8.40 | 17.2 | 0.026 | |
| 8.50 | 14.7 | 0.024 | |
| 8.60 | 12.4 | 0.022 | |
| 8.70 | 10.3 | 0.020 | −0.01 |
| 8.80 | 8.5 | 0.016 | |
| 8.90 | 7.0 | 0.014 | |

‡ Calculated.

*N-2-Hydroxyethylpiperazine-N'-ethanesulphonic acid (HEPES)*–NaOH *buffer solutions,* pH 7.2–8.2 *at* 21 °C .

25 ml 0.1 M-HEPES (23.83 g/l) + $x$ ml 0.1 M-NaOH diluted to 50 ml with $H_2O$

| pH | $x$ ml 0.1 M-NaOH | |
|---|---|---|
| | 21 °C | 37 °C |
| 7.0 | – | 7.4 |
| 7.2 | 6.6 | 9.9 |
| 7.4 | 8.7 | 12.3 |
| 7.6 | 11.2 | 14.6 |
| 7.8 | 13.7 | 17.1 |
| 8.0 | 16.3 | 19.5 |
| 8.2 | 18.8 | – |

*N-((Trishydroxymethyl)methyl)glycine* (*TRICINE*)—NaOH *buffer solutions*, pH 7.4—8.6 *at* 37°C

25 ml 0.05M-TRICINE (8.958 g/l) + $x$ ml 0.05M-NaOH diluted to 50 ml with $H_2O$

| pH | $x$ ml 0.05M-NaOH | |
|---|---|---|
| | 22°C | 37°C |
| 7.4 | – | 8.4 |
| 7.6 | 5.5 | 10.8 |
| 7.8 | 7.3 | 13.5 |
| 8.0 | 9.6 | 16.0 |
| 8.2 | 12.4 | 18.6 |
| 8.4 | 15.2 | 21.2 |
| 8.6 | 17.8 | 23.2 |
| 8.8 | 19.8 | – |

*N-2-Hydroxyethylpiperazine-N'-3-propanesulphonic acid* (*EPPS*)—NaOH *buffer solutions*, pH 7.5—8.7

25 ml of 0.1M-EPPS (25.232 g/l) + $x$ ml 0.1M-NaOH diluted to 50 ml

| pH | $x$ ml 0.1M-NaOH | |
|---|---|---|
| | 23°C | 37°C |
| 7.3 | – | 5.9 |
| 7.5 | 5.4 | 7.8 |
| 7.7 | 7.1 | 10.0 |
| 7.9 | 9.3 | 12.4 |
| 8.1 | 11.7 | 14.8 |
| 8.3 | 14.2 | 17.3 |
| 8.5 | 16.8 | 19.6 |
| 8.7 | 19.3 | – |

*2-Amino-2-methyl-1,3-propanediol*—HCl *buffer solutions*, pH 7.8—9.7

(Gomori, *PSEBM* **62**, 33 (1946))

2-Amino-2-methyl-1,3-propanediol, $C_4H_{11}NO_2$, M. wt. 105.14.
25 ml 0.2M-2-amino-2-methyl-1,3-propanediol (21.03 g/l), $x$ ml 0.2M-HCl; diluted to 100 ml with $H_2O$.

| pH | | $x$ ml 0.2M-HCl |
|---|---|---|
| 23°C | 37°C | |
| 9.7 | 9.6 | 2.5 |
| 9.6 | 9.4 | 3.75 |
| 9.4 | 9.3 | 5.0 |
| 9.3 | 9.1 | 6.25 |
| 9.1 | 9.0 | 7.5 |
| 9.0 | 8.9 | 8.75 |
| 9.0 | 8.8 | 10.0 |
| 8.9 | 8.8 | 11.25 |
| 8.8 | 8.7 | 12.5 |
| 8.7 | 8.6 | 13.75 |
| 8.6 | 8.5 | 15.0 |
| 8.5 | 8.4 | 16.25 |
| 8.4 | 8.3 | 17.5 |
| 8.3 | 8.2 | 18.75 |
| 8.2 | 8.1 | 20.0 |
| 8.0 | 7.9 | 21.25 |
| 7.8 | 7.7 | 22.5 |

*N,N-(Bis-2-hydroxymethyl)glycine (BICINE)*—NaOH *buffer solutions*, pH 7.9–8.9 *at* 22 °C

25 ml 0.1M-BICINE (16.317 g/l) + $x$ ml 0.1M-NaOH diluted to 50 ml with $H_2O$

| | $x$ ml 0.1M-NaOH | |
|---|---|---|
| pH | 22 °C | 37 °C |
| 7.7 | – | 6.5 |
| 7.9 | 5.7 | 8.6 |
| 8.1 | 7.8 | 11.0 |
| 8.3 | 10.0 | 13.9 |
| 8.5 | 12.7 | 17.0 |
| 8.7 | 15.8 | 19.4 |
| 8.9 | 18.3 | – |

*Clark and Lubs solutions*, pH 8.0–10.2*

(Bower and Bates, *J. Res. Natn. Bur. Stand.* **55**, 197 (1955))

50 ml of a mixture 0.1M with respect to both KCl and $H_3BO_3$ (7.455 g KCl and 6.184 g $H_3BO_3$/l), $x$ ml 0.1M-NaOH; diluted to 100 ml with $H_2O$.

| pH, 25 °C | $x$ | Buffer value ($\beta$) |
|---|---|---|
| 8.00 | 3.9 | |
| 8.10 | 4.9 | 0.010 |
| 8.20 | 6.0 | 0.011 |
| 8.30 | 7.2 | 0.013 |
| 8.40 | 8.6 | 0.015 |
| 8.50 | 10.1 | 0.016 |
| 8.60 | 11.8 | 0.018 |
| 8.70 | 13.7 | 0.020 |
| 8.80 | 15.8 | 0.022 |
| 8.90 | 18.1 | 0.025 |
| 9.00 | 20.8 | 0.027 |
| 9.10 | 23.6 | 0.028 |
| 9.20 | 26.4 | 0.029 |
| 9.30 | 29.3 | 0.028 |
| 9.40 | 32.1 | 0.027 |
| 9.50 | 34.6 | 0.024 |
| 9.60 | 36.9 | 0.022 |
| 9.70 | 38.9 | 0.019 |
| 9.80 | 40.6 | 0.016 |
| 9.90 | 42.2 | 0.015 |
| 10.00 | 43.7 | 0.014 |
| 10.10 | 45.0 | 0.013 |
| 10.20 | 46.2 | |

*Borate buffer solutions,* pH 8.1–9.0 *at* 25 °C*
(Bates and Bower, *Analyt. Chem.* **28**, 1322 (1956))
50 ml 0.025M-$Na_2 B_4 O_7 \cdot 10H_2O$ (9.525 g/l), $x$ ml 0.1M-HCl; diluted to 100 ml with $H_2O$.

$$I \approx 0.025.$$
$$d\text{pH}/dt \approx 0.008 \text{ unit/deg.}$$

| pH, 25 °C | $x$ | *Buffer value* ($\beta$) | $\Delta\text{pH}_{1/2}$ |
|---|---|---|---|
| 8.10 | 19.7 | 0.009 | + 0.07 |
| 8.20 | 18.8 | 0.010 | |
| 8.30 | 17.7 | 0.011 | |
| 8.40 | 16.6 | 0.012 | |
| 8.50 | 15.2 | 0.015 | + 0.05 |
| 8.60 | 13.5 | 0.018 | |
| 8.70 | 11.6 | 0.020 | |
| 8.80 | 9.4 | 0.023 | + 0.04 |
| 8.90 | 7.1 | 0.024 | |
| 9.00 | 4.6 | 0.026 | + 0.02 |

*Glycine–NaOH buffer solutions,* pH 8.6–10.6 *at* 25 °C
(Gomori, after Sørensen, *Meth. Enzymol.* **1**, 145 (1955))
Glycine (aminoacetic acid), $C_2 H_5 NO_2$, M. wt. 75.07.
25 ml 0.2M-glycine (15.01 g/l), $x$ ml 0.2M-NaOH; diluted to 100 ml with $H_2O$.

$$\frac{d\text{pH}}{dt} = -0.026 \text{ pH units/degree.}$$

| pH, 25 °C | $x$ ml 0.2M-NaOH |
|---|---|
| 8.6 | 2.0 |
| 8.8 | 3.0 |
| 9.0 | 4.4 |
| 9.2 | 6.0 |
| 9.4 | 8.4 |
| 9.6 | 11.2 |
| 9.8 | 13.6 |
| 10.0 | 16.0 |
| 10.4 | 19.3 |
| 10.6 | 22.75 |

*Sodium carbonate–sodium bicarbonate buffer solutions,* pH 9.2–10.8
(Delory and King, *BJ* **39**, 245 (1945))
$Na_2 CO_3 \cdot 10H_2O$, M. wt. 286.2; 0.1M-solution contains 28.62 g/l.
$NaHCO_3$, M. wt. 84.0; 0.1M-solution contains 8.40 g/l.
$x$ ml 0.1M-$Na_2 CO_3$ and $y$ ml 0.1M-NaHCO_3 mixed.

| pH | | $x$ ml 0.1M-$Na_2CO_3$ | $y$ ml 0.1M-NaHCO_3 |
|---|---|---|---|
| 20 °C | 37 °C | | |
| 9.2 | 8.8 | 10 | 90 |
| 9.4 | 9.1 | 20 | 80 |
| 9.5 | 9.4 | 30 | 70 |
| 9.8 | 9.5 | 40 | 60 |
| 9.9 | 9.7 | 50 | 50 |
| 10.1 | 9.9 | 60 | 40 |
| 10.3 | 10.1 | 70 | 30 |
| 10.5 | 10.3 | 80 | 20 |
| 10.8 | 10.6 | 90 | 10 |

## 18 pH, buffers, and physiological media

*Borate buffer solutions,* pH 9.3–10.7 *at* 25 °C*

(Bates and Bower, *Analyt. Chem.* **28**, 1322 (1956))

50 ml 0.025M-$Na_2B_4O_7 \cdot 10H_2O$ (9.525 g/l), $x$ ml 0.1M-NaOH; diluted to 100 ml with $H_2O$.

$$I = 0.001 (25 + x).$$

$$d\text{pH}/dt \approx -0.008 \text{ unit/deg.}$$

| pH, 25 °C | $x$ | Buffer value ($\beta$) | $\Delta\text{pH}_{1/2}$ |
|---|---|---|---|
| 9.30 | 3.6 | 0.027 | + 0.01[a] |
| 9.40 | 6.2 | 0.026 | + 0.01[b] |
| 9.50 | 8.8 | 0.025 | |
| 9.60 | 11.1 | 0.022 | + 0.01[a], + 0.01[b] |
| 9.70 | 13.1 | 0.020 | |
| 9.80 | 15.0 | 0.018 | + 0.01[b] |
| 9.90 | 16.7 | 0.016 | |
| 10.00 | 18.3 | 0.014 | |
| 10.10 | 19.5 | 0.011 | − 0.01[a] |
| 10.20 | 20.5 | 0.009 | 0.00[b] |
| 10.30 | 21.3 | 0.008 | |
| 10.40 | 22.1 | 0.007 | |
| 10.50 | 22.7 | 0.006 | |
| 10.60 | 23.3 | 0.005 | |
| 10.70 | 23.8 | 0.004 | |

[a] Measured.  [b] Calculated.

*Carbonate buffer solutions,* pH 9.7–10.9 *at* 25 °C*

(Bates and Bower, *Analyt. Chem.* **28**, 1322 (1956))

50 ml 0.05M-$NaHCO_3$ (4.20 g/l), $x$ ml 0.1M-NaOH; diluted to 100 ml with $H_2O$.

$$I = 0.001 (25 + 2x).$$

$$d\text{pH}/dt \approx -0.009 \text{ unit/deg.}$$

| pH, 25 °C | $x$ | Buffer value ($\beta$) | $\Delta\text{pH}_{1/2}$ |
|---|---|---|---|
| 9.70 | 6.2 | 0.013 | + 0.02[a], + 0.03[b] |
| 9.80 | 7.6 | 0.014 | |
| 9.90 | 9.1 | 0.015 | + 0.03[b] |
| 10.00 | 10.7 | 0.016 | + 0.04[a] |
| 10.10 | 12.2 | 0.016 | + 0.04[a] |
| 10.20 | 13.8 | 0.015 | |
| 10.30 | 15.2 | 0.014 | + 0.02[b] |
| 10.40 | 16.5 | 0.013 | |
| 10.50 | 17.8 | 0.013 | |
| 10.60 | 19.1 | 0.012 | + 0.03[a] |
| 10.70 | 20.2 | 0.010 | 0.00[b] |
| 10.80 | 21.2 | 0.009 | |
| 10.90 | 22.0 | 0.008 | |

[a] Measured.  [b] Calculated.

*Phosphate buffer solutions*, pH 11.0–11.9 *at* 25 °C*

(Bates and Bower, *Analyt. Chem.* **28**, 1322 (1956))

50 ml 0.05 M-$Na_2HPO_4$ (7.10 g/l), $x$ ml 0.1M-NaOH; diluted to 100 ml with $H_2O$

$$I = 0.001(77 + 2x).$$

$$d\text{pH}/dt \approx -0.025 \text{ unit/deg.}$$

| pH, 25 °C | $x$ | Buffer value ($\beta$) | $\Delta\text{pH}_{1/2}$ |
|---|---|---|---|
| 11.00 | 4.1 | 0.009 | |
| 11.10 | 5.1 | 0.011 | $-0.06^a, -0.07^b$ |
| 11.20 | 6.3 | 0.012 | |
| 11.30 | 7.6 | 0.014 | |
| 11.40 | 9.1 | 0.017 | $-0.09^a, -0.10^b$ |
| 11.50 | 11.1 | 0.022 | |
| 11.60 | 13.5 | 0.026 | |
| 11.70 | 16.2 | 0.030 | $-0.15^b$ |
| 11.80 | 19.4 | 0.034 | $-0.13^a, -0.17^b$ |
| 11.90 | 23.0 | 0.037 | |

[a] Measured.  [b] Calculated.

*Hydroxide–chloride buffer solutions*, pH 12.0–13.0 *at* 25 °C*

(Bates and Bower, *Analyt. Chem.* **28**, 1322 (1956))

25 ml 0.2M-KCl (14.91 g/l), $x$ ml 0.2M-NaOH; diluted to 100 ml with $H_2O$.

$$I = 0.001(50 + 2x).$$

$$d\text{pH}/dt \approx -0.033 \text{ unit/deg.}$$

| pH, 25 °C | $x$ | Buffer value ($\beta$) | $\Delta\text{pH}_{1/2}$ [b] |
|---|---|---|---|
| 12.00 | 6.0 | 0.028 | $-0.28$ |
| 12.10 | 8.0 | 0.042 | |
| 12.20 | 10.2 | 0.048 | $-0.28$ |
| 12.30 | 12.8 | 0.060 | |
| 12.40 | 16.2 | 0.076 | |
| 12.50 | 20.4 | 0.094 | $-0.28$ |
| 12.60 | 25.6 | 0.12 | |
| 12.70 | 32.2 | 0.16 | |
| 12.80 | 41.2 | 0.21 | $-0.28$ |
| 12.90 | 53.0 | 0.25 | |
| 13.00 | 66.0 | 0.30 | $-0.27$ |

[b] Calculated.

## BUFFERS FOR ELECTROPHORESIS

The buffer systems described in other sections can form the basis of electrophoretic buffers; it is preferable to use univalent buffers of known and constant ionic strength.

Numerous buffer solutions for zone electrophoresis (paper, gel, column) have been described in the literature; since many of these have been developed for a single specific purpose only a limited number are given in the tables of this section.

*Univalent buffer systems for electrophoresis*

In moving boundary electrophoresis it is important that the buffer ion of low mobility has the same sign as the protein ion. Some data on the mobilities of common buffer ions are given here.

| Weak acid or base | $pK_{25°C}$ | Ion mobility $\times 10^5$ at 0.1M (cm$^2$/V sec) |
|---|---|---|
| Glycine | 2.3 | + 15.6 |
| Lactic acid | 3.8 | − 13.1 |
| Acetic acid | 4.7 | − 16.6 |
| Cacodylic acid | 6.2 | − 10.1 |
| Diethylbarbituric acid | 7.9 | − 10.2 |
| Triethanolamine | 7.9 | + 9.1 |
| Diethanolamine | 9.0 | + 11.4 |
| { Sodium | | + 22.2 |
| { Chloride | | − 37.0 |

*Buffer solutions suitable for paper electrophoresis of proteins*

| pH | I | Components/l solution |
|---|---|---|
| 4.4 | 0.2 | Na$_2$HPO$_4$, 9.44 g |
| | | Citric acid, 10.3 g |
| 4.5 | 0.1 | NaCl, 3.51 g |
| | | NaOAc, 3.28 g |
| | | Adjust to pH 4.5 with M-HCl |
| 6.5 | 0.1 | KH$_2$PO$_4$, 3.11 g |
| | | Na$_2$HPO$_4$, 1.49 g |
| 7.8 | 0.12 | NaH$_2$PO$_4$ · H$_2$O, 0.294 g |
| | | Na$_2$HPO$_4$, 3.25 g |
| 8.6 | 0.05 | Diethylbarbituric acid, 1.84 g |
| | | Sodium diethylbarbiturate, 10.30 g |
| 8.6 | 0.075 | Diethylbarbituric acid, 2.76 g |
| | | Sodium diethylbarbiturate, 15.45 g |
| 8.6 | 0.1 | Diethylbarbituric acid, 3.68 g |
| | | Sodium diethylbarbiturate, 20.6 g |
| 8.9 | — | Tris(hydroxymethyl)aminomethane (Tris), 60.5 g |
| | | Ethylenediaminetetraacetic acid (EDTA), 6.0 g |
| | | Boric acid, 4.6 g |
| | | (0.5M in Tris; 0.021M in EDTA; 0.075M in H$_3$BO$_3$) |

*Volatile buffer solutions for high voltage electrophoresis*

The useful range of the various systems is given below, followed by a few specific reported mixtures.

| pH *range* | *System* |
|---|---|
| approx. 2 | Acetic acid–formic acid |
| 2.3–3.5 | Pyridine–formic acid |
| 3.5–6.0 | Pyridine–acetic acid |
| 3.0–6.0 | Trimethylamine–formic acid (or acetic) |
| 5.5–7.0 | Collidine–acetic acid |
| 7.0–12.0 | Trimethylamine–carbon dioxide |
| 6.0–10.0 | Ammonia–formic acid (or acetic) |
| 6.5–11.0 | Mono- (or tri-)ethanolamine–hydrochloric acid |
| 8.0–9.5 | Ammonium carbonate–ammonia |

*Typical volatile buffer mixtures*

| pH | *Constituents* |
|---|---|
| 1.9 | $CH_3COOH$ (87 ml glacial), HCOOH (25 ml 88%) to 1 l with $H_2O$ |
| 2.1 | HCOOH (25 ml 88%) to 1 l with $H_2O$ |
| 3.1 | Pyridine (5 ml), $CH_3COOH$ (100 ml glacial) to 1 l with $H_2O$ |
| 3.5 | Pyridine (5 ml), $CH_3COOH$ (50 ml glacial) to 1 l with $H_2O$ |
| 4.7 | Pyridine (25 ml), $CH_3COOH$ (25 ml glacial) to 1 l with $H_2O$ |
| 6.5 | Pyridine (100 ml), $CH_3COOH$ (4 ml glacial) to 1 l with $H_2O$ |
| 7.9 | 0.03M-$NH_4HCO_3$ |
| 8.9 | $(NH_4)_2CO_3$ (20 g/l solution) |

## APPROXIMATE pH OF SOME COMMON REAGENTS AT ROOM TEMPERATURE

Data from R. G. Bates, *Determination of* pH: *Theory and Practice,* 2nd ed., Wiley, New York (1964))

| Substance | Molarity | pH |
|---|---|---|
| Acid benzoic | Saturated | 2.8 |
| Acid boric | 0.1 | 5.3 |
| Acid citric | 0.1 | 2.1 |
| Acid hydrochloric | 0.1 | 1.1 |
| Acid oxalic | 0.1 | 1.3 |
| Acid salicylic | Saturated | 2.4 |
| Acid succinic | 0.1 | 2.7 |
| Acid tartaric | 0.1 | 2.0 |
| Acid trichloroacetic | 0.1 | 1.2 |
| Alum, ammonium | 0.05 | 4.6 |
| Alum, potassium | 0.1 | 4.2 |
| Ammonia water | 0.1 | 11.3 |
| Ammonium chloride | 0.1 | 4.6 |
| Ammonium oxalate | 0.1 | 6.4 |
| Ammonium phosphate, primary | 0.1 | 4.0 |
| Ammonium phosphate, secondary | 0.1 | 7.9 |
| Ammonium sulphate | 0.1 | 5.5 |
| Barbital sodium | 0.1 | 9.4 |
| Borax | 0.1 | 9.2 |
| Calcium hydroxide | Saturated | 12.4 |
| Potassium acetate | 0.1 | 9.7 |
| Potassium bicarbonate | 0.1 | 8.2 |
| Potassium bioxalate | 0.1 | 2.7 |
| Potassium carbonate | 0.1 | 11.5 |
| Potassium phosphate, primary | 0.1 | 4.5 |
| Sodium acetate | 0.1 | 8.9 |
| Sodium benzoate | 0.1 | 8.0 |
| Sodium bicarbonate | 0.1 | 8.3 |
| Sodium bisulphate | 0.1 | 1.4 |
| Sodium carbonate | 0.1 | 11.5 |
| Sodium hydroxide | 0.1 | 12.9 |
| Sodium phosphate, primary | 0.1 | 4.5 |
| Sodium phosphate, secondary | 0.1 | 9.2 |

# ACID–BASE INDICATORS

| Indicator (common name) | Preparation 0.1 g in 250 ml of | Acid colour | Basic colour | pH range |
|---|---|---|---|---|
| Cresol red (acid range) | water containing 2.62 ml 0.1 M-NaOH | red | yellow | 0.2–1.8 |
| m-Cresol purple (acid range) | water containing 2.72 ml 0.1 M-NaOH | red | yellow | 1.0–2.6 |
| Thymol blue (acid range) | water containing 2.15 ml 0.1 M-NaOH | red | yellow | 1.2–2.8 |
| Tropaeolin OO | water | red | yellow | 1.3–3.0 |
| Methyl yellow | 90% EtOH | red | yellow | 2.9–4.0 |
| Bromophenol blue | water containing 1.49 ml 0.1 M-NaOH | yellow | purple | 3.0–4.6 |
| Tetrabromophenol blue | water containing 1.0 ml 0.1 M-NaOH | yellow | blue | 3.0–4.6 |
| Congo red | water or 80% EtOH | violet | reddish-orange | 3.0–5.0 |
| Methyl orange | free acid: water Na salt: water containing 3 ml 0.1 M-HCl | red | orange-yellow | 3.1–4.4 |
| Bromocresol green (blue) | water containing 1.43 ml 0.1 M-NaOH | yellow | blue | 3.6–5.2 |
| Methyl red | Na salt: water free acid: 60% EtOH | red | yellow | 4.2–6.3 |
| Chlorophenol red | water containing 2.36 ml 0.1 M-NaOH | yellow | violet-red | 4.8–6.4 |
| Bromocresol purple | water containing 1.85 ml 0.1 M-NaOH | yellow | violet | 5.2–6.8 |
| Azolitmin (litmus) | water | red | blue | 5.0–8.0 |
| Bromothymol blue | water containing 1.6 ml 0.1 M-NaOH | yellow | blue | 6.0–7.6 |
| Phenol red | water containing 2.82 ml 0.1 M-NaOH | yellow | red | 6.8–8.4 |
| Neutral red | 70% EtOH | red | orange-brown | 6.8–8.0 |
| Cresol red (basic range) | water containing 2.62 ml 0.1 M-NaOH | yellow | red | 7.2–8.8 |
| m-Cresol purple (basic range) | water containing 2.62 ml 0.1 M-NaOH | yellow | purple | 7.6–9.2 |
| Thymol blue (basic range) | water containing 2.15 ml 0.1 M-NaOH | yellow | blue | 8.0–9.6 |
| Phenolphthalein | 70% EtOH (60% cellosolve) | colourless | pink | 8.3–10.0 |
| Thymolphthalein | 90% EtOH | colourless | blue | 9.3–10.5 |
| Alizarin yellow | EtOH | yellow | red | 10.1–12.0 |
| Tropaeolin O | water | yellow | orange | 11.1–12.7 |

It is usual to adjust the pH of indicators to an intermediate colour shade using 0.1 M-NaOH or 0.1 M-HCl.

## PHYSIOLOGICAL MEDIA

*Krebs mammalian Ringer solutions*

Parts by volume

| Solutions required (all approximately isotonic with serum) | Krebs–Henseleit original Ringer bicarbonate† | Krebs original Ringer phosphate | Krebs improved Ringer I† | Krebs improved Ringer II | Krebs improved Ringer III | Krebs substrate fortified serum† |
|---|---|---|---|---|---|---|
| | A | B | C | D | E | |
| 0.90% NaCl (0.154M) | 100 | 100 | 80 | 83 | 95 | |
| 1.15% KCl (0.154M) | 4 | 4 | 4 | 4 | 4 | |
| 1.22% CaCl$_2$ (0.11M) | 3‡ | 3‡ | 3‡ | | 3‡ | 100 vol. serum prepared from rapidly cooled blood |
| 2.11% KH$_2$PO$_4$ (0.154M) | 1 | 1 | 1 | 1 | 1 | |
| 3.8% MgSO$_4$·7H$_2$O (0.154M) | 1§ | 1§ | 1§ | 1§ | 1§ | |
| 1.3% NaHCO$_3$ | 21‖ | | 21‖ | 3 | 3 | |
| 0.1M-Phosphate buffer pH 7.4 (17.8 g Na$_2$HPO$_4$·2H$_2$O + 20 ml M-HCl diluted to 1 l) | | 21 | | | | |
| 0.16M-Na pyruvate (or L-lactate) | | | 4 | 4 | 4 | 3 |
| 0.1M-Na fumarate | | | 7 | 7 | 7 | 6 |
| 0.16M-Na-L-glutamate | | | 4 | 4 | 4 | 3 |
| 0.3M-(5.4%) glucose | | | 5 | 5 | 5 | 5 |
| 0.1M-Na phosphate buffer [100 vol. 0.1M-Na$_2$HPO$_4$ (1.78% Na$_2$HPO$_2$·2H$_2$O) + 25 vol. 0.1M-NaH$_2$PO$_4$ (1.38% NaH$_2$PO$_4$·H$_2$O)] | | | | 18 | 3 | |

† Gassed with 5% $CO_2$ in gas phase.
‡ Twice the conc. of ionized Ca in serum (*Nature, Lond.* **184**, 1315 (1959)).
§ For human serum-substitute replace 50% with 0.154M-MgCl$_2$.
‖ Gassed with 100% $CO_2$ for 1 hr before mixing with other solutions.

*Notes. A* and *B. Krebs and Henseleit bicarbonate and phosphate Ringer (ZPC* **210**, 33 (1932); **217**, 193 (1933)). Cl⁻ ions about 20 per cent higher than in mammalian serum.

*C. Krebs improved Ringer I (BBA* **4**, 249 (1950)). Conc. of electrolytes and organic acids similar to mammalian serum, and contains intrinsic substrate.

*D. Krebs improved Ringer II. Low bicarbonate,* Ca$^{2+}$ *free (BBA* **4**, 249 (1950)). Suitable for measurement of $CO_2$ production by direct $CO_2$ absorption. Valuable for minced tissues and homogenates as higher and steadier rates of respiration obtained in Ca-free media. Concentration of phosphate is 20 times higher and bicarbonate 10 times lower than physiological.

*E. Krebs improved Ringer III. Low phosphate, bicarbonate, and* $CO_2$. Suitable for measurement of $CO_2$ production by direct $CO_2$ absorption. Concentration of Ca about twice that of the ionized Ca of serum. Limited buffering capacity.

*Storage.* A composite solution containing the NaCl, KCl, CaCl$_2$, KH$_2$PO$_4$, and MgSO$_4$ ± 3 vols. NaHCO$_3$ solution will not precipitate Ca or Mg. The danger of microfloral contamination is avoided if the *individual* solutions are made up at five times the required concentrations and diluted before use. Solutions of organic acid salts and glucose should be sterilized, frozen, or freshly prepared.

*Other balanced salt solutions.*

The following salts and glucose in grams are dissolved in water to produce 100 ml solution. Solutions containing $NaHCO_3$ should not be sterilized by heating since the loss of $CO_2$ causes a more alkaline reaction. They may be sterilized by filtration through a bacteriological filter (e.g. cellulose nitrate (millipore) filter). For reptiles Krebs—Henseleit bicarbonate Ringer can be used.

| | NaCl | KCl | CaCl₂ anhyd. | MgSO₄·7H₂O | MgCl₂·6H₂O | NaH₂PO₄·H₂O | Na₂HPO₄·2H₂O | KH₂PO₄ | Glucose | NaHCO₃ | Gas | Remarks |
|---|---|---|---|---|---|---|---|---|---|---|---|---|
| Ringer (frog heart) | 0.65 | 0.014 | 0.012 | | | 0.001 | | | 0.2 | 0.02 | air | |
| Locke (mammalian heart) | 0.9 | 0.042 | 0.024 | | | | | | 0.1– 0.25 | 0.01– 0.03 | air | For cold blooded animals reduce NaCl to 0.65 g |
| Tyrode (rabbit intestine) | 0.8 | 0.02 | 0.02 | | 0.1 | 0.006 | | | 0.1 | 0.1 | air | Some workers have used 0.01 g MgCl₂ anhyd. |
| Gey (1) | 0.7 | 0.037 | 0.017 | 0.007 | 0.021 | | 0.015 | 0.003 | 0.1 | 0.227 | 5% CO₂ in air | |
| Gey (2) | 0.8 | 0.0375 | 0.0275 | | 0.021 | | 0.015 | 0.0025 | 0.2 | 0.025 | air | |
| Simms | 0.8 | 0.02 | 0.0147 | | 0.02 | | 0.021 | | 0.1 | 0.1 | 2% CO₂ in air | |
| Earle | 0.68 | 0.04 | 0.02 | 0.01 | | 0.0125 | | | 0.1 | 0.22 | 5% CO₂ in air | |
| Hanks | 0.80 | 0.04 | 0.014 | 0.01 | 0.01 | | 0.006 | 0.006 | 0.1 | 0.035 | air | 20 mg of indicator phenol red usually added |
| Dulbecco | 0.80 | 0.02 | 0.01 | | 0.01 | | 0.115 | 0.02 | | | air | |
| Amphibian Ringer | 0.65 | 0.025 | 0.03 | | | | | | | 0.02 | air | pH adjusted 7.0–7.4 |
| Marine mollusc saline | 2.34 | | 0.56 | | 1.62 | | | | | | air | |
| Marine crustacea saline | 2.92 | 0.075 | 0.44 | | | | | | | | air | |
| Elasmobranch saline | 1.64 | 0.089 | 0.11 | | | 0.007 | | | 0.1 | 0.038 | | Also ADD 2.16 g urea/ 100 ml |
| Locke (insects) | 0.9 | 0.042 | 0.025 | | | | | | 0.25 | 0.02 | air | |
| Wyatt (Lepidoptera) | | 0.298 | 0.081 | 0.37 | 0.304 | 0.127 | | | 0.07 | | | Fructose and sucrose added, each at 40 mg/ 100 ml |
| Carlson (grasshoppers) | 0.7 | 0.02 | 0.002 | | 0.01 | 0.023 | | | 0.08 | 0.005 | air | |
| Holtfreter (amphibia and fishes) | 0.35 | 0.005 | 0.0076 | | | | | | | 0.02 | air | |
| Cortland (trout) | 0.725 | 0.038 | 0.018 | 0.023 | | 0.041 | | | 0.1 | 0.1 | air | |

All figures are grams per 100 ml solution.

## 18  pH, buffers, and physiological media

*Artificial sea-water*

(i) Prepared from solutions isotonic with sea water. Atlantic sea-water is 3.50–3.55% saline while North Sea sea-water is 3.4–3.5%.

| | | ml |
|---|---|---|
| 0.54M | NaCl | 739.6 |
| 0.54M | KCl | 18.05 |
| 0.36M | $MgCl_2$ | 145.7 |
| 0.36M | $CaCl_2$ | 28.0 |
| 0.44M | $Na_2SO_4$ | 63.0 |
| 0.54M | $NaHCO_3$ | 4.6 |
| 0.54M | NaBr | 1.05 (for most purposes NaCl can be substituted) |

(ii) Prepared from the following salts dissolved in water and diluted to 1 litre. 24.7 g NaCl;  0.7 g KCl;  6.3 g $MgSO_4 \cdot 7H_2O$;  4.6 g $MgCl_2 \cdot 6H_2O$;  1.0 g  anhyd. $CaCl_2$; 0.2 g $NaHCO_3$.

# 19 Gel electrophoresis

The section describes some of the common procedures and reagents used in acrylamide and agarose gel electrophoresis of nucleic acids and proteins. Key literature references are also given as a source of details of the technique.

## Recrystallisation of acrylamides

**WARNING.** Acrylamide and bis-acrylamide are extremely toxic and appropriate precautions should be taken to avoid skin contact or inhalation of the light crystals.

*Acrylamide:* 200 g dissolved in 1 litre $CHCl_3$, heated to boiling and filtered without suction in warmed funnel with Whatman filter paper No. 541. Allowed to cool at room temperature and then left at $-15\,^{\circ}C$ overnight. Crystals collected with suction in cold funnel and washed with 300 ml cold $CHCl_3$. Crystals air dried in warm oven.

*Bis-acrylamide:* 100 g dissolved in 500 ml of boiling MeOH and filtered without suction in a warmed funnel. Allowed to cool at room temperature and placed at $-15\,^{\circ}C$ overnight. Crystals collected with suction in a cooled funnel and washed with 300 ml cold MeOH. Crystals are air-dried in a warm oven.

## Coomassie blue stain for proteins

0.2 g Coomassie Brilliant Blue dissolved in 90 ml of MeOH:$H_2O$ (1:1 v/v), and 10 ml glacial acetic acid. The gel is immersed in at least 5 volumes of stain for a minimum of 1 hour with gentle agitation; staining usually complete in 3 hours. Background destaining is carried out by repeated washing of the gel in 10% acetic acid in 20% MeOH–$H_2O$. Destaining can be accomplished electrophoretically very rapidly (*Anal. Biochem.* **33**, 259 (1970)).

Many slight variations in the Coomassie Blue staining reagents have been used, *JBC* **244**, 440 (1969); *J. Virol.* **12**, 241 (1973); *Biochemistry* **10**, 2606 (1971); *Anal. Biochem.* **43**, 173 (1971); *Meth. Enzymol.* **91**, 236 (1983).

## Silver stain for proteins

This method is about 100 times more sensitive than staining with Coomassie Brilliant Blue and is comparable in sensitivity to radioautography of radioactively labelled proteins. Simplifications and variations of the original method in *Anal. Biochem.* **98**, 231 (1979) are being published. See: *Anal. Biochem.* **105**, 361 (1980); *Electrophoresis* **2**, 135 (1983); *Anal. Biochem.* **129**, 277 (1983), **130**, 353 (1983), **131**, 46 (1983).

## Staining for RNA

*Toluidine blue:* 0.01–0.5% toluidine blue in $H_2O$. The more intensely a gel is stained, the longer is the destaining period required. The time of staining can be varied from 1 min to several hours depending on the amount of RNA on the gels. Destaining is carried out in water with repeated changes and gentle agitation.

Other basic dyes such as methylene blue have been used and many procedures have been reported in the literature, *Anal. Biochem.* **59**, 599 (1974).

Concentrations of methylene blue greater than 0.1% stains agarose so tightly that several days destaining is necessary. Breakdown of RNA by a light-dependent dye-catalysed reaction has been reported to occur with toluidine blue, methylene blue, and several others, but not with ethidium bromide* staining (q.v.) *Anal. Biochem.* **65**, 331 (1975).

* **WARNING** This is a powerful mutagen and should accordingly be handled with great care.

## 19 Gel electrophoresis

*Ethidium bromide:* Gel stained in 0.01% ethidium bromide* in 0.02-M sodium acetate pH 7.8. RNA bands visible in U.V. light without destaining, *Anal. Biochem.* **65**, 331 (1975); also visualizes DNA.

*Silver stain*: This is more sensitive than ethidium bromide or toluidine blue. However, the biological activity of the RNA is likely to be impaired. Simplifications and variations of the original staining method as originally used for proteins are in *Anal. Biochem.* **134**, 184 (1983); *J. Virol. Methods* **7**, 185 (1983).

### Ethidium bromide staining for DNA

The gel is immersed in a dilute solution of ethidium bromide* in water or electrophoresis buffer (0.5 µg/ml is satisfactory) for 1−2 hours and examined under U.V. light (*JMB* **98**, 583 (1971)). A brief wash in water may be helpful in detecting small amounts of DNA.

Strong visible light is reported to cause single-strand scissions in presence of ethidium, *J. Virol.* **9**, 317 (1972). RNA also is stained.

### Fluorography of acrylamide slab gels

The original method (*EJB* **46**, 83 (1974)) used 22% PPO. Based on a thin layer procedure (*Anal. Biochem.* **89**, 247 (1978)), a modified procedure using naphthalene has been developed which is less expensive and equally efficient, *Virology* **113**, 1 (1981).

The gel is fixed in 10% acetic acid−10% isopropanol (minimum of 1 hour) and then soaked twice for 30-min periods in DMSO, followed by 3 hours in freshly prepared 20% (w/v) naphthalene (technical grade)−0.5% (w/v) PPO in DMSO. The reagent is poured off and DMSO removed by at least 2 washes in $H_2O$ for 1−2 hours each. Complete removal of DMSO is essential to avoid sticky gels after drying.

The gel is dried on Whatman 3 mm paper under vacuum at 100 °C (details of the apparatus and procedure in *Methods in Virology* **5**, 179 (1971); a commercial apparatus is also available).

The gel is exposed to Kodak Xomat RP film at − 80 °C. Preflashing of the film can increase sensitivity − *EJB* **46**, 83 (1974). As a rough guide, 100 c.p.m. of $^{14}C$ in a 1 cm band is visible after overnight exposure (without preflashing).

A more rapid method makes use of sodium salicylate as fluor (*Anal. Biochem.* **98**, 132 (1979)). However the bands produced are slightly more diffuse than with PPO or naphthalene.

The gel is soaked in 10 volumes of 1 M sodium salicylate, pH 5−7, for 30 min. The gel is dried under vacuum for 2 hours at 80 °C and exposed to X-ray film at − 70 °C.

### References to techniques in gel electrophoresis

#### A. Nucleic acids

RNA and DNA ranging in size from mononucleotides to double-strand DNAs with molecular weights over $100 \times 10^6$ can be fractionated on the basis of size by electrophoresis in a solid support of either cross-linked polyacrylamide and/or agarose. For DNA of large M. wt. agarose must be used. Both tube gels and slab gels are commonly used. Although tube gels are very convenient to use, slab gels have the advantage of better resolution, better comparison of different nucleic acid samples, and greater ease of autoradiography. Slab gels are more suitable for the large scale purification of nucleic acids.

Since it is impossible to summarize briefly the various techniques used in the gel electrophoresis of nucleic acids, a number of key references have been given

---

* **WARNING** This is a powerful mutagen and should accordingly be handled with great care.

which will provide the necessary details. The article by H. Gould and H.R. Mathews (1976) on Separation methods for nucleic acids and oligonucleotides in Volume 4 of *Laboratory techniques in biochemistry and molecular biology* (eds. T.S. Work and E. Work, North-Holland Publishing Co.) is a comprehensive reference. See also *Gel electrophoresis of nucleic acids: a practical approach* (eds. D. Rickwood and B. D. Hames). IRL Press, Oxford (1982).

*RNA*
*Basic techniques:*                    *BJ* **102**, 251 (1967)
                                       *Methods in Virology* **5**, 125 (1971)
                                       *Meth. Enzymol.* **21**, 167 (1971)
                                       *JMB* **79**, 237 (1973)
                                       *Biochemistry* **12**, 3055 (1973)
                                       *Biochemistry* **12**, 4361 (1973)
                                       *Anal. Biochem.* **59**, 599 (1974)
                                       *Biochemistry* **16**, 2763 (1977)
                                       *FEBS Lett.* **87**, 107 (1978)

*Estimation of molecular weight under denaturing conditions:*
Formamide:                             *Nature, New Biol.* **235**, 108 (1972)
                                       *Biochemistry* **13**, 5373 (1974)
                                       *EJB* **62**, 313 (1976)
Urea:                                  *BBA* **324**, 320 (1973)
                                       *Virology* **60**, 515 (1974)
Formaldehyde:                          *BBA* **240**, 448 (1971)
Glyoxal:                               *PNAS* **74**, 4835 (1977)
Methyl mercury:                        *Anal. Biochem.* **70**, 75 (1976)
                                       *Biochemistry* **16**, 4743 (1977)
*Elution of RNA from gels:*            *JMB* **63**, 41 (1972)
                                       *JMB* **87**, 377 (1974)
                                       *Anal. Biochem.* **68**, 36 (1975)
                                       *Anal. Biochem.* **74**, 198 (1976)
                                       *Aust. J. Biol. Sci.* **31**, 25 (1978)
                                       *FEBS Lett.* **98**, 319 (1979)


*DNA*
*Basic techniques:*                    *Anal. Biochem.* **79**, 1 (1977)
                                       *JMB* **110**, 119 (1977)
                                       *Nucleic Acids Res.* **5**, 653 (1978)
                                       *FEBS Lett.* **87**, 107 (1978)
                                       *Meth. Enzymol.* **68**, 152 (1979)
                                       *Meth. Enzymol.* **65**, 299, 305, 319 (1980)
*Molecular weight estimation:*         *Biochemistry* **12**, 3055 (1973)
                                       *Biochemistry* **14**, 3787 (1975)
                                       *JMB* **110**, 119 (1977)
*Elution of DNA from gel:*             *Anal. Biochem.* **66**, 213 (1975)
                                       *Anal. Biochem.* **79**, 1 (1977)
                                       *JMB* **110**, 119 (1977)
                                       *BBA* **520**, 498 (1978)
                                       *Gene* **4**, 213 (1978)
                                       *Meth. Enzymol.* **68**, 176 (1979)
                                       *Meth. Enzymol.* **65**, 371, 499 (1980)
*Separation of DNA strands:*           *Virology* **49**, 342 (1972)
                                       *Anal. Biochem.* **83**, 666 (1977)
                                       *PNAS* **74**, 560 (1977)

*B. Proteins*

Proteins in either the undissociated or denatured form can be fractionated by electrophoresis on cross-linked polyacrylamide gels. Both tube gels and slab gels are commonly used although slab gels have the advantage of better comparison of protein samples and greater ease of autoradiography or fluorography. The article by Maizel, *Methods in Virology* **5**, 179 (1971) is a comprehensive basic reference. See also *Gel electrophoresis of proteins: a practical approach* (eds. B. D. Hames and D. Rickwood). IRL Press, London (1981)

| | |
|---|---|
| *Basic techniques:* | *Nature* **227**, 680 (1970) |
| | *Methods in Virology* **5**, 179 (1971) |
| | *Meth. Enzymol.* **22**, 412 and 565 (1971) |
| | *JMB* **79**, 237 (1973) |
| | *Meth. Enzymol.* **91**, 190 and 214 (1983) |
| | *Anal. Biochem.* **133**, 545 (1983) |
| *Molecular weight estimation:* | *JBC* **244**, 4406 (1969) |
| | *Meth. Enzymol.* **26**, 3 (1972) |
| | *Meth. Enzymol.* **48**, 3 (1978) |

*Low molecular weight proteins ($M_r$ less than 10 000):*

| | |
|---|---|
| | *Anal. Biochem.* **39**, 462 (1971) |
| | *Biochemistry* **15**, 2930 (1976) |
| | *Anal. Biochem.* **129**, 192 (1983) |
| *Electrophoresis of nucleoproteins:* | *J. Gen. Virol.* **12**, 325 (1971) |
| | *Virology* **60**, 476 (1974) |
| *Two-dimensional gel electrophoresis:* | *Meth. Enzymol.* **30**, 497–506 (1974) |
| | *JBC* **250**, 4007 (1975) |
| | *Cell* **12**, 1133 (1977) |
| | *Anal. Biochem.* **93**, 329 (1979) |
| | *Meth. Enzymol.* **91**, 190 (1983) |
| *Autoradiography and fluorography:* | *Methods in Virology* **5**, 179 (1971) |
| | *EJB* **46**, 83 (1974) |
| | *FEBS Lett.* **82**, 314 (1977) |
| | *Virology* **113**, 1 (1981) |
| | *Anal. Biochem.* **98**, 132 (1979) |
| *Elution of protein from gels:* | *Anal. Biochem.* **77**, 168 (1977) |
| | *Anal. Biochem.* **128**, 7 (1983) |
| | *Virology*, **123**, 284 (1982) |
| | *Meth. Enzymol.* **91**, 227 and 263 (1983) |

*'Fingerprinting' of proteins isolated on SDS gels:*

*JBC* **252**, 1102 (1977)

# 20 Methods for the detection of biochemical compounds on paper and thin layer chromatograms with some notes on separation

## 1 ACIDS

### VOLATILE FATTY ACIDS

Volatile fatty acids are now largely separated by GLC. If paper chromatography or TLC are used they are almost always separated with a solvent containing volatile base e.g. $NH_3$, ethylamine. With an ethanol/3M-$NH_3$ (95/6) solvent typical $R_F$s would be formic 0.31, acetic 0.33, propionic 0.44, butyric 0.54, valeric 0.60, caproic 0.68. They are detected by pH indicator methods. The formation of heavy-metal soaps, which can be used for the higher fatty acids, is not applicable as the soaps of the volatile fatty acids are too soluble in water.

### 1 Indicators

Spray with 0.04% bromocresol green in EtOH or $H_2O$, adjusted to a blue colour (pH 7.5) with NaOH. Anions give yellow spots and cations deep blue spots on a pale blue background, or if bromothymol blue is used, a green background. Sensitivity is 5 µg. If the chromatogram has been run in a solvent containing $NH_3$ or ethylamine these colours are given only if, before spraying, the paper is dried at 95 °C for 5 min to decompose salts. If the paper is dried at RT for a short time and then sprayed with 2% bromocresol green in EtOH, ammonium or ethylamine salts give blue spots on a greenish-yellow background.

### 2 Modified procedures

(i) Spray with 0.04% bromocresol purple in formalin–EtOH (1:5) adjusted to pH 5 with NaOH. Expose sprayed paper to $NH_3$. Acids give yellow spots on a purple background.

(ii) Spray with 0.1% aq. thymol blue, adjusted to a deep blue colour (pH 10) with NaOH. Ammonium salts give yellow spots on a blue ground.

## 20 Detection of biochemical compounds

### HIGHER FATTY ACIDS

Higher fatty acids are now more generally separated by GLC although geometric isomers of unsaturated acids are commonly examined using TLC plates coated with silicic acid–$AgNO_3$ mixtures.

#### 1 *Indicator*

Spray with 0.4% bromothymol blue in methyl cellosolve. Acids give yellow spots on a blue ground.

#### 2 *Lipophilic dyes*

Spray with 0.1% Rhodamine B in $H_2O$ or 0.5M-HCl. In u.v. light fatty acids show a clear red fluorescence. Sensitivity $10-100\,\mu g$. Nile blue is also used as well as fluorescent indicators, quinine, acridine orange.

#### 3 *Metallic soaps*

Dip in 1% aq. Pb acetate and wash in water. After drying, expose to $H_2S$. Acids give brown spots on a white or pale tan ground. $0.5\,\mu g$ of stearic acid may be detected. Instead of exposing to $H_2S$ the paper may be dipped in sat. aq. solution of the K salt of rhodizonic acid followed by washing in water until the water is colourless. Purple spots of Pb rhodizonate on a pale pink background result. This is slightly less sensitive than the $H_2S$ treatment.

#### 4 *Reaction with unsaturated centres*

Spray with 0.5% osmic acid. Unsaturated acids slowly give black spots.
*See also* Lipids, 5. $I_2$ vapour can be used for detecting unsaturated fatty acids: saturated acids react far less readily.

### DETECTION OF ACIDS INVOLVED IN CARBOHYDRATE METABOLISM

Various solvents have been described but *n*-propanol–2 M-$NH_3$ (7:3 v/v) is very useful for paper separation. $R_F$s citric and isocitric 0.11, *cis* or *trans*-aconitic 0.14, oxalic 0.17, tartaric 0.18, malic 0.20, succinic 0.23, fumaric 0.27, glutaric 0.27, adipic 0.30, glyceric 0.37, glycollic 0.38, lactic 0.47, 2-hydroxybutyric 0.54.

### GENERAL METHODS

#### 1 *Indicators*

After strongly acid chromatographic solvents, papers are dried for 1 hr at $60^{\circ}$C, then at RT for 2–3 hr. Spray with 0.04% bromophenol blue in 95% EtOH, adjusted to a purple tint (pH 5) with NaOH, or with bromocresol green indicator adjusted to a blue tint. A few drops of $NH_4OH$ added just before spraying assists in giving a vivid contrast. Bromothymol blue is more sensitive but the colour is less stable.

After alkaline solvents, when acids are separated as ammonium salts:
(i) Heat the paper at $95^{\circ}$C for 5 min and then spray with 0.04% aq. chlorophenol red, pH 4.7. Anions give bright yellow spots on a mauve ground.
(ii) Spray with a solution containing 50 mg phenol red in 20 ml 96% EtOH + 2 ml M-NaOH, diluted to 100 ml with $H_2O$. Acids give bright yellow spots on a red ground.

#### 2 *Dimethylglyoxime–nickel biuret*

The paper is first allowed to dry in air and then well steamed to remove all traces of volatile acidic solvent. Dip in (*a*) 1% dimethylglyoxime in 95% ethanol. Partially dry and then spray with (*b*) freshly prepared alkaline nickel biuret solution: 1 g nickel sulphate heptahydrate is dissolved in 50 ml $H_2O$, and 1 g biuret then dissolved, with warming. Add 10 ml 1M-NaOH and allow to stand 30 min before being filtered to remove precipitated nickel hydroxide. The acids appear as stable pink to red spots on a colourless background. After 2 min wash twice in 400—500 ml ethanol—0.88 $NH_3$ (1:1) for 2 min. Sensitivity 10 $\mu$g.

### 3 Mercurochrome

Spray with 0.1% mercurochrome in EtOH. Acids give white spots on a pink ground; in u.v. light, violet spots on a greenish-yellow fluorescent ground.

### 4 Multiple spray for amino acids + acids + sugars

Spray with (a) 0.2% ninhydrin in BuOH saturated with water and dry at 70°C. Mark amino acids (1—5 $\mu$g) and then spray with (b) 0.1% methyl red in EtOH adjusted with NaOH to the pH where the soln. just turns orange on paper. Dry in air. Organic acids (25 $\mu$g) give red spots. Then spray with (c) 3:5-dinitrosalicylate (see Carbohydrates). Dry in air, then heat at 105°C until dark spots of reducing sugars (15 $\mu$g) appear. Store in the dark at RT for 2 weeks. Non-reducing sugars give grey-green spots (60 $\mu$g).

### 5 Semicarbazide hydrochloride

Spray with 0.1% semicarbazide hydrochloride in 0.15% aq. Na acetate. Heat at 110°C. Free keto acids appear as dark spots on a faintly fluorescent background in u.v.

### 7 o-Phenylenediamine

Spray with 0.05% o-phenylenediamine in 10% aq. trichloroacetic acid. Heat at 100°C for 2 min. In u.v. $\alpha$-keto compounds show a yellow-green fluorescence.

### PHENOLIC AND AROMATIC ACIDS

### 8 2,6-Dibromoquinone-4-chloroimide*

Spray with a 0.33% solution of 2:6-dibromoquinone-4-chloroimide in dry dioxan—acetone (4:1). Then spray with dilute ammonia. Phenolic compounds give blue, green, and grey colours.

**Warning**: This compound can be an explosive risk at temperatures of 50°C and above.

### 9 Ferric chloride

Spray with 2% $FeCl_3 \cdot 6H_2O$ in water or with a saturated solution of anhydrous ferric chloride in anhydrous dioxan or chloroform. Most phenolic compounds give red-violet spots. Pyrocatechol derivatives give green spots.

### 10 Fluorescent hydroxy derivatives

Spray with 0.3% hydrogen peroxide. Irradiate the wet chromatogram with u.v. light. Within a few minutes some aromatic acids give blue fluorescent spots.

### TRICARBOXYLIC ACIDS

### 11 Furth—Hermann reagent

Spray with acetic acid—pyridine (1:9). Heat at 100°C for 5 min. Tricarboxylic acids give yellow to red spots showing fluorescence in u.v. Glucuronic and ascorbic acids give yellow spots; aconitic, brown; itaconic, orange.

## 2 ALDEHYDES AND KETONES

### DETECTION

#### 1 2:4-*Dinitrophenylhydrazine*

Spray with 0.4% 2:4-dinitrophenylhydrazine in 2M-HCl. Carbonyl compounds give yellow spots which turn red-brown when treated with 10% NaOH and α-dicarbonyl compounds give a purple colour.

#### 2 *Orcinol*

Spray with 0.5 g orcinol + 15 g trichloroacetic acid in 100 ml $H_2O$-saturated *n*-BuOH. Different coloured spots are given by aldehydes depending on the time and temp. of heating (e.g. heat at $25°C$ for $5-10$ min; $50°C$, 1 or 10 min; $100°C$, 1 or 5 min). Characteristic colours, mostly pinks, are given with vanillin and other aromatic aldehydes.

*2:4-Dinitrophenylhydrazone derivatives of volatile aldehydes and ketones*

#### 3 *Sodium hydroxide*

Spray with 10% NaOH. The yellow coloured spots of 2:4-dinitrophenylhydrazones turn red-brown.

## 3 AMINES

It is not possible to give a comprehensive list of the solvents which have been employed for the separation of amines on paper or thin layers but the following have proved useful: (a) *n*-butanol–acetic acid–water 4:1:1 or 12:3:5; (b) *iso*-propanol–conc. $NH_3$–water 8:1:1 or 20:1:2; (c) *tert* amyl alcohol–17% aqueous methylamine 4:1; (d) *sec* butanol–pyridine–acetic acid–$H_2O$ 604:10:41:100; (e) ethanol–water–$NH_3$ 18:1:1; (f) methanol–water–pyridine 20:5:1; (g) *tert* butanol–water–methylethylketone–diethylamine 10:10:5:1.

### GENERAL METHODS OF DETECTION

#### 1 *Inspection in short-wave* (253 nm) *and long-wave* (366 nm) *ultraviolet light*

Fluorescent amines include kynurenine (pale blue), *o*-aminoacetophenone (pale blue), 3-hydroxykynurenine (green), anthranilic acid (purple), aminosalicylic acid (blue), xanthopterine (yellow-green), many drugs and alkaloids.

Other compounds, possessing single or condensed aromatic rings, may be visible as dark spots on a faintly fluorescent background.

By reacting a primary amine with fluorescamine (see amino acids 2) spots are produced with fluoresce strongly in u.v. light (sensitivity 1 nmole).

#### 2 *Indicators, for the detection of non-volatile bases*

Thoroughly remove basic or acidic solvents in current of hot air. Spray with one of the following reagents:

(i) 0.05% bromocresol green in 95% ethanol, adjusted to green colour (pH $6-7$) with dilute NaOH.

(ii) mixture (1:1) of saturated ethanolic solutions of methyl orange and congo red.

If spots do not show up, expose paper alternately to vapours of $NH_3$ and HCl.

(iii) Spray with 1% solution of tetraphenylborosodium in butanone saturated with water. Dry, then spray with 0.015% solution of a flavon-3-ol in methanol (e.g. fisetin, quercetin, hyperin, or rutin). Spots are orange to red.

## PRIMARY AMINES

### 3 *Ninhydrin*

One of the following ninhydrin sprays may be used:

(i) 0.1% in *n*-butanol saturated with water or in acetone. Heat at $105^{\circ}$C for 5 min.

(ii) 0.2% in *iso*propanol–pyridine (80:20). Heat at $105^{\circ}$C for 2–3 min. Aliphatic amines blue-red, tyramine purple, tryptamine purple-brown, histamine red-brown, noradrenaline and 5-hydroxytryptamine brown.

(iii) 0.2% in mixture of abs. ethanol, acetic acid and 2:4:6-collidine (50:10:2). Immediately before use, mix 25 parts with 1.5 parts of a 1% solution of $Cu(NO_3)_2 \cdot 3H_2O$ in abs. ethanol. Spray and dry for 1.5–2 min at $105^{\circ}$C. Polychromatic spots are obtained with a mixture of amino acids.

Ninhydrin is specific for the aliphatic or alicyclic primary amino group. Secondary, tertiary, and quaternary amines, amides, and amino-substituted aromatic compounds give weak or no reaction. Exception – proline gives yellow spot, probably due to opening of ring. Amino ketones initially yellow turning purple.

### 4 *o-Acetoacetylphenol or* 2-*acetoacetyl*-4-*methylphenol*

Spray with 0.1% solution of *o*-acetoacetylphenol or 2-acetoacetyl-4-methylphenol in *n*-butanol. Primary aliphatic or alicyclic amines show brilliant greenish-yellow fluorescence in u.v. Does not react with secondary amines, primary aromatic amines, or amino acids.

## SECONDARY AMINES

### 5 *Sodium nitroprusside–acetaldehyde*

Immediately before spraying mix equal volumes of 5% sodium nitroprusside in 10% aqueous acetaldehyde and 2% sodium carbonate. Alternatively, spray first with nitroprusside–acetaldehyde solution, then, when the paper is almost dry, with 2% sodium carbonate. Secondary amines appear as blue spots.

### 6 *Fluorescamine*

Spray with 0.05% fluorescamine in acetone. Wet the paper successively with 0.1M-acetic acid in acetone and then 0.1M *N*-chlorosuccinimide in acetone. Leave 5 min – wash with acetone and heat for 5–10 min at $110^{\circ}$C. Secondary amines are converted to primary amines which react with fluorescamine and fluoresce in u.v. light (very sensitive).

## TERTIARY AMINES, QUATERNARY AMMONIUM COMPOUNDS, AND ALKALOIDS

### 7 *Iodoplatinate*

Mix 5 ml of 5% platinum chloride in 1M-HCl with 45 ml 10% potassium iodide and 100 ml water. Protect the reagent against light. After spraying wash out excess from paper with water. For TLC, a mixture (1:1) of 0.3% $PtCl_4$ and 6% KI may be used. Blue or black spots. Sensitivity $10\,\mu$g.

8 *Dragendorff's reagent*

Stock solutions:

Soln. I: Dissolve 17 g basic bismuth nitrate and 200 g tartaric acid in 800 ml water.

Soln. II: Dissolve 160 g potassium iodide in 400 ml water.

Mix solutions I and II. Protect from light. For spraying mix 50 ml stock, 100 g tartaric acid and 500 ml water.

Alkaloids appear as orange spots (sensitivity about 5 μg).

Modification for TLC: Stock solution: boil 2.6 g bismuth carbonate, 7 g sodium iodide and 25 ml acetic acid for a few minutes. After 12 hr filter from precipitate of sodium acetate. Mix 20 ml of filtrate with 8 ml ethyl acetate and store in dark bottle.

Spray solution: mix 10 ml stock, 25 ml acetic acid, and 60 ml ethyl acetate.

Sensitivity can be enhanced by a second spray with $0.025-0.5\text{M-H}_2\text{SO}_4$. The most favourable concentration and amount of acid should be ascertained in a trial experiment.

9 *Iodine*

Paper: 2% solution in ethanol or treat with iodine vapour.

For TLC: 0.5% solution in chloroform, or treat with iodine vapour.

Iodine is a relatively unspecific reagent which forms brown spots with many organic compounds, but especially with bases and lipids.

## SPECIAL METHODS

Many reagents used for the detection of particular amines or groups of amines interact with functions other than the amino group and will, therefore, be found in other sections. To avoid undue duplication only a few selected reagents which are less commonly used for the detection of other classes of compounds will be described here.

### ETHANOLAMINE

10 *Benzoquinone*

Spray with 0.5 g benzoquinone in 10 ml pyridine + 40 ml *n*-butanol. Ethanolamine gives a brown-red spot at room temperature. Serine reacts feebly at 100°C, choline not at all.

### CHOLINE

11 *Phosphomolybdic acid*

Spray with (*a*) 2% aq. phosphomolybdic acid. Wash the paper in a large vol. *n*-butanol for 5 min, then in running water. Dip in (*b*) freshly prepared 0.4% stannous chloride in 3M-HCl. Spots of choline phosphomolybdate are reduced to molybdenum blue. Sensitivity 5−10 μg. This method is also positive for sphingosine.

Modification for TLC: spray with (*a*) 1% phosphomolybdic acid in 1:1 mixture of ethanol−chloroform. Dry for 3 min. Then spray with (*b*) 1% stannous chloride in 3M-HCl. Dry for 10 min.

12 *Potassium ferrocyanide−cobalt chloride*

Spray with (*a*) 1% aq. $K_4\text{Fe(CN)}_6$. Then spray with (*b*) 0.5% aq. cobalt chloride. Choline gives a green spot. Sensitivity 10 μg. Suitable for TLC.

CHOLINE ESTERS

### 13 Hydroxylamine—ferric chloride

Hydroxylamine solution: (a) dissolve $20\,g$ $NH_2OH \cdot HCl$ in $50\,ml$ water and dilute to $200\,ml$ with 95% ethanol; (b) dissolve $50\,g$ KOH in minimum amount of water and dilute to $500\,ml$ with 95% ethanol. Mix 1 vol. of (a) with 2 vol. of (b) and filter from precipitated KCl. The mixture is stable for 2 weeks in the cold. It is best kept at $-10^{\circ}C$.

Ferric chloride solution: dissolve $10\,g$ of finely powdered $FeCl_3 \cdot 6H_2O$ in $20\,ml$ conc. HCl. Shake with $200\,ml$ ether until a homogeneous solution is formed.

Spray first with $NH_2OH$ solution, dry at room temp., then spray with $FeCl_3$-solution. Any organic ester gives a purple spot on a yellow ground. Sensitivity for carboxylic esters, $0.5-2\,\mu g$. Suitable for TLC.

GLUTARIMIDES, CARBAMATES, UREIDES

### 14 Sodium hypochlorite

Dilute a solution of NaOCl containing 10–13% available chlorine with 4 vol. water. Spray and dry paper in current of air for 1 hr to remove excess chlorine. Then spray with 2% starch solution containing 1% KI. Spots appear blue-black on colourless or pale blue background.

o-AMINOPHENOLS, INDOLES

### 15 Urorosein test

Expose damp paper to nitrous fumes generated in beaker from $NaNO_2$ and HCl. o-Aminophenols give yellow spots. The reaction is also positive for indoles.

o-, m-, AND p-AMINOPHENOLS

### 16 Ammoniacal silver nitrate

Spray with 1:1 mixture of $0.1\,M$-$AgNO_3$ and $5M$-$NH_3$, prepared immediately before use. Dark spots on light brown background.

### 17 Salicylaldehyde

Spray with 1% soln. of salicylaldehyde in ethanol containing 5% (v/v) acetic acid. Dry at room temp. Yellow fluorescent spots appear.

AROMATIC AMINES, SULPHONAMIDES

### 18 Coupling with diazonium salts

(i) *Diazotized sulphanilic acid: see* Amino acids, 12, for method. This reagent has been used for the detection of histamine, tyramine, tryptamine, and 5-hydroxytryptamine. Some phenols develop a colour after spraying with diazotized sulphanilic acid, whereas the majority do so only after a second spray with alkali.

(ii) *Diazotized p-nitroaniline.* To a stock solution of 0.2% p-nitroaniline in $1M$-HCl (5 ml) add $50\,ml$ $0.1M$-HCl, then $1\,ml$ 5% $NaNO_2$. When the solution has become colourless, leave in ice for a few minutes. Keep cold until ready to spray. Immediately afterwards spray with ice-cold 20% $K_2CO_3$. Metanephrine, normetanephrine, N-methylmetanephrine, tyramine, hordenine, give purple spots; p-sympatol and octopamine, red; 3-O-methyldopamine, olive; phenylethylamine and phenylethanolamine, crimson; 5-hydroxytryptamine, dark red. This spray has also been used for sulphonamides.

(iii) *Diazotized p-anisidine.* Mix equal volumes of 1% soln. of p-anisidine in ethanol containing $0.11M$-HCl and 10% (v/v) soln. of amyl nitrite in ethanol. Allow to stand for some minutes before spraying. Dry the paper in current of air. While still slightly damp expose it to $NH_3$ vapours or spray with ethanolic KOH.

Modification: replace half of the *p*-anisidine with sulphanilamide.

### 19 *Diazotization of amines on paper, followed by coupling reaction*

Spray with 0.2% $NaNO_2$ in 0.1M-HCl *or* 0.1% $NaNO_2$ in acetic acid containing 0.05 ml conc. HCl per 100 ml. (0.2% $NaNO_2$ in 10% trichloroacetic acid has been used before reagent vii). Wait 1—3 min, then spray with one of the following coupling reagents:

(i) *N-Ethyl-α-naphthylamine.* 0.2% soln. of *N*-ethyl-α-naphthylamine hydrochloride in ethanol. Aromatic amines give red-violet spots.

(ii) *N-(1-Naphthyl)ethylenediamine.* Spray with 5% ammonium sulphamate soln. to decompose excess nitrite. Then spray with 1% aq. soln. of *N*-(1-naphthyl)ethylenediamine hydrochloride. Spots: kynurenine purple, tryptophan yellow, 4-amino-imidazole-5-carboxamide magenta, creatinine orange, urocanic acid pale brown, 2-aminohippuric acid purple. Sulphonamides give intensely coloured compounds.

(iii) *Dimethyl-α-naphthylamine.* Spray with 1% aq. solution. This has been used for sulphonamides which give red or pink spots. Sensitivity 1 $\mu$g.

(iv) *Alkaline β-naphthol.* Spray with 1% soln. in M-NaOH. Aminophenols give red to red-violet spots. This spray has also been used for sulphonamides.

Modification for TLC: Spray with (*a*) 1% $NaNO_2$ in 1M-HCl. Then spray with (*b*) 0.2% β-naphthol in 1M-KOH. Dry at $60^{\circ}$C.

(v) *Phenol.* Spray with 1% phenol in M-NaOH. *o*-Aminobenzoic acid gives an orange colour; *m*- and *p*-aminobenzoic acids and sulphonamides give yellow spots.

(vi) *Hexylresorcinol.* Spray with 0.5% soln. in 2M-NaOH. Various colours are given by aromatic amines.

(vii) *1-Amino-8-naphthol-5:6-disulphonic acid.* Spray with 0.2% soln. Sulphonamides give red colours.

### INDOLEAMINES

### 20 *p-Dimethylaminobenzaldehyde (Ehrlich's reagent)*

Spray with 2% *p*-dimethylaminobenzaldehyde in either 1.3M-HCl or 6M-HCl.

With the weaker acid aromatic amines appear immediately, while indoles appear slowly. In the strongly acid solution indole colours appear rapidly, but the aromatic amines appear more gradually, as the excess HCl evaporates from the paper. Modifications:

(i) 2 g *p*-dimethylaminobenzaldehyde (or *p*-dimethylaminocinnamaldehyde) dissolved in 80 ml 95% ethanol + 20 ml conc. HCl.

(ii) 0.1% *p*-dimethylaminocinnamaldehyde in 1M-HCl. *p*-Dimethylaminocinnamaldehyde is more sensitive but less specific than *p*-dimethylaminobenzaldehyde. A purple, red, or blue spot appearing after spraying with Ehrlich's reagent is presumptive evidence for the presence of a substance with an indole or pyrrole ring. Urea, aromatic amines, sulphonamides, allantoin, xanthurenic, and urocanic acids give yellow to orange colours.

### 21 *Ninhydrin—acetic acid*

Dip paper in 0.25% solution of ninhydrin in acetone containing 10% (v/v) acetic acid. Heat for 2—3 min at $90-100^{\circ}$C.

Tryptamine and 5-hydroxytryptamine give blue-green fluorescent spots. Very sensitive test, capable of revealing 0.02 $\mu$g 5-HT.

### 22 *α-Nitroso-β-naphthol*

Spray with (*a*) 0.1% α-nitroso-β-naphthol in 95% ethanol. Dry and apply (*b*) 2.5% $NaNO_2$:2M-HCl = 4:100, mixed immediately before spraying. The reagent is specific for 5-hydroxyindoles, sensitivity 10—20 $\mu$g.

### 23 *Tetrazotized di-o-anisidine*

Dissolve 100 mg tetrazotized di-*o*-anisidine in 30 ml water. Immediately before spraying, add 20 ml borate buffer, pH 9.0. Hydroxyindoles and xanthurenic acid give blue colour; indoles, indoxyl, adrenochrome, and many aromatic amines do not react.

### 24 *Formaldehyde—HCl, for TLC*

Spray with freshly prepared mixture of 10 ml 35% formaldehyde soln., 10 ml 25% HCl and 20 ml ethanol. Dry at $100^\circ$C for 5 min. Indoles form yellow or green fluorescent spots. The sensitivity of the reaction (0.005—0.01 $\mu$g) is intensified by exposure to vapours of conc. HCl—conc. $HNO_3$, 3:1.

## CATECHOLAMINES

The tendency of catecholamines to undergo oxidation, particularly at a pH above 6, is the overriding consideration in their chromatography. Basic solvent systems have to be avoided for this reason. Phenol and *n*-butanol, with the addition of aqueous solutions of various acids, are the solvents most frequently used. Especially with phenol as solvent, the chromatograms are run in an atmosphere of $SO_2$, $CO_2$, or nitrogen and, as a further protection against oxidation, the paper may be treated with a dilute solution of ascorbic acid (50 mg per 100 ml) before use.

Catecholamines may form complexes or compounds with trichloroacetic acid or with lactic acid during the processing of tissue extracts and these may appear on the chromatogram as separate spots.

Acetylation of catecholamines prior to their separation on paper or by TLC has been recommended.

Methods for the detection of catecholamines on paper chromatograms fall into three groups: (1) those based on oxidation to coloured 'chromes' (e.g. adreno-chrome) or their decomposition products, (2) those based on the formation of fluorescent condensation products with formaldehyde or ethylenediamine, and (3) those based on reactions with the phenolic or amino-function of the molecule or simply on its reducing power. The reactions of the third group are generally less specific and sensitive, and since the reagents (ammoniacal silver nitrate, ferric chloride, diazonium salts, etc.) are described in other sections, they will not be considered here.

### 25 *Potassium ferricyanide*

Spray with 0.44% $K_3Fe(CN)_6$ in 0.2M-phosphate buffer, pH 7.8 or, when the chromatogram has been run in an acidic solvent, in 0.2M-$Na_2HPO_4$ soln. to give pH 8.3. Colours may be intensified by exposure to ammonia vapour. Adrenaline forms a pink spot turning yellow, noradrenaline a lavender spot turning brown, and dopamine a lavender spot. Limit of sensitivity about 2 $\mu$g. Smaller quantities may be detected by green fluorescence in u.v.

*N*-Methyladrenaline gives no colour when oxidized since no indole ring closure is possible, but the ferricyanide is bleached by reduction. The reduced ferrocyanide may be demonstrated by a drop of very dilute copper sulphate solution resulting in a red colour. The surrounding, unreduced ferricyanide turns brown.

Ferrocyanide formation may also be demonstrated by the Prussian blue reaction: spray with soln. containing 5 g ferric sulphate, anhyd., and 75 ml 85% $H_3PO_4$ per litre. This reaction, indicating merely the presence of a reducing compound, is less specific than the colour formation observed after the single ferricyanide spray.

### 26 *Exposure to ammonia vapour*

Adrenaline shows apple-green fluorescence in u.v. light. Sensitivity 10 $\mu$g.

### 27 *Exposure to vapours of iodine and ammonia*

Adrenaline and noradrenaline form brilliant red spots turning brown. Sensitivity, about 25 $\mu$g/3 cm$^2$.

### 28 *Iodine, for TLC*

Spray with solution of 0.5 g iodine in 100 ml chloroform and observe fluorescence in u.v. light. Sensitivity 0.005 $\mu$g.

### 29 *Potassium iodate*

Spray with 1% aq. KIO$_3$. Heat at 100–110°C for not more than 2 min. Like the two preceding ones this test is based on the formation of iodo-chromes. Adrenaline (1 $\mu$g) gives a pink spot, turning brown, noradrenaline (2 $\mu$g) a violet spot, turning brown, dopamine an orange-brown spot. Isopropyl noradrenaline red, epinine orange.

### 30 *Ferricyanide–formaldehyde*

Spray with a freshly prepared mixture of 0.66% K$_3$Fe(CN)$_6$ and 40% formaldehyde (9:1), and heat at 100°C for 5 min. In a modification the K$_3$Fe(CN)$_6$–formaldehyde solution is made up in 0.6M-phosphate buffer, pH 5.9.

Adrenaline, noradrenaline, dopamine, isopropyl noradrenaline, and epinine give red to purple spots (sensitivity 1–2 $\mu$g) which show yellow-green fluorescence in u.v. light (sensitivity 0.2 $\mu$g).

### 31 *Ferricyanide or iodine, followed by Ehrlich's reagent*

Following oxidation of catecholamines to indoles, blue pigments are formed by reaction with Ehrlich's reagent.

First spray: 0.2% K$_3$Fe(CN)$_6$ in water or 0.0005M-iodine in 0.2M-acetate buffer pH 6 or 0.005M-iodine in 0.6M-phosphate buffer, pH 5.9. Dry in current of cold air for 3–5 min.

Second spray: 4 g *p*-dimethylaminobenzaldehyde in 380 ml ethanol + 80 ml conc. HCl. Detects 0.2 $\mu$g adrenaline or noradrenaline.

### 32 *Ethylenediamine–ammonia*

Spray with 2:8 mixture of redist. ethylenediamine and 2M-ammonia or 10% (w/v) ammonia. Catecholamines, as well as other catechol derivatives, give yellow to brown spots showing brilliant yellow fluorescence in u.v. light. Sensitivity 0.1 $\mu$g adrenaline.

### 33 *Ferricyanide or iodine–ethylenediamine*

This combination is intended to accelerate the oxidative step preceding the condensation with ethylenediamine and thereby minimize side reactions.

Spray with solution of 0.1% K$_3$Fe(CN)$_6$ or 0.05M-I$_2$, both in 5% (v/v) aq. ethylenediamine. Dry for 5 min at 50°C.

Dip reagents: Dip in 1% solution of iodine in carbon tetrachloride, blot and before the paper is completely dry, dip in 1% solution of ethylenediamine in *iso*propanol. Blot and dry at RT for 24 hr. Detects 0.05 $\mu$g of catecholamines.

CATECHOLAMINE TRIACETATES

### 34 *Ferric chloride–potassium ferricyanide*

Spray with (*a*) 10% KOH in methanol–water (1:1). Then spray with (*b*) freshly prepared mixture of 1% FeCl$_3$ and 2% K$_3$Fe(CN)$_6$.

35 *Blue tetrazolium reagent*

Spray with (*a*) 10% KOH in methanol–water (1:1). Then spray with (*b*) 0.2% aq. soln. of triphenyltetrazolium chloride.

36 *TLC of catecholamine triacetates*

Spray with 40% $H_3PO_4$. Heat for 7 min at $110^\circ C$. Then spray with 5% phosphomolybdic acid in ethanol and heat for 2 min at $110^\circ C$.

Alternative method: dissolve 3 g vanillin in 100 ml abs. ethanol and add dropwise 3 ml conc. $H_2SO_4$. Spray and heat plate at $110^\circ C$ for 7 min.

---

# 4 AMINO ACIDS AND PEPTIDES

Amino acids and peptides can readily be separated on paper or cellulose-type thin layers using small amounts of material. Table 20.I gives examples of the types of solvents or buffer for ionophoresis which can be used and the separation of the amino acids achieved in one-dimensional runs. Ambiguities can often be resolved by a second run at right-angles or ionophoresis at a different pH.

*Detection*

Some of the general reagents for amino acids are non-destructive and allow the subsequent estimation or re-running of the spots concerned.

In the methods below, dipping is to be preferred to spraying as it gives a more even result. However the treatments are often interchangeable although dipping cannot be applied where the substances on the paper are soluble in the reagents—for example, when the latter are aqueous solutions.

GENERAL REAGENTS

1 *Ninhydrin*

(i) For general use as a locating agent use 0.25% w/v ninhydrin in acetone. The spots may be developed by heating at $100^\circ C$ for 5 min, or for a lighter background, by leaving at room temperature for a few hours. The amino acids give purple spots except for histidine and glycine (red-grey); phenylalanine, tyrosine, and aspartic acid (blue); tryptophan (brown); asparagine (dirty yellow); proline (yellow). The sensitivity ranges from 0.2 $\mu$g for glycine to about 2 $\mu$g for histidine.

(ii) For identification by colour use 50 ml of 0.1% ninhydrin in ethanol plus 2 ml collidine. Some workers add 10 ml $CH_3COOH$. The less pure the collidine the better the colours. Heat, observing the colours as they come up. The colours given by each amino acid are best learnt by experience, but note particularly that tyrosine changes colour a few seconds after it comes up and that many of the colours fade within a few minutes to purple and blue.

(iii) Some workers prefer a modification of 1 (ii) incorporating copper ion. It is claimed that the colour differences are such as to enable identification of all amino acids.

The reagent consists of (*a*) 0.2% ninhydrin in 50 ml ethanol + 10 ml of glacial acetic acid + 2 ml of collidine. (*b*) 1% $Cu(NO_3)_2 \cdot 3H_2O$. A fresh mixture of 25 ml of (*a*) and 1.5 ml of (*b*) is sprayed onto the paper which is dried and heated for 1.5 to 2 min at $105^\circ C$. This reagent has been used on thin layer plates. The plates are dried, the reagent is sprayed on and the plates are reheated so that the colours may be seen as they come up.

(iv) For the detection of *N*-methyl amino acids (which normally give a very weak colour with ninhydrin) in the presence of free amino acids use the following reagent.

Table 20.I    *Separation of amino acids by paper chromatography and ionophoresis*

| Amino acid | *n-Butanol* 12 *acetic acid* 3 $H_2O$ 5 $R_F$ | *Phenol saturated with* $H_2O$ $R_F$ | *Phenol sat.* $H_2O$ 15 *ethanol* 4 $H_2O$ 1 $R_F$ | *n-Butanol* 1 *pyridine* 1 $H_2O$ 1 $R_F$ | *Electrophoresis in 8% aqueous formic acid pH 1.6; mobility towards cathode in cm (45 min, 40 V/cm)* |
|---|---|---|---|---|---|
| γ-aminobutyric acid | 0.40 | 0.78 | 0.56 | 0.26 | 59 |
| alanine | 0.30 | 0.58 | 0.41 | 0.37 | 47 |
| asparagine | 0.12 | 0.40 | 0.22 | 0.20 | 35 |
| aspartic acid | 0.23 | 0.20 | 0.06 | 0.20 | 26 |
| arginine | 0.15 | 0.83 | 0.66 | 0.15 | 59 |
| cysteine | 0.08 | 0.22 | 0.05 | 0.14 | – |
| cysteic acid | 0.07 | 0.06 | 0.05 | 0.26 | 1 |
| cystine | 0.05 | 0.15 | 0.16 | 0.15 | 36 |
| ethanolamine | 0.38 | 0.72 | 0.83 | 0.43 | 73 |
| glutamine | 0.17 | 0.27 | 0.29 | 0.23 | 33 |
| glutamic acid | 0.28 | 0.33 | 0.12 | 0.20 | 33 |
| glycine | 0.23 | 0.42 | 0.26 | 0.29 | 53 |
| histidine | 0.11 | 0.65 | 0.50 | 0.24 | 58 |
| hydroxyproline | 0.22 | 0.67 | 0.44 | 0.30 | 31 |
| leucine | 0.70 | 0.85 | 0.73 | 0.60 | 36 |
| isoleucine | 0.67 | 0.85 | 0.71 | 0.56 | 36 |
| lysine | 0.12 | 0.42 | 0.57 | 0.13 | 64 |
| methionine | 0.50 | 0.82 | 0.62 | 0.53 | 36 |
| methionine sulphone | 0.22 | 0.60 | 0.55 | 0.31 | – |
| phenylalanine | 0.60 | 0.84 | 0.72 | 0.63 | 33 |
| proline | 0.34 | 0.90 | 0.75 | 0.34 | 40 |
| serine | 0.22 | 0.35 | 0.22 | 0.33 | 41 |
| taurine | 0.20 | 0.35 | 0.28 | 0.38 | 8 |
| threonine | 0.26 | 0.48 | 0.33 | 0.36 | 38 |
| tyrosine | 0.45 | 0.60 | 0.43 | 0.60 | 30 |
| tryptophan | 0.50 | 0.77 | 0.58 | 0.62 | 25 |
| valine | 0.51 | 0.78 | 0.62 | 0.48 | 39 |

Mix equal vols. of 0.33% ninhydrin in *tert*-butanol and glacial acetic–water–pyridine (1:5:5). Spray, and heat for 10–15 min at 100–10°C. Primary and *N*-methyl amino acids give purple spots of comparable intensity. *N*-methyl amino acids are distinguished by their feeble colour on spraying with ninhydrin in water saturated *n*-butanol, 2% with respect to acetic acid.

Ninhydrin stained papers fade on exposure to air and light. A permanent record may be made by respraying with a $Cu(NO_3)_2$ reagent. To 1 ml of saturated solution of $Cu(NO_3)_2$ add 0.2 ml of 10% $HNO_3$ and make up to 100 ml in 95% ethanol. It is best to varnish the papers by dipping in a saturated solution of perspex in chloroform.

## 2 Fluorescamine

This reagent reacts with primary amino groups in amino acids and peptides. Spray with 0.05% fluorescamine in acetone and observe fluorescing spots. A preliminary and following spray of the chromatogram with 10% triethylamine in methylene chloride improves the sensitivity and stability of the fluorescent spots produced (1 nmole). Proline and hydroxyproline spots appear slowly on heating at 110°C for 3 hr or after 2 days at room temperature. Alternatively, wet the fluorescamine-treated paper or plate successively with 0.1M-acetic acid in acetone and 0.1M *N*-chlorosuccinimide in acetone. Stand 5 min, wash with acetone and heat for 5–10 min at 110°C.

### 3 *Isatin*

*See also* proline and hydroxyproline, Amino acids, 22.

One disadvantage of ninhydrin is the ease with which proline can be masked by other spots. Two reagents have been described which overcome this difficulty, and also provide a range of colours for the amino acids.

(i) Dissolve 1 g isatin + 1.3 g zinc acetate in 70–80 ml warm *iso*propanol. After cooling add 1 ml pyridine.

(ii) Dissolve 1 g isatin + 1.5 g zinc acetate in 93 ml warm *iso*propanol + 3 ml of water. Add 1 ml of glacial acetic acid on cooling.

The two reagents give slightly different ranges of colour. With both reagents spray, dry, and heat at 80–85°C for 10 min. The background may be washed out by a quick rinse in water without displacing the amino acid colours.

### 4 *Ultraviolet light*

(i) The amino group can react with free aldehyde groups in the paper. The resulting Schiff's bases fluoresce blue in u.v. light. Heat the paper at 100°C for 30 min. *N*-substituted amino acids give dark spots. The sensitivity is somewhat lower than ninhydrin, and some of the amino acid may be destroyed.

(ii) Spray with 0.2% salicylaldehyde in acetone. The Schiff's bases may be decomposed by spraying with water and exposure to air.

(iii) Soak the paper in 0.01% 1:2-naphthoquinone-4-sulphonate (Folin's reagent) in methanol. Heat at 110°C–120°C for 10 min.

### 5 *Iodine*

A non-destructive but non-specific method. The paper, or thin layer plate, is exposed to $I_2$ vapour produced by a few crystals in a glass tank. After 10–30 sec it is removed and the rapidly fading brown spots marked with pencil. Alternatively, the paper may be sprayed with petroleum ether (60–80°C fraction) saturated with $I_2$.

### 6 *Chlorine*

Useful for amino acids, N blocked amino acids (q.v.) and peptides (q.v.). The test is said to be specific for the N–C bond and so solvents such as pyridine and collidine must be removed. The paper or thin layer plate is washed with ether and then acetone–ethanol, 1:1, in which amino acids and most peptides are insoluble. Expose for 5 min to $Cl_2$ from a tray containing equal volumes of satd. $KMnO_4$ and 10% HCl. Remove, allow excess $Cl_2$ to disappear and dip in a solution of equal volumes saturated *o*-tolidine* in 2% acetic acid and 0.05M-KI. Blue-black spots are given on a lighter background. It is claimed that background colour is reduced if the chlorinated paper is exposed to ammonia vapour for 10 sec before dipping.

*N*-chloro derivatives can also be formed by spraying with 1% *t*-butylhypochlorite (*Org. Syn.* **32**, 1–20) in cyclohexane followed by spraying with 1% starch in 1% KI. The sensitivity to amino acids varies. Methionine, cysteine, cystine, and tyrosine are scarcely detected at all.

* Warning: *o*-tolidine has been listed as carcinogenic. The 1% starch–1% KI mixture may be used in its place with only slightly inferior results.

## D-AMINO ACIDS

### 7 D-*Amino acid oxidase (to distinguish between* D- *and* L-*amino acids)*

Run two duplicate papers. Spray one with a solution of D-amino acid oxidase in 0.06 M-pyrophosphate buffer, pH 8.3. Incubate for $2\frac{1}{2}$ hr at 37°C in moist oxygen. Dry and spray both papers with ninhydrin. Only L-amino acids and glycine will remain on the treated paper. Alternatively the α-keto acids (q.v.) formed from the D-amino acids may be detected by the use of a 2:4-dinitrophenylhydrazine spray.

## SPECIFIC REAGENTS

Where, for some reason, it has not been possible to identify a spot by position and colour with one of the general tests, reagents exist which are specific for single amino acids or groups of amino acids.

### TYROSINE

#### 8 α-Nitroso-β-naphthol

Dip in (a) 0.1% α-nitroso-β-naphthol in acetone. Dry at room temperature. Dip in (b) acetone to which has been added 10% by volume conc. $HNO_3$. Allow to dry and heat progressively from one edge in a position where the paper can be seen. The yellow colour of the paper lightens when any area has been heated sufficiently. Tyrosine is indicated by a red colour, with a sensitivity of the order of 1 μg. Tryptophan gives a grey or brown colour with less sensitivity. Phenol and collidine should be removed by washing with acetone—diethyl ether, 1:1. Tyrosine is also detected in the Pauly test (see Histidine, 12).

### TRYPTOPHAN AND RELATED COMPOUNDS

#### 9 Ehrlich's reagent

(i) Dip in 1% w/v p-dimethylaminobenzaldehyde in acetone—conc. HCl (9:1). Stand at room temperature for a few minutes. Tryptophan gives a purple spot, pyrroles and related compounds give red spots.

(ii) Alternatively, spray with 2% p-dimethylaminobenzaldehyde in 5% HCl. Dry at room temperature. Tryptophan gives a purple colour, aromatic amines and citrulline yellow; hydroxykynurenine, kynurenine, and 2-amino-3-hydroxyacetophenone give orange spots.

#### 10 Ultraviolet light

(i) Dry the paper at room temperature. Examine under u.v. Tryptophan gives little or no colour (what little there is is due to decomposition products and is usually slightly ahead of the true spot). Some related compounds due to interaction with the paper are readily seen, for example, kynurenine (blue); kynurenic acid (blue-green); hydroxykynurenic acid (greenish-yellow); aminoacetophenone (sky-blue); 2-amino-3-hydroxyacetophenone (yellow); xanthurenic acid (blue); anthranilic acid (blue-violet); hydroxyanthranilic acid (sky-blue). Aromatic solvents sometimes interfere.

(ii) Spray with perchloric acid (70–72%)–water (6:1).* Tryptophan gives a stable and intense green-blue fluorescence within 10 min. Subsequent spraying with 1% $FeCl_3$ gives a reddish-yellow colour. Indoleacetic acid responds to this test with a faint pinkish fluorescence.

#### 11 Acid terephthalaldehyde

Spray with 0.2% terephthalaldehyde in acetone, 10% with respect to acetic acid. Heat at 105°C for 3 min. Tryptophan gives a blue spot, tryptamine yellow-green. This reagent is extremely sensitive (see also Histidine, 13).

### HISTIDINE

#### 12 Pauly reagent

Solution I (1% sulphanilic acid in M-HCl) and solution II (5% $NaNO_2$ aq.) are kept in the refrigerator. Equal volumes are mixed, still being kept cold, 5 min. before

*Inflammable and potentially explosive!

use. Spray, taking care not to displace the spots by flooding the paper. Then spray with 15% $Na_2CO_3$. Histidine and other imidazoles give red colours at once. Coloured spots are also given with reduced sensitivity by histamine (rose-brown); tyrosine (rose); xanthine, diiodotyrosine (orange); thiamin, tryptophan, hordenine, hydroxy-kynurenine (orange-red); adenine (pink); guanine (orange-purple); catechol (purple); ergothionine (red); thiolhistidine (light orange). A modification reduces interference by tyrosine. Spray with 0.1% $p$-anisidine in ethanolic 0.11M-HCl— 10% ethanolic amyl nitrite (1:1). Dry in air at RT. Spray with 1% KOH in ethanol. Recryst. $p$-anisidine may not work.

Residual solvents such as phenol and collidine must be washed out with acetone and ether.

### 13 *Terephthalaldehyde*

Spray with 0.2% terephthalaldehyde in acetone. Heat at $105°C$ for 10 min. Histidine gives a yellow-green spot. Tryptophan gives a brown spot in the u.v. The reagent is very sensitive, especially for histidine.

### PHENYLALANINE

### 14 *Ninhydrin*—$NaHCO_3$

Stain the chromatogram with ninhydrin (1 (i)). On spraying the heated paper with dilute (0.15 to 10%) $NaHCO_3$, only the phenylalanine spot is stable.

### SULPHUR-CONTAINING AMINO ACIDS

### 15 *Platinic iodide*

(i) Dip in 0.002M-chloroplatinic acid—M-KI—2M-HCl—acetone (4:0.25:0.4:76). Intensify with HCl vapour after drying at room temperature. Bleached areas on a pink ground are given by cystine, cysteine, methionine, cystathionine, lanthionine, djenkolic acid, methionine sulphoxide, etc. After using a phenol or collidine solvent papers must first be washed in acetone—ether (1:1).

(ii) For greater contrast (the background is dark brown) replace the 0.002M $H_2PtCl_6$ solution in (i) with 0.002M-$PdCl_2$ in 0.1M-HCl.

### 16 *Azide*—*iodine*

Spray with 0.025M-$I_2$ in 50% ethanol containing 1.5% $NaN_3$. White spots on a light brown ground are given by cysteine immediately, then cystine (15 min), then methionine (60 min). The spots are best seen in u.v. This spray also detects thiamin.

### 17 *Nitroprusside*

Reagent (*a*): mix together 1.5 g Na nitroprusside in 5 ml M-$H_2SO_4$ + 95 ml MeOH + 10 ml 28% $NH_3$. Filter. Dip in this soln. Red colours are given with —SH compounds. While the paper is still damp dip in (*b*) 2% NaCN in 95% MeOH. The cleavage of —S—S— bonds by this reagent causes red colours to appear in a few seconds to 10 min. Sensitivity for cystine, 1 $\mu$g. If the detection of —SH compounds is not required use an equal vol. of (*a*) and (*b*) made up in double concentrations. Arginine gives an orange spot on a pale yellow ground, turning grey-blue on an intense green ground.

### GLYCINE

### 18 *o-Phthalaldehyde*

Spray with 0.2% *o*-phthalaldehyde in acetone. Heat at $50°C$ for 10 min. A green spot is given with glycine, chocolate brown in u.v. (at 365 nm); $NH_4^+$ ion gives a dark grey spot; histidine and tryptophan show intense yellow fluorescence at

365 nm. This spray cannot be used after aromatic solvents.

### ARGININE

#### 19 *Sakaguchi*

Dip in 0.1% 8-hydroxyquinoline in acetone. Dry in air. Spray carefully with a soln. of 0.2 ml $Br_2$ in 100 ml 0.5M-NaOH. Orange-red spots are given by arginine and other guanidines. Taurocyamine and glycocyamine give only transient colours.

### GUANIDINES

#### 20 *α-Naphthol–diacetyl*

Spray with 0.1 ml diacetyl + 15 ml 1% α-naphthol in 6% NaOH, freshly mixed. Let stand for 2–10 min. Blue-violet spots on a beige ground are given by guanidine, its disubstituted derivatives (e.g. creatine), and monosubstituted derivatives (e.g. arginine, glycocyamine) with less sensitivity. Creatinine does not react.

### ORNITHINE

#### 21 *Vanillin*

Spray with 0.2% vanillin in acetone followed by 0.1% KOH in ethanol. Heat at 110°C for 10 min. Ornithine gives a red spot, as do proline and hydroxyproline.

### IMINO ACIDS (*proline and hydroxyproline*)

#### 22 *Isatin*

(i) Spray with 0.2% isatin in *n*-butanol, 4% with respect to acetic acid. Heat at 105°C for 15 min. Stable spots are given by proline and hydroxyproline (blue) and pipecolinic acid (blue-green). Many amino acids give colours in this range which fade after a few hours at room temperature.

To obtain only the blue spots of proline and hydroxyproline, wash the paper, after developing, in M-HCl and then in water.

(ii) To distinguish between proline and hydroxyproline, dip as above and then in Ehrlich's reagent (*see* 9). All the colours given by isatin are removed except that of hydroxyproline which turns from blue to cerise.

### MULTIPLE SPRAYING

Ninhydrin (1 (i)) may be followed by α-nitroso-β-naphthol (8) or Ehrlich's reagent (9). It may also be followed, with diminished sensitivity, by the Pauly test (12) or the Sakaguchi (19). Isatin may be preceded by ninhydrin or followed by Ehrlich's reagent or α-nitroso-β-naphthol, the latter with diminished sensitivity. Ehrlich's reagent may be followed by the Sakaguchi even if it was preceded by ninhydrin or isatin. Ultra-violet and iodine do not interfere with any subsequent test.

## AMINO ACID DERIVATIVES

### DNP-AMINO ACIDS

#### 1 *Visual inspection*

Quite small quantities of these compounds can be seen by their yellow colour. They may be distinguished from the common artefact dinitrophenol by inspection in the u.v. (dinitrophenol appears much more black than any other spot).

### PHENYLTHIOHYDANTOINS AND HYDANTOINS

#### 2 *Iodine–azide*

Before running the chromatogram, dip the paper in 0.5% starch solution and dry. After running, dry at room temp. and spray with a mixture of equal volumes of

0.01M-I$_2$ in 0.5M-KI and 0.5M-sodium azide. Phenylthiohydantoins and hydantoins give bleached areas on a dark ground.

### 'DANSYL' AMINO ACIDS

#### 3 *Ultraviolet light*

'Dansyl' amino acids in extremely small amounts can be seen as yellow spots in u.v. light. Dansyl-OH gives a blue-green spot.

### PEPTIDES

#### *Separation*

Electrophoresis is to be preferred to chromatography as it gives sharper spots and is less dependent on changes in conditions. Several pHs are used, including pH 1.9 (basic groups fully ionized, nearly all carboxyls completely suppressed, the sulphonic acid group partly charged); pH 3.5 (the terminal carboxyl group and the carboxyls of aspartic and glutamic acids are discharged to an extent depending on neighbouring groups); pH 6.5 (all carboxyls fully charged save in exceptional cases, most $\alpha$-NH$_2$ groups fully charged, basic side chains fully charged except that of histidine, which is charged to an extent depending upon neighbouring groups). The most generally used chromatographic systems are butanol—acetic acid—water (3:1:1 for most applications, 4:1:5 gives better separation for basic peptides but is more troublesome).

It is often valuable to combine electrophoretic with chromatographic separations. For preparative work electrophoresis should be used last in order to sharpen up the bands, and to avoid the risk of the partial destruction of some amino acids during acid hydrolysis after elution from the paper.

#### *Detection*

#### 1 *Ninhydrin*

Method 1 (i), (*see* Amino acids) is recommended. Heating is to be avoided if possible. Some peptides, particularly large, cyclic, or acetylated ones, give poor colour yields. Most glycine and some asparagine N-terminal peptides give yellow colours. Valine and isoleucine N-terminal peptides are slow to come up and sometimes give a low colour yield. Proline N-terminal peptides give a very faint yellow colour which is usually missed.

#### 2 *Ultraviolet light*

*See* Amino acids, 4.

Ultraviolet methods can be used for peptides with free amino groups. Heating is to be avoided, as some peptides cannot then be eluted in good yield. Spraying with fluorescamine (Amino acids 2) allows a very sensitive location of peptides with free amino groups under u.v.

#### 3 *Iodine*

*See* Amino acids, 5

#### 4 *Chlorine*

*See* Amino acids, 6.

This method is of especial value for those peptides which do not give good ninhydrin colours. The intensity of colour given is roughly proportional to the number of peptide bonds although sometimes the sensitivity may vary widely from that expected. Peptides largely consisting of those amino acids not detected will themselves often not be detected.

### 5 Phenylisothiocyanate

Spray with pyridine−water−triethylamine−phenylisothiocyanate (150:50:6:2) and leave in an atmosphere of the same mixture for 3 hr to allow conversion of peptides to phenylthiocarbamyl derivatives. Wash three times with benzene,* twice with ethylene chloride. Dry 30 min at RT. Locate spots with u.v. light by the use of a fluorescent screen. Prewashing of papers is necessary before running chromatograms.

   * **Warning**: Vapour is extremely toxic.

### 6 More specific reagents for peptides

Some of the specific reagents for amino acids will show the presence of the amino acid concerned in a peptide. The remarks above about multiple staining apply equally to the use of these reagents for peptides. The numbers given below are those of the reagent in the section on amino acids.

   Tyrosine peptides will be detected by α-nitroso-β-naphthol (8); tryptophan peptides are detected by the Ehrlich's reagent (9); histidine by the Pauly (12) (N-terminal histidine in a peptide gives a more brown colour than the usual pink); sulphur-containing peptides by platinic iodide (15); arginine by the Sakaguchi (19); proline and hydroxyproline, if N-terminal, by isatin (22).

---

# 5 CARBOHYDRATES

Sugars are commonly separated by chromatography on cellulose (paper sheets or thin layer), less frequently on silica gel (either in the free form or as the sugar acetates).

   Although a wide variety of solvents have been used, Table 20.2 gives an indication of three useful solvents and the separations achieved. Identity of sugar should only be assumed after its running behaviour in several solvents and reaction to various sprays have been established.

### GENERAL METHODS

### 1 Silver nitrate−sodium hydroxide

Dip in $AgNO_3$ (0.1 ml saturated aq. soln. diluted to 20 ml with acetone and water added dropwise until $AgNO_3$ redissolves), dry, and spray with 0.5M-NaOH in aq. EtOH (made by diluting saturated aq. NaOH with EtOH). Reducing substances appear immediately, at RT, as black spots (sensitivity, $1-2\,\mu g$), and non-reducing substances (including non-reducing oligosaccharides, methyl glycosides, hexitols, and glycerol; sensitivity, $2-10\,\mu g$) appear more slowly. Sugar acetates can be detected if they are saponified by a prior exposure to diethylaminomethanol vapour. Better control and differentiation of reducing and non-reducing substances are obtained by using the above $AgNO_3$ solution at half-strength, when reducing substances appear in under 1 min and non-reducing compounds in $5-10$ min. Papers may be fixed by dipping in strong aq. $NH_3$, washing well in water, and drying. This spray has largely replaced the older *Ammoniacal silver nitrate* (spray with $0.1M-AgNO_3:5M-NH_3 = 1:1$, heat at $105°C$ for $5-10$ min) which gives similar reactions with reducing and non-reducing carbohydrates. A spray used for locating sugar derivatives on thin-layer chromatograms consists of a 5:1:2 freshly prepared mixture of (a) 0.3% $AgNO_3$ in methanol, (b) methanol saturated with $NH_3$, (c) 7% solution of sodium in methanol. The plate is dipped or sprayed when reducing and non-reducing carbohydrates and their acyl derivatives produce brown, yellowish-brown or greenish spots on a beige background.

**Table 20.2**  *Paper chromatographic behaviour of some sugars  in three useful solvents*

Descending chromatography. Values are compared to the running of glucose = 1.0.

| | isopropanol 4<br>Water          1 | Ethyl acetate 12<br>Pyridine          5<br>Water          4 | n-Propanol          7<br>Ethyl acetate 1<br>Water          2 |
|---|---|---|---|
| Arabinose | 1.12 | 1.32 | 1.17 |
| Cellobiose | 0.45 | 0.61 | 0.50 |
| Deoxyglucose | 1.46 | — | — |
| Deoxyribose | 1.50 | 2.02 | 1.94 |
| Dulcitol | 1.05 | 0.86 | 1.02 |
| Fructose | 1.05 | 1.18 | 1.09 |
| Fucose | 1.35 | 1.46 | 1.28 |
| Galactose | 0.90 | 0.86 | 0.91 |
| Galacturonic acid | 0.15 | 0.14 | — |
| Glucuronic acid | 0.20 | 0.14 | 0.23 |
| Glucose | 1.00 | 1.00 | 1.00 |
| Inositol | 0.35 | 0.32 | 0.34 |
| Lactose | 0.32 | 0.47 | 0.41 |
| Maltose | 0.47 | 0.63 | 0.56 |
| Mannitol | 1.10 | 0.92 | 1.02 |
| Mannose | 1.05 | 1.20 | 1.06 |
| Melibiose | 0.35 | 0.42 | 0.39 |
| Raffinose | 0.30 | 0.37 | 0.33 |
| Rhamnose | 1.52 | 1.72 | 1.78 |
| Ribose | 1.37 | 1.89 | 1.42 |
| Ribulose | 1.42 | 2.00 | 1.52 |
| Sorbitol | 1.05 | 0.86 | 0.98 |
| Sorbose | 1.02 | 1.20 | 1.03 |
| Xylose | 1.30 | 1.58 | 1.28 |
| Xylulose | 1.55 | 2.14 | 1.58 |

### 2 Alkaline potassium permanganate

Spray with 1% aq. $KMnO_4$ containing 2% $Na_2CO_3$. Dry at RT or rapidly at $100°C$. Yellow spots on a purple ground, then grey spots on a brown ground are given by sugar alcohols, glycosides, reducing and non-reducing sugars. Not given by methyl or acetyl sugars.

### 3 Periodate–potassium permanganate; periodate–p-anisidine

(*a*) Spray with 2% aq. Na metaperiodate:1% $KMnO_4$ in 2% aq. $Na_2CO_3$ = 4:1, freshly mixed. Wash in $H_2O$ after the spots develop. Brown spots on a white ground are produced. Sensitivity for glucose, $3\,\mu g$; mannitol, 3-methylglucose, $5-8\,\mu g$; substances which reduce periodate only slowly, e.g. sucrose and trehalose, need $10-15\,\mu g$, and 40–60 min may be necessary for the colour to appear.

(*b*) Spray with 0.01M-Na metaperiodate, and after 2 min spray with 1% *p*-anisidine HCl in BuOH. White spots appear on a pink ground with polyols or any substance reacting with periodate. Sensitivity $25\,\mu g$.

### 4 Iodine

Expose for 15 min to $I_2$ vapour. Brown spots are given by sugar mercaptals and alcohols, glycosides, hexonic acids, N-acylamino sugars, neutral and acidic poly-saccharides. Do not use this method after solvents containing pyridine, collidine, or other N-compounds.

### 5 p-Aminodimethylaniline

Spray with a 0.3% soln. of the $ZnCl_2$ double salt of p-aminodimethylaniline in EtOH. General reagent for reducing and non-reducing mono- and oligo-saccharides giving various colours.

### 6 Ultraviolet light

Bright yellow fluorescence is shown by tetroses in u.v. light.

## REDUCING SUGARS

### 7 p-Anisidine

3% p-anisidine hydrochloride in $BuOH-EtOH-H_2O$ (4:1:1) plus a trace of $SnCl_2$. Spray and heat at $100-110°C$ for 3–5 min. Aldohexoses and methylpentoses, green to brown; ketohexoses, brilliant lemon yellow; uronic acids, red-brown; pentoses, cherry red; methylated aldohexoses, brown; methylated aldopentoses, intense red. Sensitivity $1-5\,\mu g$. Reducing oligosaccharides react as their reducing unit. Non-reducing substances, except acid-labile oligosaccharides such as sucrose and raffinose, do not react. p-Anisidine phosphate (0.5 g p-anisidine in 2 ml $H_3PO_4$ (Sp. G. 1.75) + EtOH to 50 ml) may also be used to give essentially similar reactions. Also used in conjunction with u.v. to detect sugar sulphates.

### 8 Aniline–diphenylamine

Reagent: aniline (4 g), diphenylamine (4 g), and syrupy $H_3PO_4$ (20 ml) in EtOH or acetone (200 ml), freshly prepared. Spray or dip (acetone) and heat for 5 min at $60-65°C$ (pentoses) or $80°C$ (all other sugars). Aldohexoses, grey to brown; ketoses, yellow-brown; methyl pentoses, orange; aldoheptoses, bright purple; uronic acids, bright red brown; pentoses, green-blue. A split version of the reagent can also distinguish between fructose and sorbose. In this, one reagent contains diphenylamine (4 g) phosphoric acid (20 ml) and acetone (200 ml) while the second has aniline (4 ml) substituted for the diphenylamine. Spraying in succession with either reagent first, with drying and heating after each spray, produces characteristic colours. Oligosaccharides give similar colours except those containing a 1→4 linked reducing aldohexose (maltose), bright blue or 1→2 linked reducing aldohexose (sophorose), orange.

### 9 Triphenyltetrazolium chloride (TTC)

Spray with 2% aq. TTC:M-NaOH = 1:1, freshly mixed. Heat at $40°C$ in a damp atmosphere for 20 min. Red spots on a white-pink ground are given by reducing sugars, especially fructose and xylose ($5\,\mu g$). Reducing oligosaccharides also react except those with a 2-substituted reducing aldohexose or 1-substituted reducing fructofuranose. Alternatively, 0.5% TTC in $CHCl_3$ can be used with the dipping technique followed by a spray with alcoholic NaOH (0.5M).

### 10 Benzidine*

Spray with 0.5 g benzidine in 20 ml glacial $CH_3COOH$ + 80 ml EtOH. Heat at $100-5°C$ for 15 min. Pentoses give chocolate brown spots in 5 min; lactose, maltose, galactose, glucose, fructose, dark brown spots in 10 min. Sensitivity $5\,\mu g$. Ascorbic acid gives a pale brown spot after 10 min. Sensitivity $10\,\mu g$. Inositol, and other polyols, sucrose, and raffinose do not react. Sensitivity and specificity are extended if the chromatogram is further sprayed with either HCl (0.3M) or phosphoric acid (0.3M) in 95% ethanol followed by heating for 15 min at $70°C$.

A modification giving brown spots with $1\,\mu g$ glucose (free or combined) is a spray containing 0.5 g benzidine in 10 ml $CH_3COOH$ + 10 ml 40% aq. trichloroacetic acid + 80 ml EtOH. Yellow colours are given with free or combined fructose but the reaction is much less sensitive than with glucose. Disaccharides with an aminosugar reducing unit give different colours depending on the position of the glycosidic link.

  * **Warning**: Benzidine is carcinogenic

### 11  *p-Anisidine–diphenylamine*

Mix equal vols. of 2% diphenylamine and 2% *p*-anisidine, each in acetone containing 10% (v/v) conc. $H_3PO_4$, shake well, spray, and heat 2–3 min at 90–95°C. Aldopentoses and aldohexoses, green to blue-green; methylpentoses, pale yellow; uronic acids, red-brown. ketohexoses, yellow-brown; ketoheptoses, bright red-brown. Disaccharides with a reducing aldose unit give similar colours but those with a reducing ketose unit give different colours according to the position of the glycosidic link.

### 12  *Acid potassium permanganate*

Spray with 0.03 to 0.15M-$KMnO_4$ containing 3% $H_2SO_4$. Organic compounds give white or light yellow spots. If this spray is applied after aniline oxalate (which gives brown spots with fructose, glucose, and maltose (*see* 22)), and the paper heated at 90°C, the paper loses its background colour, fructose, sucrose, and melizitose turn grey-black, and glucose and maltose remain brown.

### 13  *p-Aminophenol*

Reagent: 0.5 g *p*-aminophenol + 2 g $H_3PO_4$ + 50 ml 96% EtOH. Filter. Spray and then heat at 105–10°C for 5 min. Glucose gives dark brown spots; fructose, lemon yellow; sucrose and maltose, brownish-yellow; raffinose, light-brown.

### 14  *m-Phenylenediamine*

Spray with 0.2M *m*-phenylenediamine dihydrochloride in 76% EtOH. Heat at 105°C for 5 min. Bright fluorescent spots are given in u.v., yellow with glucose, orange with ribose. Sensitivity 10 $\mu$g. Pentoses give pink-brown spots; disaccharides yellow; uronic acids pink. Phenol, morpholine, diethylene glycol, and dioxan interfere with the fluorescence.

### 15  *p-Aminohippuric acid*

Spray with 0.3% *p*-aminohippuric acid in EtOH. Heat at 140°C for 8 min. In u.v. most hexoses and pentoses give orange fluorescent spots. Sensitivity 1 $\mu$g.

### 16  *Phthalic acid*

Spray with 3% phthalic acid in ethanol. Detects 0.25 $\mu$g glucose, 1 $\mu$g fructose by orange fluorescence in u.v. In visible light four to five times these amounts give orange-red spots. Also detects reducing disaccharides and acid-labile non-reducing oligosaccharides. 4-Aminoantipyrene may be used in place of phthalic acid but it has slightly lower sensitivity and the paper must be heated at 150°C for 10 min.

### 17  *α-Naphthylamine*

Spray with a 2% soln. of α-naphthylamine in BuOH–MeOH (1:1), containing 5% trichloroacetic acid. General spray for sugars giving a variety of colours.

### 18  *β-Naphthylamine**

Reagent: 0.1 g pure β-naphthylamine in 50 ml EtOH + 50 ml *n*-BuOH + 0.4 ml 3.8M-HCl + 0.2 ml $H_2O$ + 0.05 ml 10% ferric sulphate. Spray and heat at 160–70°C for 10 min. Fructose gives a yellow colour at first, later turning yellow-brown; the same results are given with oligosaccharides which give fructose on hydrolysis;

methylpentoses give duller yellow spots; pentoses, bright pink-red; aldoses, light brown.

    * **Warning**: $\beta$-naphthylamine is extremely carcinogenic.

### 19 *Dinitrosalicylic acid*

Spray with 0.5% 3:5-dinitrosalicylic acid in 4% NaOH. Reducing sugars give brown spots on a pale yellow ground.

### 20 *Dinitrobenzoic acid*

Spray with 1% 3:4-dinitrobenzoic acid in $1\text{M-Na}_2\text{CO}_3$. Heat 5 min at $100^\circ$C. Reducing sugars give blue spots turning brown. Ketoses react faster than aldoses; ascorbic acid reacts in the cold. Sensitivity 1 $\mu$g.

### 21 *Ammonium molybdate*

Reagents: 20 ml 10% $NH_4$ molybdate is mixed with 3 ml HCl. Then 5 g $NH_4$Cl is added. Spray the paper. Any inorganic phosphate or readily hydrolysable organic phosphate gives yellow spots immediately. Heat at $75^\circ$C for 15 min. Reducing substances give blue spots on a white ground due to reduction of molybdate to molybdenum blue. Sensitivity for glucose, 2 $\mu$g. Ketoses are more easily detected than aldoses. Sucrose also gives a positive reaction.

## ALDOSES

### 22 *Aniline*

Many variations of this reagent have been reported, the most useful being the following:

    (i) Spray with 0.93 g aniline + 1.66 g phthalic acid in 100 ml water-saturated *n*-BuOH. Heat at $105^\circ$C for 5 min. Aldopentoses give bright red spots, with red fluorescence in u.v.; aldohexoses, deoxysugars, and uronic acids give various shades of green and brown with yellow fluorescence. The colour given by ketoses is very weak. Oligosaccharides need longer heating. Sensitivity for maltose is 10 $\mu$g; maltotriose, 20 $\mu$g; glucose, 2 $\mu$g.

    (ii) Spray with a mixture of equal vols. of $0.1\text{M}$-aniline and $0.1\text{M-H}_3\text{PO}_4$, each in water-saturated *n*-BuOH. Heat as in (i). Detects a wider range of sugars and is more sensitive, particularly for reducing oligosaccharides.

    (iii) Aniline hydrogen oxalate spray is prepared by shaking 100 ml $0.1\text{M}$-oxalic acid with 0.9 ml aniline. Pentoses (5 $\mu$g) bright red in 5 min; glucose brown in 10 min. In u.v. light tetroses (1 $\mu$g) show a bright fluorescence. Aldopentoses and hexoses also give this but not ketohexoses or dihydroxyacetone.

    (iv) Spray with 2.5% aniline trichloroacetate in glacial acetic acid. This gives coloured spots with methylated aldohexoses (brown), pentoses (brown), ketohexoses (brown), and uronic acids (red), but not with polyols. Sensitivity 1$-$5 $\mu$g.

    (v) Dip ionophoretograms in acetone containing $0.1\text{M}$-aniline and $0.2\text{M}$-picric acid and heat at $100^\circ$C. Sugars develop as dark brown spots on a yellow ground.

    (vi) Any of the following aromatic bases in conjunction with HCl, HCOOH, trichloroacetic or toluenesulphonic acids, give colours with methylated sugars after heating at $100-103^\circ$C: aniline; *p*-aminodimethyl-(or diethyl-)aniline; the colours with these depending on the degree of methylation and position of methyl group on the sugar; *p*-phenylenediamine; *N*-(1-naphthyl)-ethylenediamine; the latter is useful for methyl derivatives of ketoses.

### 23 *Diphenylamine*

Spray with 2% diphenylamine in BuOH–MeOH (1:1), containing 5% trichloroacetic acid. Heat at $100^\circ$C for 10 min. Aldohexoses give brown spots; aldopentoses, purple.

## KETOSES AND PENTOSES

### 24 *Naphthoresorcinol*

Spray with 0.2% naphthoresorcinol in EtOH—2% aq. trichloroacetic acid (1:1), mixed just before use. Heat at 100°C for 5—10 min. Fructose, sorbose, sucrose, raffinose give red colours; pentoses, uronic acids, blue on standing; aldoses, non-reactive. α-Naphthol and resorcinol can also be used.

An alternative procedure is to spray with 1% of any of the above phenols in EtOH—2M-HCl (1:9). Heat at 90°C for 10 min. Ketohexoses give red and brown colours. Sensitivity 10 $\mu$g.

Phosphoric acid can also be used as the acid, detecting a wider range of sugars and attacking the paper less. In this spray a 0.2% soln. of resorcinol, naphthoresorcinol, α-naphthol, phloroglucinol, or orcinol in EtOH is mixed with 0.1 vol. $H_3PO_4$ (sp. gr. 1.85). The naphthoresorcinol version of this spray is very sensitive and excellent for locating higher sucrose oligosaccharides. Used also on thin-layer chromatograms. A modification of the spray is 1% α-naphthol in EtOH—$H_3PO_4$ (10:1). Spray and air-dry for 30 min. Then heat at 90°C for 5 min. Used for detecting raffinose, 2 $\mu$g.

### 25 *Urea or anthraquinone*

(i) To 100 ml of 1M-$H_3PO_4$ in water-saturated *n*-BuOH add 3 g of urea then 5 ml of EtOH to eliminate the water phase which forms when the urea dissolves, spray and heat at 100—110°C. Free or acid-labile bound ketoses (sucrose, etc.), bright blue, highly sensitive; acid-stable oligosaccharides with a reducing fructose grey-brown. Aldoses only react, brown, if present in very high concentration.

(ii) 3% urea or anthraquinone in 5% HCl in EtOH give similar reactions. If applied after aniline—phthalic acid (*see* 22 (i)) glucose turns brown-red; fructose and fructosans green-black.

### 26 *2:5-Diphenyl-3-p-styrylphenyltetrazolium chloride*

Dissolve 20 mg of the above substance in 10 ml EtOH. Mix, immediately before spraying, with an equal vol. of 0.1M-NaOH. After a few minutes at RT or slight warming free ketoses and oligosaccharides with a reducing ketose (not sucrose) appear as purple spots on a yellow ground. Sensitivity 5 $\mu$g. Aldoses only react if the paper is heated strongly.

### 27 *Phloroglucinol*

Spray with 0.2 g phloroglucinol in 80 ml 90% EtOH + 20 ml 25% aq. trichloroacetic acid. Heat at 110°C. Ketoses (5 $\mu$g) give orange-brown spots; pentoses (20 $\mu$g), green-blue after long heating; aldoses, no reaction.

### 28 *Orcinol*

Spray with water-saturated *n*-BuOH containing 0.5% orcinol and 15% trichloroacetic acid. Heat at 105°C for 20 min. Specific for ketoheptoses, sedoheptulose and mannoheptulose, which give bluish-green spots; ketohexoses, yellow; no colour with aldoheptoses or hexoses. If followed by aniline—phthalic acid (see 22 (i)) with no further heating, D-xylulose gives a purple colour; D-ribulose, pink; aldopentoses, negative. A modification is the spray 3% orcinol in 5% HCl in EtOH. Ketoses and methylketoses give red colours.

### 29 *Urea—diphenylamine*

Mix equal vols. of 1% diphenylamine in acetone containing 10% $H_3PO_4$ and 3% urea in water-saturated *n*-BuOH also containing 10% $H_3PO_4$. Spray and heat 2—3 min at 90°C, observe colours immediately and 1 hr after heating. Fructose and sorbose, brown to grey-black; mannoketoheptose, purple-blue. Disaccharides with a reducing ketose give colours which are dependent on the position of the glycosidic link. If the diphenylamine is increased to 2% and the papers heated for 4–5 min at 95–100°C most aldoses give bright red or pink colours.

### 30 Anthrone

Spray with 300 mg anthrone in 10 ml warm glacial acetic acid and 20 ml EtOH + 3 ml $H_3PO_4$ (sp. gr. 1.6) + 1 ml $H_2O$. Heat at 108°C for 5–6 min. Mono-, di-, tri-, and polysaccharides containing ketohexoses give bright yellow spots; ketopentoses, purple; ketoheptoses, orange-yellow. In u.v., ketoses, brown; aldoses may show a light blue fluorescence. Stronger acid conditions, e.g. $H_2SO_4$, give green spots with both aldo- and keto-sugars.

### 31 2:4-Dinitrophenylhydrazine

Spray with a saturated soln. of 2:4-dinitrophenylhydrazine in 95% EtOH containing 1% conc. HCl. Heat at 70°C for 3–5 min. Fructose, sucrose, and raffinose give orange spots on a light yellow ground.

### 32 Diazouracil

Dissolve 15 mg diazouracil in 10 ml 0.1 M-NaOH. Spray paper immediately, partly dry at 60–80°C for 3 min, dip in 2% aq. $MgCl_2$ and dry by blotting. Sucrose and substituted sucroses (e.g. raffinose) appear as blue spots provided that the sucrose is not substituted on the fructose portion. Sensitivity 100 μg. Aldoses and monosaccharides do not react.

## KETOSE-AMINO ACIDS

### 33 Ferricyanide—ferric sulphate

Spray with (a) 0.1% K ferricyanide in 80% EtOH:10% NaOH in 80% EtOH = 10:1, mixed just before use. Leave at RT for 5 min. Then spray with (b) ferric sulphate—gum ghatti—$H_3PO_4$ soln. (Prep. in JBC **83**, 115 (1929)). Dark blue spots on a colourless or light blue ground are given by ketose-amino acids. Sensitivity 10 μg.

## SUGAR ALCOHOLS, GLYCOLS, DEOXY-SUGARS, AND GLYCALS

See also Inositol in Vitamins.

### 34 Potassium periodocuprate

Dissolve 12.5 g $CuSO_4 \cdot 5H_2O$ in 400 ml boiling water, add 23 g K periodate plus a conc. aq. soln. of 56 g KOH followed by 20 g K persulphate (in small portions at 1 min intervals). Boil 20 min, dilute to 500 ml and add 500 ml 2 M-KOH. Stable. On spraying, sugars, polyhydric alcohols, esters, and other non-reducing substances appear as white spots on a brown ground. Highly sensitive.

### 35 Vanillin

Spray with 1% vanillin in EtOH:3% aq. perchloric acid = 1:1, mixed just before use. Heat at 85°C for 3–4 min. Polyhydric sugar alcohols give pale blue spots, turning lilac then pale grey-blue on a sandy ground. Sensitivity, hexitols, 15 μg; pentitols, 20 μg; erythritol, 25 μg; glycerol, 30 μg. Inositol, dihydroxyacetone, aldopentoses, and aldohexoses do not react except rhamnose (20 μg) which gives a brick red spot; sorbose and fructose (5 μg) give deep grey-green spots. Phenols and some indolic compounds react. A greater range of compounds may be detected by examining the sprayed, heated, paper under u.v. light.

36 *Periodate oxidation — (nitroprusside/piperazine) or (nitroaniline/NaOH)*

Spray with (*a*) saturated aq. Na metaperiodate:$H_2O$ = 1:2. Leave at RT for 10 min and then spray with (*b*) saturated Na nitroprusside: $H_2O$:EtOH saturated with piperazine = 1:3:20. Methylpentoses, deoxysugars and glycals give blue spots in 5—10 min, later fading.

Oxidize with periodate as above, spray with (*b*) 1% *p*-nitroaniline in EtOH—conc. HCl (4:1). Deoxysugars and glycals give deep yellow spots on a pale yellow ground and, in u.v., a yellow fluorescence on a brown ground. Then spray with (*c*) 5% NaOH in MeOH. The spots turn green. Methylpentoses do not react.

37 *Periodate oxidation—Schiff's reagent*

Spray with (*a*) 2% aq. Na metaperiodate. Heat at 60°C for 7 min in an atmosphere of $N_2$ then place in an atmosphere of $SO_2$ to reduce iodate and excess periodate. Then spray with (*b*) Schiff's reagent (prepared by dissolving 1 g rosaniline in 50 ml $H_2O$ followed by decolorization with $SO_2$; the solution is treated with charcoal, filtered and diluted to 1 l with $H_2O$). Heat at 60°C for 10 min. Aldehydes arising during oxidation give blue and purple spots. Sensitivity is 10 $\mu$g for all 1:2-glycols tested. Carbohydrates containing the 1:2:3 triol-system are distinguished from 1:2-diols because they also give HCOOH on periodate oxidation; the latter gives a brown iodine stain with 5% KI, sprayed after excess periodate has been destroyed with 10% aq. ethylene glycol.

Reducing oligosaccharides containing a 1 → 2 linked reducing unit (e.g. kojibiose, sophorose) give a specific yellow colour with the periodate-rosaniline spray reagent.

38 *Periodate—$MnSO_4$—aromatic base*

Spray with (*a*) 0.5% $KIO_4$. Leave for 1—5 min. Then spray with (*b*) 15% aq. $MnSO_4$: saturated soln. di-(*p*-dimethylaniline)methane in 2M-$CH_3COOH$ = 1:1. $\alpha$-Glycols give white spots on a blue ground. Sensitivity 5—50 $\mu$g.

39 *Periodate—thiobarbiturate*

Spray with (*a*) 0.02M-Na periodate. After 15 min spray with (*b*) ethylene glycol: acetone:conc. $H_2SO_4$ = 50:50:0.3 and, after 10 min, spray with (*c*) aq. 6% Na-2-thiobarbiturate. Heat at 100°C for 5 min when 2-deoxysugars give red spots. Sensitivity 0.5 $\mu$g.

40 *Lead tetra-acetate oxidation*

Spray with xylene. Immediately spray with 1% Pb tetra-acetate in benzene, the reagent being decolorized with charcoal and filtered if necessary before spraying. White spots on a brown ground are given by all 1:2-glycols (10 $\mu$g), $\alpha$-hydroxyacids, pyruvic acid, and dihydroxyacetone. For locating sugar alcohols on ionophoretograms sensitivity is improved by subsequently spraying with rosaniline (see 37).

41 *Hydrochloric acid*

Spray with conc. HCl:EtOH = 1:4. Heat at 90°C. Glycals give pink spots turning brown. If alcoholic $FeCl_3$ soln. is used instead of the HCl spray, sensitivity is slightly less.

42 *Carbazole—cysteine*

Spray with 0.12% carbazole in EtOH:1.5% cysteine·HCl:EtOH:12.5M-$H_2SO_4$ = 1:1:5:0.2. Heat at 65—70°C for 5 min. Xylulose and ribulose give violet spots turning grey (3 $\mu$g) or black (15 $\mu$g) on a colourless ground; xylose (15 $\mu$g) gives a very faint colour. Also given by glycals.

### 43 p-Dimethylaminobenzaldehyde

Spray with 1% p-dimethylaminobenzaldehyde in EtOH:conc. HCl = 4:1. Heat at 90°C for 30 sec. Deoxypentoses, deoxypentosides, D-ribal give bluish- or purplish-grey spots; deoxyhexoses, deoxyhexosides, glucal, galactal, pinkish-grey. After 2 min, xylose and arabinose give grey spots; acetylglucosamine, violet. Ninhydrin may be substituted for p-dimethylaminobenzaldehyde, giving more bluish colours.

## SUGAR ACIDS

### 44 o-Phenylenediamine

Spray with 2% o-phenylenediamine dihydrochloride in 80% EtOH. Heat at 100°C for several min. 2-Ketohexonic acids (50 $\mu$g) give greenish-grey spots; 10—20 $\mu$g detected by fluorescence in u.v. light. Some aldoses may react but give different colours.

A spray of 0.05% o-phenylenediamine in 10% aq. trichloroacetic acid has also been used for uronic acids but m-phenylenediamine as described in 14 is more sensitive, although it may not be as specific as o-phenylenediamine.

### 45 Hydroxylamine—ferric chloride

Spray with (a) M-NH$_2$OH·HCl in MeOH:1.1M-KOH in MeOH = 1:1, freshly prepared. Leave at RT for 10 min. Then spray with (b) 1—2% FeCl$_3$ in 1% aq. HCl. Esters, lactones, or ester lactones give blue or mauve spots. Also given with certain amides and methylamides of sugar acids and most esters.

A modification of this spray in which soln. (b) is strongly acid Fe(NO$_3$)$_3$ gives purple colours with sugar acetates and inositol acetates on thin-layer chromatograms.

## HEXOSAMINES

### 47 Acetylacetone—p-dimethylaminobenzaldehyde

Component solutions of first spray: (a) 0.5 ml acetylacetone in 50 ml n-BuOH, (b) 50% aq. KOH:EtOH = 5:20. (a):(b) = 10:0.5, mixed just before use and a few drops 50% EtOH added to redissolve any crystals. Spray. Heat at 105°C for 5 min. Spray with (c) 1 g p-dimethylaminobenzaldehyde in 30 ml EtOH + 30 ml conc. HCl + 180 ml n-BuOH. Heat at 90°C for 5 min. Free hexosamines give cherry red spots except fructosamine, red-purple and sialic acids, salmon pink. N-Acetylglucosamine gives an intense purple-violet colour with (c) alone, without previous treatment with acetylacetone; cf. 43. With the complete reagent 1 → 6 and 1 → 3 linked disaccharides with an N-acetyl aminosugar reducing unit give a purple colour but similar 1 → 4 linked compounds do not react.

### 48 Ninhydrin

Spray with 0.05% ninhydrin in n-BuOH. Heat at 105—110°C for 10 min. Aminosugars give red colours. This spray may be followed by aniline hydrogen oxalate (22iii) for free sugars.

### 49 Periodate—thiobarbiturate

Spray with (a) 0.05M-Na metaperiodate in 0.025M-H$_2$SO$_4$, then with reagents (b) and (c) of 39. Red colour with sialic acids after heating for 10 min at 100°C. Sensitivity 3 $\mu$g.

## POLYSACCHARIDES

### 50 Copper sulphate—phosphomolybdate

Spray with (a) 40 g Na$_2$CO$_3$ (anhyd.) + 20 g NaHCO$_3$ + 25 g Rochelle salt + 7.5 g CuSO$_4$·5H$_2$O + H$_2$O to 1 l. Heat at 105°C for 5 min. Then spray with reagent (*b*) prepared by dissolving 150 g molybdic acid + 75 g $Na_2CO_3$ (anhyd.) in 500 ml $H_2O$; heat and filter; add 300 ml 85% $H_3PO_4$ + $H_2O$ to 1 l. Reducing polysaccharides give blue spots on a white ground.

51 *Toluidine blue*

For acidic mucopolysaccharides, fix polysaccharides by dipping in EtOH–ether (95:5). Dry. Then dip in 0.06% toluidine blue 0 in 0.5% aq. $CH_3COOH$. Finally rinse in 2% aq. $CH_3COOH$. Heparin gives a bright pink colour; chondroitin sulphate and hyaluronate, purple, on a light blue ground; dextran sulphate gives purple colour on a light blue ground. Azure blue (0.05%) is also used as a metachromatic stain for sulphated acid mucopolysaccharides. Other stains used for acid polysaccharides are Alcian blue, mucicarmine, and azur A7.

52 *Carmine*

Stock solution: 1 g carmine + 0.5 g anhyd. $AlCl_3$ + 2 ml $H_2O$ are heated in a porcelain crucible for 2–3 min. Dissolve in 100 ml 50% EtOH. Filter after 24 hr. Store at 5°C. Spray with the mixture, stock solution:EtOH:$H_2O$ = 5:17:3. Rinse in $H_2O$ containing a small amount of $CH_3COOH$. Both acid and neutral mucopolysaccharides give bright pink spots on a very light pink or colourless ground.

---

# 6 THYROXINE AND RELATED COMPOUNDS

1 *Ninhydrin*

Spray with 0.2% ninhydrin in *n*-BuOH saturated with $H_2O$, containing 5% $CH_3COOH$. Sensitivity for thyroxine, 20 μg. This spray is suitable for iodothyronines and iodotyrosines but unsuitable for the deaminated analogues or when amino acid contamination is high. See amino acids 1

2 *Pauly reaction*

(i) *Diazotized sulphanilic acid. See* Amino acids, 12.

(ii) *Diazotized N', N'-diethylsulphanilamide.* Mix equal vols. cold 0.05M-*N'*, *N'*-diethylsulphanilamide in 9% HCl and cold 4% $NaNO_2$. Let stand for 10 min at 4°C. Spray and let stand 5 min. Then spray with 10% aq. $Na_2CO_3$. Purple colours are given with compounds containing diphenolic ethers (e.g. thyroxine) and orange with compounds possessing a single benzene ring (e.g. diiodotyrosine). Sensitivity for iodothyronines and analogues is 20–30 μg and 10–15 μg for iodotyrosines. The Pauly reaction is particularly suitable for the deaminated analogues and for iodothyronines and iodotyrosines in the presence of large amounts of amino acids. Unsuitable for phenolic conjugates, i.e. β-glucuronides and sulphate esters.

3 *Ceric sulphate–arsenious acid*

(i) Component solutions of the spraying reagent: (*a*) 10 g $Ce(SO_4)_2 \cdot 4H_2O$ is suspended in 100 ml 0.5M-$H_2SO_4$ at 0–5°C. Filter after 1 hr. (*b*) 5 g Na arsenite in 100 ml 0.5M-$H_2SO_4$ at 0°C. (*a*):(*b*) = 1:1, mixed just before use. The reagent is applied by thoroughly wetting a blank paper on a glass plate; the chromatogram is then placed on top and covered with another glass plate for 30 min. Dry in an $I_2$-free atmsophere. Iodine-containing compounds give white spots on a yellow ground. If photographed in u.v. these show as black spots on a white ground. Sensitivity for KI, 0.01 μg; diiodotyrosine, 0.02 μg; thyroxine and triiodothyronine, 0.1 μg. To prevent fading of the background colour due to traces of $I_2$ in the atmosphere, spray with (c) 1% aq. o-phenylenediamine before drying in air. A stable chocolate-coloured ground is produced by the reaction of excess ceric sulphate with the amine.

(ii) Modification of Robbins. Stock solutions: (a) 10 g $Ce(SO_4)_2 . 4H_2O$ in 100 ml 10% (v/v) $H_2SO_4$; (b) 5 g $NaAsO_2$ in 100 ml $H_2O$; (c) 0.025M-aq. o-phenanthroline ferrous sulphate ('Ferroine'). One part of solution (a) is added to 6 parts of solution (b), giving a clear orange-yellow solution. One part of 'Ferroine' solution (c) is then added giving a turbid, dark green suspension which is kept shaken. The dried chromatogram paper is sprayed lightly on each side (about 8 ml of reagent to spray 30 × 30 cm). Spots of iodine-containing substances turn orange at a rate depending on their concentration. The green background is unstable, first turning orange and then decolorized. Storage in dark increases stability. Sensitivity 0.2 μg for iodothyronines and 0.02 μg for iodotyrosines.

### 4 Ferric chloride—ferricyanide—arsenite

Stock solutions: (a) 2.7 g $FeCl_3 \cdot 6H_2O$ in 100 ml 2M-HCl. (b) 3.5 g $K_3Fe(CN)_6$ per 100 ml $H_2O$. (c) 5 g $NaAsO_2$ in 30 ml 1M-NaOH (under cooling) and then add 65 ml 2M-HCl under vigorous stirring. Store in a cool, dark place. Before use, mix (a):(b):(c) = 5:5:1. Dried paper chromatograms are sprayed evenly from both sides and placed between 2 glass plates for 15 min under dim light or in a dark room. The paper is then washed well in distilled $H_2O$ and dried. Iodide, iodotyrosines and iodothyronines give blue spots which can be quantitated photometrically (Zeiss filter FE-54). Sensitivity is 0.01—0.07 μg for the above compounds.

### 5 Starch—iodate

Dried papers are first sprayed with 1% starch solution and then with 1% $KIO_3$ or $KBrO_3$ solution. While still wet, the paper is exposed for 3—4 min to u.v. light. Positions of iodinated substances appear as blue spots which later fade away. Sensitivity 0.5 μg for thyroxine, 0.05 μg for diiodotyrosine.

---

# 7 LIPIDS

Complex lipids are now almost universally examined by thin layer chromatography.

## GENERAL SPRAYS OR DIPS

### 1 Sulphuric acid

Spray TLC plates or glass papers with conc. or 50% $H_2SO_4$ or sat. chromic—$H_2SO_4$. Heat in oven or on hot plate; diagnostic colours appear with increasing temperature, especially with steroids. Most non-volatile compounds eventually give black spots. As little as 0.1 μg lipid is detected by the charring technique, although completely saturated lipids are less reactive.

### 2 Dichlorofluorescein

0.2% 2′:7′-dichlorofluorescein in 95% ethanol. View under u.v. at 366 nm.

### 3 Phosphomolybdic acid

10% phosphomolybdic acid in absolute ethanol. Spray hot chromatogram immediately after removal from oven at 160—180°C. Intense blue spots appear immediately on pale yellow background.

### 4  *Rhodamine 6G or Rhodamine B*

0.001% aq. Rhodamine 6G in $0.25\text{M-K}_2\text{HPO}_4$. View wet under u.v. light. Purple, blue, and yellow spots against rose background. Optimal length of time of immersion in stain varies with compound and type of chromatogram (0.2–10 min).

### 5  *Iodine vapour*

Detects all lipids, nitrogenous compounds, non-reducing carbohydrates. Compounds recovered unchanged after detection. Expose to crystals of $I_2$ in closed chamber, see Steroids 32. Test the day chromatograms are developed. Ultraviolet light enhances feeble staining. If the chromatography solvent contained acid it must first be removed from chromatograms in a vacuum dessicator or with $NH_3$.

### 6  *Hydroxylamine-ferric chloride for acyl esters*

Spray plates or papers with alkaline hydroxylamine reagent, dry briefly, spray with ethereal acid ferric chloride reagent prepared as below. Purple spots appear quickly on a yellow background.

    *Alkaline hydroxylamine*. Dissolve $10\,\text{g}\ NH_2OH\cdot HCl$ in 25 ml water, dilute to 100 ml with ethanol, mix with 26 ml of saturated aq. NaOH diluted to 200 ml with ethanol. Filter off NaCl ppt.

    *Acid ferric chloride*. Grind $10\,\text{g}\ FeCl_3\cdot6H_2O$ and 20 ml HCl (37% w/v) in pestle and mortar, shake resulting solution with 300 ml ether.

## SPECIFIC SPRAYS OR DIPS

### 7  *Ninhydrin*

For lipids containing free amino groups.

    (i) Spray or dip in 0.25% solution of ninhydrin in acetone. Develop at RT for several hours or heat in oven at $85°\text{C}$ for a few minutes.

    (ii) Stock ninhydrin in *n*-butanol (1 mg/ml) diluted with 2:4-lutidine (20% by volume) immediately before use. Develop at $120°\text{C}$ for 5 min. Intensify colour by dipping chromatogram in 2M-HCl for 2 min, washing and drying before spraying with reagent.

### 8  *Fluorescamine*

A sensitive detection reagent for lipids containing free amino groups. Spray with 0.5% fluorescamine in acetone. Examine plate under u.v. to detect fluorescing spots.

### 9  *2:4-Dinitrophenylhydrazine*

For aldehydogenic lipids, spray plate with 30% $H_2SO_4$, then after 5 min with reagent containing 1.2 g 2:4-dinitrophenylhydrazine, 260 ml methanol, 40 ml conc. HCl and 20 ml $CHCl_3$. Aldehydogenic lipids – pale yellow spots against almost white background.

### 10  *4-Amino-5-hydrazino*-1,2,4-*triazole-3-thiol (AHTT)*

Spray plate with freshly prepared 2% AHTT in 1M NaOH. Free aldehydes rapidly show as purple spots with full intensity after 45 min (palmitaldehyde 1 $\mu$g). Ketones no reaction —autoxidized unsaturated fatty acid and lipids can show a reaction. For aldehydogenic lipids, expose solvent-developed plate to HCl vapour to release free aldehyde before using spray reagent.

### 11  *Periodate–Schiff's reagent*

For phosphatidylglycerol, inositol phosphatides, and cerebrosides. Wash chromatogram with distilled water and dry. Immerse in 2% aqueous sodium periodate for

1 min. Rinse with water, immerse in 2% aqueous sodium bisulphite for 25 min. Dip in Schiff's reagent (1% p-rosaniline decolorized with $SO_2$ and filtered through charcoal) for 30 sec. Purple spot develops in 10–15 min.

### 12 Dragendorff's reagent

To detect choline. Mix 4 ml solution (a), 1 ml solution (b), and 20 ml distilled water. Solution (a) 1.7 g $Bi(NO_3)_3 \cdot 5H_2O$ diluted to 100 ml with 20% (v/v) acetic acid. Solution (b) 40 g KI in 100 ml water. Dry at RT. Free choline. purple spot; choline containing compounds, orange spots. See amines 11, 12.

### 13 Bial's orcinol–$FeCl_3$–HCl reagent

For glycolipids. Heat chromatograms for $1\frac{1}{2}$ hr at 80°C in HCl atmosphere. Treat with Bial's reagent and replace in HCl vapour at 80°C. Violet spots develop on a white background. Bial's reagent: 40.7 ml conc. HCl, 0.1 g orcinol, 1 ml 1% $FeCl_3$, and distilled water to 50 ml.

### 14 Molybdenum blue reagent

For phospholipids. Reagent (a) shake 40 ml conc. HCl + 10 ml metallic mercury + 80 ml 13.3% ammonium molybdate solution for 30 min. Reagent (b) add 200 ml conc. $H_2SO_4$ carefully to 40 ml 13.3% ammonium molybdate. Mix solution (a) (minus Hg) and solution (b), dilute to 1000 ml and cool. Spray on TLC plate at R.T.; phospholipids are revealed as blue spots on white ground. Sensitivity 0.5 $\mu$g P. May be used after ninhydrin spray (7). Heating at 100°C for 30 min will char all lipids.

### 15 Sudan black

For lipoproteins and histochemistry. Dissolve 0.1 g of Sudan black B in 1 ml ethyl acetate at RT. Dilute after solution with 9 ml propylene glycol. Stain for 15 min. Ratio stain: lipoprotein = 1:5.

---

# 8 PHENOLS AND RELATED COMPOUNDS

Although some chemically simple phenols are involved in animal metabolism, the widest variety of phenolic compounds which occur in Nature are found in plants (i.e. flavonoid compounds, cinnamic acids, coumarins, and tannins), usually in a combined form (e.g. glycosides). The majority of the phenolic compounds or their derivative (e.g. glucuronides) which are present in normal urine arise from these two sources, but administration of drugs and other foreign organic compounds containing an aromatic nucleus can lead to the formation of phenols even though the original substance contained no phenolic groups. Thus there is a wide range of compounds of different reactivities and polarities included in the term phenolic, and the choice both of solvent for separation and of reagent for detection depends therefore on the class of compounds under examination.

As most of the compounds encountered both in plants and in urine are combined, it is desirable to examine the extract before and after hydrolysis (with acid, base (usually in an atmosphere of $N_2$) or an enzyme).

By far the most useful solvents for the separation of less polar compounds (i.e. simple phenols) are combinations of benzene (or toluene or chloroform), acetic (or formic) acid and water (e.g. Bz–HAc–$H_2O$, 125:72:3). Such water-poor solvents are usually temperature sensitive and also require pre-equilibration.

For the more polar compounds (i.e. the majority of those present in plant extracts and the phenolic derivatives in urine) the most useful solvents are those based on combinations of alcohols, water, and acetic (or formic) acid (e.g. $n$-BuOH–HAc–$H_2O$, 6:1:2; $n$-BuOH–EtOH–$H_2O$, 4:1:2.2; 2% aqueous HAc; HAc–conc. HCl–$H_2O$, 30:3:10). Basic solvents have been used for separating certain classes (especially phenolic acids), but since many phenols are readily oxidized at high pH, such solvents should be avoided if possible.

## DETECTION BY COLOUR OR FLUORESCENCE

### 1  *Colour in visible light and fluorescence in u.v.*

The majority of phenolic compounds occurring in plant extracts are either coloured or more usually fluoresce strongly under a long wave u.v. lamp ($\sim 300$ nm). However, simple phenols are both colourless and non-fluorescent. They may, however, be detected by their absorption (i.e. appear dark) when examined under short wave u.v. ($\sim 250$ nm).

The major classes of compounds which are coloured are anthocyanins (orange to mauve), flavonols and some nitrophenols (pale yellow), and chalkones and aurones (deep yellow). The shade and depth of colour changes with increase in the number of suitably oriented phenolic groups. Fluorescence is usually brown (flavones, flavonol-3-glycosides, and chalkones), varying shades of yellow (flavonols and aurones) or varying shades of blue or purple (cinnamic acids, coumarins, methylated flavones, and stilbenes), but there is a wide overlap depending on orientation or substitution of the phenolic hydroxyl groups.

When the chromatogram is exposed to $NH_3$ vapour (best) or sprayed with base (0.05 to 1 M aq. $Na_2CO_2$ is suitable) usually both the visible colour and fluorescence undergo characteristic changes due to the ionization of phenolic hydroxyl groups and subsequent increase in conjugation. It can generally be taken that a reversible change in colour or fluorescence on exposure to ammonia indicates the presence of a phenolic compound. Anthocyanins go to bluer shades, and flavonols, etc., deeper yellow. Some compounds, colourless before exposure to alkaline pH (e.g. chlorogenic acid), may also appear yellow. Exposure to base also induces oxidation of certain compounds leading to the formation of permanent brown spots. Changes in the fluorescence colour in the presence of base are usually to longer wavelengths (i.e. blue → green → yellow). Absence of change in visible or fluorescence colour probably indicates methylation or other forms of substitution of the phenolic groups.

## SUBSTITUTION REAGENTS

### 2  *Diazotized amines*

All compounds containing phenolic hydroxyl groups which have a free *para* or *ortho* position and which do not contain strongly deactivating substituents or sterically hindering groups react with diazotized amines at a suitable pH to give coloured azo dyestuffs. Imidazoles also react. Many different amines have been used for the coupling reaction but the most useful is $p$-nitroaniline since the azo dyes produced often show variation of colour with pH.

#### (i) *Diazotized p-nitroaniline*

*(a)* A solution of the amine (5 ml, 0.5% w/v) in 2M-HCl is mixed with aq. sodium nitrite (0.5 ml, 5% w/v), and sodium acetate (15 ml, 20%) added *(b)* $Na_2CO_3$ (20% w/v). The two sprays are used successively, the colour reaction with each being noted. If required a further overspray with 0.1M-NaOH can be used. Spraying with the first reagent should be light and even, or excessive background develops.

#### (ii) *Diazotized sulphanilic acid and benzidine**

Both these amines are used at 0.5% w/v in 2M-HCl and after diazotization the first is made alkaline with sodium carbonate solution (3 vol. 20% w/v).

*Carcinogenic

## OTHER SUBSTITUTION REAGENTS

The most useful reagent of those which have been used are 2:6-dibromoquinone-4-chloroimide, *p*-dimethylaminobenzaldehyde, vanillin and toluene-*p*-sulphonic acid, and nitrous acid. The first reagent reacts only with phenols that have a free *para* position; the next two react most strongly with *meta* substituted dihydric undeactivated phenols and thus can be used to detect catechins and leuco-anthocyanins in the presence of other compounds. Nitrous acid, on the other hand, reacts with many phenolic compounds but the nitroso phenols produced do not all give coloured quinonoid salts with base.

### 3 2:6-Dibromoquinone-4-chloroimide*

The reagent (0.5%) in ethanol is sprayed first, followed by a spray of any suitable base ($\sim$ pH 10) or exposure of the paper to ammonia. Blue colours are formed with most phenols that react; some other compounds also react (e.g. thiol-imidazoles).

 * **Warning**: This compound can be an explosive risk at temperatures of 50°C and above.

### 4 *p-Dimethylaminobenzaldehyde*

A solution of *p*-dimethylaminobenzaldehyde (10% w/v) in conc. HCl is diluted fivefold with acetone or EtOH. If the reagent is dissolved in acetic anhydride instead of conc. HCl it is somewhat selective for aryl glycines (e.g. hippuric acid) which give orange or red colours; some organic acids also react. Catechins and similar compounds give magenta spots either slowly in the cold or on heating. Indoles, pyrroles and aromatic amines react more readily but may be differentiated from phenols with other groups.

### 5 *Vanillin—p-toluenesulphonic acid*

The aldehyde (2 g) and acid (1 g) are dissolved in EtOH (100 ml), and after spraying the paper is heated to 100°C for 10 min. Catechins and related compounds give pink to violet-red colours.

### 6 *Nitrous acid*

Sodium nitrite (1%) in M-acetic acid is sprayed first, followed by 0.1M-NaOH. Red colours with many phenols including chlorogenic acid.

## OXIDIZING AGENTS

Most phenols, except those which are highly substituted, are readily oxidized, especially at high pH, but compounds containing vicinal di- or tri-hydric groups are the most reactive.

   Although certain phenols may be detected, usually as brown spots, either by allowing them to autoxidize after spraying with base, it is better to select reagents which themselves change colour. The most useful is the ferric chloride-potassium ferricyanide reagent, which is fairly specific for phenolic compounds. Monohydric phenols, however, react very slowly. Alkaline silver nitrate can also be used but it reacts with a wide variety of other compounds. Advantage can be taken of autoxidation of vicinal di- or tri-hydric phenols at high pH by condensing the quinones formed with ethylenediamine.

### 7 *Ferric chloride—potassium ferricyanide*

Aqueous 1% solutions of each salt (AR quality) are mixed in equal proportions before spraying or dipping (the solution should be orange-brown with no trace of blue). Reactive phenols give blue spots immediately in the cold. After development the paper must be washed with 0.1M-HCl followed by water if a permanent record is required.

### 8 *Alkaline silver nitrate*

See Carbohydrates, 1.

### 9 *Ethylenediamine*

Equal volumes of ethylenediamine (10% v/v) and 0.5M-$Na_2CO_3$ are mixed, and after spraying the paper is heated to $100°C$ for 5 min. Vicinal tri-hydroxy compounds give immediate colour of various shades which go brown on heating and usually have a yellow fluorescence; *ortho*-dihydroxy compounds give either dark colours on heating or yellow spots with a blue fluorescence.

## CHELATING AGENTS

These reagents are rather insensitive but have the advantage that the phenols can be recovered after use. The formation of all the chelates is pH-dependent.

### 10 *Ferric salts*

Phenols having two or more vicinal hydroxy groups, or *ortho* (or *para*) hydroxy-carbonyl groups, give coloured chelates with ferric salts. The chelates with di-hydroxy compounds are usually green, those with tri-hydroxy compounds blue, and others brown or red. Ferric ammonium sulphate (0.2%) or ferric chloride (2%) are suitable reagents.

### 11 *Aluminium salts*

Aluminium salts (e.g. 1% ethanolic aluminium chloride) form coloured or fluorescent chelates with flavonols, and other compounds. Blueing of anthocyanin colours by aluminium salts indicates the presence of vicinal hydroxy groups.

### 12 *Molybdates*

Molybdates (e.g. 0.1M-sodium molybdate) give yellow-coloured chelates in the cold, with vicinal di- and tri-hydroxy phenols.

---

# 9 PHOSPHATE ESTERS

Separation methods in general involve chromatography in mixtures of aqueous and organic solvents or electrophoresis, or both, on paper. Chromatography is the slower of the two methods, while electrophoresis at high voltage may be accomplished in about 30 min. The *detection* of phosphates on paper varies with the compounds studied, the non-phosphate moiety of the compound may afford a rapid and non-destructive means of detection. e.g. u.v. absorption of nucleotides.

### 1 *Molybdate—perchloric acid*

(i) Spray with the mixture 60% (w/v) perchloric acid:M-HCl:4% ammonium molybdate:$H_2O$ = 5:10:25:60. Inorganic phosphate gives a yellow spot. Dry the paper at $85°C$ for 1 min. Glucose 1-phosphate and other readily labile phosphate esters give yellow spots. Expose the paper to u.v. radiation. All organic phosphates, including those hydrolysed with difficulty (e.g. phosphoglyceric acid), now give blue spots. Inorganic phosphate, yellow-green. Citric acid may give a blue spot. Remove background colour by exposing the paper to $NH_3$ vapour.

(ii) Spray with molybdate–perchloric acid. Heat at 85°C for 10 min. Then spray with a fresh soln. containing 3 vol. 60% perchloric acid and 1 vol. reducing agent (1 g $p$-methylaminophenol sulphate + 3 g Na bisulphite in 100 ml $H_2O$). Sugar phosphates give blue spots on a white ground.

(iii) Dip in mixture of 3 ml 5% w/v ammonium molybdate, 7 ml 5M-HCl, and 90 ml acetone. Air-dry. Then dip in mixture of 10 ml of 1% vanadyl chloride in 1.0M-HCl and 90 ml acetone. The mixture is freshly reduced by shaking with 0.2 g of Zn powder. Orthophosphate, phosphite, pyrophosphate, and a number of phosphate esters and phosphonates produce spots varying from green to purple on a white background.

### 2 Ferric chloride–salicylsulphonic acid

Spray with (a) 0.1% $FeCl_3 \cdot 6H_2O$ in 80% EtOH. Dry at RT. Ferric ion is fixed by phosphate esters. Then spray with (b) 1% salicylsulphonic acid in 80% EtOH, which reacts with free iron. Phosphate esters give white spots on a pale mauve ground.

### 3 Quinine

Dip or spray paper in 0.025% quinine sulphate. $2H_2O$ in ethanol. Wash twice with ethanol to remove excess quinine, dry paper and examine under u.v. Phosphate esters show as light areas on grey-blue background. Sensitivity $< 1\,\mu g\,P$.

Inorganic salts on paper can interfere.

---

# 10 PURINES, PYRIMIDINES, NUCLEOSIDES, AND NUCLEOTIDES

Identification of purine and pyrimidine bases is usually achieved by comparing the $R_F$ values of the unknown in a number of solvents with those of marker compounds. Comparison of the u.v. absorption spectrum of the chromatographically purified compound with that of appropriate reference compounds should as a rule give fairly conclusive identification.

## GENERAL METHODS

### 1 Absorption in ultraviolet light

Purine and pyrimidine derivatives show as dark spots on the faintly fluorescing paper backing when viewed under u.v. light. This is the most sensitive method of detection ($1\,\mu g$) and permits location of the compound without chemical modification. Caution should be taken not to expose the naked eyes to the u.v. light. The compounds may be directly visualized or photographed by contact printing. If phenol or collidine solvents have been used they must first be removed by exhaustive washing with ether. A preliminary spray of 0.5M-NaOH is used for barbituric acids. To increase background fluorescence and thereby the contrast, a spray of 0.005% fluorescein in 0.5M-$NH_3$ may be used. This is not recommended, however, if the compound is to be subsequently eluted from the paper for spectrophotometry.

### 2 Fluorescence in ultraviolet light

Certain purine and pyrimidine derivatives may fluoresce when exposed to u.v. light. This may be seen directly or photographed by contact printing. A sheet of nitrocellulose film (0.08 mm) placed between the chromatogram and the photographic paper excludes the u.v. light but permits the transmission of the visible fluorescent light. The compound is thus shown as a black spot on a grey-white background. Sensitivity 0.1 μg.

## PURINES

### 3 *Silver chromate*

Spray with (a) 2% $AgNO_3$. Then dip in (b) 0.5% Na dichromate. This gives a red Ag chromate precipitate. Dip in (c) 0.5M-$HNO_3$. In this bath the red precipitate slowly dissolves leaving red deposits (purine–Ag chromate complexes) at the purine positions. Remove from the $HNO_3$ while the background is still slightly pink. Wash in $H_2O$. 0.5 μg guanine or adenine detected. Pyrimidines do not react.

### 4 *Mercury salt*

Spray with (a) 0.25% mercuric acetate in 95% ethanol containing a few drops of glacial acetic acid. Air-dry and spray with (b) 0.05% diphenylcarbazone in 95% ethanol. Purines containing one ionizable hydrogen will react. Sensitivity 5 μg. Spots should be immediately obvious but will stand out more after 24–48 hr. If phenol or pyridine have been used they must first be removed by washing the paper in ether.

### 5 *Bromine*

Expose paper to $Br_2$ vapour for 2 min and then to steam over a boiling water bath for 1 min. Dry paper for 5 min at 110°C. A rose pink spot which becomes reddish-purple when exposed to $NH_3$ is given by caffeine, theobromine, and theophylline. Sensitivity 10–20 μg.

## PYRIMIDINES

### 6 *Mercury salt*

Immerse the paper for 30 sec in (a) 0.1M-mercuric acetate:M-Na acetate:$H_2O$ = 1:3:6. Then immerse for exactly 20 sec in slowly renewed water. Finally dip in (b) ammonium sulphide soln. Uracil and cytosine (5 μg) and thymine (10 μg) give black spots.

### 7 *p-Dimethylaminobenzaldehyde*

Spray with 2% p-dimethylaminobenzaldehyde in 30% HCl. Yellow-orange spots are given with sulphapyrimidines.

## RIBONUCLEOSIDES

### 8 *Periodate oxidation–Schiff's reagent*

Ribonucleosides and 5′-ribonucleotides after periodate oxidation of the *cis*-glycol groups give Schiff's reaction for dialdehydes; *see* Carbohydrates, 37. Sensitivity for ribonucleotides, 20–50 μg.

## DEOXYRIBONUCLEOSIDES

### 9 *Cysteine hydrochloride*

Spray with 0.5% cysteine·HCl in 1.5M-$H_2SO_4$. Heat at 85°C for 5–10 min. Deoxyribose and deoxyribosides give pink spots. Sensitivity, 10–20 μg. Purine compounds react more quickly than pyrimidines. Not given by ribose or the ribonucleosides.

### 10 *Dische reaction*

Reagent: 1% diphenylamine in glacial acetic acid to which 2.75% by vol. $H_2SO_4$ has been added is diluted with 0.5 vol. $H_2O$. Spray. Clamp the paper between glass and heat at 90°C. Purine deoxyribonucleosides (10 $\mu$g) give purplish blue-spots in 5–10 min; pyrimidine deoxyribonucleosides (40–80 $\mu$g) give blue spots in 25–30 min. Deoxyribose reacts. Sensitivity of the pyrimidine derivatives increased 4-fold by bromination. Lightly spray with $Br_2$:water:acetic acid = 1:50:10 and heat between glass plates at 100°C for 5 min prior to diphenylamine reaction.

### 11 *Feulgen reaction for purine deoxyribonucleosides*

Spray with Schiff's reagent as in Carbohydrates, 37, made 0.05M with respect to $H_2SO_4$. Heat at 60°C for 6 min, then leave at RT for 24 hr. Purine deoxyribonucleosides give purple colours; sensitivity 10 $\mu$g.

## NUCLEOTIDES

### 12 *Molybdate–perchloric acid, etc.*

*See* Phosphate esters, 1.

### 13 *Uranyl acetate–ferrocyanide*

Dip in (*a*) 0.15% aq. uranyl acetate. Wash 20 sec in $H_2O$, then dip in (*b*) 3% aq. K ferrocyanide, made acid with HCl. Nucleotides give brown spots.

## PYRIDINE NUCLEOTIDES

### 14 *Ultraviolet light*

Fluorescence in u.v. light is shown by reduced pyridine nucleotides. Sensitivity 3 $\mu$g. (A spray of 2% $Na_2S_2O_4$:4% $NaHCO_3$ = 1:1 will reduce NAD and NADP to dihydro forms.)

### 15 *Ultraviolet light–potassium cyanide*

The paper is streaked with M-KCN from a Pasteur pipette. Addition compounds with intense fluorescence under u.v. light are formed by oxidized pyridine nucleotides, nicotinamide mononucleotide, and nicotinamide riboside.

### 16 *Sulphuric acid*

For use on thin-layer chromatograms. Spray with 50% $H_2SO_4$ and heat at 200°C for about 10 min until charring occurs.

### 17 *Iodine vapour*

Iodine vapour is used for transitory location on TLC if it is required to elute the spots for estimation.

## FLAVINS

### 18 *Ultraviolet light*

Yellow-green fluorescence is shown by flavins, especially after spraying with 0.05M-NaOH. Sensitivity, 0.01 $\mu$g. Remove any residual phenol solvent from the paper with an ether wash since it quenches fluorescence.

---

# 11 STEROIDS

Steroids vary in properties from the lipid-like, monofunctional cholesterol to the hydrophilic sapogenins and corticosteroids. Both adsorption and partition chromatographic procedures have been widely used to separate out the individual steroids but the use of adsorption is frequently precluded by the occurrence of decomposition of the polyoxygenated derivatives. Whilst conventional partition procedures are generally satisfactory, reversed phase conditions are required for the monofunctional steroids.

The location procedures described in this section may be assumed to be satisfactory for both paper and TLC procedures unless otherwise stated. It is, however, simple enough to test each reaction under the circumstances under which it will be used, and this is doubly necessary because reactions may be upset by both adsorbants and binders.

The following *abbreviations* will be used in this section; **St** = steroid; **keto** = oxo; **ol** = hydroxy; **al** = aldehyde; **3ol** = 3α- and/or 3β-hydroxy.

## UNSATURATED CENTRES

### 1 *Osmic acid*

Expose to the vapours from a 1% aq. soln. of osmic acid (very toxic!). Grey to black spots are produced with unsaturated steroids; 9(11)-ene, $10 \mu g$; 5-ene, $5 \mu g$; 4-en-3-one, $2 \mu g$. Oestrogens, negative.

### 2 *Ultraviolet light (for conjugated double bonds)*

(i) Absorption of 254 nm u.v. light. The weak fluorescence of the paper is quenched by absorption centres consisting of two or more double bonds in conjugation, e.g. 3:5 and 5:7-dienes; 4-en-3-one, 5-en-7-one, 16-en-20-one, 4-ene-3:6-dione, etc., $0.5 \mu g$. The sensitivity is increased five-fold by photography on document paper or by impregnating the paper with a fluorescing substance, e.g. 0.01% anthracene (Au) in light petroleum (40–60°C). The anthracene is inert and does not interfere with subsequent operations.

(ii) Absorption of 360 nm u.v. light. A similar quenching of fluorescence is shown by three or more double bonds in conjugation (but not aromatic centres), e.g. 4-ene-3:6-dione, $5 \mu g$. The increased sensitivity on anthracene treatment is available as above.

## KETONES

### 3 *Alkaline m-dinitrobenzene (Zimmerman reaction)*

(i) Reagents: (*a*) Dilute 1 vol. of stock 15M-KOH (80 g KOH + 60 ml $H_2O$) with 5 vol. ethanol, mix well ($N_2$ stream). (*b*) 2% ethanolic *m*-dinitrobenzene. Dip through (*a*), blot, dip through (*b*), blot, and warm gently with a hair drier.

17-one (no 15, 16 or 18-oxy) and 6-ol-4-en-3-one purple, $1 \mu g$; 3-one blue, $5 \mu g$; 4-en-3-one blue, $2 \mu g$; 4-ene-3:6-dione yellow (*see* procedure 5(i)) becoming black, $0.5 \mu g$; 20-one brown, $10 \mu g$; 21-deoxy-17-ol-20-one red, $2 \mu g$. Butenolides of the digitalis series, blue or purple, $1-5 \mu g$.

### 4 *2:4-Dinitrophenylhydrazine*

Dip through 0.3% dinitrophenylhydrazine in 0.3% HCl (v/v) in methanol. Heat 5 min at 90°C. Wash by drawing through 2M-NaOH in water, and 2M-HCl.

Most ketones give yellow spots, $2-5 \mu g$; but 4-en-3-ones give orange spots, $1 \mu g$.

### 5 *Alkali*

(i) Dip through M-NaOH. 4-ene-3:6-dione gives yellow colour, $2 \mu g$, and yellow fluorescence under 365 nm u.v. light, $0.5 \mu g$ 4-en-3-one-6-ol gives this reaction weakly on standing for some hours.

(ii) A yellow fluorescence, and weaker colour, appearing after warming, indicates 4-en-3-one, usually with three or more oxygen functions. Use of 50% methanolic NaOH with the paper sandwiched between glass plates to avoid evaporation makes

## 20 Detection of biochemical compounds

the results more reliable, 0.5 µg. Inclusion of a tetrazolium derivative suppresses background fluorescence and thus increases sensitivity.

### 6 *Nitroprusside (for aceto-derivatives)*

Reagent: Make a paste as follows in a quantity proportional to the area of the dish. Mix 0.5 g Na nitroprusside, 10 g $Na_2CO_3$ and 10 g $NH_4$ acetate with 10 ml methanol for each 100 cm$^2$ area of the dish to be used. Spread the paste to cover the floor of the dish, lay the chromatogram on the paste, and gently press into contact. The spots appear in 5 to 10 min, and intensify in the course of 1 hr. Methyl-ketones give violet spots; 21-deoxy-20-one, progesterone, (2 µg) 17- and other hydroxylic substituents do not interfere but 16-ene or 16-one does.

## ALDEHYDES

### 7 *Schiff's reaction*

Reagent: Dissolve 1 g basic fuchsin in 100 ml boiled-out distilled water, cool to 60°C, add 2 g K metabisulphite, mix to dissolve, and slowly add 20 ml M-HCl. Stopper, leave overnight, add animal charcoal, mix, and filter. This reagent remains colourless if stored in the dark at 4°C.
Dip, blot, heat at 60°C for 10 min, and suspend in a tank gassed out with $SO_2$. This preserves the colours; alternatively enclose between glass or polythene sheet to keep out the air. Free aldehydes react quickly, 2 µg; some involved in hemi-acetal condensation may react slowly.

## ALCOHOLS

Most reagents described in the earlier literature for the location of 'sterols' also detect 'sterones' and are largely unspecific. They are, of course, none the less useful and will be found in the miscellaneous section.

### 8 *Tert-butyl chromate oxidation (for β:γ-unsaturated alcohols)*

Reagent: Add 5 g $CrO_3$ to a cold mixture of 10 ml *tert*-butanol and 10 ml $CCl_4$, stir 10 min, add 65 ml $CCl_4$, and filter through 10 g $Na_2SO_4$ (anhyd.) on a sintered filter. Store at 4°C over $Na_2SO_4$; keeps 2 months or more. Immediately before use dilute 1 ml with a mixture of 80 ml xylene and 20 ml pyridine; shake the cloudy solution well. Spray evenly, heat at 100°C for 5 min. Dip through M-NaOH and dry at 100°C. 3β-ol-5-enes give yellow colours, 5 µg, and yellow fluorescences under 360 nm u.v. lamp, 1 µg, due to conversion to 4-ene-3:6-diones which also react if originally present. The colour and fluorescence may be slow to develop if the oxidation was incomplete, resulting in the 6-ol instead of the 6-one.

2α-Hydroxytestosterone gives a yellow colour during the heating with *tert*-butyl chromate, 5 µg, which fades on treatment with alkali. 7-Ketodehydro*epi*androsterone gives a blue fluorescence on alkali treatment.

### 9 *Tert-butyl chromate oxidation (for α-substituted ethanols)*

Use the *tert*-butyl chromate oxidation described in procedure 8. After heating at 100°C proceed as for procedure 6. Violet spots appear from 17:21-deoxy-20-ols, 10 µg, the 20-one also reacts and must be differentiated using procedure 6 without the oxidation.

### 10 *Phenol red (for α-glycols)*

Reagent: Dilute 2 ml of 0.1% phenol red in ethanol, and 1 ml of 0.15M-$H_3BO_3$ with 20 ml methanol. Titrate with 0.1M-NaOH to pH 11 on the pH meter. Spray the paper; yellow spots appear on a pink ground from acids and *cis*-α-diols. 16:17 diols, 5 µg. N.B. 2-ol-3-one-4-ene, 10 µg. Pregnane side-chain diols are negative.

## ACIDS

### 11 *Indicators*

pH indicator reagents which locate the long-chain fatty acids work well provided that neutral solvents are used in the chromatography.

To 0.1% bromocresol green in ethanol add 0.1 M-NaOH until bluish-green. Dilute 1:4 with acetone for use. Dip or spray. The background is green upon which the acids appear as yellow spots, bases are blue. The spots more stable if covered with plastic film to keep out $CO_2$.

### 12 *Salt formation*

Dip through 1% ammoniacal $AgNO_3$. Wash well with distilled water, irradiate with u.v. light for 10–20 sec, and immerse in photographic developer. Silver salts give black spots, $2\,\mu g$, which may be preserved by the photographic fixing process. Reducing substances do not interfere unless the paper is heated.

## ESTERS AND LACTONES

### 13 *Hydroxamic reaction*

Reagents: (*a*) $14\,g\,NH_2OH\cdot HCl$ in $100\,ml\,CH_3OH$; (*b*) 3.5 M-KOH in $CH_3OH$; (*c*) $2\,g\,FeCl_3$ in $100\,ml$ 10% HCl (v/v). Mix (*a*):(*b*) = 5:4, shake, and filter off the KCl. Spray (not dip), stand 10 min, and spray with (*c*). If brown $Fe(OH)_3$ appears, leave to dry and spray again with (*c*). Acetates and propionates, but not formates, of steroid alcohols, methyl and ethyl esters of steroid acids, and steroid lactones give purple spots, $2\,\mu g$.

### 14 *Nitroprusside ( for α:β-unsaturated lactones)*

Legal's reagent: 1% nitroprusside in 50% ethanolic M-NaOH. Dip; the cardenolides with α:β-unsaturated lactone rings give red to violet colours, e.g. digitonin, $5\,\mu g$.

## PHENOLS

These are all general reagents for phenols and thus care must be taken in interpreting the results purely in terms of phenolic steroids, the oestrogens.

### 15 *Diazo reaction*

Reagent: (*a*) 0.5% Brentamine Fast Blue B base (ICI Ltd.) in water. (*b*) $NaHCO_3$ adjusted to pH 9.0 (pH meter) with 10% NaOH. Stable indefintely in cold. For use mix equal volumes of (*a*) and (*b*). Dip and blot. All phenols give orange to red spots. Oestrogens, $5-10\,\mu g$.

### 16 *Sodium p-phenolsulphonate*

Spray with 2% Na *p*-phenolsulphonate in 85% $H_3PO_4$. Oestrogens give light green or orange colours, with blue-green, violet-pink, or yellow-orange fluorescence in u.v. light, $10\,\mu g$.

## REDUCING CENTRES

The principal reducing centre of the steroids is the α-ketol although α:β-unsaturated ketones also react weakly.

### 17 *Blue tetrazolium*

Reagents: (*a*) stock BTT, 0.2% dianisole-*bis*diphenyl-tetrazolium chloride (Merck) in water. (*b*) 2 M-NaOH. Mix (*a*):(*b*):EtOH = 3:10:5 immediately before use. Dip and blot. Blue spots appear at room temperatures above 20°C. Clear blue spots on a yellow ground are obtained if styryl tetrazolium (M & B 1767) is used.

Blue spots appear immediately for 21-ol-20-one, 16-ol-17-one, 1 $\mu$g. 2-ol-3-one reacts slowly, 1 $\mu$g. 4-en-2-one reacts slowly on warming, 10 $\mu$g.

The background does not develop and the spots are preserved by washing in 5% acetic acid in water.

### 18 *Triphenyltetrazolium chloride*

Reagent: 0.2% triphenyltetrazolium chloride (TPT) in water. Mix with $\frac{1}{2}$ vol. of 10% NaOH. Dip or spray and warm. Red spots appear on a pink ground from 21-ol-20-ones, 5 $\mu$g.

To differentiate 17-hydroxylated side chains precede the above by dipping through M-NaOH. Lay on a sheet of glass, cover with another sheet of glass, and heat at 100°C for 5 min. The 17-ols are destroyed by this procedure so that only 17-deoxy-21-ol-20-ones give the reddish spots.

### 19 *Ammoniacal silver nitrate*

Spray with 0.1M-AgNO$_3$:conc. NH$_3$:10% NaOH = 100:5:50, mixed just before use. After 5−10 min fix the spots in a bath of 25 g Na$_2$S$_2$O$_3$ + 15 g KAl(SO$_4$)$_2$ · 12H$_2$O in 1.5 lH$_2$O. After 30 min rinse for 30 min in H$_2$O. Dry at RT. Black or brown spots are given by cardiac aglycones containing the $\alpha$:$\beta$-unsaturated lactone ring. 2−25 $\mu$g. This test is also given by the $\alpha$-ketol group on C$_{17}$ characteristic of the corticosteroids, 10−15 $\mu$g. $\alpha$-Ketoaldehydes also give brown spots, but glycols do not.

### 'OGENIC REACTIONS

This group consists of reactions for the conversion of one chemical type into another for detection by one of the above reactions, or for detection of a small molecular fragment. The reactions for steroid moieties should be carried out on duplicate chromatograms, with and without the 'ogenic conversion, so that a distinction may be drawn between the preformed and formed reactors.

### 20 *Formaldehydogenic*

Reagent: Dissolve 15 g NH$_4$ acetate in 85 ml of 80% methanol. Add 1 ml acetyl-acetone, 0.3 ml gl. acetic acid, and 0.1 ml HIO$_4$ (50% aq. solution). Prepare the reagent and use it in diffuse light. Dip and blot. After 10 min the greenish-yellow fluorescent spots appear, becoming most intense after an hour when yellow colours will have developed. 21-ols with 20-ol or 20-one react, sens. 5 $\mu$g by colour and 1 $\mu$g by fluorescence. The reagent is generally specific for $\alpha$-substituted primary alcohols. It is ineffective on chromatograms prepared by impregnation with glycols.

### 21 *Acetaldehydogenic*

Reagents: (*a*) Dilute 5 ml of 50% aqueous HIO$_4$ solution with 5 ml water and 90 ml *tert*-butanol. (*b*) 2 g Na nitroprusside and 15 ml piperidine diluted to 100 ml with methanol. Dip through (*a*), blot, hang up for 5−10 min to react. Spray with (*b*). After 10 min blue spots appear on the pale yellow ground where acetaldehyde has been liberated. Among the steroids, only pregnane-17:20-diols react, 2 $\mu$g. This procedure is not applicable after a chromatographic run involving impregnation of the paper with a glycol.

An extension of the above procedure is as follows. Reagent: Freshly prepared 0.1% solution of Na (or K) BH$_4$ in 0.01M-NaOH in methanol (dilute aqueous M-NaOH). Dip, blot, hang in the room atmosphere 30 min to react, and proceed as above. 21-Deoxy-17-ol-20-ones now react in addition to the 17:20-diols, 10 $\mu$g.

### 22 *Specific 17-ketogenic*

Reagent: Freshly prepared 2.5% lead tetra-acetate in warm gl. acetic acid containing 10% acetic anhydride (lachrymatory). Dip, blot, and hang in air for 15 min.

Blow off the excess acid with a hair dryer and detect the ketones by procedure 3(i). The reagent is positive for the ketones listed under 3 (i) and with 17:20-diols, 5 μg.

An alternative oxidizing agent is 1% $HIO_4$ and 1% $H_2SO_4$ in 75% ethanol. Hang for 30 min to react and use procedure 3 (i) as described above. This reactions is sometimes accompanied by iodine liberation and the spots diffuse more than with $PbAc_4$.

### 23 *Non-specific* 17-*ketogenic*

Use *tert*-butyl chromate oxidant as described in procedure 8. Follow with procedure 3 (i) to detect ketones. Ketones listed under 3 (i) are detected together with all 17-ols, with or without the side chain, 2 μg. Side chains without 17-ol, 5–20 μg, mainly by detection of blue reacting 3-substituent.

### 24 *Aldehydogenic*

Dip through reagent (*a*) of procedure 21 and blot. Hang to react for 10 min, then suspend in an $SO_2$ atmosphere 15 min. Apply the aldehyde reagent of procedure 7. Steroid aldehydes present before oxidation and formed on oxidation give red to blue colours. 17-deoxy-20:21-diols, 10 μg. 17:20:21-triol, negative due to further oxidation. 16:17-diol, oestriol, 5 μg.

### 25 *Acidogenic*

Reagent: 1 vol. 0.7% $KIO_4$ in water diluted with 3 vol. ethanol. Dip, blot, and hang for an hour. Spray with reagent 11 for acids. Yellow spots indicate acids formed on oxidation or present before oxidation. 17-deoxy-21-ol-20-ones, 5 μg; 17:21-diol-20-ones, 10 μg; 16-ol-17-one, 5 μg; but 2-ol-3-one-4-ene, negative. Does not work on chromatograms impregnated with glycols.

## SAPOGENINS

### 26 *Haemolysis*

Spray with 2% suspension of guinea pig blood cells in physiological saline. Haemolysis by sapogenins causes lighter or darker spot on a tan ground. Sensitivity is less than 60 μg.

See also 39ii, 44i and 43.

## CONJUGATES

Steroid conjugates are compounds of steroids with another moiety and are formed during metabolism. Products of synthesis are not included in this term. The steroid portion may be detected by the steroid reagents provided that the position of conjugation does not block the reaction. Reactions for the non-steroid portion may be dependent on hydrolytic liberation from combination with the steroid. Whilst the conjugates are acidic in themselves, indicator reagents (procedure 11) are rarely of use since acidic solvents are used in the chromatographic procedure.

### 27 *Naphthoresorcinol* (*for glucuronides*)

Reagent: To 100 ml of 0.2% naphthoresorcinol in ethanol add 10 ml phosphoric acid. Dip, blot, and hang in warm air $\frac{1}{2}$–1 hr. Heat at 90°C, 5 min. Glucuronides give blue spots, 10 μg (free glucuronic acid, 1 μg).

The procedure is rendered more sensitive by using glucuronidase hydrolysis. Dip in 5000 units per ml glucuronidase in pH 4.5, 0.1M-acetate buffer. After hanging in an incubator for an hour at 37°C—preferably in a moist atmosphere—dry and apply the naphthoresorcinol reagent. Proceed directly to the 90°C heating. Glucuronides give blue spots, 2 μg, but they are rather more diffuse after the enzymic hydrolysis.

## 20 Detection of biochemical compounds

### 28 *Rhodizonic acid test (for sulphate)*

Reagents: (*a*) 20 ml conc. HCl diluted with 180 ml dioxan. (*b*) 20 mg $BaCl_2$ in 100 ml 75% methanol. (*c*) 12 mg K rhodizonate in 15 ml water, diluted with 10 ml 0.880 ammonia and 25 ml ethanol. Suspend the chromatogram in an enclosed chamber saturated with the vapours from (*a*) for 3 hr. Dry in an air stream in the fume cupboard for 1 hr. Dip through (*b*), dry in the air stream for 10 min. Dip through (*c*) and blot. Sulphates appear as yellow spots on a pink ground; sens. 10 $\mu$g for $DHASO_4$. This reaction is specific for all organic sulphates.

### 29 *Methylene blue test (for sulphate)*

Reagent: 20 mg methylene blue (922) histological stain and 5 g $Na_2SO_4$ are dissolved in 100 ml water, and 1 ml conc. $H_2SO_4$ is carefully added immediately before use. Dip and blot. Suspend in chloroform and agitate gently for 1–2 min. Large quantities of sulphate appear as pinkish-white zone on the blue ground before the $CHCl_3$ wash. Small quantities appear as white zones during the wash; sens. 1 $\mu$g for $DHASO_4$. This reaction is positive for all organic sulphates and also for organic phosphates. Counterstaining by 0.01% rhodamine-6G in chloroform produces reddish spots on a blue ground and a yellow fluorescence under 360 nm u.v. light, (0.1 $\mu$g).

## MISCELLANEOUS

All the following are unspecific procedures and care must be taken in interpreting the results since very different steroids may produce the same reaction and non-steroidal substances likewise.

### 30 *Phosphotungstic acid*

Reagent: 15% phosphotungstic acid in ethanol. Dip, blot, and heat in an oven at 80°C. A variety of colours are produced, especially from cholestane derivatives. 3$\beta$-ol-5-enes produce pink colours, 3 $\mu$g.

### 31 *Phosphomolybdic acid*

Reagent: 10% *dodeca*-molybdophosphoric acid in *n*-propanol, filter if cloudy (reject if not almost entirely dissolved). Use within an hour. Dip, blot, and heat whilst watching (infra-red lamps or oven with glass door). Blue spots on a yellow ground indicate substances such as steroids with a low degree of oxygenation. All steroids with mono- or di-oxygenated nuclei react; trioxygenated nuclei react on quick heating in the oven, 2–5 $\mu$g. Red colours are given by *cis*-testosterone and the 17-alkyl-testosterone derivatives. Does not work on adsorption TLC.

### 32 *Iodine*

(i) Dip in a saturated soln. of $I_2$ in pet. ether (60–80°C) to detect many steroids. Sensitivity for oestrogens, 1 $\mu$g. Yellow or brown spots.

(ii) Spray with 0.3% $I_2$ in 5% aq. KI followed by a $H_2O$ rinse. $\Delta^4$-3-Ketones (20–50 $\mu$g) give yellow spots; cortisone (15 $\mu$g), a blue spot.

(iii) Spray with a cold saturated soln. of $I_2$ in EtOH. This gives a blue colour with cholic acid.

(iv) Stock reagent: Hydriodic acid (sp. gr. 1.5) saturated with $I_2$. This solution is diluted ten times with tap-water just before use. Immerse the paper. Rinse with tap-water until the background is free of colour. Functional groups giving a reaction with this reagent are $\alpha$:$\beta$-unsaturated ketones, 17-ketones, and $C_3$-hydroxyl groups on a molecule containing a methyl ketone or $\alpha$-ketol side chain. Brown, orange, and blue colours are given; 8–20 $\mu$g.

Of these procedures (i) is the most satisfactory if other reagents are to be applied in sequence. The other procedures give colours with a wider variety of steroids and may be most satisfactory in particular problems.

### 33 *Bromine*

Spray with a saturated aq. soln. of $Br_2$. A crimson spot is given by the non-steroid diethylstilboestrol. $5 \mu g$.

A modified method for detecting sterols is as follows. Expose to $Br_2$ vapour for 30 sec. Spray with (*a*) saturated KI in MeOH. Then spray with (*b*) 20% starch soln. Sterols give dark blue spots on a colourless or light blue ground; $10 \mu g$.

### 34 *Potassium permanganate*

Spray with 0.2% $KMnO_4$ in 5% $Na_2CO_3$. Rinse in $H_2O$ until the background is colourless. Corticosteroids give brown colours. Groups which react with this spray are 4-en-3-one, $\alpha$-ketol, 17:20:21-triol; $30-70 \mu g$.

### 35 *Sulphuric acid*

(i) Concentrated $H_2SO_4$ is applied in a thin layer to a glass plate and the filter paper is laid on this. Vivid green fluorescence is shown with compounds containing an 11-hydroxyl group, especially compound F. The reaction is useful for characterization of $C_{19}O_3$ steroids.

(ii) An alternative method using (15% $SO_3$) fuming $H_2SO_4$ gives orange-yellow to red-brown colours with oestrogens in visible light and yellow-green or red-brown fluorescence in u.v. light. Sensitivity, $5 \mu g$. This method is sensitive, but non-specific for $C_{19}$ and $C_{21}$ steroids. Sensitivity range: pregnanediols (orange spots), $5 \mu g$; androstanedione (pink), $50 \mu g$.

(iii) Reagent: 1% $H_2SO_4$ in ethanol. Dip, blot, and heat at $100-120°C$. Watch carefully and remove from the oven at the first signs of charring. 4-en-3-ones give red colours with orange fluorescence, sensitivity $1 \mu g$; most steroids react, e.g. THE yellow and THF blue fluorescence, sensitivity $2 \mu g$.

### 36 *Phosphoric acid*

(i) Dip through 70% $H_3PO_4$ in water, lay on a glass plate, and heat at $90°C$. A great variety of colours are produced including purples from pregnanetriols, $1-2 \mu g$. 360 nm u.v. light produces various fluorescent emissions. 85% ethanolic $H_3PO_4$ has been used for bile acids.

(ii) Dip through 20% $H_3PO_4$ in water and heat at $90°C$ for 20 min. Most steroids give colours which differ from those of procedure 35iii.

### 37 *Hydrochloric acid*

Dip through conc. HCl, lay on a glass sheet and heat at $60°C$ for 5 min. 17 $\alpha$-alkylated steroids give characteristic colours and fluorescence emissions.

### 38 *Formic acid*

Dip through cold formic acid (98–100%). A green colour changing to blue is produced after a few minutes by 7 $\alpha$-hydroxydehydro*epi*androsterone.

### 39 *Trichloroacetic acid*

(i) Reagent: 10 g TCA in 20 ml ethanol. Dip, blot, and heat at $70°C$ for 10 min. Many steroids give yellow or pink fluorescences (360 nm u.v. light) but the pregnane-3:17:20-triols give characteristic blue fluorescences, $2 \mu g$.

(ii) 25% TCA in $CHCl_3$ heated at $100°C$ for 20 min gives colours and fluorescences with cardiac glycosides and sapogenins.

### 40 *Liebermann—Burchard reaction*

Reagent: Add 5 ml conc. $H_2SO_4$ slowly and with agitation to 20 ml ice-cold acetic anhydride (lachrymatory). Dip rapidly and lay out on a glass sheet. Alternatively, lay on a glass sheet and spread the reagent with the aid of a glass rod used as a roller. Cover with another glass or plastic sheet. Within a few minutes green colours appear from cholesterol or its esters, which slowly change to blue; 5 μg.

### 41 *Phosphomolybdotungstic acid*

Spray with Folin's phenol reagent (BDH), freshly diluted with 5 vol. $H_2O$. Expose to $NH_3$ vapour for 5 min. Oestrogens (0.5 μg) give blue spots. Other steroids with an α-ketol side chain give intense blue colours.

### 42 *Aniline phthalate*

*See* Carbohydrates, 22(i). Yellow, orange, or brown spots on a white ground are given by steroids with a $\Delta^4$-3-keto group in the A ring. Sensitivity is increased 10 times when *p*-phenylenediamine is substituted for aniline in the spray. Sensitivity, 2—3 μg.

### 43 *Aromatic aldehydes*

Spray with 0.5 ml anisaldehyde in 50 ml $CH_3COOH$ + 1 ml conc. $H_2SO_4$. Heat at 90°C for 2—5 min. Corticosteroids give coloured spots.

The following method detects steroidal sapogenins. Spray with (*a*) 1% soln. in EtOH of one of the aldehydes mentioned below. Dry for 5 min. Then spray with (*b*) acetic anhydride: conc. $H_2SO_4$ = 12:1. Heat at 85—90°C until spots appear. Vanillin, anisaldehyde, cinnamaldehyde, and salicylaldehyde give rise to yellow spots on a white-grey ground with steroid sapogenins; *p*-dimethylaminobenzaldehyde gives rise to rose spots on a yellow ground; 4-acetoxy-2-naphthaldehyde is the most sensitive reagent giving red spots with sapogenins. Suitable for TLC.

### 44 *Antimony trichloride*

This reagent is very poisonous.

(i) Spray with 10—20% $SbCl_3$ in $CHCl_3$. Heat at 70—90°C for 4 min. Various colours in visible and u.v. light are given by corticosteroids, oestrogens (brown, yellow, and pink spots); $C_{19}$ and $C_{21}$ steroids containing an —OH group (20—50 μg); *Digitalis* glycosides ($<0.5$ μg); sterols: ergosterol (0.5 μg) and cholesterol (5 μg); and steroidal sapogenins (mainly yellow or reddish orange spots; sens. 2—5 μg).

(ii) Spray with 25 g anhyd. $SbCl_3$ in 5 ml nitrobenzene. This has been used as a general spray for non-ketonic, hydroxylated steroids (1—2 μg).

(iii) A fresh solution of 380 g $SbCl_3$ in 100 ml acetic anhydride is sprayed after exposing the paper for 20 min to an atmosphere of $Cl_2$. Heat at 90—100°C to dry the paper. Spots both fluorescent and non-fluorescent in u.v. light are obtained. 0.5—5 μg except cortisone.

(iv) Spray with 50% $SbCl_3$ in gl. acetic acid. Heat at 90—96°C for 3—5 min. Rose, purple, and yellow colours are given by bile acids.

### 45 *Antimony pentachloride*

This reagent is very poisonous.

Spray with 20—40% $SbCl_5$ in $CHCl_3$. Various colours, mainly brown and red, are given by oestrogens (15 μg); vitamin D sterols; ergosterol (0.5 μg); cholesterol (5 μg).

### 46 *Ferric chloride*

Spray with 2% $FeCl_3$ in MeOH. Oestrogens give purple spots; 20 μg. Alternatively a spray containing 1% $FeCl_3$ + 1% K ferricyanide may be used. Oestrogens, corticosteroids, and androgens give blue spots. A permanent record is obtained by washing the paper in 0.1 M-HCl and then in $H_2O$.

### 47 *Zinc chloride*

(i) Spray with 30% anhyd. $ZnCl_2$ in MeOH. Heat at 130°C for 1 hr. Various colours in visible light and fluorescence in u.v. light are given by hydroxysteroids, $2-10\,\mu g$.

(ii) A modification of this spray is 40% $ZnCl_2$ in gl. $CH_3COOH$:benzoyl chloride: $CHCl_3 = 5:7:12$. Heat at 90°C for 5 min. Mainly orange, pink, or brown colours with yellow or pink fluorescence in u.v. are given by corticosteroids and oestrogens, sensitivity $5\,\mu g$. Suitable for TLC.

(iii) Reagent: $4\,g\ ZnCl_2$ mixed with 0.5 ml water. Slowly add 25 ml acetyl chloride with careful mixing. Use within an hour. Dip through the reagent, lay on a glass plate, and heat at 100°C. A great variety of colours are produced by a wide range of steroids, $2-5\,\mu g$.

### 48 *Stannous chloride*

Reagent: Dissolve $0.3\,g\ SnCl_2$ and $4\,g$ urea in 10 ml 40% $H_2SO_4$. Dip, blot, and heat on glass at 80°C. Fluorescent emissions (360 nm u.v. light) are produced by oestrogens, $2-5\,\mu g$ and corticosteroids, $10\,\mu g$.

---

# 12 VITAMINS

## FAT-SOLUBLE VITAMINS

### VITAMIN A

#### 1 *Antimony trichloride*

This reagent is the most specific one known for vitamin A. Spray with a saturated solution of $SbCl_3$ in $CHCl_3$. Blue colours are given by vitamin A, its esters, retinene, and anhydro-vitamin A. The reagent is very poisonous!

#### 2 *Ultraviolet light*

Vitamin A fluoresces with a bright, golden-brown colour under short-wave light (256 nm).

### VITAMIN D

#### 1 *Potassium permanganate*

On silica gel layers, spray with alkaline $KMnO_4$ to give brown spots.

#### 2 *Ultraviolet light*

On paper chromatograms, vitamins D show as dark spots on a fluorescent ground under short-wave light (256 nm). Under long-wave light (365 nm), vitamins and provitamins appear fluorescent.

#### 3 *Antimony trichloride*

Spray with 24% $SbCl_3$ in $CHCl_3$ and heat the paper. Vitamins D give brown spots, whereas provitamins D and cholesterol have a violet tinge. Reagent very poisonous!

## 4 *Other colour reactions*

Vitamins D give well-defined colours with many acidic reagents, most of them non-specifically. Antimony pentachloride* (20% in $CHCl_3$) is very sensitive for chromatographic detection (brown-blue colours). Brown colours are also given with 33% bismuth trichloride in ethanol, or 15% silicotungstic or phosphotungstic acid in ethanol. Dimethyl-*p*-phenylene-diamine in water gives blue colour. After being sprayed with the appropriate reagent, the chromatograms are generally heated for some time at 60°C. 1 $\mu$g quantities are detectable.

*Very poisonous.

### VITAMIN E (TOCOPHEROLS)

## 1 *Dipyridyl-ferric chloride*

Spray with a freshly-prepared mixture of 2:2′-dipyridyl (0.5%) and $FeCl_3 \cdot 6H_2O$ (0.2%) in EtOH. Tocopherols give bright red spots. Sensitivity 2−5 $\mu$g. The sensitivity of the reagent can be considerably increased by the use of other Fe-complexing reagents instead of 2:2′-dipyridyl. 4:7-Diphenyl-1:10-phenanthroline is especially effective, increasing the depth of colour $2\frac{1}{2}$ times.

## 2 *Ultraviolet light*

If $ZnCO_3$-impregnated paper contains a few ppm of sodium fluorescein, tocopherols can be observed as dark spots on a fluorescent ground under short-wave light (256 nm). Spraying chromatograms with an aqueous solution of sodium fluorescein is also effective.

## 3 *Potassium ferricyanide*

Spray with (*a*) 2% HCl in EtOH. Dry and then spray with (*b*) 0.05% aq. $K_3Fe(CN)_6$. Tocopherols give deep blue colours. Sensitivity 1 $\mu$g. Wash in $H_2O$ and dry in the dark.

## 4 *Diazo reaction*

Spray with an excess of 2% $Na_2CO_3$, followed by 0.5% diazotized *o*-dianisidine. Tocopherols lacking a methyl group at C-5 give blue or violet colours, readily distinguishable from each other. Tocopherols lacking a methyl group at C-7 give pale reddish-amber spots. Fully substituted tocopherols give no reaction.

## 5 *Antimony pentachloride*

Spray thin-layer chromatograms with 20% $SbCl_5$* in $CHCl_3$ and observe after 3 min. The known tocopherols give widely differing colours, which depend also on the adsorbent being used. Limit of detection, 2 $\mu$g. Optimal colour with 20−50 $\mu$g.

*Very poisonous.

### VITAMIN K

## 1 *Ultraviolet light*

Vitamins K show as dark spots on a fluorescent ground under short-wave u.v. light.

## 2 *Diazo reaction*

Spray with a mixture of *p*-nitroaniline (0.4% in 0.33M-HCl), $NaNO_2$ (1% in $H_2O$), urea or ammonium sulphamate (5% in $H_2O$) and $H_2O$ in the following proportions, 1:1:1:7. Vitamin K gives a reddish spot.

### 3 Leucomethylene blue

The reagent is prepared by dissolving 100 mg of methylene blue in 100 ml of EtOH, adding 1 ml of acetic acid and 1 g of zinc dust, and swirling until the blue is discharged. Vitamins K give blue spots (about 1 $\mu$g detectable) when sprayed with the reagent, but the reaction is given by many other quinones, especially the ubiquinones and plastoquinones.

## WATER-SOLUBLE VITAMINS

### THIAMIN AND DERIVATIVES

### 1 Ultraviolet light

Strong absorption is shown by thiamin and its derivatives at 250−60 nm. Chromatographic solvents which absorb u.v. cannot be used, e.g. phenol, $p$-toluenesulphonic acid.

### 2 Potassium ferricyanide

Spray with 2.5% $K_3Fe(CN)_6$ :10% NaOH:55% EtOH = 0.1:5:5. Thiamin and its esters are oxidized to thiochromes which have a blue fluorescence in u.v. light. Sensitivity 0.5 $\mu$g.

### 3 Potassium bismuth iodide

Reagent: 5 g K bismuth iodide is added to 100 ml $H_2O$ containing 0.5 ml conc. HCl. Boil and filter when cold. On spraying with this reagent thiamin derivatives give red-purple to orange spots. Remove background colour by washing in ether saturated with $H_2O$. Sensitivity 0.1 $\mu$g.

### PYRIDOXINE

### 1 Ultraviolet light

Pyridoxine absorbs at 297 nm in u.v. light.

### 2 2:6-Dichloroquinone chloroimide (Gibbs' reagent)*

Spray with 0.1% 2:6-dichloroquinone chloroimide in benzene. Then expose the paper to $NH_3$ vapour. A blue spot is given by vitamin $B_6$. Sensitivity 1 $\mu$g.

  * **Warning**: Closely related compounds are explosive above 50°C.

### 3 Phenylhydrazine

Spray with a saturated soln. of phenylhydrazine in 95% EtOH containing 10% $CH_3COOH$. A yellow spot is given with pyridoxine (1 $\mu$g).

### 4 Diazotized p-aminoacetophenone

Component solutions of spraying reagent: (a) 3.18 g $p$-aminoacetophenone in 45 ml conc. HCl diluted to 1 l with $H_2O$. (b) 2.25% $NaNO_2$. (c) 25% Na acetate. Spray with (a):(b):(c) = 2:10:10, freshly mixed. Heat at 50−60°C for 10 min. Pink, orange, and yellow colours are given by pyridoxine, pyridoxal, and pyridoxamine and their phosphates.

### NICOTINIC ACID AND RELATED COMPOUNDS

### 1 König reaction

Hang the paper in a closed vessel over cyanogen bromide crystals for 30−60 min. isoNicotinic acid hydrazide, nicotinic acid hydrazide, and isopropylisonicotinic acid hydrazide give a specific blue fluorescence in u.v. light. Follow the CNBr treatment by spraying with one of the following aromatic amines:

(i) Spray with 2 g *p*-aminobenzoic acid in 75 ml 0.75M-HCl diluted to 100 ml with 96% EtOH. Nicotinic acid gives a yellow spot; nicotinamide, deep yellow; nicotinuric acid, orange; diethylnicotinamide (coramine), pink. Sensitivity 0.1 μg. Little or no colour is given with *iso*nicotinic derivatives.

(ii) Spray with 0.25% benzidine in 50% EtOH. Nicotinic acid gives a red-violet spot; *iso*nicotinic acid, grey-lavender; nicotinamide, red-violet; coramine, violet. Sensitivity 5 μg. Warning: Benzidine is carcinogenic.

## 2 *Picryl chloride*

Dip in 1.5% picryl chloride in EtOH. Dry. Hang in $NH_3$ vapour. Red spots are given with pyridine, nicotinic acid, *iso*nicotinic acid, nicotinamide, and *iso*nicotinamide, but only the red-purple spots of *iso*nicotinic acid hydrazide, nicotinic acid hydrazide, and *iso*propyl *iso*nicotinic acid hydrazide remain after exposure to acetic acid vapour. Sensitivity 5 μg.

## PANTOTHENIC ACID AND DERIVATIVES (COENZYME A)

### 1 *Ninhydrin*

*See* Amino acids, 1. Pantoic acid derivatives give purple spots. Pantothenic acid, no colour.

### 2 *β-Naphthoquinone-4-sulphonate (Folin's reagent)*

Spray with 0.5% β-naphthoquinone-4-sulphonate, adjusted to pH 9.2 to 9.4 with Na tetraborate. Heat at 100°C for 10 min. Pantothenic acid gives an intense yellow spot; β-alanine, reddish orange. Allow to stay in the light for several hours to bleach the background.

### 3 *Ultraviolet light*

Quenching of the natural fluorescence of the paper is shown by CoA and acetyl-CoA due to the adenine constituent.

### 4 *Nitroprusside*

Spray with (*a*) 3% NaOH in 95% MeOH. Then spray with (*b*) nitroprusside reagent, Amino acids, 17 (*a*). This gives a positive test for the −SH group of alkyl mercaptans.

An alternative method is to spray with (*a*) 5% NaCN and 5% $Na_2CO_3$ in 25% EtOH, then after a few minutes spray with (*b*) 2% Na nitroprusside in 75% EtOH. This method detects the −S−S− link of oxidized CoA, etc.

## INOSITOL

### 1 *Alkaline silver nitrate*

Detected as a non-reducing substance by either the acetone-$AgNO_3$−alcoholic NaOH or ammoniacal $AgNO_3$ reagents (Carbohydrates, 1). These sprays, and those listed under 2 (below) react with other sugar compounds. Failure of the suspected $AgNO_3$-inositol spot to react with the specific sprays for various classes of reducing sugars will at least eliminate these types of compounds.

### 2 *Other carbohydrate sprays*

Many of the more general carbohydrate sprays, based on reagents such as periodate will detect inositol.

### 3 *Rhodizonic acid reaction*

Reagents: (*a*) 10 ml conc. $HNO_3$ in 90 ml EtOH. (*b*) *n*-BuOH:glacial acetic:10% (w/v) aq. Ba acetate:$CaCl_2$ = 40:10:10:0.5 g. (*c*) 5% (w/v) $CaCl_2$ in 50% aq. EtOH. Dip in (*a*), heat 95–100°C for 10 min, expose to $NH_3$ vapour 1–2 sec then dip in (*b*). Inositol gives an orange colour on a white ground; sensitivity 8–10 µg. For greater sensitivity, spray with (*c*) and heat at 95–100°C for 2 min; orange spots turning pink; sensitivity 1 µg. A modification will also detect inositol phosphate. Amino acids and aldohexoses do not interfere and the reagent may be used following ninhydrin detection of amino acids.

### ASCORBIC ACID

### 1 *Alkaline silver nitrate*

Detected by the various alkaline $AgNO_3$ spray reagents (*see* Carbohydrates, 1).

### 2 *2:6-Dichlorophenol indophenol (Tillmann's reagent)*

Reagent: 0.8 g 2:6-dichlorophenol indophenol is dissolved in 1 l $H_2O$ and diluted with an equal volume of EtOH. Spray. Ascorbic acid and related dienols give colourless spots on a dark blue ground. Sensitivity 1–2 µg.

### 3 *Ferric salt–o-phenanthroline*

Spray with 0.15% ferric ammonium sulphate:2% *o*-phenanthroline HCl = 1:9. Dry at 80–100°C. Uric acid (0.5 µg) and ascorbic acid reduce $Fe^{3+}$ to $Fe^{2+}$, which reacts giving a red spot.

# 21 Ion exchange, gel filtration, and affinity chromatography media

## 1 ION EXCHANGE RESINS

Ion exchange resins consist of a cross-linked polymer matrix to which ionized or ionizable groups are attached. Most ion exchange resins are based on a polystyrene (S in the tables) or polymethacrylic acid (A) matrix, cross-linked by incorporating a proportion of divinylbenzene. The resin is formed into spherical beads, or in a few cases is granular, and has a relatively rigid gel-like structure. The size of the pores in gel-type resins, and so the size of molecule that can diffuse into the resin beads, depends on the degree of crosslinking of the resin, which in turn depends on the divinylbenzene content. Resins of relatively high crosslinkage (8–12%) are suitable for the chromatography of small ions, whereas resins of low crosslinkage (2–4%) are suitable for larger molecules. Resins of low crosslinkage swell more on hydration and have a lower physical stability than those of higher crosslinkage.

More recently a number of macroporous (MP) or macroreticular (MR) ion exchange resins have been introduced. These are also based on polystyrene or polyacrylic polymers but have large discrete pores penetrating a rigid structure. The large pores facilitate the access of large molecules, such as proteins, to the ionizable groups in the interior of the beads.

Many ion exchange resins are available in 'analytical' or 'chromatographic' grades, which have been specially purified and carefully sized within specified limits. The properties given in the tables refer to these grades of resin where they are available.

*Stability.* The maximum working temperatures of the various resins are given in the tables. Most resins show good stability to organic solvents, such as alcohols, and to all but the strongest oxidizing and reducing agents. Most are also stable, though not necessarily effective ion exchangers (see below), over a wide range of pH.

*Particle size.* As the particle size of an ion exchange resin is decreased, the time required to reach equilibrium decreases, leading to an increased efficiency of a given volume of resin and to sharper separations. The sharpness of the separation also depends on the range of particle sizes present in the resin. For column operation, 100–200 mesh or finer particles are recommended, whereas coarser grades are more suitable for batch operation. For desalting, particle size is not critical.

*Exchange capacity.* The exchange capacity of an ion exchange resin will depend not only on the concentration of ionizable groups on the resin, but also on their state of ionization. Exchangers bearing strongly acidic or basic groups are effective over a wide range of pH. Those with weakly acidic or basic groups will have a more limited useful range (as indicated in the tables), depending on the $pK_a$ of the functional group.

*Suppliers.* The tables give details of ion exchange resins from the following manufacturers:

(i) Dow Chemical Company, Midland, Michigan, USA: Dowex resins.

(ii) Bio-Rad Laboratories, Richmond, California, USA: AG resins, which are analytical grade equivalents of Dowex resins; Bio-Rex resins; Chelex resin.

(iii) Rohm and Haas Company, Philadelphia, Pennsylvania, USA: Amberlite resins.

(iv) Dia-Prosim Ltd.: Duolite resins – supplied by BDH Chemicals Ltd., Poole, Dorset, UK. These resins are the successors to Zerolit, Zeo-Karb, and De-Acidite resins.

# 21 Ion exchange, gel filtration, and affinity chromatography media

**(a) ANION EXCHANGE RESINS**

| Designation | Polymer type[*] | Basicity and functional group | Crosslinkage (%) | Particle size (US standard mesh range) | |
|---|---|---|---|---|---|
| Dowex 1-X2 (AG 1-X2) | S | Strong base $-CH_2 \cdot N^+(CH_3)_3$ | 2 | Dry | 50–100, 100–200, 200–400, minus 400 |
| Dowex 1-X4 (AG 1-X4) | S | Strong base $-CH_2 \cdot N^+(CH_3)_3$ | 4 | Dry | 20–50, 50–100, 100–200, 200–400, minus 400 |
| Dowex 1-X8 (AG 1-X8) | S | Strong base $-CH_2 \cdot N^+(CH_3)_3$ | 8 | Dry | 20–50, 50–100, 100–200, 200–400, minus 400 |
| AG MP-1 | MP | Strong base $-CH_2 \cdot N^+(CH_3)_3$ | | Dry | 20–50, 50–100, 100–200, 200–400 |
| Amberlite IRA-401 | S | Strong base $-CH_2 \cdot N^+(CH_3)_3$ | 4 | Wet | 16–50 |
| Amberlite IRA-402 | S | Strong base $-CH_2 \cdot N^+(CH_3)_3$ | 6 | Wet | 16–50 |
| Amberlite IRA-400 | S | Strong base $-CH_2 \cdot N^+(CH_3)_3$ | 8 | Wet | 16–50 |
| Amberlite CG-400 | S | Strong base $-CH_2 \cdot N^+(CH_3)_3$ | 8 | Dry | 100–200, 200–400 |
| Amberlite IRA-904 | MR | Strong base $-CH_2 \cdot N^+(CH_3)_3$ | | Wet | 20–50 |
| Duolite 113 | S | Strong base $-CH_2 \cdot N^+(CH_3)_3$ | 2–3 | Wet | 16–50 |
| | S | Strong base $-CH_2 \cdot N^+(CH_3)_3$ | 3–5 | Wet | 16–50 |
| | S | Strong base $-CH_2 \cdot N^+(CH_3)_3$ | 7–9 | Wet | 16–50, 50–100 |
| Duolite A161 | MP | Strong base $-CH_2 \cdot N^+(CH_3)_3$ | | Wet | 16–45 |
| Dowex 2-X8 (AG 2-X8) | S | Strong base $-CH_2 \cdot N^+(CH_3)_2 C_2H_4OH$ | 8 | Dry | 20–50, 50–100, 100–200, 200–400 |
| Dowex 2-X10 (AG 2-X10) | S | Strong base $-CH_2 \cdot N^+(CH_3)_2 C_2H_4OH$ | 10 | Dry | 100–200 |
| Amberlite IRA-410 | S | Strong base $-CH_2 \cdot N^+(CH_3)_2 C_2H_4OH$ | 8 | Wet | 16–50 |
| Duolite A116 | S | Strong base $-CH_2 \cdot N^+(CH_3)_2 C_2H_4OH$ | | Wet | 16–50 |
| Duolite A162 | MP | Strong base $-CH_2 \cdot N^+(CH_3)_2 C_2H_4OH$ | | Wet | 16–45 |
| Bio-Rex 9 | | Strong base | | Dry | 20–50, 50–100, 100–200, 200–400 |
| Bio-Rex 5 | AA | Mixed weak and strong basic groups, tertiary amine plus $-CH_2 \cdot N^+(CH_3)_2 C_2H_4OH$ | | Dry | 20–50, 50–100, 100–200, 200–400 |
| Duolite A303 | S | Mixed weak and strong basic groups, tertiary amine plus quaternary ammonium | 7–9 | Wet | 16–50 |
| Doulite A378 | MP | Mixed weak and strong basic groups, tertiary amine plus quaternary ammonium | | Wet | 16–50 |
| Dowex 3-X4A (AG 3-X4A) | S | Weak base $-CH_2 \cdot NR_2$ | 4 | Dry | 20–50, 100–200, 200–400 |

*Footnotes.* See p. 506.

504

| Wet exchange capacity (meq/ml) | Water content (%) | Max. operating temp. (°C) | Comments |
|---|---|---|---|
| 0.7 | 70–78 | 50 (OH⁻ form)<br>150 (Cl⁻ form) | Order of selectivity for monovalent anions:<br>I > phenolate > $HSO_4$ > $NO_3$ > Br > CN > Cl<br>> $HCO_3$ > formate > acetate > OH > F. |
| 1.2 | 59–65 | 50 (OH⁻ form)<br>150 (Cl⁻ form) | |
| 1.4 | 39–45 | 50 (OH⁻ form)<br>150 (Cl⁻ form) | |
| 1.2 | 56–64 | | |
| 1.0 | 59–65 | 60 (OH⁻ form)<br>77 (Cl⁻ form) | |
| 1.25 | 53–60 | 60 (OH⁻ form)<br>77 (Cl⁻ form) | |
| 1.4 | 42–48 | 60 (OH⁻ form)<br>77 (Cl⁻ form) | |
| 1.4 | | 60 (OH⁻ form)<br>77 (Cl⁻ form) | Chromatographic grade of IRA-400. |
| 0.7 | 56–62 | 60 (OH⁻ form)<br>77 (Cl⁻ form) | |
| 1.3 | 1.5–2.0† | 60 | Equivalent to Zerolit FF(ip) and De-Acidite FF(ip). |
| 1.3 | 1.0–1.5† | 60 | |
| 1.3 | 0.6–1.0† | 60 | |
| 1.1 | 53–57 | 60 (OH⁻ form)<br>100 (Cl⁻ form) | Equivalent to<br>Zerolit MPF. |
| 1.4 | 34–40 | 30 (OH⁻ form)<br>150 (Cl⁻ form) | Order of selectivity for monovalent anions:<br>phenolate > I > $HSO_4$ > $NO_3$ > Br > CN > Cl > OH ><br>formate > acetate > F. |
| 1.5 | 28–36 | 30 (OH⁻ form)<br>150 (Cl⁻ form) | |
| 1.4 | 40–45 | 40 (OH⁻ form)<br>77 (Cl⁻ form) | |
| 1.4 | 43–50 | 35 (OH⁻ form)<br>75 (Cl⁻ form) | Equivalent to Zerolit N(ip) and<br>De-Acidite N(ip). |
| 1.1 | 48–53 | 35 (OH⁻ form)<br>75 (Cl⁻ form) | Equivalent to Zerolit MPN. |
| 1.3 | 46–54 | 50 (OH⁻ form)<br>100 (Cl⁻ form) | Very resistant to strong<br>oxidizing agents<br>eg. hot conc. $HNO_3$. |
| 2.8 | 50–58 | 60 | |
| 1.3 | 46–51 | 70 | Equivalent to<br>Zerolit H(ip) and<br>De-Acidite H(ip). |
| 1.6 | 55–61 | 60 (OH⁻ form)<br>100 (Cl⁻ form) | Equivalent to Zerolit MPH. |
| 1.9 | 40–45 | 65 | Use at or below pH 7. |

| Designation | Polymer type* | Basicity and functional group | Crosslinkage (%) | Particle size (US standard mesh range) | |
|---|---|---|---|---|---|
| Amberlite IR-45 | S | Weak base, tertiary amine | | Wet | 16–50 |
| Amberlite IRA-67 | A | Weak base, tertiary amine | | Wet | 18–50 |
| Amberlite IRA-93 | MR | Weak base, tertiary amine | | Wet | 16–50 |

## (b) CATION EXCHANGE RESINS

| Designation | Polymer type* | Acidity and functional group | Crosslinkage (%) | Particle size (US standard mesh range) | |
|---|---|---|---|---|---|
| Dowex 50W-X2 (AG 50W-X2) | S | Strong acid $-SO_3^-$ | 2 | Dry | 50–100, 100–200, 200–400 |
| Dowex 50W-X4 (AG 50W-X4) | S | Strong acid $-SO_3^-$ | 4 | Dry | 20–50, 50–100, 100–200, 200–400, minus 400 |
| Dowex 50W-X8 (AG 50W-X8) | S | Strong acid $-SO_3^-$ | 8 | Dry | 20–50, 50–100, 100–200, 200–400, minus 400 |
| Dowex 50W-X12 (AG 50W-X12) | S | Strong acid $-SO_3^-$ | 12 | Dry | 50–100, 100–200, 200–400, minus 400 |
| Dowex 50W-X16 (AG 50W-X16) | S | Strong acid $-SO_3^-$ | 16 | Dry | 200–400 |
| Amberlite IR-120 | S | Strong acid $-SO_3^-$ | 8 | Wet | 16–50 |
| Amberlite CG-120 | S | Strong acid $-SO_3^-$ | 8 | Dry | 100–200, 200–400 |
| Duolite 225 | S | Strong acid $-SO_3^-$ | 4 | Wet | 16–50, 50–100 |
| | S | Strong acid $-SO_3^-$ | 8 | Wet | 16–50, 50–100, 100–200, over 200 |
| | S | Strong acid $-SO_3^-$ | 12 | Wet | 16–50, 50–100 |
| Duolite C255 | S | Strong acid $-SO_3^-$ | 10 | Wet | 16–35 |
| Duolite C26C | MP | Strong acid $-SO_3^-$ | High | Wet | 16–50 |
| Amberlite IRC-50 | A | Weak acid $-COO^-$ | 5 | Wet | 16–50 |
| Amberlite CG-50 | A | Weak acid $-COO^-$ | 5 | Dry | 100–200, 200–400 |
| Duolite 436 | A | Weak acid $-COO^-$ | 2.5 | Wet | 16–50 |
| Bio-Rex 70 | MR, A | Weak acid $-COO^-$ | 10 | Dry | 20–50, 50–100, 100–200, 200–400, minus 400 |
| Chelex 100 | S | Weak acid $-CH_2N \big\langle {}^{CH_2COO^-}_{CH_2COO^-}$ | | Dry | 50–100, 100–200, 200–400, minus 400 |

* Polymer type:
S, polystyrene resin, crosslinked with divinylbenzene;
A, polymethacrylic resin, crosslinked with divinylbenzene;
AA, polyalkyleneamine resin;
MP, macroporous resin;
MR, macroreticular resin.

† Water regain:
   Anion exchange resins, weight of water associated with 1.0 g of dry resin chloride, measured by drying the resin after centrifuging to remove interstitial water.
   Cation exchange resins, weight of water associated with 1.0 g of dry hydrogen resin, measured as above.

| Wet exchange capacity (meq/ml) | Water content (%) | Max. operating temp. (°C) | Comments |
|---|---|---|---|
| 1.9 | 40—45 | 100 | Useful pH range 1—9. |
| 1.6 | 56—62 | 75 | Replacement for Amberlite IRA-47. Useful pH range 0—7. |
| 1.4 | 50—58 | 100 | Useful pH range 1—7. |

| Wet exchange capacity (meq/ml) | Water content (%) | Max. operating temp. (°C) | Comments |
|---|---|---|---|
| 0.7 | 75—83 | 150 | Order of selectivity for monovalent cations: $Ag > Rb > Cs > K > NH_4 > Na > H > Li$. Divalent: $Zn > Cu > Ni > Co$ |
| 1.2 | 64—72 | 150 | |
| 1.7 | 50—56 | 150 | |
| 2.3 | 42—48 | 150 | |
| 2.6 | 36—44 | 150 | |
| 1.9 | 49—55 | 120 | |
| 1.9 | | 120 | Chromatographic grade of Amberlite IR-120. |
| 4.5—5.0 meq/g (dry) | 1.2—1.6[†] | 120 | Equivalent to Zerolit 225 and Zeo-Karb 225. |
| 4.5—5.0 meq/g (dry) | 0.68—0.85[†] | 120 | |
| 4.5—5.0 meq/g (dry) | 0.46—0.7[†] | 120 | |
| 2.0 | 45—49 | 140 | Equivalent to Zerolit 325 and Zeo-Karb 325. |
| 1.8 | 41—47 | 140 | Equivalent to Zerolit 625 and Zeo-Karb 625. |
| 3.5 | 40—50 | 120 | Useful pH range 5—14. |
| 3.5 | | 120 | Chromatographic grade of Amberlite IRC-50. Useful pH range 5—14. |
| 3.7 | 1.1—1.5[†] | 100 | Useful pH range 6—9; stable pH 1—14. Equivalent to Zerolit 236. |
| 3.3 | 65—74 | 100 | Order of selectivity for monovalent cations: $H \gg Ag > K > Na > Li$. Divalent: $H \gg Fe > Ba > Sr > Ca > Mg$. |
| 0.4 | 68—76 | 75 | Chelating resin, strong selectivity for divalent ions over monovalent. Order of selectivity: $Cu > Fe^{3+} > Ni > Zn > Ag^+ > Co > Fe^{2+} > Mn > Ba > Ca \gg Na^+$. Monovalent cations: $H \gg Li > Na > K$. Most effective above pH 4. |

## 2 CELLULOSE ION EXCHANGERS

*Manufacturers.* Cellulose ion exchangers manufactured by the following companies are included in the table below:

Whatman Chemical Separation Ltd, Maidstone, Kent, UK
Bio-Rad Laboratories, Richmond, California, USA (Cellex)
Serva Feinbiochemica, Heidelberg, Fed. Rep. of Germany (Servacel)
Pharmacia Fine Chemicals, Uppsala, Sweden (Sephacel)

*Cellulose type.* Three main types of cellulose are used:
(**F**) Cellulose fibres, made from wood or cotton celluloses, treated to reduce the proportion of fines and, in some cases (Serva), cross-linked with diepoxides. Range of fibre size may be quite large.
(**M**) Microgranular cellulose. Cellulose treated to increase the proportion of micro-crystalline cellulose and cross-linked. It consists of short rod-shaped particles of more uniform dimensions giving improved chromatographic characteristics and more uniform behaviour.
(**B**) Bead-form cellulose. Microcrystalline cellulose stabilized by cross-linking and formed into spherical beads.

*Exchange capacity.* The figures quoted represent approximate maximal values obtainable with small ions. The exchange capacity for macromolecules may be influenced by other factors, for example pH, ionic strength, molecular exclusion effects, etc.

More detailed information on these exchangers, methods of use and particular applications is available from the manufacturers or other suppliers.

## (a) ANION EXCHANGERS

| Designation | Chemical constitution | Cellulose type | Exchange capacity (meq/g) | Bed volume (ml/dry g) | Comments |
|---|---|---|---|---|---|
| **AE-Cellulose** | Aminoethyl cellulose $\xi$—O·CH$_2$·CH$_2$·NH$_2$ | | | | |
| Servacel AE | | | 0.3—0.4 | | Weak base. Most frequent use is as the matrix to which to couple ligands (to —NH$_2$ group) for affinity chromatography. Particle size 50—200 μm. |
| **BD-Cellulose** | Benzoylated diethylaminoethyl-(DEAE)-cellulose | | | | |
| Cellex BD | | F | 0.38 ± 0.08 | 16 | Weak base. pK$_a$ 9. Prepared by benzoylating all the hydroxyl groups of DEAE-cellulose, rendering the exchanger strongly hydrophobic. Supplied hydrated. Moist particle size 50—300 μm. |
| Servacel BD | | F | 0.35 | | |
| **BND-Cellulose** | Benzoylated naphthoylated DEAE-cellulose | | | | |
| Servacel BND | | F | 0.2—0.3 | | Weak base. Similar to BD-cellulose, but substituted with a mixture of benzoyl and naphthoyl (~10%) groups, making it more strongly hydrophobic. Moist particle size 50—300 μm. |
| **DEAE-Cellulose** | Diethylaminoethyl cellulose $\xi$—O·CH$_2$·CH$_2$·NEt$_2$ | | | | |
| Whatman DE23 | | F | 1.0 | 8.3 (pH 6.0) 9.1 (pH 7.5) | Intermediate strength base. pK$_a$ 9.5. |
| Whatman DE51 | | M | 0.22 | | |
| Whatman DE52/DE32 | | M | 1.0 | 6.0—6.3 | Supplied preswollen as citrate. DE52 preswollen; DE32 dry form of same material. |
| Whatman DE53 | | M | 2.0 | | Supplied preswollen as chloride. |
| Cellex D (low capacity) | | F | 0.4 ± 0.1 | 8 | |
| Cellex D (standard capacity) | | F | 0.7 ± 0.1 | 6.25 | |
| Cellex D (high capacity) | | F | 0.9 ± 0.05 | 7.8 | |
| Servacel DEAE 23 SN | | F | 0.4—0.55 | 8.5 | Particle size 50—200 μm. |
| Servacel DEAE 23 SS | | F | 0.55—0.75 | 7.5 | Particle size 50—200 μm. |
| Servacel DEAE 23 SH | | F | 0.75—0.9 | 6.5 | Particle size 50—200 μm. |
| Servacel DEAE 52/32 | | M | 0.9—1.0 | 5.5 | DEAE 52 supplied preswollen, DEAE 32 dry form of same material. Particle size 100—200 μm. |
| Servacel DEAE 80 | | B | 0.8—1.0 | | Bead diameter 50—150 μm. |
| DEAE-Sephacel | | B | 1.4 ± 0.1 | | Supplied preswollen. Bead diameter 40—160 μm. |

(a) ANION EXCHANGERS (continued)

| Designation | Chemical constitution | Cellulose type | Exchange capacity (meq/g) | Bed volume (ml/dry g) | Comments |
|---|---|---|---|---|---|
| ECTEOLA-Cellulose | Condensation product of epichlorohydrin, triethanolamine and cellulose. Structure undefined. | | | | Weak base, $pK_a$ 7.5. |
| Cellex E | | F | 0.3 ± 0.05 | 3.5 | |
| Servacel ECTEOLA 23 | | F | 0.3–0.4 | 7.5 | Particle size 50–200 µm. |
| PAB-Cellulose | p-Aminobenzyl cellulose $\sim$O·CH₂—⟨benzene⟩—NH₂ | | | | Weak base. Can be diazotized and coupled to proteins, nucleic acids, etc. for affinity chromatography. Particle size 50–200 µm. |
| Servacel PAB 23 | | F | 0.15–0.2 | 9 | |
| PEI-Cellulose | High mol. wt. polyethylene-imine adsorbed onto very weakly phosphorylated cellulose fibres. | | | | |
| Servacel PEI | | F | 0.1 | 7 | Particle size 50–100 µm. |
| QAE-Cellulose | Quaternary aminoethyl cellulose $\sim$O·CH₂·CH₂·N⁺·CH₂·CH(OH)·CH₃ with CH₂·CH₃ and CH₂·CH₃ | | | | Strong base. |
| Cellex QAE | | F | 0.7–0.9 | 8 | Counterion Br⁻. |
| TEAE-Cellulose | Triethylaminoethyl cellulose $\sim$O·CH₂·CH₂·N⁺Et₃ | | | | Intermediate strength base, $pK_a$ 9.5. As well as quaternizing the amine group, residual carboxyl gps. are esterified. |
| Cellex T | | F | 0.4–0.6 | 6 | |
| Servacel TEAE 23 | | F | 0.55–0.75 | 6 | Counterion Br⁻. Particle size 50–200 µm. |

## (b) CATION EXCHANGERS

| Designation | Chemical constitution | Cellulose type | Exchange capacity (meq/g) | Bed volume (ml/dry g) | Comments |
|---|---|---|---|---|---|
| CM-Cellulose | Carboxymethyl cellulose $\rangle$O–CH$_2$·COOH | | | | Weak acid. p$K_a$ 4. |
| Whatman CM23 | F | 0.6 | 9.1 | | Counterion Na$^+$. |
| Whatman CM52/CM32 | M | 1.0 | 6.7 | | CM 52 preswollen; CM 32 is dry form of same material. Counterion Na$^+$. |
| Cellex CM | F | 0.7 ± 0.1 | 7 | | Particle size 50–200 $\mu$m. |
| Servacel CM 23 | F | 0.6 ± 0.1 | 9.5 | | CM 52 preswollen; CM 32 is dry form of same product. |
| Servacel CM52/CM32 | M | 1.0 | 5 | | Particle size 100–200 $\mu$m. |
| Servacel CM 80 | B | 1.0 ± 0.1 | ~ 12 | | Bead diameter 50–150 $\mu$m. |
| Hydroxyphenylazonaphthyl cellulose | | | | | Weak cation exchanger having chelating action. High selectivity for heavy metals. Particle size ~ 70 $\mu$m. |
| Servacel CHEL | F | 0.4–0.5 | | | |
| P-Cellulose | Phospho cellulose $\rangle$O–PO$_3$H$_2$ | | | | Dibasic acid. p$K_a$ 1.5 and 6. |
| Whatman P1 | Floc | 3.7 (1st dissoc.) 5.7 (complete) | | | Counterion mono-NH$_4^+$. |
| Whatman P11 | F | 3.2 (1st dissoc.) 5.2 (complete) | | | Counterion mono-NH$_4^+$. |
| Cellex P | F | 0.85 ± 0.1 | 4.5 | | Particle size 50–200 $\mu$m. |
| Servacel P23 | F | 0.8–0.9 | 4.5 | | |
| Servacel P80 | B | 1.0 ± 0.1 | ~ 6 | | Bead diameter 50–150 $\mu$m. |
| SE-Cellulose | Sulphoethyl cellulose $\rangle$O·CH$_2$·CH$_2$·SO$_3^-$ | | | | Strong acid. |
| Whatman SE 53 | M | 2.3 | | | Counterion Na$^+$. Supplied preswollen. |
| Servacel SE 23 | F | 0.2–0.3 | 5.5 | | Particle size 50–200 $\mu$m. |
| Servacel SE 80 | B | 0.2–0.3 | ~ 10 | | Bead diameter 50–150 $\mu$m. |

## 3 DEXTRAN AND AGAROSE ION EXCHANGERS

These exchangers are prepared from gel filtration media composed of cross-linked dextran (Sephadex) or agarose (Sepharose CL, Bio-Gel A). They combine ion-exchange and gel-filtration properties and will have a much reduced exchange capacity for molecules larger than the exclusion limit of the exchanger under the experimental conditions used. Because of the presence of charged groups, the degree of swelling, and hence the exclusion limit, will vary with pH and ionic strength, in a manner not found with the unmodified gel filtration media.

| Designation | Chemical constitution | Matrix | Exchange capacity (meq/g) | Bed volume (ml/dry g) | Comments |
|---|---|---|---|---|---|
| **A Anion exchangers** | | | | | |
| DEAE | $\text{\}-O\cdot CH_2\cdot CH_2\cdot NEt_2$ | | | | Intermediate strength base. $pK_a$ 9.5. |
| DEAE-Sephadex A-25 | | Sephadex G-25 | $3.5 \pm 0.5$ | 5† | |
| DEAE-Sephadex A-50 | | Sephadex G-50 | $3.5 \pm 0.5$ | 28† | |
| DEAE-Sepharose CL-6B | | Sepharose CL-6B | $0.15 \pm 0.02$* | Preswollen | |
| DEAE-Bio-Gel A | | Bio-Gel A (4% agarose) | $0.02 \pm 0.005$* | Preswollen | Exclusion limit $\sim 1 \times 10^6$. |
| QAE | $\text{\}-O\cdot CH_2\cdot CH_2\cdot \overset{Et}{\underset{Et}{N^+}}-CH_2\cdot CH(OH)\cdot CH_3$ | | | | Strong base. |
| QAE-Sephadex A-25 | | Sephadex G-25 | $3.0 \pm 0.4$ | 6† | |
| QAE-Sephadex A-50 | | Sephadex G-50 | $3.0 \pm 0.4$ | 38† | |
| **B Cation exchangers** | | | | | |
| CM | $\text{\}-O\cdot CH_2\cdot COOH$ | | | | Weak acid, $pK_a$ 4. |
| CM-Sephadex C-25 | | Sephadex G-25 | $4.5 \pm 0.5$ | 10† | Counterion Na$^+$. |
| CM-Sephadex C-50 | | Sephadex G-50 | $4.5 \pm 0.5$ | 45† | Counterion Na$^+$. |
| CM-Sepharose CL-6B | | Sepharose CL-6B | $0.12 \pm 0.02$* | Preswollen | |
| CM-Bio-Gel A | | Bio-Gel A (4% agarose) | $0.02 \pm 0.005$* | Preswollen | Exclusion limit $\sim 1 \times 10^6$. |
| SP (Sulphopropyl) | $\text{\}-O\cdot CH_2\cdot CH_2\cdot CH_2\cdot SO_3^-$ | | | | Strong acid. |
| SP-Sephadex C-25 | | Sephadex G-25 | $2.3 \pm 0.3$ | 7† | Counterion Na$^+$. |
| SP-Sephadex C-50 | | Sephadex G-50 | $2.3 \pm 0.3$ | 38† | Counterion Na$^+$. |

* Exchange capacity in meq/ml of **wet** gel.

† Bed volumes may vary with the ionic strength and pH of the buffer used. Values quoted are for $I = 0.05$ and pH 8 (anion exchangers) or pH 6 (cation exchangers). The most significant effects are those of ionic strength on Sephadex 50 exchangers where the bed volume falls quite sharply with increasing ionic strength up to about $I = 0.1$. For details see the manufacturer's literature, *Ion exchange chromatography: principles and methods* (Pharmacia).

## 4 GEL FILTRATION MEDIA

### (a) Sephadex and Bio-Gel P media

*Sephadex*. (Pharmacia Fine Chemicals, Uppsala, Sweden.) *G series*: Bead-form dextran gels cross-linked with epichlorohydrin. Strongly hydrophilic, swells in water and aqueous salt solutions. Different gel types have different degrees of cross-linking and hence differ in their degree of swelling, pore size, and fractionation range. The degree of swelling is largely independent of salts and detergents, though the fractionation range will change if the conformation of the substances being fractionated is altered, e.g. by salts, chaotropic agents, detergents. Stable in pH range 2−12, in urea and detergents, and in organic solvents. Degraded in strong acid and by prolonged exposure to oxidizing agents. May be sterilized by autoclaving at 120°C; above 120°C begins to caramelize.

*LH Series*: LH-20 and LH-60 are prepared from G-25 and G-50 respectively by hydroxypropylation. Separations may depend not only on gel filtration but also on adsorption chromatography and phase partition chromatography. Stability similar to G series. May be used in organic solvents or in water-solvent mixtures. The degree of swelling and hence the effective fractionation range depends upon the solvent used and the conformation of the substances being fractionated.

*Bio-Gel P*. (Bio-Rad Laboratories, Richmond, California, USA) Polyacrylamide beads, prepared by copolymerizing acrylamide and $N,N'$-methylenebisacrylamide. Pore size is regulated by the proportion of cross-linking reagent used. Stable in organic solvents (but does not swell in most and so cannot be used in such solvents), salt solutions, detergents, 8M-urea, 6M-guanidine·HCl. Stable in pH range 2−10; amide groups are hydrolysed at higher and lower pHs. Oxidized by strong oxidizing agents. May be autoclaved at 120°C and pH 5.5−6.5.

| Type | Bead diameter* ($\mu m$) | Fractionation range and exclusion limit (M.wt.)† Peptides/proteins | Dextrans | Water regain (g of $H_2O$/ g of dry gel) | Bed volume (ml/g of dry gel) | Max. recommended operating pressure (cm $H_2O$) | Approx. max. flow rate‡ (cm/h) |
|---|---|---|---|---|---|---|---|
| **Sephadex G** | (dry bead diam.) | | | | | | |
| G-10 | 40–120 | up to 700 | up to 700 | 1.0 ± 0.1 | 2–3 | No limit | — |
| G-15 | 40–120 | up to 1500 | up to 1500 | 1.5 ± 0.2 | 2.5–3.5 | No limit | — |
| G-25 Coarse | 100–300 | 1000–5000 | 100–5000 | 2.5 ± 0.2 | 4–6 | No limit | — |
| Medium | 50–150 | | | | | | |
| Fine | 20–80 | | | | | | |
| Superfine | 10–40 | | | | | | |
| G-50 Coarse | 100–300 | 1500–30 000 | 500–10 000 | 5.0 ± 0.3 | 9–11 | No limit | — |
| Medium | 50–150 | | | | | | |
| Fine | 20–80 | | | | | | |
| Superfine | 10–40 | | | | | | |
| G-75 | 40–120 | 3000–80 000 | 1000–50 000 | 7.5 ± 0.5 | 12–15 | 160 | 77 |
| Superfine | 10–40 | 3000–70 000 | | | | 160 | 18 |
| G-100 | 40–120 | 4000–150 000 | 1000–100 000 | 10.0 ± 1.0 | 15–20 | 96 | 50 |
| Superfine | 10–40 | 4000–100 000 | | | | 96 | 12 |
| G-150 | 40–120 | 5000–300 000 | 1000–150 000 | 15.0 ± 1.5 | 20–30 | 36 | 23 |
| Superfine | 10–40 | 5000–150 000 | | | 18–22 | 36 | 6 |
| G-200 | 40–120 | 5000–600 000 | 1000–200 000 | 20.0 ± 2.0 | 30–40 | 16 | 12 |
| Superfine | 10–40 | 5000–250 000 | | | 20–25 | 16 | 3 |
| **Sephadex LH** | | | | | | | |
| LH-20 | 40–120 | 100–4000 (EtOH)¶ 100–2000 (CHCl₃)¶ | | | 4 (H₂O, EtOH, CHCl₃)§ | | |
| LH-60 | 40–120 | 400–10 000 (H₂O, MeOH)¶ 400–20 000 (CHCl₃)¶ | | | 12–13(H₂O, EtOH, CHCl₃)§ | | |
| **Bio-Gel P** | (wet bead diam.) | | | | | | |
| P-2 Coarse | 150–300 | 100–1800 | | 1.5 ± 0.2 | 3.5 | >100 | |
| Medium | 80–150 | | | | | | |
| Fine | 40–80 | | | | | | |
| Extra fine | <40 | | | | | | |
| P-4 Coarse | 150–300 | 800–4000 | | 2.4 ± 0.2 | 5 | >100 | |
| Medium | 80–150 | | | | | | |
| Fine | 40–80 | | | | | | |
| Extra fine | <40 | | | | | | |
| P-6 Coarse | 150–300 | 1000–6000 | | 3.7 ± 0.4 | 7 | >100 | |
| Medium | 80–150 | | | | | | |
| Fine | 40–80 | | | | | | |
| Extra fine | <40 | | | | | | |

| Type | Bead diameter* (μm) | Fractionation range and exclusion limit (M.wt.)† Peptides/proteins | Fractionation range and exclusion limit (M.wt.)† Dextrans | Water regain (g of H₂O / g of dry gel) | Bed volume (ml/g of dry gel) | Max. recommended operating pressure (cm H₂O) | Approx. max. flow rate‡ (cm/h) |
|---|---|---|---|---|---|---|---|
| P-10 Coarse | 150–300 | 1500–20 000 | | 4.5 ± 0.5 | 9 | >100 | |
| Medium | 80–150 | | | | | | |
| Fine | 40–80 | | | | | | |
| Extra fine | <40 | | | | | | |
| P-30 Coarse | 150–300 | 2500–40 000 | | 5.7 ± 0.6 | 11 | >100 | |
| Fine | 80–150 | | | | | | |
| Extra fine | <80 | | | | | | |
| P-60 Coarse | 150–300 | 3000–60 000 | | 7.2 ± 0.7 | 14 | 100 | |
| Fine | 80–150 | | | | | | |
| Extra fine | <80 | | | | | | |
| P-100 Coarse | 150–300 | 5000–100 000 | | 7.5 ± 0.7 | 15 | 100 | |
| Fine | 80–150 | | | | | | |
| Extra fine | <80 | | | | | | |
| P-150 Coarse | 150–300 | 15 000–150 000 | | 9.2 ± 1.0 | 18 | 100 | |
| Fine | 80–150 | | | | | | |
| Extra fine | <80 | | | | | | |
| P-200 Coarse | 150–300 | 30 000–200 000 | | 14.7 ± 1.5 | 25 | 75 | |
| Fine | 80–150 | | | | | | |
| Extra fine | <80 | | | | | | |
| P-300 Coarse | 150–300 | 60 000–400 000 | | 18.0 ± 2.0 | 30 | 60 | |
| Fine | 80–150 | | | | | | |
| Extra fine | <80 | | | | | | |

* Dry bead diameter for Sephadex; wet bead diameter for Bio-Gel P.
† The higher figure in each pair is the exclusion limit. Fractionation ranges have been measured with (a) peptides or globular proteins, and (b) dextrans representing macromolecules in more extended configuration.
‡ Approximate maximum flow rate measured in columns of 2.5 cm diameter and a bed height of 30 cm.
¶ With Sephadex LH-20 and LH-60, fractionation range, solvent regain, and bed volume depend markedly on the solvent used. Fractionation range measured with polyethylene glycol and polystyrene.
§ The bed volume depends on the solvent used. See manufacturer's literature for information on other solvents.

**Swelling or hydration times (hr)**

| | Sephadex | | | Bio-Gel P | | | |
|---|---|---|---|---|---|---|---|
| | G-10–G-50 | G-75 | G-100–G-200 | P-2–P-10 | P-30–P-60 | P-100–P-150 | P-200–P-300 |
| At 20°C | 3 | 24 | 72 | 4 | 12 | 24 | 48 |
| At 90–100°C | 1 | 3 | 5 | 2 | 3 | 5 | 5 |

## (b) Agarose Media

*Bio-Gel A*. (Bio-Rad). Spherical bead-form agarose gel containing very few charged groups. The fractionation range is determined by the concentration of agarose in the beads. Compatible with all common buffers. Gels containing more than 2% agarose tolerate 6M-guanidine·HCl and 7M-urea, though slight shrinkage may occur; gels with less than 2% agarose liable to structural disruption by these reagents. Stable over pH range 4–10; will tolerate exposure to 0.1M-NaOH or M-HCl for periods up to 2–3 h. Liable to degradation by oxidizing agents. Operating temperature range, 2–30°C; softens above 40°C. Freezing causes collapse of gel structure. Supplied pre-swollen.

*Sepharose*. (Pharmacia). Bead-form agarose gel containing very few charged groups. The fractionation range is governed by the agarose concentration in the beads. Stable in aqueous solutions, pH 4–9. Can be used with high concentrations of salts, urea, guanidine HCl, though Sepharose CL is to be preferred under strongly dissociating conditions. Degraded by oxidizing agents. Melts on heating, do not use above 40°C. Can be chemically sterilized, e.g. with diethylpyrocarbonate, but not by autoclaving. Do not freeze; freezing destroys the bead structure.

Sepharose CL is a cross-linked agarose gel, prepared by reacting the corresponding Sepharose type with 2,3-dibromopropane. Cross-linking gives improved chemical, thermal, and mechanical stability. Stable over pH range 3–14, in 8M-urea, 6M-guanidine·HCl, 3M-KSCN. Can be used in many organic solvents and at temperatures up to 70°C; stable to autoclaving at 120°C and pH 7. Liable to degradation under oxidizing conditions.

Sepharose and Sepharose CL are supplied pre-swollen.

| Type | % Agarose in gel | Wet bead diameter ($\mu m$) | Fractionation range and exclusion limit (M. wt.)* | | Max. recommended operating pressure (cm $H_2O$) | Approx. max. flow rate† (cm/h) |
|---|---|---|---|---|---|---|
| | | | Proteins | Polysaccharides | | |
| **Bio-Gel A** | | | | | | |
| A-0.5m Coarse | 10 | 150–300 | $<10\,000$–$500\,000$ | | $>100$ | |
| Medium | | 80–150 | | | | |
| Fine | | 40–80 | | | | |
| A-1.5m Coarse | 8 | 150–300 | $<10\,000$–$1.5\times10^6$ | | $>100$ | |
| Medium | | 80–150 | | | | |
| Fine | | 40–80 | | | | |
| A-5m Coarse | 6 | 150–300 | $10\,000$–$5\times10^6$ | | $>100$ | |
| Medium | | 80–150 | | | | |
| Fine | | 40–80 | | | | |
| A-15m Coarse | 4 | 150–300 | $40\,000$–$15\times10^6$ | | 90 | |
| Medium | | 80–150 | | | | |
| Fine | | 40–80 | | | | |
| A-50m Coarse | 2 | 150–300 | $100\,000$–$50\times10^6$ | | 50 | |
| Fine | | 80–150 | | | | |
| A-150m Coarse | 1 | 150–300 | $1\times10^6$–$>150\times10^6$ | | 30 | |
| Fine | | 80–150 | | | | |
| **Sepharose** | | | | | | |
| 6B | 6 | 45–165 | $10\,000$–$4\times10^6$ | $10\,000$–$1\times10^6$ | 90 | 14 |
| 4B | 4 | 60–140 | $60\,000$–$20\times10^6$ | $30\,000$–$5\times10^6$ | 60 | 11.5 |
| 2B | 2 | 60–200 | $70\,000$–$40\times10^6$ | $100\,000$–$20\times10^6$ | 30 | 10 |
| **Sepharose CL** | | | | | | |
| CL–6B | 6 | 45–165 | $10\,000$–$4\times10^6$ | $10\,000$–$1\times10^6$ | $>120$ | 30 |
| CL–4B | 4 | 60–140 | $60\,000$–$20\times10^6$ | $30\,000$–$5\times10^6$ | 120 | 26 |
| CL–2B | 2 | 60–200 | $70\,000$–$40\times10^6$ | $100\,000$–$20\times10^6$ | 50 | 15 |

* The higher figure in each pair is the exclusion limit.
† Approximate maximum flow rate measured in columns of 2.5 cm diameter and a bed height of 30 cm.

### (c) Sephacryl

*Sephacryl.* (Pharmacia). Gel beads prepared by covalently cross-linking allyl dextran with $N,N'$-methylenebisacrylamide. Cross-linking gives good chemical, thermal, and mechanical stability. Can be used in aqueous buffer systems in pH range 2–11, in SDS, 8M-urea and 6M-guanidine·HCl, and in a number of organic solvents (though these may cause some shrinkage compared with gel volume in water). Unaffected by heat, can be autoclaved repeatedly at 120°C and pH 7. Supplied pre-swollen. The rigid structure allows operating pressures up to very high values (150–300 cm $H_2O$) and flow rates up to 25–40 cm/hr can be used and are recommended for column packing. For fractionations requiring average resolution, flow rates about 10 cm/hr are recommended; for high resolution, lower flow rates should be used.

| Type | Wet bead diameter (μm) | Fractionation range and exclusion limit (M. wt.)[*] | |
|---|---|---|---|
| | | *Protein* | *Polysaccharides* |
| **Sephacryl** | | | |
| S-200 Superfine | 40–105 | 5000–250 000 | 1000–80 000 |
| S-300 Superfine | 40–105 | 10 000–1.5×10⁶ | 1000–400 000 |
| S-400 Superfine | 40–105 | 20 000–8×10⁶ | 10 000–2×10⁶ |
| S-500 Superfine | 40–105 | | 40 000–20×10⁶ |
| S-1000 Superfine | 40–105 | | 500 000– >10⁸ (exclusion limit for particles – diam. of 300–400 nm) |

[*] The higher figure in each pair is the exclusion limit.

## 5 AFFINITY CHROMATOGRAPHY

Affinity chromatography relies on the specific interaction of proteins (or other biological molecules) with ligands immobilized by covalent binding to an insoluble matrix. For example an enzyme may interact with an immobilized substrate or substrate analogue, an immobilized lectin may interact with the carbohydrate moiety of a glycoprotein or a receptor protein with its specific ligand. Elution of the adsorbed protein may use specific eluants, for example the ligand or an analogue, or non-specific factors such as salt concentration or pH.

Affinity chromatography adsorbents usually consist of three covalently-linked components, the insoluble matrix, a spacer and the specific ligand.

*Insoluble matrix.* Much the most frequently used matrix is beaded 4% or 6% agarose, which may be stabilized by cross-linking with epichlorohydrin, divinyl-sulphone or a bisepoxide (bisoxirane). A cellulose matrix is commonly used for oligonucleotide ligands, e.g. oligo dT-cellulose. Other supports which have been used include cross-linked dextran, polyacrylamide, hydroxyalkylmethacrylate polymers, coated glass and silica.

*Spacer.* If a low molecular weight ligand is attached directly to the matrix, steric effects may reduce the interaction between the ligand and the protein for which it is specific. To counteract this, a 'spacer' is introduced between the matrix and the ligand. A hydrocarbon chain 6 or 8 carbon atoms long, which places the ligand 5–10 Å from the matrix, is often used for this purpose, but longer spacers, up to 17 atoms in length, are sometimes employed. Hydrocarbon spacers may interact hydrophobically with certain macromolecules and affect their adsorption; for this reason spacers containing hydrophilic groups are sometimes preferred. When the ligand is a macromolecule, for example a protein, it is not usually necessary to include a spacer; the macromolecular ligand can be attached directly to the solid matrix.

The table of 'Materials for the preparation of affinity adsorbents' (p. 522) includes the structures of some of the spacers commonly used and shows the mode of attachment of the spacer molecule to the matrix and the terminal reactive group through which it can be covalently linked to the ligand.

*Ligand.* Any molecule, whether of low molecular weight or macromolecular, which interacts specifically with the protein, nucleic acid or other molecule that is to be purified, is potentially useful as a ligand in affinity chromatography. Many ligands, such as enzyme substrates, lectins or antigens, will interact with only a single type of protein or, at most, a very limited range. Others, such as coenzymes (NAD, NADP), nucleotides (ATP, AMP, cAMP, etc.) and immobilized dyes, interact specifically with a wider, though still limited, range of macromolecules, and so are known as group-specific ligands.

A wide range of immobilized ligands is available commercially. The table of 'Ligands used in commercially-available affinity adsorbents' (p. 526) lists, with examples, the principal classes of ligand that are available from commercial suppliers. For full details, it is always advisable to consult the manufacturers' literature which often includes information about applications.

*Preparation of affinity adsorbents.* It is sometimes necessary, or convenient, to prepare an affinity adsorbent for a specifc purpose. This can be done by reacting the chosen ligand either with an activated derivative of agarose or other solid support or with a derivatized agarose carrying a spacer which terminates in a reactive group. The table of 'Materials for the preparation of affinity adsorbents' lists activated agaroses and agaroses with spacers attached, which are available commercially. Using these as starting materials, the attachment of the ligand to complete the affinity adsorbent is readily achieved, requiring mild experimental conditions and straightforward procedures.

*Suppliers.* The principal suppliers of complete affinity adsorbents and materials for their preparation are:

I   Pharmacia P-L Biochemicals, Uppsala, Sweden and Milton Keynes, UK.
II  Sigma Chemical Company, St Louis, Missouri, USA and Poole, UK.
III Bio-Rad Laboratories, Richmond, California, USA and Watford, UK.
IV  Pierce Chemical Company, Rockford, Illinois, USA and Chester, UK.

*References*

*Meth. Enzymol.* vol. **34** (1974) and **104** (1984).

*Laboratory Techniques in Biochemistry and Molecular Biology*, ed. T. S. Work, vol. 7, p. 267, Elsevier-North Holland (1979).

*Techniques in the Life Sciences*, vol. BS1/1, *Techniques in Protein and Enzyme Biochemistry*, Part 1 Supplement, section BS103, Elsevier (1984).

**MATERIALS FOR THE PREPARATION OF AFFINITY ADSORBENTS**

**A Activated Agaroses**

| Type of activation | Reactive group of activated gel | Reactive group of ligand | Mode of coupling of ligand to the gel | Suppliers | Comments |
|---|---|---|---|---|---|
| Carbonyl-diimidazole-activated | (structure: —O—C(=O)—N⟍N imidazole) | R-NH₂ | (structure: —O—C(=O)—NH—R) | IV (Reacti-Gel (6X)) | Alternative to CNBr-activation for coupling proteins directly to agarose. Coupled product is more stable than with CNBr-activation, so reducing leakage of ligand, and substituted carbamate coupling group is uncharged. Imidazolyl-carbamate group of activated gel is only slowly hydrolysed at mildly alkaline pHs (half-life in hours). Also available with cross-linked beaded dextran, controlled-pore glass beads or Fractogel TSK HW-65F as the insoluble matrix. |
| Cyanogen bromide (CNBr)-activated | (structure: —O—C≡N); (structure: cyclic —O—C(=NH)—O); plus minor components | R-NH₂ | (structures: —O—C(=NH)—NH—R; —O—C(—O)=N—R cyclic; —O—C(=O)—NH—R) | I, II | Most widely used and best documented method for coupling proteins and nucleic acids directly to agarose. Prepared by reaction of CNBr (Caution – highly toxic and can become explosive) with agarose. Chemistry of activation and of coupling is complex, only the principal reactive groups and products are shown. In CNBr-activated agarose, the cyanate ester groups are reactive but unstable under alkaline conditions (stable below pH 4), whereas cyclic imidocarbonate groups are stable to alkali but less reactive. In the coupled product, the *N*-substituted isourea groups are not completely stable, causing a small leakage of ligand. The isourea group also carries a positive charge (p$K_a$ ~ 9.5), giving the adsorbent ion exchange properties. See *Biochem. Int.* **4**, 629 (1982); *Meth. Enzymol* **34**, 96 (1974); **104**, 3 (1984), for discussion of these problems. |
| *N*-Hydroxy-succinimide-activated | (structure: N-hydroxysuccinimide ester —O—C(=O)—O—N(C=O)₂) | R-NH₂ (R-SH) | (structure: —O—C(=O)—NH—R) | II | Prepared by reaction of *N*-hydroxysuccinimido-chloroformate with agarose. The *N*-hydroxy-succinimide ester bond in the activated gel is rapidly hydrolysed above pH 8.5. Coupled product is more stable (less leakage of ligand) than with CNBr-activation and the coupling group is uncharged. |

| Type | Structure | Reactive group of ligand | Mode of coupling of ligand | Suppliers | Comments |
|---|---|---|---|---|---|
| $p$-Nitrophenyl-activated | $\sim\!O\!-\!\overset{\displaystyle O}{\overset{\|}{C}}\!-\!O\!-\!C_6H_4\!-\!NO_2$ | $R\text{-}NH_2$ | $\sim\!O\!-\!\overset{\displaystyle O}{\overset{\|}{C}}\!-\!NH\!-\!R$ | II | Prepared by reaction of $p$-nitrophenyl chloroformate with agarose. Coupled product is more stable (less leakage of ligand) than with CNBr-activation and the coupling group is uncharged. |
| Tresyl-activated | $\sim\!CH_2\!-\!O\!-\!SO_2\!-\!CH_2\!-\!CF_3$ | $R\text{-}NH_2$ $R\text{-}SH$ | $\sim\!CH_2\!-\!NH\!-\!R$ $\sim\!CH_2\!-\!S\!-\!R$ | I | Prepared by reaction of 2,2,2-trifluoroethane-sulphonyl chloride (tresyl chloride) with agarose. Activated gel stable in the cold, overnight at pH 7.5, for several weeks in 1mM-HCl. Activated gel reacts with sulphydryl groups, as well as amino groups, forming stable bonds. |

**B. Agarose with spacers attached**

| Type | Structure | Reactive group of ligand | Mode of coupling of ligand | Suppliers | Comments |
|---|---|---|---|---|---|
| Spacer terminating in amino group $-NH_2$ | $\sim\!NH\!\cdot\!(CH_2)_n\!\cdot\!NH_2$ | $R\text{-}COOH$ | $-NH\!-\!CO\!-\!R$ | I, II | Products with $n = 2,3,4,5,6,8,10$ and 12 are available commercially. Spacer can be extended by reaction with succinic anhydride. Coupling is usually carried out with a water-soluble carbodiimide, such as 1-ethyl-3-(3-dimethylaminopropyl)-carbodiimide (EDAC). |
| | $\sim\!O\!\cdot\!CH_2\!\cdot\!CO\!\cdot\!NH\!\cdot\!(CH_2)_2\!\cdot\!NH_2$ | $R\text{-}COOH$ | $-NH\!-\!CO\!-\!R$ | III (Affi-Gel 102) | Six-atom hydrophilic spacer. |
| | $\sim\!CH_2\!\cdot\!NH\!\cdot\!(CH_2)_3\!\cdot\!NH\!\cdot\!(CH_2)_3\!\cdot\!NH_2$ | $R\text{-}COOH$ | $-NH\!-\!CO\!-\!R$ | IV | Nine-atom spacer. |
| | $\sim\!O\!\cdot\!CH_2\!\cdot\!CHOH\!\cdot\!CH_2\!\cdot\!O\!\cdot\!(CH_2)_4$ $\cdot\!O\!\cdot$ $H_2N\!\cdot\!(CH_2)_n\!\cdot\!NH\!\cdot\!CH_2\!\cdot\!CHOH\!\cdot\!CH_2$ | $R\text{-}COOH$ | $-NH\!-\!CO\!-\!R$ | II | Diaminoalkane is attached to epoxy-activated agarose, giving a spacer containing $13 + n$ atoms. Products with $n = 2,3,6$ and 10 are commercially available. |
| Spacer terminating in carboxyl group $-COOH$ | $\sim\!O\!\cdot\!CH_2\!\cdot\!COOH$ | $R\text{-}NH_2$ | $\sim\!O\!\cdot\!CH_2\!\cdot\!CO\!-\!NH\!-\!R$ | III | Coupling is usually carried out with a water-soluble carbodiimide, such as 1-ethyl-3-(3-dimethylamino-propyl)carbodiimide (EDAC). |
| | $\sim\!NH\!\cdot\!(CH_2)_5\!\cdot\!COOH$ | $R\text{-}NH_2$ | $\sim\!NH\!\cdot\!(CH_2)_5\!\cdot\!CO\!-\!NH\!-\!R$ | I (CH-Sepharose), II | |
| | $\sim\!O\!\cdot\!CH_2\!\cdot\!CO\!\cdot\!NH\!\cdot\!(CH_2)_2\!\cdot\!NH$ $\quad\quad HOOC\!-\!(CH_2)_2\!\cdot\!CO$ | $R\text{-}NH_2$ | $-CO\!-\!NH\!-\!R$ | III (Affi-Gel 202) | Hydrophilic 10-atom spacer. |

523

| Type | Structure | Reactive group of ligand | Mode of coupling of ligand | Suppliers | Comments |
|---|---|---|---|---|---|
| Spacer terminating in epoxy group $-CH-CH_2$ over O (Epoxy-activated agarose) | ⁀O·CH₂·CHOH·CH₂·O—(CH₂)₄—O·CH₂·CHOH·CH₂·O ; CH₂-CH-CH₂-O with epoxide O | R-NH₂ R-OH R-SH | $-CH-CH_2 \longrightarrow$ over O $-CHOH-CH_2-NH-R$ $-CHOH-CH_2-O-R$ $-CHOH-CH_2-S-R$ | I, II | Prepared by reaction of agarose with the bisepoxide (bisoxirane), 1,4-bis(2,3-propoxy)-butane (1,4-butanediol diglycidyl ether). Forms a 12-atom spacer on coupling with ligand. Coupling with ligand requires high pHs, e.g. pH 12–13, but spacer is not cleaved from agarose under these conditions. Couples with amino, hydroxyl and sulphydryl groups forming stable secondary amine, ether and thioether bonds respectively. Useful for ability to couple to hydroxyl-containing ligands, e.g. carbohydrates. |
| Spacer terminating in hydrazide group $-NH.NH_2$ | ⁀NH·NH·CO·(CH₂)₄·CO·NH·NH₂ | R-CHO | $-NH-N=CH-R$ $\downarrow NaBH_4$ $-NH-NH-CH_2-R$ | I, II | Useful for coupling with aldehyde groups, e.g. those formed in carbohydrates and nucelotides by periodate oxidation. |
| Spacer terminating in N-hydroxy-succinimide ester (N-Hy·lroxy-succin·mide-activated agarose) | ⁀NH·(CH₂)₅·CO·O·N (succinimide ring) | R-NH₂ | $-CO-NH-R$ | I (Activated CH-Sepharose), II | Forms six-atom hydrophobic spacer. N-Hydroxysuccinimide ester is rapidly hydrolysed at pHs above 8.5. |
| | ⁀O·CH₂·CO·NH·(CH₂)₂·NH·CO·(CH₂)₂·N·O·CO·(CH₂)₂ (succinimide ring) | R-NH₂ | $-CO-NH-R$ | III (Affi-Gel 10) | Hydrophilic, uncharged 10-atom spacer. |
| | ⁀O·CH₂·CO·NH·(CH₂)₃·NH⁺(CH₃)(CH₂)₃·NH·CO·(CH₂)₂·CO·N·O (succinimide ring) | R-NH₂ | $-CO-NH-R$ | III (Affi-Gel 15) | Hydrophilic, cationic 15-atom spacer. |

| | Structure | Reactant | Product | Code | Notes |
|---|---|---|---|---|---|
| Spacer terminating in thiol group –SH | ~NH·CH₂·CH₂·SH | R-SH | –S–S–R | I, II | Reversible coupling of ligand by disulphide bond. |
| | –NH·(CH₂)₂·NH·CO·CH₂·CH₂·SH | R-SH | –S–S–R | I (Agthiol) | |
| | –O·CH₂·CO·NH·(CH₂)₂·NH / HS·(CH₂)₂·CH·CO / CH₃·CO·NH | R-SH | –S–S–R | III (Affi-Gel 401), IV | Formed by coupling N-acetylhomocysteine to spacer. |
| Spacer terminating in groups which react with thiol groups | –O·CH₂·CHOH·CH₂·S·S-[pyridyl] | R-SH | –S–S–R | I (Thiopropyl-Sepharose), II | Couples reversibly with thiol compounds, including proteins containing thiol groups, by disulphide exchange. |
| | HOOC·CH₂·NH·CO / –NH·CH·(CH₂)₂·CO·NH·CH / COOH / [pyridyl]-S-S-CH₂ | R-SH | –S–S–R | I (Activated thiol-Sepharose), II | Spacer group is glutathione. Couples reversibly with thiol compounds, including proteins, by disulphide exchange. |
| Multivalent spacers: Poly-L-lysine | –NH–Lys / (Lys)ₙ–NH₂ / –NH–Lys | R.COOH | –NH–CO–R | II, IV | Poly-L-lysine attached at multiple sites to agarose through ε-amino groups. Multi-point attachment reduces ligand leakage. |
| Polyacryl-hydrazido-agarose | –NH·NH·CO·(CH₂)₂·CH / NH / CO / NH / CH·(CH₂)₂·CO·NH·NH₂ / CO / NH / –NH·NH·CO·(CH₂)₂·CH / CO | | | | Multipoint attachment limits ligand leakage. For preparation and ligand attachment, see *Meth. Enzymol.* **34**, 72 (1974), **104**, 14 (1984). |

## LIGANDS USED IN COMMERCIALLY-AVAILABLE AFFINITY ADSORBENTS

| Class of ligand | Examples | Comments |
|---|---|---|
| Nucleotides | ATP, ADP, 5'-AMP, 2'-AMP, 3',5'-cAMP, 2',5'-ADP, 3',5'-ADP, dATP, $Ap_5A$, adenosine<br>CTP, CDP, 5'-CMP<br>GTP, GDP, 5'-GMP, 7-methyl-GTP<br>UTP, UDP, 5'-UMP, UDP-glucuronic acid | Commonest mode of coupling is via a $C_6$ hydrazide spacer linked to aldehyde groups formed by periodate oxidation of the ribose moiety of the nucleotide. Adsorbents with adenine nucleotides linked via N-6 amino group or via C-8 to spacers of various lengths are also available. In a few adsorbents coupling is through the phosphate group to a $p$-aminophenol spacer. 2',5'-ADP and 3',5'-ADP are group specific ligands for NADP- and CoA-requiring enzymes respectively. |
| Oligonucleotides and polynucleotides | Oligo dT, oligo dA, oligo dC, oligo dG, oligo dI, DNA (native and denatured) | Attached via 5'-phosphate to a cellulose matrix. Oligonucleotides less than 20 nucleotide residues in length. |
|  | Poly rA, poly rC, poly rG, poly rI, poly rU, poly rI · poly rC, DNA (denatured) | Attached to an agarose matrix. |
| Coenzymes and vitamins | NAD, NADP, FMN<br>CoA, HMG-CoA<br>Biotin, desthiobiotin, iminobiotin, other biotin analogues<br>Methotrexate | NAD and NADP are available linked to 6 or 8-atom spacers through N-6 amino, C-8 or periodate-oxidized ribose residue of adenine moiety. CoA may be linked through —SH group or have a free —SH. Biotin and analogues are generally linked to a spacer through the carboxyl group on the side chain. |
| Amino acids, peptides and amines | All 20 L-amino acids found in proteins<br>D-Arginine, D-phenylalanine, D-tryptophan<br>L-Thyroxine<br>Glutathione (reduced and oxidised), hexylGSH, sulphobromophthalein-S-GSH<br>5-Hydroxytryptamine, histamine, spermine, cysteamine<br>Pepstatin | Coupled via amino group directly to CNBr-activated agarose. A few amino acids are available linked via a spacer. |

| Class of Ligand | Examples | Comments |
| --- | --- | --- |
| Proteins: Lectins | Many lectins, including: Concanavalin A, Peanut lectin, Anti-Protein A lectin (*Dolichos biflorus*), *Helix pomatia* lectin, Soybean lectin, Lentil lectin, Erythrocyte agglutinating phytohaemagglutinin (*Phaseolus vulgaris*), Pea lectin, Wheat germ lectin | In almost all cases, lectin is directly linked to CNBr-activated agarose. Use of alternative methods of agarose activation should reduce leakage of ligand. |
| Proteins: other proteins | Immunoglobulins, Protein A (*Staph. aureus*), Avidin (tetramer and monomer), Trypsin inhibitor (soybean and lima bean), Calmodulin, Parvalbumin, Gelatin, Haemoglobin, Ovalbumin, $\alpha$-Lactalbumin, Protamine, Insulin Many enzymes | Most proteins can be immobilised by reaction under mild conditions with agarose activated by CNBr or by an alternative method. |
| Carbohydrates | D-Xylose, L-fucose D-Glucose, D-galactose, D-mannose D-Glucosamine, *N*-acetyl-D-glucosamine, D-galactosamine, *N*-acetyl-D-galactosamine D-Lactose, D-melibiose, D-maltose Heparin | Mono- and disaccharides are most commonly coupled by glycosidic (or thioglycosidic) links to a *p*-aminophenol spacer: Agarose—NH—⟨benzene ring⟩—O—$C^1$ of sugar or by a glycosylamine link to an aminohexanoic acid spacer: Agarose-NH-$(CH_2)_5$-CO-NH-$C^1$ of sugar. With both of these types of link the configuration of the sugar at C-1 will be specified ($\alpha$ or $\beta$). Other modes of coupling include linking via C-6 hydroxyl to epoxy-activated agarose, coupling of C-1 to a divinyl sulphone spacer, and coupling of aminosugars through the amino group to an aminohexanoic acid spacer. Affinity adsorbents with sugar ligands are usually prepared by first attaching the spacer to the sugar and then reacting with activated agarose. |

| Class of Ligand | Examples | Comments |
|---|---|---|
| Dyes | Cibacron Blue F3G-A, Procion Red HE 3B, other unspecified dyes | These dyes have been found to be useful group-specific ligands for nucleotide-requiring enzymes, as well as for a number of other proteins. Procion Red HE 3B shows higher affinity for NADP-enzymes than for NAD-enzymes. Review, *Dye-Ligand Chromatography* (Amicon Ltd.). |
| Hydrophobic | Agarose-NH-$(CH_2)_n$-$CH_3$ where $n = 0, 1, 2, 3, 4, 5, 7, 9$ and $11$<br><br>Agarose-NH-$(CH_2)_4$ —⟨phenyl⟩<br><br>Agarose-O-$CH_2 \cdot CHOH \cdot CH_2 \cdot O \cdot R$<br><br>where $R = -(CH_2)_7 \cdot CH_3$ or —⟨phenyl⟩ | Effective in protein separation as a result of hydrophobic interaction with proteins. Diamino-alkane derivatives of agarose: Agarose-NH-$(CH_2)_n$-$NH_2$ can also be used as adsorbents for hydrophobic chromatography. |
| Miscellaneous ligands | Aminophenylboronic acid | Affinity for *cis*-diols, such as sugars. |
| | *m*- and *p*-Aminobenzamidine<br>Chloramphenicol<br>Cholesteryl hemisuccinate, oestradiol hemisuccinate<br>Cholic acid, deoxycholic acid<br>Choline phosphate, ethanolamine phosphate | |
| | *p*-Hydroxymercuribenzoate | Forms mercaptides with thiol compounds, including thiol-containing proteins. |
| | Iminodiacetic acid, triscarboxymethylethylene diamine | Metal chelating properties. |
| | Oxamic acid<br>Phenothiazine<br>Tartaric acid | Specific for calmodulin. |

# 22 Isotopic data

## DEFINITIONS

***curie (milli-, micro-).*** The quantity of radon in radioactive equilibrium with 1 g of radium. Equivalent to the amount of an isotope undergoing $3.7 \times 10^{10}$ nuclear disintegrations per second ($2.22 \times 10^{12}$ per minute). 1 curie equals $3.7 \times 10^{10}$ becquerels.

***becquerel.*** The SI unit of radioactivity. 1 becquerel (Bq) = $2.70 \times 10^{-11}$ curies (Ci)

$$1 \,\mu\text{Ci} = 37\,000 \,\text{Bq} \equiv 37 \,\text{kBq (kilo Bq)}$$
$$1 \text{mCi} = 37 \times 10^6 \,\text{Bq} \equiv 37 \,\text{MBq (mega Bq)}$$
$$1 \,\text{Ci} = 37 \times 10^9 \,\text{Bq} \equiv 37 \,\text{GBq (giga Bq)}$$

***atom per cent excess.*** The concentration of an isotope in a sample of the element expressed as the difference between the per cent of the atoms existing as the isotope in the sample and the per cent of the atoms existing as the isotope in the element found in its natural state.

***specific activity.*** The radioactivity of an element per unit mass of element.

***carrier-free isotope.*** Theoretically the isotope under consideration free from all other isotopes of the same element.

***electron volt (eV, or MeV = $10^6$ eV).*** The energy acquired by an electron when accelerating along a potential gradient of 1 volt = $1.6 \times 10^{-12}$ erg.

***half-value thickness.*** The depth of material which reduces the intensity of a radiation beam by one-half.

***röntgen (r).*** That quantity of X- or gamma-radiation such that the associated corpuscular emission per 0.001293 g of air produces, in air, ions carrying 1 electrostatic unit of quantity of electricity of either sign (1 ml air at 0°C, dry, 760 mm Hg). 1 r corresponds to the absorption of $5.24 \times 10^{13}$ eV of energy or 83.8 erg per g of air. 3876 rontgens = 1 coulomb/kg (SI units).

***röntgen-equivalent physical.*** The dose of radiation which produces, when absorbed in tissue, the same amount of energy dissipation per g of tissue as the absorption of 1 r in 1 g of dry air, i.e. 83.8 erg per g of tissue.

***relative biological effectiveness (RBE)*** of a particular radiation dose is the ratio of the body damage it causes to that produced by the same dose of X-rays with an average specific ionization of 100 ion pairs/micron of water.

The ***rad*** is a unit of absorbed dose. 1 rad is an absorbed dose of 100 erg/g of tissue. The SI unit is the **gray (Gy)** equal to one joule/kg. 1 gray equals 100 rads.

The ***rad equivalent man*** (rem) is defined as (dose in rem) = (dose in rad) $\times$ (RBE). In SI units 100 rem equal one joule/kg = 1 sievert (SV).

***electron charge, e*** = $1.6 \times 10^{-19}$ coulombs.

***beta-ray absorption half thickness*** = max. range/7 approx.

## FORMULAE, ETC.

*Dead time correction*

$$N = \frac{N_0}{1 - N_0 t}, \quad \text{or} \quad N - N_0 = N_0\{N_0 t + (N_0 t)^2 + (N_0 t)^3 + \ldots\},$$

where $N$ = true counting rate,
  $N_0$ = observed counting rate,
   $t$ = dead time of the counter (period during which the counter is insensitive to incoming pulses).

(This correction is subject to an error of the order $\frac{1}{2} N_0 (N_0 t)^2$.)

## 22 Isotopic data

*Statistical formulae*

Standard deviation (%) of a count $= \pm (10^4/N_t)^{1/2}$ where $N_t =$ total number of counts recorded. For example, if $10^4$ counts are recorded, the probability of the error being less than $\pm 1\%$ is 2 to 1, and less than $\pm 2\%$ 19 to 1.

Standard deviation (SD) of the difference between two counts

$$= \pm \{(SD_1)^2 + (SD_2)^2\}.^{1/2}$$

Therefore the accuracy of background counting will only be of importance when the counting rate of the sample is low.

The difference between two counting rates ($N_1$, $N_2$) is obtained with maximum accuracy by counting for times $t_1$ and $t_2$ such that

$$t_1/t_2 = (N_1/N_2)^{1/2}$$

*Autoradiography*

The response of an emulsion to a series of exposures to X-rays or electrons is given by $a = A(1 - e^{-\epsilon r})$,

where  $a =$ number of developed grains,
$A =$ total number of grains per unit area,
$r =$ exposure in röntgens or number of electrons,
$\epsilon =$ factor of proportionality depending on the emulsion.

As a rough guide a satisfactory autoradiograph may be obtained with $10^7$ $\beta$-particles $cm^{-2}$ or $2 \times 10^6$ $\alpha$-particles $cm^{-2}$.

*Weight radionuclide/microcurie*

This can be calculated from the formulae $W = 3.19 \times 10^{10} N(T_{1/2})M$,

where  $W =$ wt. in micrograms;
$N =$ number of microcuries;
$T_{1/2} =$ half-life in hours;
$M =$ molecular weight.

*Radioactive decay correction*

$$\log_{10} \frac{N_0}{N_t} = 0.3010(t/h)$$

$$\text{Percentage isotope remaining} = \frac{100}{\text{antilog}\{0.3010\,(t/h)\}}, \text{ or } 100 \times e^{-0.6931\left(\frac{t}{h}\right)}$$

where  $t =$ time of decay
$h =$ half-life or time taken for radioactivity to decay to 50% of original activity,
$N_0 =$ radioactivity at zero time,
$N_t =$ radioactivity at time t.

After $x$ half-lives the percentage of original isotope remaining $= 2^{-x} \times 100$.
Thus, $x = 1, 50\%; x = 2, 25\%; x = 3, 12.5\%; x = 4, 6.25\%; x = 5, 3.13\%; x = 6, 1.56\%; x = 7, 0.78\%; x = 8, 0.39\%; x = 9, 0.20\%; x = 10, 0.1\%$

| $^{24}$Na (half-life 14.8 hr) | | $^{32}$P (half-life 14.3 days) | | $^{35}$S (half-life 87.1 days) | | $^{42}$K (half-life 12.4 hr) | | $^{131}$I (half-life 8.1 days) | |
|---|---|---|---|---|---|---|---|---|---|
| Time (hr) | % activity remaining | Time (days) | % activity remaining | Time (days) | % activity remaining | Time (hr) | % activity remaining | Time (days) | % activity remaining |
| 1 | 95.4 | 1 | 95.3 | 2 | 98.4 | 1 | 94.6 | 0.2 | 98.3 |
| 2 | 91.1 | 2 | 90.8 | 5 | 96.1 | 2 | 89.5 | 0.4 | 96.6 |
| 3 | 86.9 | 3 | 86.5 | 10 | 92.3 | 3 | 84.5 | 0.6 | 95.0 |
| 4 | 82.9 | 4 | 82.4 | 15 | 88.7 | 4 | 80.0 | 1.0 | 91.8 |
| 5 | 79.1 | 5 | 78.5 | 20 | 85.3 | 5 | 75.6 | 1.6 | 87.2 |
| 6 | 75.5 | 6 | 74.8 | 25 | 82.0 | 6 | 71.5 | 2.3 | 81.2 |
| 7 | 72.1 | 7 | 71.2 | 31 | 78.1 | 7 | 67.6 | 3.1 | 76.7 |
| 8 | 68.7 | 8 | 67.8 | 37 | 74.5 | 8 | 63.9 | 4.0 | 71.0 |
| 9 | 65.6 | 9 | 64.7 | 43 | 71.0 | 9 | 60.5 | 5.0 | 65.2 |
| 10 | 62.6 | 10 | 61.5 | 50 | 67.0 | 10 | 57.2 | 6.1 | 59.3 |
| 11 | 59.7 | 11 | 58.7 | 57 | 63.6 | 11 | 53.9 | 7.3 | 53.4 |
| 12 | 57.0 | 12 | 55.9 | 65 | 59.6 | 12 | 51.2 | 8.1 | 50.0 |
| 13 | 54.4 | 13 | 53.2 | 73 | 56.0 | 12.4 | 50.0 | | |
| 14 | 51.9 | 14 | 50.7 | 81 | 52.5 | | | | |
| 14.8 | 50.0 | 14.3 | 50.0 | 87.1 | 50.0 | | | | |

| $^{3}$H (half-life 12.3 yr) | | $^{125}$I (half-life 60 days) | | $^{45}$Ca (half-life 165 days) | | $^{51}$Cr (half-life 28 days) | |
|---|---|---|---|---|---|---|---|
| Time (yr) | % activity remaining | Time (days) | % activity remaining | Time (days) | % activity remaining | Time (days) | % activity remaining |
| 1 | 94.5 | 4 | 95.5 | 10 | 95.9 | 2 | 95.2 |
| 2 | 89.3 | 8 | 91.2 | 20 | 91.9 | 4 | 90.6 |
| 3 | 84.4 | 12 | 87.1 | 30 | 88.2 | 6 | 86.2 |
| 4 | 79.8 | 16 | 83.1 | 40 | 84.5 | 8 | 82.0 |
| 5 | 75.4 | 20 | 79.4 | 50 | 81.1 | 10 | 78.1 |
| 6 | 71.3 | 24 | 75.8 | 60 | 77.7 | 12 | 74.3 |
| 7 | 67.4 | 28 | 72.4 | 70 | 74.5 | 14 | 70.7 |
| 8 | 63.7 | 32 | 69.1 | 80 | 71.5 | 16 | 67.3 |
| 9 | 60.2 | 36 | 66.0 | 90 | 68.5 | 18 | 64.0 |
| 10 | 56.9 | 40 | 63.0 | 100 | 65.7 | 20 | 61.0 |
| 11 | 53.8 | 44 | 60.2 | 110 | 63.0 | 22 | 58.0 |
| 12 | 50.9 | 48 | 57.4 | 120 | 60.4 | 24 | 55.2 |
| 12.3 | 50.0 | 52 | 54.8 | 130 | 57.9 | 26 | 52.5 |
| | | 56 | 52.4 | 140 | 55.5 | 28 | 50.0 |
| | | 60 | 50.0 | 150 | 53.3 | | |
| | | | | 160 | 51.1 | | |

## SOME RADIOACTIVE ISOTOPES USED IN BIOCHEMICAL INVESTIGATIONS

| Element (mass no.) | Radiation | Half-life | Energy of radiation (MeV) | | Scintillator for detection |
|---|---|---|---|---|---|
| | | | Particles | γ-rays | |
| $^3$H | β— | 12.3 yr | 0.0185 | . . | LSC |
| $^{11}$C | β+ | 20.5 min | 0.95 | . . | LSC |
| $^{14}$C | β— | 5760 yr | 0.156 | . . | LSC |
| $^{22}$Na | β+,γ | 2.6 yr | 0.58 (90%) | 1.3 | LSC or NaI(Tl) |
| $^{24}$Na | β—,γ | 14.8 hr | 1.39 | 1.38, 2.76 | LSC or NaI(Tl) |
| $^{28}$Mg | β— | 21.4 hr | 0.459 | . . | LSC |
| $^{31}$Si | β— | 170 min | 1.8 | . . | Cerenkov |
| $^{32}$P | β— | 14.3 days | 1.71 | . . | LSC or Cerenkov |
| $^{35}$S | β— | 87.J days | 0.169 | . . | LSC |
| $^{36}$Cl | β+,κ,β— | $3.1 \times 10^5$ yr | 0.71 | . . | LSC |
| $^{38}$Cl | β—,γ | 38.5 min | 1.19 (36%) 2.70 (11%) 5.20 (53%) | 1.60 (43%) 2.12 (57%) | LSC or Cerenkov or NaI (Tl) |
| $^{42}$K | β—,γ | 12.4 hr | 2.04 (25%) 3.58 (75%) | 1.4, 2.1 | LSC or Cerenkov or NaI(Tl) |
| $^{45}$Ca | β— | 165 days | 0.260 | . . | LSC |
| $^{51}$Cr | κ,γ | 28 days | . . | 0.323, 0.237 | LSC or NaI(Tl) |
| $^{52}$Mn | β+ (35%) κ (65%) | 5.8 days | 0.58 | 1.0, 0.73 0.94, 1.46 | LSC |
| $^{54}$Mn | κ,γ | 310 days | . . | 0.835 | NaI (Tl) |
| $^{55}$Fe | κ only | 2.94 yr | . . | . . | LSC |
| $^{57}$Co | γ | 270 days | . . | 0.136 (10%) 0.122 (88%) | NaI (Tl) |
| $^{58}$Co | β+(14.5%),γ | 72 days | 0.472 | 0.805 | LSC or NaI (Tl) |
| $^{59}$Fe | β—,γ | 46.3 days | 0.46 (50%) 0.26 (50%) | 1.3 (50%) 1.1 (50%) | LSC |
| $^{60}$Co | β—,γ | 5.3 yr | 0.31 | 1.16, 1.32 | LSC or NaI (Tl) |
| $^{64}$Cu | κ (54%) β—(31%) β+(15%) γ+κ(1.5%) | 12.8 hr | 0.57 (β—) 0.66 (β+) | 1.35 (2.5%) | LSC |
| $^{65}$Zn | β+ (1.3%) κ(98.7%) | 250 days | 0.32 | 1.14(46% of κ) | LSC |
| $^{76}$As | β—,γ | 26.8 hr | 3.04 (60%) 2.49 (25%) 1.29 (15%) | 1.705 1.20 0.55 | LSC or NaI (Tl) |
| $^{75}$Se | κ,γ | 121 days | . . | 0.076–0.405 | NaI (Tl) |
| $^{82}$Br | β—,γ | 36 hr | 0.465 | 0.547, 0.787 1.35 | LSC or NaI (Tl) |
| $^{86}$Rb | β—,γ | 18.7 | 1.822 (80%) 0.716 (20%) | 1.081 | LSC or Cerenkov or NaI (Tl) |
| $^{89}$Sr | β— | 51 days | 1.46 | . . | LSC or Cerenkov |
| $^{90}$Sr | β— | 28.5 yr | 0.61 | . . | LSC |
| $^{99}$Mo | β—,γ | 68 hr | 1.3 | 0.75, 0.24 | LSC or Cerenkov |
| $^{125}$Sb | β—,γ | 2.7 yr | 0.3 (65%) 0.7 (35%) | 0.55 | LSC |
| $^{125}$I | γ,EC con. cl. | 60 days | . . | 0.035 | NaI(Tl), LSC |
| $^{131}$I | β—,γ | 8.1 days | 0.605 (86%) 0.25 (14%) | 0.637, 0.363 0.282, 0.08 | LSC or NaI (Tl) |

## ATTENUATION OF β-PARTICLES AND γ-RAYS

### *β -Particles*

The attenuation of β-particles depends on the density of the shielding material and is largely independent of its atomic weight.

| | | *Thickness of material in mm required to reduce intensity by one-half* | | | |
|---|---|---|---|---|---|
| *Energy β-particles (MeV)* | *Weight material $cm^{-2}$ to reduce intensity by one-half (mg)* | *Water* | *Glass (d = 2.5)* | *Lead* | *Perspex* |
| 0.1 | 1.3 | 0.013 | 0.005 | 0.0011 | 0.0125 |
| 1.0 | 48 | 0.48 | 0.192 | 0.042 | 0.38 |
| 2.0 | 130 | 1.3 | 0.52 | 0.115 | 1.1 |
| 5.0 | 400 | 4.0 | 1.6 | 0.35 | 4.2 |

### *γ- Rays*

| | *Thickness of material in centimeters required to attenuate broad beam of γ-rays by a factor of 10* | | | |
|---|---|---|---|---|
| *Energy of γ-rays (MeV)* | *Water* | *Aluminium* | *Iron* | *Lead* |
| 0.5 | 54.6 | 20.3 | 6.1 | 1.8 |
| 1.0 | 70 | 25.4 | 8.2 | 3.8 |
| 2.0 | 76 | 32 | 11.0 | 5.9 |
| 3.0 | 89 | 37 | 12.0 | 6.4 |
| 4.0 | 97 | 40 | 12.7 | 6.3 |
| 5.0 | 107 | 44 | 13.0 | 6.1 |

## LIQUID SCINTILLATION COUNTING

### *Cerenkov counting*

Cerenkov radiation can be used for measuring isotopes which emit a hard β-radiation e.g. $^{32}P$. No scintillator is required and since chemical quenching is absent, the sample can simply be dissolved in a wide variety of solvent systems ranging from organic solvents, perchloric acid, water, etc. and counted directly in a scintillation counter. Efficiency is dependent on the energy of β-particles so in practice, weak β-emitters cannot be counted. Approximate efficiency: maximum β-particle energy in MeV/detection efficiency

0.6 MeV 1–2%, 1.0 MeV 12%, 1.5 MeV 19%, 2 MeV 32%, 2.5 MeV 44%

Colour quenching operates and coloured substances have to be removed or the quenching allowed for. Added wavelength shifters e.g. 4-methyllumbelliferone 100 mg/l have been used for increasing the counting efficiency but such compounds can be influenced by substances present in the sample and the pH.

### *Counting of solvent-soluble substances*

Radioactive samples soluble in hydrocarbon solvents can be directly introduced into mixtures such as (1) scintillation-grade toluene or xylene containing 5 g/litre 2,5-diphenyloxazole (PPO) and 0.1 g/litre 1,4-di{2-(5-phenyloxazolyl)}-benzene (POPOP); (2) scintillation-grade toluene or xylene containing 10 g/litre 2-phenyl-5-(4-biphenylyl)-1,3,4-oxadiazole (PBD) or 15 g/litre 2-(4′-*t*-butylphenyl)-5-(4″-biphenylyl)-1,3,4-oxadiazole (butyl PBD).

Scintillation fluid 2 is better for use in the more recent scintillation counters containing bialkali photocathodes. Chemical quenching and colour quenching both occur.

*Counting of aqueous samples*

(a) water-miscible solvent

Aqueous samples can be introduced into scintillation cocktails containing 1,4-dioxan which can take up to 30% by volume water.

(1)  Brays (1960)

| | | |
|---|---|---|
| Naphthalene | 60 g | |
| PPO | 4 g | |
| POPOP | 0.2 g | for chemical names see previous section |
| Methanol | 100 ml | |
| Ethylene glycol | 20 ml | |
| p-Dioxan | to 1 litre | |

(2)  Naphthalene    60 g
butyl PBD    15 g (or PBD) for chemical name see previous section.

p-dioxan to 1 litre

Cocktail 2 is more suitable for more recent scintillation counters containing bialkali photocathodes. p-Dioxan is readily oxidized during storage, forming peroxides which quench severely. They can be removed by passage of the dioxan through a molecular sieve column or by refluxing with metallic sodium, and their formation during storage may be prevented by adding an antioxidant e.g. di-*t*-butyl-4-hydroxytoluene (BHT). If the radioactive aqueous sample is alkaline, intense chemiluminescence is produced which interferes with counting.

(b) emulsion counting

Aqueous samples can also be counted in hydrocarbon-based scintillation fluids using a polyethoxylate surfactant to produce an emulsion.

e.g. 660 ml toluene or xylene (scintillation grades)
340 ml surfactant (Triton X-100, Triton X-114, Sterox DJ,
Igepal CA 720, Fiscint)

5 g PPO      Can be replaced by 15 g butyl PBD or 10 g PBD
0.1 g POPOP   with advantage for more recent counters
containing bialkali photocathodes

The disadvantage of such systems is that separation into two phases can occur with marked reduction in counting efficiency (*Anal. Biochem.* **74**, 25 (1976)). Sometimes the phase separation cannot be observed visually and it cannot be detected by external standard measurements. Consequently each cocktail mix has to be examined for the stability of counting rate with time at the counting temperature with various percentages of aqueous sample incorporated.

It is claimed that a modified Tritosol cocktail (*Anal. Biochem.* **63**, 555 (1975)) can accept up to 23% of water with no phase separation and a linear relationship between counting efficiency and external standard ratio over wide quenching ranges. This contains:

| | | |
|---|---|---|
| Ethylene glycol | 35 ml | |
| Ethanol | 140 ml | |
| Triton X-100 (X-114) | 250 ml | |
| Xylene | 575 ml | |
| PPO | 3 g | (see previous |
| POPOP | 0.2 g | section) |

Numerous commercial emulsifying cocktails are also available but it is wise to examine the counting efficiency and emulsion stability under the precise conditions being used, e.g. percentage of aqueous sample incorporated, the presence of solutes, and the pH.

Such surfactant cocktails can often be used directly for the counting of radio-active samples on solid supports or suspension counting. Thus spots on TLC plates may often be counted if the gel is scraped off and introduced into the counting vial along with the detergent scintillation cocktail and some water (10% by vol). Spots on paper may be cut out and the paper arranged round the perimeter of the vial and wetted with the scintillation fluid.

Solid tissues and other biological samples can be solubilized before counting by incubating with quarternary bases such as hyamine hydroxide (p-diisobutylcresoxy-ethoxyethyl)dimethylbenzylammonium hydroxide. However this often produces strong phosphorescence with tissue proteins and various commercial stabilizers have been developed based on quarternary N bases which do not have this disadvantage. During digestion of the sample, frequent agitation or ultrasonic vibration is required: heating to $50°C$ helps, but higher temperatures cause excessive coloration and quenching.

# 23 Biochemical procedures

## 1 PROCEDURES USED IN PROTEIN FRACTIONATION

(a) AMMONIUM SULPHATE

*Chart for ammonium sulphate additions*

The chart shows the amount of solid $(NH_4)_2SO_4$ required to bring a solution of known initial saturation to a desired final saturation. In this chart, *the saturation is relative to full saturation at $0°C$,* which requires the addition of 706.8 g of $(NH_4)_2SO_4$ to 1 l of water (molarity, 3.90M). A similar chart based on saturation at 25 °C is given in *Meth. Enzymol.* **1**, 76 (1955). Nomograms for the calculation of $(NH_4)_2SO_4$ additions are given in *BJ* **54**, 457 (1953) (for room temperature, about 22 °C) and *JBC* **243**, 2022 (1968) (for 0 °C).

*This chart is slightly different from that in the 2nd edition of this work.* It has been recalculated to take account of the fact that full saturation at $0°C$ requires the addition of 70.7 g of solid $(NH_4)_2SO_4$ (rather than 69.7 g) to 100 ml of water.

Final concentration of ammonium sulphate, % saturation at 0 °C

| Initial concentration of ammonium sulphate, % saturation at 0°C. | g solid ammonium sulphate to add to 100 ml of solution | | | | | | | | | | | | | | | | |
|---|---|---|---|---|---|---|---|---|---|---|---|---|---|---|---|---|---|
| | 20 | 25 | 30 | 35 | 40 | 45 | 50 | 55 | 60 | 65 | 70 | 75 | 80 | 85 | 90 | 95 | 100 |
| 0 | 10.7 | 13.6 | 16.6 | 19.7 | 22.9 | 26.2 | 29.5 | 33.1 | 36.6 | 40.4 | 44.2 | 48.3 | 52.3 | 56.7 | 61.1 | 65.9 | 70.7 |
| 5 | 8.0 | 10.9 | 13.9 | 16.8 | 20.0 | 23.2 | 26.6 | 30.0 | 33.6 | 37.3 | 41.1 | 45.0 | 49.1 | 53.3 | 57.8 | 62.4 | 67.1 |
| 10 | 5.4 | 8.2 | 11.1 | 14.1 | 17.1 | 20.3 | 23.6 | 27.0 | 30.5 | 34.2 | 37.9 | 41.8 | 45.8 | 50.0 | 54.4 | 58.9 | 63.6 |
| 15 | 2.6 | 5.5 | 8.3 | 11.3 | 14.3 | 17.4 | 20.7 | 24.0 | 27.5 | 31.0 | 34.8 | 38.6 | 42.6 | 46.6 | 51.0 | 55.5 | 60.0 |
| 20 | 0 | 2.7 | 5.6 | 8.4 | 11.5 | 14.5 | 17.7 | 21.0 | 24.4 | 28.0 | 31.6 | 35.4 | 39.2 | 43.3 | 47.6 | 51.9 | 56.5 |
| 25 | | 0 | 2.7 | 5.7 | 8.5 | 11.7 | 14.8 | 18.2 | 21.4 | 24.8 | 28.4 | 32.1 | 36.0 | 40.1 | 44.2 | 48.5 | 52.9 |
| 30 | | | 0 | 2.8 | 5.7 | 8.7 | 11.9 | 15.0 | 18.4 | 21.7 | 25.3 | 28.9 | 32.8 | 36.7 | 40.8 | 45.1 | 49.5 |
| 35 | | | | 0 | 2.8 | 5.8 | 8.8 | 12.0 | 15.3 | 18.7 | 22.1 | 25.8 | 29.5 | 33.4 | 37.4 | 41.6 | 45.9 |
| 40 | | | | | 0 | 2.9 | 5.9 | 9.0 | 12.2 | 15.5 | 19.0 | 22.5 | 26.2 | 30.0 | 34.0 | 38.1 | 42.4 |
| 45 | | | | | | 0 | 2.9 | 6.0 | 9.1 | 12.5 | 15.8 | 19.3 | 22.9 | 26.7 | 30.6 | 34.7 | 38.8 |
| 50 | | | | | | | 0 | 3.0 | 6.1 | 9.3 | 12.7 | 16.1 | 19.7 | 23.3 | 27.2 | 31.2 | 35.3 |
| 55 | | | | | | | | 0 | 3.0 | 6.2 | 9.4 | 12.9 | 16.3 | 20.0 | 23.8 | 27.7 | 31.7 |
| 60 | | | | | | | | | 0 | 3.1 | 6.3 | 9.6 | 13.1 | 16.6 | 20.4 | 24.2 | 28.3 |
| 65 | | | | | | | | | | 0 | 3.1 | 6.4 | 9.8 | 13.4 | 17.0 | 20.8 | 24.7 |
| 70 | | | | | | | | | | | 0 | 3.2 | 6.6 | 10.0 | 13.6 | 17.3 | 21.2 |
| 75 | | | | | | | | | | | | 0 | 3.2 | 6.7 | 10.2 | 13.9 | 17.6 |
| 80 | | | | | | | | | | | | | 0 | 3.3 | 6.8 | 10.4 | 14.1 |
| 85 | | | | | | | | | | | | | | 0 | 3.4 | 6.9 | 10.6 |
| 90 | | | | | | | | | | | | | | | 0 | 3.4 | 7.1 |
| 95 | | | | | | | | | | | | | | | | 0 | 3.5 |
| 100 | | | | | | | | | | | | | | | | | 0 |

*Formulae for ammonium sulphate additions*

The amount (in g) of solid $(NH_4)_2SO_4$ to be added to 1 l of a solution of initial saturation $S_1$ to produce a final saturation $S_2$ is given by the formula

$$\text{Weight (in g) of } (NH_4)_2SO_4 \ = \ \frac{G(S_2 - S_1)}{1 - \dfrac{\bar{v}G}{1000} S_2},$$

where $G$ is the weight (in g) of $(NH_4)_2SO_4$ contained in 1 l of saturated solution, $\bar{v}$ is the partial specific volume of $(NH_4)_2SO_4$ in the saturated solution, and $S_1$ and $S_2$ are expressed as fractions of complete saturation, e.g. $S_1 = 0.5$ and $S_2 = 0.7$. Values of $\bar{v}$ and $G$ are given in the table below. This formula ignores the change in partial specific volume with $(NH_4)_2SO_4$ concentration.

For the addition of saturated $(NH_4)_2SO_4$ solutions, the volume changes on mixing are small. The volume (in ml) of saturated $(NH_4)_2SO_4$ solution required to increase the initial saturation $S_1$ of 1 l of solution to a final saturation of $S_2$ is given by the equation

$$\text{Vol. of saturated soln.} \ = \ \frac{1000(S_2 - S_1)}{1 - S_2},$$

where $S_1$ and $S_2$ are expressed as fractions of complete saturation.

Formulae for calculating the required quantities of solid $(NH_4)_2SO_4$ or of a saturated solution are given in *JBC* **208**, 149 (1954), *J. gen. Physiol.* **35**, 423 (1952), and *The proteins*, eds. Neurath and Bailey, 1st ed., vol. 1, part A, p. 55, Academic Press (1953). A chart based upon the formulae in the first reference and expressing $(NH_4)_2SO_4$ concentration as a molarity is given in *Manometric Techniques*, eds. Umbreit *et al.*, 4th ed., p. 158, Burgess (1964).

*Saturated ammonium sulphate solutions at various temperatures*

| | Temperature (°C) | | | | |
|---|---|---|---|---|---|
| | 0 | 10 | 20 | 25 | 30 |
| Moles $(NH_4)_2SO_4$ per 1000 g $H_2O$ | 5.35 | 5.53 | 5.73 | 5.82 | 5.91 |
| Percentage by weight | 41.42 | 42.22 | 43.09 | 43.47 | 43.85 |
| g $(NH_4)_2SO_4$ required to saturate 1000 ml $H_2O$ | 706.8 | 730.5 | 755.8 | 766.8 | 777.5 |
| g $(NH_4)_2SO_4$ per l of saturated solution $(G)$ | 514.7 | 525.1 | 536.1 | 541.2 | 545.9 |
| Molarity of saturated solution | 3.90 | 3.97 | 4.06 | 4.10 | 4.13 |
| Density (in g/cm³) | 1.2428 | 1.2436 | 1.2447 | 1.2450 | 1.2449 |
| Apparent specific volume in saturated soln. $(\bar{v})$ | 0.5281 | 0.5357 | 0.5414 | 0.5435 | 0.5458 |

## (b) PREPARATION OF ALUMINA $C_\gamma$ GEL

Willstätter and Kraut, *Ber.* **56**, 1117 (1923); see also *Meth. Enzymol.* **1**, 97 (1955); **2**, 823 (1957); **6**, 169 (1963).

Dissolve 300 g of $(NH_4)_2SO_4$ in 6.5 l of water, heat to 60 °C, and add 420 ml of 20% (w/w) $NH_3$ (this contains 77.5 g of $NH_3$ which provides a small excess necessary to keep the fluid slightly alkaline during the addition of $Al_2(SO_4)_3$). Maintaining the temperature at not less than 60°C and stirring vigorously, rapidly pour a hot solution of 500 g of $Al_2(SO_4)_3 \cdot 18H_2O$ in 1 l of water into the $(NH_4)_2SO_4 - NH_3$ solution. Continue stirring for 15 min after the addition is complete, still keeping the temperature at not less than 60°C. When the initial voluminous precipitate becomes flocculent dilute to 40 l with water. Allow the precipitate to settle and decant (or siphon off) the supernatant. Repeat the washing of the gel and on the fourth wash add 80 ml of 20% $NH_3$ to the water to precipitate any residual $Al_2(SO_4)_3$. Between the 12th and 20th washes the wash water will remain turbid. After this point is reached wash twice more; these washings generally require a period of 2 days.

The gel should be free from sulphate when tested with HCl and $BaCl_2$. It is usual to allow the gel to stand for 3 months before use in order to convert the $C_\alpha$ form into the $C_\gamma$ form.

## (c) PREPARATION OF HYDROXYAPATITE

Methods of preparing hydroxyapatite (or hydroxylapatite) and the properties of various preparations have been examined by Spencer et al., J. Chromatogr. **166**, 423, 435, 447 (1978).

(i) Method of Tiselius et al. (ABB **65**, 132 (1956)), modified by Levin, Meth. Enzymol. **5**, 28 (1962). A similar preparation on a larger scale is described in Biochem. Preps. **9**, 83 (1962).

Two litres of 0.5M-$CaCl_2$ and 2 l of 0.5M-$Na_2HPO_4$ are allowed to run at equal rates (12-15 ml per min) into a 5-l beaker and the mixture stirred constantly. The resulting precipitate is allowed to settle and the supernatant sucked off with a water pump. The precipitate is washed four times with 3-l quantities of water, complete settling being allowed each time. The final suspension is diluted to 3 l with distilled water and 100 ml of freshly prepared 40% (w/v) NaOH solution added with stirring. Bring the mixture to the boil over about 45 min and boil gently for 1 hr, stirring slowly throughout. Allow to settle for 5 min and suck off the very turbid supernatant. The precipitate is then washed four times with 3-l quantities of water as before, allowing 5 min settling each time. Add 4 l of 0.01M-sodium phosphate buffer, pH 6.8, to the precipitate and heat the suspension just to boiling with stirring. Allow to settle for 5 min and then suck off supernatant. Repeat this procedure twice with 0.01M- and twice with 0.001M-sodium phosphate buffer, pH 6.8, but allowing 15 min boiling each time. Make up the final suspension in 0.001M-buffer. It is stable for at least a year. Slow stirring and gentle boiling are essential to give a product which is sufficiently coarse-grained to allow reasonable rates of flow through columns.

(ii) Method of Spencer, J. Chromatogr. **166**, 435 (1978). Variations on the method described here (details are in the reference) give preparations having either a higher flow rate or better resolving power.

To prepare brushite, 2.0 l of 0.5M-$CaCl_2$ are added to 2.4 l of 0.5M-sodium phosphate buffer, pH 6.7, at a rate of 50 ml/min. The mixing is done in a 9-l bucket fitted with a bath recirculator having an impeller pump; the impeller orifice is adjusted to give a circulation rate of about 4 l/min. The $CaCl_2$ solution is fed in just above the impeller orifice. (Before use, the apparatus should be washed briefly with 0.1M-HCl to remove brushite crystallites which might prematurely seed the preparation. This factor and the vigour with which the mixture is circulated by the impeller pump markedly affect the size of the crystal clusters of brushite, and hence the flow characteristics of the final hydroxyapatite preparation.) After mixing is complete the crystals are allowed to settle (settled vol. about 700 ml) and washed in 5 l of distilled $H_2O$ to remove soluble salts.

In order to convert it into hydroxyapatite, the brushite suspension is transferred, after removal of the supernatant, to a well-lagged 5-l beaker. Boiling distilled water (2.5 l) is rapidly added while the mixture is stirred with a 50 × 100 mm paddle stirrer at 200 r.p.m. After the addition the temperature is 70–75°C and the pH

5.0–5.5. The stirrer is stopped, the sediment allowed to settle and the supernatant is removed by suction without delay. 5.0 ml of M-HCl are added. A further 2.5 l of boiling water are then added as before, followed by about 72 ml of 20% NaOH, added through a tube reaching to the bottom of the beaker. The pH is monitored continuously using high-temperature electrodes and the addition of alkali is regulated so that the pH stays at $7.0 \pm 0.2$ after the first 0.5 min, during which there is an initial drop to pH 5.5–6.0. Typical delivery rates for the NaOH soln. are: 0–0.5 min, 35 ml/min; 0.5–1.0 min, 50 ml/min; 1.0–2.0 min, 30 ml/min. During this time the temperature falls by about $6\,°C$ from an initial value of $85–90\,°C$. Delivery of NaOH soln. is stopped when the pH stays steady at 7.2. After allowing the sediment to settle and removing the supernatant, the material is twice washed in 2.5-l quantities of boiling water. After the final addition, the beaker is covered and transferred, without removing the supernatant, to an insulated cabinet, where it is allowed to cool slowly overnight; the initial cooling rate should be about $0.3\,°C/min$. The settled volume of the hydroxyapatite is about 750 ml.

## 2 METHODS FOR PROTEIN ESTIMATION

Methods for determining protein concentration have been reviewed by:

C.J.R. Thorne, in *Techniques in Protein and Enzyme Biochemistry*, Part I, Section B104, Elsevier–North Holland (1978).

E. Layne, *Meth. Enzymol.* **3**, 447 (1957).

### (a) BY ABSORBANCE AT 260 nm AND 280 nm

Method of Warburg and Christian, *BZ* **310**, 384 (1941).

*Procedure.* Using a 1-cm path-length cell, measure the absorbance $A$ (extinction, optical density) of an appropriately diluted protein solution at 260 nm and at 280 nm.

*Calculation of protein concentration.* (i) Calculate the ratio $A_{280}/A_{260}$. From the table on p. 542 (or a graph constructed from the figures) read off the factor corresponding to the calculated $A_{280}/A_{260}$ ratio. The protein concentration is given by:

$$\text{Protein conc. (mg/ml)} = A_{280} \times \text{Factor}$$

(ii) Protein concentration is given by the formula:

$$\text{Protein conc. (mg/ml)} = 1.55A_{280} - 0.76A_{260}$$

*Comment.* The values in the table and the equation were calculated from the absorbance values of crystalline yeast enolase (for a concentration of 1 mg/ml, $A_{260}$ 0.512, $A_{280}$ 0.894) and purified yeast nucleic acid (for 1 mg/ml, $A_{260}$ 22.1, $A_{280}$ 10.8). The method will be strictly accurate only for mixtures of proteins and nucleic acids having these absorbance values.

Absorbance values for many proteins have been tabulated in *Handbook of biochemistry and molecular biology*, ed. G. D. Fasman, vol. II, p. 383, 3rd ed., CRC Press (1976); *Anal. Biochem.* **68**, 464 (1975), **80**, 193 (1977), **81**, 220 (1977), **82**, 83 (1977), **87**, 223 (1978), **90**, 309 (1978); *Int. J. Pept. Protein Res.* **13**, 479 (1979); *Int. J. Biochem.* **11**, 487 (1980), **13**, 621 (1981). $A_{280}$ values for most proteins at a concentration of 1 mg/ml fall in the range 0.5 to 2.0, though there are significant numbers of proteins with values either above or below this range.

*Factor for Calculation of Protein Concentration*

| $A_{280}/A_{260}$ | Nucleic acid (%)[†] | Factor |
|---|---|---|
| 1.75 | 0 | 1.118 |
| 1.60 | 0.30 | 1.078 |
| 1.50 | 0.56 | 1.047 |
| 1.40 | 0.87 | 1.011 |
| 1.30 | 1.26 | 0.969 |
| 1.25 | 1.49 | 0.946 |
| 1.20 | 1.75 | 0.921 |
| 1.15 | 2.05 | 0.893 |
| 1.10 | 2.4 | 0.863 |
| 1.05 | 2.8 | 0.831 |
| 1.00 | 3.3 | 0.794 |
| 0.96 | 3.7 | 0.763 |
| 0.92 | 4.3 | 0.728 |
| 0.90 | 4.6 | 0.710 |
| 0.88 | 4.9 | 0.691 |
| 0.86 | 5.2 | 0.671 |
| 0.84 | 5.6 | 0.650 |
| 0.82 | 6.1 | 0.628 |
| 0.80 | 6.6 | 0.605 |
| 0.78 | 7.1 | 0.581 |
| 0.76 | 7.8 | 0.555 |
| 0.74 | 8.5 | 0.528 |
| 0.72 | 9.3 | 0.500 |
| 0.70 | 10.3 | 0.470 |
| 0.68 | 11.4 | 0.438 |
| 0.66 | 12.8 | 0.404 |
| 0.64 | 14.5 | 0.368 |
| 0.62 | 16.6 | 0.330 |
| 0.60 | 19.2 | 0.289 |

[†] Nucleic acid is expressed as a percentage of the total (protein + nucleic acid).

## (b) BIURET METHOD

Method of Gornall, Bardawill, and David, *JBC* **177**, 751 (1949).

*Reagent.* Dissolve 1.5 g of $CuSO_4 \cdot 5H_2O$ and 6 g of sodium potassium tartrate (Rochelle salt, $NaKC_4H_4O_6 \cdot 4H_2O$) in 500 ml of water. Add, mixing thoroughly, 300 ml of 10% (w/v) sodium hydroxide solution (carbonate free). Potassium iodide (1 g) may also be added to prevent the formation of a precipitate of cuprous oxide. Make up to 1 l with water and store in a plastic bottle.

*Method.* Mix 4.0 ml of biuret reagent and 1.0 ml of protein solution (diluted if necessary) containing 1–10 mg of protein, and allow the mixture to stand at room temperature for 30 min. Read the absorbance at a wavelength between 540 nm and 560 nm.

Protein concentration is obtained by comparison with a calibration curve (usually linear) prepared with 1-10 mg of a suitable standard protein. Different proteins give somewhat different absorbance values, but the range is less (not more than two-fold) than for other methods.

*Interfering substances.* Peptides, tris, sucrose, and bile pigments give a colour in the biuret reaction; ammonium salts, tris, sucrose, and glycerol affect the colour given by proteins. Lipids and detergents may cause turbidity.

(c) LOWRY−FOLIN METHOD

Method of Lowry, Rosebrough, Farr and Randall, *JBC*, **193**, 265 (1951); see also *Anal. Biochem.* **100**, 201 (1979).

*Reagents.* Solution A: 2% $Na_2CO_3$ in 0.1M-NaOH.

Solution B: 0.5% $CuSO_4 \cdot 5H_2O$ in 1% sodium or potassium tartrate or trisodium citrate.

Solution C: Mix 50 ml of solution A with 1 ml of solution B. Renew daily.

Solution D: Commercial Folin−Ciocalteu reagent (store in refrigerator) diluted with water to make it 1M in acid (an approximately 2-fold dilution is usually required).

*Method.* Use a protein sample containing $25-500\,\mu g$ of protein in 1.0 ml. Add 5.0 ml of solution C, mix well and allow to stand for 10 min or longer at room temperature. Add 0.5 ml of solution D rapidly with immediate mixing. Stand for 30 min and then read absorbance at 750 nm (for low protein concentrations) or 500 nm (for high protein concentrations). Multiples or fractions of these quantities may be used.

Protein concentration is obtained by comparison with a calibration curve (usually slightly curved) prepared with a suitable standard protein. Different proteins give markedly different absorbance values in the Lowry−Folin assay, depending in part on their tyrosine and tryptophan content.

*Interfering substances.* Many widely used biochemical reagents interfere with the estimation, usually by increasing the blank value or by decreasing the colour yield with protein. They include tyrosine, tryptophan and phenolic substances, buffers (e.g. tris, Hepes, glycine, histidine, citrate), sugars (e.g. sucrose, glucose, glycerol), gradient-forming materials (Ficoll, metrizamide, polyvinyl pyrrolidone), thiol compounds, reducing agents, EDTA, $(NH_4)_2SO_4$, Triton X-100. For full lists and details of suitable precautions, see *Anal. Biochem.* **70**, 241 (1976), **100**, 201 (1979), and Thorne (ref. on p. 541).

(d) DYE-BINDING METHOD

Method of Bradford, *Anal. Biochem.* **72**, 248 (1976); see also *Anal. Biochem.* **86**, 142 (1978).

*Reagent.* Coomassie Brilliant Blue G-250 (100 mg) dissolved in 50 ml of 95% EtOH. Add 100 ml of 85% (w/v) phosphoric acid. Dilute to 1 l with $H_2O$.

*Method.* Use a sample (diluted if necessary) containing $10-100\,\mu g$ of protein in 0.1 ml. Add 5.0 ml of dye reagent and mix well. After 5 min and before 1 hr read the absorbance at 595 nm against a reagent blank.

For micro assay, use a sample containing $1-10\,\mu g$ of protein in 0.1 ml, add 1.0 ml of dye reagent, mix and read at 595 nm as before.

Protein concentration is calculated by comparison with a standard curve, which is slightly curved, prepared using a suitable protein (see below). Different proteins show considerable variation in their dye-binding capacities and so give different responses in the assay. In particular, bovine serum albumin gives a high $A_{595}$ value and so it is not suitable as a standard protein for general use with this assay.

*Interfering substances.* Strongly alkaline buffers and detergents such as SDS and Triton X-100 reduce the colour yield.

## 3 METHODS FOR NUCLEIC ACID ESTIMATION

(a) RNA ESTIMATION − ORCINOL METHOD

*Reagents.* Solution A: 1% orcinol in water. This solution will keep for several weeks in a refrigerator.

Solution B: Conc. HCl.

Solution C: 10% $FeCl_3 \cdot 6H_2O$ in water. A trace of HCl may be neccesary to obtain a clear solution.

*Method.* Mix 10 ml of solution A, 40 ml of solution B and 1 ml of solution C just before use. Add 3.0 ml of this solution to 0.5 ml of the RNA-containing solution and heat in a boiling water bath (with marbles on top of the tubes) for 25 min. Cool and read absorbance at 660 nm against a reagent blank.

*Comments.* The range of this assay is 0–200 μg of RNA. Any pure RNA can be used as a standard. Solid RNA always contains an indeterminate amount of water and it is normally necessary to determine the concentration of the standard by measuring its absorbance at 260 nm. A solution with $A_{260}$ of 24.0 contains 1 mg of RNA/ml.

### (b) DNA ESTIMATION – DIPHENYLAMINE METHOD

Method of Burton, *BJ* **62**, 315 (1956); *Meth. Enzymol.* **12B**, 163 (1968).

*Diphenylamine reagent.* 1.5% (w/v) diphenylamine in redistilled glacial acetic acid with 1.5 ml of conc. $H_2SO_4$ added per 100 ml. Aqueous acetaldehyde (0.1 ml, 16 mg/ml) is added to each 20 ml of reagent. (It is essential that the glacial acetic acid is redistilled for the reagent to remain colourless.)

*Method.* Add $HClO_4$ to the DNA sample to bring the $HClO_4$ concentration to 0.5M. Add two volumes of diphenylamine reagent to one volume of sample containing 10–100 μg of DNA/ml of 0.5M-$HClO_4$. At the same time, set up DNA standards and a reagent blank. Incubate for 16-20 hr at 30°C and read the absorbance at 600 nm.

*Comments.* Any pure DNA can be used as standard. Solid DNA always contains an indeterminate amount of water and it is necessary to determine the concentration of the standard by measuring its absorbance at 260 nm. A solution containing 1 mg of DNA/ml has $A_{260}$ of 20.0.

This method is particularly useful for the estimation of DNA extracted from tissues with dilute $HClO_4$. The $HClO_4$ concentration must lie between 0.25M and 0.65M. Trichloroacetic acid up to a concentration of 10% has no effect on the assay. The presence of RNA in manifold excess seems to have no effect on colour development.

## 4 DENSITY GRADIENT SOLUTIONS

### (a) SUCROSE

Molecular weight: 342.30

| Conc. of sucrose | | | Density (g/ml) | | Refractive index $(n_D)$* | Viscosity (centipoise) | |
| --- | --- | --- | --- | --- | --- | --- | --- |
| % (w/w) | g/l of soln. at 20°C | Molarity (M) | 0°C | 20°C | 20°C | 0°C | 20°C |
| 0 | – | – | 1.000 | 0.998 | 1.3330 | 1.78 | 1.00 |
| 1 | 10.02 | 0.029 | 1.004 | 1.002 | 1.3344 | 1.83 | 1.03 |
| 2 | 20.12 | 0.059 | 1.008 | 1.006 | 1.3359 | 1.88 | 1.06 |
| 4 | 40.55 | 0.119 | 1.016 | 1.014 | 1.3388 | 2.00 | 1.12 |
| 6 | 61.31 | 0.179 | 1.024 | 1.022 | 1.3418 | 2.13 | 1.18 |
| 8 | 82.40 | 0.241 | 1.033 | 1.030 | 1.3448 | 2.29 | 1.25 |
| 10 | 103.81 | 0.303 | 1.041 | 1.038 | 1.3478 | 2.46 | 1.34 |
| 12 | 125.6 | 0.367 | 1.050 | 1.046 | 1.3509 | 2.65 | 1.43 |
| 14 | 147.7 | 0.431 | 1.058 | 1.055 | 1.3541 | 2.88 | 1.53 |
| 16 | 170.2 | 0.497 | 1.067 | 1.063 | 1.3573 | 3.13 | 1.65 |
| 18 | 193.0 | 0.564 | 1.076 | 1.072 | 1.3605 | 3.43 | 1.79 |
| 20 | 216.2 | 0.632 | 1.085 | 1.081 | 1.3638 | 3.81 | 1.96 |
| 22 | 239.8 | 0.701 | 1.094 | 1.090 | 1.3672 | 4.21 | 2.14 |
| 24 | 263.8 | 0.771 | 1.104 | 1.099 | 1.3706 | 4.69 | 2.35 |
| 26 | 288.1 | 0.842 | 1.113 | 1.108 | 1.3740 | 5.26 | 2.59 |
| 28 | 312.9 | 0.914 | 1.123 | 1.118 | 1.3775 | 5.93 | 2.87 |
| 30 | 338.1 | 0.988 | 1.133 | 1.127 | 1.3811 | 6.74 | 3.21 |
| 32 | 363.7 | 1.063 | 1.143 | 1.137 | 1.3847 | 7.70 | 3.61 |
| 34 | 389.8 | 1.139 | 1.153 | 1.146 | 1.3883 | 8.90 | 4.08 |
| 36 | 416.2 | 1.216 | 1.163 | 1.156 | 1.3920 | 10.38 | 4.65 |
| 38 | 443.2 | 1.295 | 1.173 | 1.166 | 1.3958 | 12.25 | 5.35 |
| 40 | 470.6 | 1.375 | 1.184 | 1.176 | 1.3997 | 14.65 | 6.21 |
| 42 | 498.4 | 1.456 | 1.194 | 1.187 | 1.4036 | 17.8 | 7.28 |
| 44 | 526.8 | 1.539 | 1.205 | 1.197 | 1.4076 | 21.9 | 8.64 |
| 46 | 555.6 | 1.623 | 1.216 | 1.208 | 1.4117 | 27.4 | 10.37 |
| 48 | 584.9 | 1.709 | 1.227 | 1.219 | 1.4158 | 34.8 | 12.60 |
| 50 | 614.8 | 1.796 | 1.238 | 1.230 | 1.4200 | 45.1 | 15.54 |
| 52 | 645.1 | 1.885 | 1.249 | 1.241 | 1.4242 | 59.5 | 19.5 |
| 54 | 676.0 | 1.975 | 1.261 | 1.252 | 1.4285 | 80.5 | 24.9 |
| 56 | 707.4 | 2.067 | 1.272 | 1.263 | 1.4329 | 112 | 32.4 |
| 58 | 739.4 | 2.160 | 1.284 | 1.275 | 1.4373 | 160 | 43.1 |
| 60 | 771.9 | 2.255 | 1.296 | 1.286 | 1.4418 | 237 | 58.9 |
| 62 | 804.9 | 2.351 | 1.308 | 1.298 | 1.4464 | 367 | 83.0 |
| 64 | 838.6 | 2.450 | 1.320 | 1.310 | 1.4509 | 596 | 121 |
| 66 | 872.8 | 2.550 | 1.332 | 1.322 | 1.4555 | 1020 | 183 |

* Refractive index for the sodium D line, 589 nm $(n_D)$.

Additional data are given in *Prog. Biophys. Biophys. Chem.* **9**, 357 (1959); *International Critical Tables*, vol. 2, p. 343 (1927); F.J. Bates, *Polarimetry, Saccharimetry and the Sugars*, Circular 440, National Bureau of Standards, Washington, D.C. (1942).

The density of sucrose solutions at any temperature between 0°C and 30°C may be calculated using the equation of Barber, *Natl. Cancer Inst. Monograph* **21**, 219 (1966). (This paper also contains equations for calculation of density at higher temperatures and for calculation of viscosity):

$$\rho_T = (B_1 + B_2 T + B_3 T^2) + (B_4 + B_5 T + B_6 T^2) Y + (B_7 + B_8 T + B_9 T^2) Y^2$$

where $\rho_T$ = density of a sucrose solution.

$T$ = temperature ($^\circ$C),

$Y$ = weight fraction of sucrose in the solution,

and $B_{1-9}$ are constants with the following values:

| | | |
|---|---|---|
| $B_1$ 1.00037 | $B_2$ 3.96805 × 10$^{-5}$ | $B_3$ −5.85133 × 10$^{-6}$ |
| $B_4$ 0.389824 | $B_5$ −1.05789 × 10$^{-3}$ | $B_6$ 1.23928 × 10$^{-5}$ |
| $B_7$ 0.170976 | $B_8$ 4.75301 × 10$^{-4}$ | $B_9$ −8.92397 × 10$^{-6}$ |

## (b) CAESIUM CHLORIDE

Molecular weight: 168.37

| Conc. of CsCl | | | Density (g/ml) | | Refractive index $(n_D)$* |
|---|---|---|---|---|---|
| % (w/w) | g/l of soln. at 25°C | Molarity (M) | 0°C | 25°C | 25°C |
| 0 | — | — | 1.000 | 0.997 | 1.3326 |
| 1 | 10.05 | 0.056 | 1.008 | 1.005 | 1.3333 |
| 2 | 20.25 | 0.119 | 1.016 | 1.013 | 1.3340 |
| 3 | 30.61 | 0.182 | | 1.020 | 1.3348 |
| 4 | 41.14 | 0.244 | 1.032 | 1.028 | 1.3356 |
| 5 | 51.83 | 0.308 | | 1.037 | 1.3364 |
| 6 | 62.68 | 0.373 | 1.049 | 1.045 | 1.3372 |
| 7 | 73.72 | 0.438 | | 1.053 | 1.3380 |
| 8 | 84.92 | 0.504 | 1.066 | 1.062 | 1.3388 |
| 9 | 96.30 | 0.572 | | 1.070 | 1.3397 |
| 10 | 107.88 | 0.641 | 1.084 | 1.079 | 1.3405 |
| 11 | 119.6 | 0.710 | | 1.088 | 1.3414 |
| 12 | 131.6 | 0.782 | 1.102 | 1.097 | 1.3423 |
| 13 | 143.8 | 0.854 | | 1.106 | 1.3431 |
| 14 | 156.1 | 0.927 | 1.121 | 1.115 | 1.3441 |
| 15 | 168.7 | 1.002 | | 1.124 | 1.3450 |
| 16 | 181.4 | 1.077 | 1.140 | 1.134 | 1.3459 |
| 17 | 194.4 | 1.155 | | 1.144 | 1.3469 |
| 18 | 207.6 | 1.233 | 1.160 | 1.154 | 1.3478 |
| 19 | 221.1 | 1.313 | | 1.164 | 1.3488 |
| 20 | 234.8 | 1.395 | 1.181 | 1.174 | 1.3498 |
| 21 | 248.7 | 1.477 | | 1.184 | 1.3508 |
| 22 | 262.9 | 1.561 | 1.203 | 1.195 | 1.3518 |
| 23 | 277.3 | 1.647 | | 1.205 | 1.3529 |
| 24 | 291.9 | 1.734 | 1.225 | 1.216 | 1.3539 |
| 25 | 306.9 | 1.823 | | 1.227 | 1.3550 |
| 26 | 322.1 | 1.913 | 1.247 | 1.239 | 1.3561 |
| 27 | 337.6 | 2.005 | | 1.250 | 1.3572 |
| 28 | 353.3 | 2.098 | 1.271 | 1.262 | 1.3584 |
| 29 | 369.4 | 2.194 | | 1.274 | 1.3595 |
| 30 | 385.7 | 2.291 | 1.296 | 1.286 | 1.3607 |
| 31 | 402.4 | 2.390 | | 1.298 | 1.3619 |
| 32 | 419.5 | 2.492 | | 1.311 | 1.3632 |
| 33 | 436.9 | 2.595 | | 1.323 | 1.3644 |
| 34 | 454.2 | 2.698 | | 1.336 | 1.3657 |
| 35 | 472.4 | 2.806 | 1.361 | 1.350 | 1.3670 |

| Conc. of CsCl | | | Density (g/ml) | | Refractive index $(n_D)$* |
|---|---|---|---|---|---|
| % (w/w) | g/l of soln. at 25°C | Molarity (M) | 0°C | 25°C | 25°C |
| 36 | 490.7 | 2.914 | | 1.363 | 1.3683 |
| 37 | 509.5 | 3.026 | | 1.377 | 1.3696 |
| 38 | 528.6 | 3.140 | | 1.391 | 1.3709 |
| 39 | 548.3 | 3.257 | | 1.405 | 1.3722 |
| 40 | 567.8 | 3.372 | 1.432 | 1.420 | 1.3736 |
| 41 | 588.4 | 3.495 | | 1.434 | 1.3749 |
| 42 | 609.0 | 3.617 | | 1.450 | 1.3763 |
| 43 | 630.0 | 3.742 | | 1.465 | 1.3777 |
| 44 | 651.6 | 3.870 | | 1.481 | 1.3792 |
| 45 | 673.6 | 4.001 | 1.511 | 1.497 | 1.3807 |
| 46 | 696.0 | 4.134 | | 1.513 | 1.3822 |
| 47 | 718.6 | 4.268 | | 1.530 | 1.3837 |
| 48 | 742.1 | 4.408 | | 1.547 | 1.3853 |
| 49 | 766.4 | 4.552 | | 1.565 | 1.3869 |
| 50 | 791.3 | 4.700 | 1.598 | 1.582 | 1.3886 |
| 51 | 816.5 | 4.849 | | 1.601 | 1.3902 |
| 52 | 841.9 | 5.000 | | 1.619 | 1.3920 |
| 53 | 868.1 | 5.156 | | 1.638 | 1.3937 |
| 54 | 895.3 | 5.317 | | 1.658 | 1.3955 |
| 55 | 922.8 | 5.481 | 1.695 | 1.678 | 1.3973 |
| 56 | 951.4 | 5.651 | | 1.698 | 1.3992 |
| 57 | 980.4 | 5.823 | | 1.719 | 1.4011 |
| 58 | 1009.8 | 5.998 | | 1.740 | 1.4031 |
| 59 | 1040.2 | 6.178 | | 1.762 | 1.4051 |
| 60 | 1070.8 | 6.360 | 1.804 | 1.785 | 1.4072 |
| 61 | 1102.9 | 6.550 | | 1.808 | 1.4093 |
| 62 | 1135.8 | 6.746 | | 1.831 | 1.4115 |
| 63 | 1167.3 | 6.945 | | 1.855 | 1.4137 |
| 64 | 1203.2 | 7.146 | | 1.880 | 1.4160 |
| 65 | 1238.4 | 7.355 | | 1.905 | 1.4183 |

* Refractive index for the sodium D line, 589 nm $(n_D)$.

Additional data are given in *International Critical Tables,* vol. 3, p. 94 (1927); *BBA* **108**, 18 (1965) — this paper includes viscosity data; *Biopolymers* **9**, 597 (1970).

The concentration of CsCl solution corresponding to any desired density between 1.29 and 1.80 (30–60% (w/w) of CsCl) at 25°C can be calculated from the formula:

$$\text{Weight \% of CsCl} = 137.48 - 138.11(1/\rho_{25})$$

where $\rho_{25}$ is the desired density at 25°C.

The relationship between density $(\rho_{25})$ and refractive index for the sodium D line $(n_D^{25})$, both at 25°C, of CsCl solutions is given by the following relationships:

$$\rho_{25} = 10.2402n_D^{25} - 12.6483 \qquad \text{(for } \rho_{25} < 1.37)$$

$$\rho_{25} = 10.8601n_D^{25} - 13.4974 \qquad \text{(for } \rho_{25} = 1.25 - 1.90)$$

$$\rho_{25} = 1.1584 - 10.2219n_D^{25} + 7.5806(n_D^{25})^2 \qquad \text{(for } \rho_{25} = 1.00 - 1.90)$$

## 23  Biochemical procedures

### (c) OTHER SALTS

Expressions relating density to refractive index or concentration of various salt solutions are given in *Fortschr. Chem. Org. Naturst.* **20**, 372 (1962) and *Biopolymers* **9**, 597 (1970). Expressions for some salts which have been used to make density gradients are given below. Density data for these and other salts are given in *International Critical Tables*, vol. 3, pp. 51–95 (1928).

| Salt | Expression to calculate density at 25°C | Applicable to densities in the range: |
|---|---|---|
| $Cs_2SO_4$ | $12.1200 n_D^{25} - 15.1662$ | 1.15–1.40 |
| | $13.6986 n_D^{25} - 17.3233$ | 1.40–1.70 |
| | $1.0047 + 0.28369 m - 0.017428 m^2$ | 1.14–1.80 |
| | $0.9945 + 11.1066 (n_D^{25} - n_0) - 26.4460 (n_D^{25} - n_0)^2$ | 1.14–1.80 |
| CsBr | $9.9667 n_D^{25} - 12.2876$ | 1.25–1.35 |
| | $2.7798 - 12.2102 n_D^{25} + 8.1615 (n_D^{25})^2$ | 1.05–1.50 |
| CsI | $8.8757 n_D^{25} - 10.8381$ | 1.20–1.55 |
| | $4.5245 - 13.5833 n_D^{25} + 8.2067 (n_D^{25})^2$ | 1.05–1.55 |
| NaCl | $4.23061 n_D^{25} - 4.64125$ | 1.00–1.19 |
| KBr | $6.4786 n_D^{25} - 7.6431$ | 1.10–1.35 |
| RbCl | $21.7661 - 39.2834 n_D^{25} + 17.7843 (n_D^{25})^2$ | 1.05–1.35 |

$n_D^{25}$ = refractive index for sodium D line at 25°C.
$n_0$  = refractive index of water at 25°C.
$m$  = molality (moles/1000 g of solution).


### (d) PROPRIETARY GRADIENT FORMING SUBSTANCES

*Metrizamide* (Nyegaard & Co., Oslo, Norway)
  2-(3-Acetamido-5-*N*-methylacetamido-2,4,6-triiodobenzamido)-2-deoxy-D-glucose.

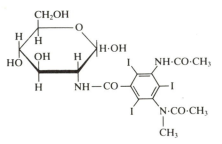

M. wt. 789. Non-ionic. Wh. powder, v.s. $H_2O$, s. dil. aq. acids, s. 75% EtOH. Strong u.v. absorbance, $\lambda_{max}$ 242 nm. Solns. stable indefinitely in the dark at $-20°C$, stable in the dark at room temperature and pH 3–8. Light and temperatures above 55°C cause decomposition with release of $I_2$.
  Max. density of aqueous soln. 1.46. Viscosity lower than sucrose solns. of same density, but rises rapidly above $\rho = 1.30$. REVIEW. *FEBS Lett.* **50**, 102 (1975)

| Conc. (w/v) | 10 | 20 | 30 | 40 | 50 | 60 | 70 | 80 |
|---|---|---|---|---|---|---|---|---|
| $\rho$ at 20°C | 1.025 | 1.106 | 1.160 | 1.214 | 1.268 | 1.322 | 1.376 | 1.430 |

$$\rho \text{ at } 20°C = 3.350 n_D^{20} - 3.462$$

$$\rho \text{ at } 5°C = 3.453 n_D^{20} - 3.601$$

where $\rho$ is the density and $n_D^{20}$ the refractive index for sodium D line at 20°C.

*Urograffin* (Schering Chemicals, Berlin)
Mixed Na and 1-deoxy-1-(methylamino)-D-glucitol (methylglucamine) salts of diatrizoic acid.

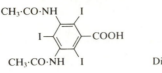

Diatrizoic acid

M.wt. of free acid 614. Strong u.v. absorbance. Store in the dark, light causes loss of $I_2$.
Max. density of aq. soln. 1.45. Low viscosity, considerably less than sucrose solns. of the same density.

*Ficoll 400* (Pharmacia)
Highly branched copolymer of sucrose and epichlorohydrin.
Wt. av. M. wt. 400 000. No ionizable groups. Soluble in $H_2O$ up to 50% (w/v). Stable in alkaline and neutral solns. Hydrolysed at pHs below 3, esp. at elevated temps. In neutral soln. can be sterilized by autoclaving at 110°C for 30 min without degradation. Liable to degradation by strong oxidizing and reducing agents.
Max. density of aq. soln. 1.23. Osmotic pressure of Ficoll solns. very low compared with sucrose solns. of the same density, but viscosity of Ficoll solns. is very much higher.

| Conc. % (w/v) | 10 | 20 | 30 | 40 | 50 |
|---|---|---|---|---|---|
| $\rho$ at 20°C | 1.033 | 1.068 | 1.103 | 1.138 | 1.171 |
| Viscosity ($\eta_{rel}$) at 20°C | 5 | 20 | 60 | 180 | 600 |

Full tables of density and viscosity of Ficoll solns. at 4°C, 15°C, and 25°C are given in *Anal. Biochem.* **29**, 230 (1969).

*Percoll* (Pharmacia)
Colloidal silica particles coated with polyvinylpyrrolidone (PVP). PVP content of coated particles approx. 12%; 1-2% free PVP. Average diameter of coated particles 21-22 nm (range 15-30 nm). In absence of added salt or sucrose, can be sterilized by autoclaving at 120°C for 20 min without deterioration.
Max. density possible in gradients 1.30 g/ml. Low osmotic pressure. Low viscosity, affected by ionic strength. At a density of 1.20, viscosity in 0.15M-NaCl is approx. 10 cP, in 0.25M-sucrose approx. 30 cP. Supplied as 23% (w/v) colloidal sol with density of 1.130 ± 0.005.
REVIEW. *Anal. Biochem.* **88**, 271 (1978).


## 5 PROTEIN PRECIPITANTS

(a) TUNGSTIC ACID

*JBC* **38**, 81 (1919); **182**, 29 (1950).
Solution A. 10% (w/v) sodium tungstate ($Na_2WO_4 \cdot 2H_2O$) in water.
Solution B. 0.335M-$H_2SO_4$.
Homogenize tissue sample with water to required dilution, then add tungstate solution, followed by an equal volume of sulphuric acid dropwise with thorough

mixing. Alternatively equal volumes of solution A and solution B may be mixed before adding to the sample. The mixed reagent is not stable; it should be kept not more than two weeks and renewed if any precipitate appears. The filtrate obtained by tungstic acid precipitation has a pH of approx. 6.5.

Approximate amounts required for complete precipitation of protein (rat tissues):

| Tissue | Amount | Homogenize with (ml $H_2O$) | Solution A | Solution B |
|---|---|---|---|---|
| Whole blood | 1 ml | 7 ml | 1 ml | 1 ml |
| Plasma | 1 ml | 8 ml | 0.5 ml | 0.5 ml |
| Liver | 1 g | 7.5 ml | 0.75 ml | 0.75 ml |
| Brain | 1 g | 3.4 ml | 0.3 ml | 0.3 ml |
| Muscle | 1 g | 2.8 ml | 0.6 ml | 0.6 ml |
| Spleen | 1 g | 8.1 ml | 0.45 ml | 0.45 ml |

### (b) ZINC SULPHATE–ALKALI

*JBC* **86**, 655 (1930); **160**, 69 (1945).

Cadmium sulphate may be used in place of $ZnSO_4$, but offers no particular advantage as a protein precipitant.

(i) Solution A. 10% $ZnSO_4 \cdot 7H_2O$
Solution B. 0.5M-NaOH

10 ml A diluted with 70 ml $H_2O$ should require approx. 11 ml B when titrated using phenolphthalein (permanent pink).

Dilute 1 ml whole blood to 8 ml, add 1 ml solution A, mix, add 1 ml solution B, mix and filter. Quantities for other tissues similar to those for tungstic acid.

(ii) Solution A. 12.5 g $ZnSO_4 \cdot 7H_2O$ plus 125 ml 0.125M-$H_2SO_4$. Dilute to 1 l.
Solution B. 0.75M-NaOH

50 ml A should require 6.7–6.8 ml B when titrated using phenolphthalein (permanent pink).

Mix 1 ml whole blood with 8 ml solution A. Add 1 ml solution B, mix, and filter. Use similar proportions for other tissues.

(iii) Solution A. 5% $ZnSO_4 \cdot 7H_2O$
Solution B. 0.15M-Ba(OH)$_2$

10 ml A diluted with 100 ml $H_2O$ should require 10 ml B when titrated using phenolphthalein (permanent pink).

Dilute 1 ml whole blood with 5 ml $H_2O$. Add 2 ml solution A, mix, and then add 2 ml solution B. Mix and filter. Use same proportions for other tissues.

### (c) TRICHLOROACETIC ACID

For blood, mix 1 ml blood with 9 ml 10% (w/v) trichloroacetic acid and then centrifuge or filter. For tissue extracts, enzyme incubation mixtures, etc., a final concentration of 3–5% (w/v) is normally sufficient to ensure complete precipitation of proteins. Non-protein N remains in the supernatant. After removal of the protein precipitate, the trichloroacetic acid can be largely removed from the supernatant by extracting several times with water-saturated diethyl ether.

### (d) PERCHLORIC ACID

For tissue extracts, enzyme incubation mixtures, etc., add sufficient perchloric acid to give a final concentration of 3–5% (0.3–0.5M). After centrifuging, excess perchloric acid may be precipitated as the potassium salt by neutralizing the supernatant with KOH, $K_2CO_3$, or $K_3PO_4$ solution, and then cooling to $0°C$ before removing the precipitate of $KClO_4$ by centrifuging. Do not allow the mixture to warm up during centrifuging since $KClO_4$ is appreciably more soluble at room temperature than at $0°C$.

(e) ETHANOL

Add sufficient ethanol to give a final concentration of 75–80% (v/v), heat the mixture (preferably to boiling for 1–2 min), cool, centrifuge, and decant the supernatant. Ethanol may be removed, together with lipid material, by the addition of 3 volumes of $CHCl_3$. Mix thoroughly and centrifuge. The ethanol dissolves in the $CHCl_3$ (lower) layer.

# 24 Definitions, formulae, and general information

## 1 APPROXIMATE MOLARITIES AND SPECIFIC GRAVITIES OF CONCENTRATED ACIDS AND AMMONIA

|  | M. wt. | Percentage by weight | Approx. molarity M | ml per 1 to prepare M-soln. | Sp.gr. |
|---|---|---|---|---|---|
| Acetic acid | 60.05 | 99.6 | 17.4 | 57.5 | 1.05 |
| Ammonia | 17.03 | 25 | 13.3 | 75.1 | 0.91 |
|  |  | 35 | 18.1 | 55.2 | 0.88 |
| Formic acid | 46.03 | 90 | 23.6 | 42.4 | 1.205 |
|  |  | 98 | 25.9 | 38.5 | 1.22 |
| Hydrochloric acid | 36.46 | 36 | 11.6 | 85.9 | 1.18 |
| Nitric acid | 63.01 | 70 | 15.7 | 63.7 | 1.42 |
| Perchloric acid | 100.46 | 60 | 9.2 | 108.8 | 1.54 |
|  |  | 72 | 12.2 | 82.1 | 1.70 |
| Phosphoric acid | 98.00 | 85 | 14.7 | 67.8 | 1.70 |
| Sulphuric acid | 98.07 | 98 | 18.3 | 54.5 | 1.835 |

## 2 PRESSURE–TEMPERATURE TABLE FOR AUTOCLAVES

| Pressure (lb/in²) | (kPa) | Temperature °C | °F | Pressure (lb/in²) | (kPa) | Temperature °C | °F |
|---|---|---|---|---|---|---|---|
| 0 | 0 | 100.0 | 212.0 | 16 | 110.32 | 122.0 | 251.6 |
| 1 | 6.89 | 101.9 | 215.4 | 17 | 117.21 | 123.0 | 253.4 |
| 2 | 13.79 | 103.6 | 218.5 | 18 | 124.11 | 124.1 | 255.4 |
| 3 | 20.68 | 105.3 | 221.5 | 19 | 131.00 | 125.0 | 257.0 |
| 4 | 27.58 | 106.9 | 224.4 | 20 | 137.90 | 126.0 | 258.8 |
| 5 | 34.47 | 108.4 | 227.1 | 25 | 172.37 | 130.4 | 266.7 |
| 6 | 41.37 | 109.8 | 229.6 | 30 | 206.84 | 134.5 | 274.1 |
| 7 | 48.26 | 111.3 | 232.3 | 35 | 241.32 | 138.1 | 280.6 |
| 8 | 55.16 | 112.6 | 234.7 | 40 | 275.79 | 141.5 | 286.7 |
| 9 | 62.05 | 113.9 | 237.0 | 45 | 310.26 | 144.6 | 292.3 |
| 10 | 68.95 | 115.2 | 239.4 | 50 | 344.74 | 147.6 | 297.7 |
| 11 | 75.84 | 116.4 | 241.5 | 60 | 413.69 | 153.0 | 307.4 |
| 12 | 82.74 | 117.6 | 243.7 | 70 | 482.63 | 157.8 | 316.0 |
| 13 | 89.63 | 118.8 | 245.8 | 80 | 551.58 | 162.1 | 323.8 |
| 14 | 96.53 | 119.9 | 247.8 | 90 | 620.53 | 166.2 | 331.2 |
| 15 | 103.42 | 121.0 | 249.8 | 100 | 689.48 | 169.9 | 337.8 |

Conversion factors for units of pressure:

$$1 \, lbf/in^2 = 6895 \, Pa$$

$$1 \, atmosphere = 101325 \, Pa$$

$$1 \, mm \, Hg = 133.3 \, Pa$$

## 3 CENTRIFUGAL FIELD (g)

Centrifugal field or $g$ value may be calculated by the following formulae:

$$\text{Centrifugal field } (g) = 1118 \times 10^{-8} \times R \times N^2$$

where $R$ = radius in **cm** from the centre of the rotor to the point at which the centrifugal field is required, and $N$ = speed of rotor in revolutions/min.

$$\text{Centrifugal field } (g) = 284 \times 10^{-7} \times R \times N^2$$

where $R$ = radius in **inches** from the centre of the rotor to the point at which the centrifugal field is required, and $N$ = speed of rotor in revolutions/min.

## 4 SPECTROPHOTOMETRIC TERMS

The following definitions are recommended by IUPAC:

$$A = -\log_{10} T = \log_{10} I_0/I = \epsilon lc,$$

where $A$ = absorbance,
$T$ = transmittance (transmission),
$I_0$ = intensity of incident light,
$I$ = intensity of transmitted light,
$\epsilon$ = molar absorption coefficient,
$c$ = concentration (mol/litre),
$l$ = length of optical path (cm).

Under this definition $\epsilon$ is numerically equal to the absorbance of a 1M-solution (i.e. 1 mol/litre) using a 1-cm light path. It has the dimensions litre. $mol^{-1}.cm^{-1}$ or $M^{-1}.cm^{-1}$ (*not* $cm^2.mol^{-1}$) and, for substances which absorb visible or u.v. light strongly, e.g. purines, pyrimidines, flavins, porphyrins, nictotinamide nucleotides, etc., is of the order of magnitude $10^3$ to $10^5$.

An alternative definition, once widely employed, expresses $c$ (concentration) in mol/ml. In this case, $\epsilon$ is numerically equal to the absorbance of a solution containing 1 mol/ml using a 1-cm light path; it has the dimensions $cm^2.mol^{-1}$ and is of the order of magnitude $10^6$ to $10^8$.

## 5 OPTICAL ROTATION

$$[\alpha] = 100\alpha/lc,$$

where $[\alpha]$ = specific rotation, defined as the rotation of a 10-cm thickness of a solution containing 1 g of solute/ml. Temperature is denoted by a superscript and the wavelength of light used by a subscript (D indicates the D line of sodium at 589 nm),
$\alpha$ = observed rotation,
$l$ = length of light path in **decimeters**,
$c$ = concentration in g/100 ml solution.

$[M]$, the molar rotation, is the rotation of a 10-cm thickness of a solution containing 1 mol of solute in 100 ml. It is calculated from the equation

$$[M] = (\text{M. wt.}/100)[\alpha],$$

where M.wt. = molecular weight.

## 6 OXIDATION–REDUCTION POTENTIAL

The oxidation–reduction potential is the electrode potential of a half-cell containing a mixture of oxidized and reduced forms of an oxidation–reduction system,

$$E = E_0 + \frac{RT}{nF}\ln\frac{a_{ox}}{a_{red}},$$

where
- $E$ = observed potential,
- $E_0$ = the standard potential, defined as the potential of the system when all the reactants are present at unit activity,
- $R$ = gas constant,
- $T$ = absolute temperature,
- $n$ = number of equivalents involved in the reaction,
- $F$ = the faraday (96 494 coulombs),
- $a_{ox}$ = activity of the oxidized form of the oxidation – reduction system,
- $a_{red}$ = activity of the reduced form of the system.

In practice, $E_0$ is often taken to be the electrode potential when the concentrations of oxidized and reduced forms are equal, and not necessarily unity.

Note that, for reactions involving a proton, $E_0$ is the standard electrode potential at unit activity of hydrogen ions, i.e. pH 0. For such reactions the term $E_0'$ is used to indicate measurements made at stated pHs other than 0. In biochemical work this pH is usually 7.

## 7 UNITS OF ENZYME ACTIVITY

The commonest way of expressing enzyme activity is as the rate of the reaction catalysed, for example in units of $\mu$mol of substrate transformed/min or $\mu$mol of product formed/min.

There are, in addition, two defined units of enzyme activity currently in use, the standard unit (U), which was defined in *Enzyme Nomenclature, Recommendations 1964*, and the katal (kat), which was introduced in *Enzyme Nomenclature, Recommendations 1972* to take account of the practice in chemical kinetics and of the introduction of SI units. They are defined as follows:

One unit (U) of any enzyme is defined as that amount which will catalyse the transformation of 1 $\mu$mol of substrate per minute, or, where more than one bond of each substrate molecule is attacked, 1 micro-equivalent of the group concerned per minute, under defined conditions.

One katal (kat) is that catalytic activity that will raise the rate of reaction by one mole per second in a specified assay system. [This definition is given with comments in *EJB* **97**, 319 (1979)].

In both cases it is important that the conditions employed, such as temperature, pH, substrate concentration, should be stated.

Specific activity is usually expressed, in the first two cases, as $\mu$mol.min$^{-1}$.(mg of protein)$^{-1}$ or U.(mg of protein)$^{-1}$ respectively. When enzyme activity is expressed in katals, specific activity should be given in kat.(kg of protein)$^{-1}$

In order to convert between the three systems:

$$1\,\mu mol.min^{-1} \equiv 1\,U \equiv 16.67\,nkat$$

## 8 SOLUBILITIES OF GASES: BUNSEN COEFFICIENTS

The Bunsen coefficient ($\alpha$) is defined as the volume of gas in ml reduced to $0\,^{\circ}C$ and 760 mm pressure dissolved in 1 ml of water (or other fluid) when the gas pressure is 760 mm Hg.

(a) IN WATER

| Temp. (°C) | $O_2$ | $H_2$ | $N_2$ | $CO_2$ |
|---|---|---|---|---|
| 0 | 0.049 | 0.021 | 0.024 | 1.713 |
| 5 | 0.043 | 0.020 | 0.021 | 1.424 |
| 10 | 0.038 | 0.020 | 0.019 | 1.194 |
| 15 | 0.034 | 0.019 | 0.017 | 1.019 |
| 20 | 0.031 | 0.018 | 0.015 | 0.878 |
| 25 | 0.028 | 0.018 | 0.014 | 0.759 |
| 30 | 0.026 | 0.017 | 0.013 | 0.665 |
| 35 | 0.024 | 0.017 | 0.013 | 0.592 |
| 37 | 0.024 | 0.017 | 0.012 | 0.567 |
| 38 | 0.023 | 0.017 | 0.012 | 0.550 |
| 40 | 0.023 | 0.016 | 0.012 | 0.530 |
| 45 | 0.022 | 0.016 | 0.011 | 0.479 |
| 50 | 0.021 | 0.016 | 0.011 | 0.436 |

(b) IN SALT SOLUTIONS, ETC.

(1) Carbon dioxide. Van Slyke et al.—JBC **78**, 765 (1928)—give values for $\alpha_{CO_2}$ at 38°C in various salt solutions, including the following (compared with $\alpha_{CO_2}$ at 38°C in water = 0.546):

| Conc. | NaCl | KCl | Na lactate | $KH_2PO_4$ | $NaH_2PO_4$ |
|---|---|---|---|---|---|
| 0.15M | 0.529 | 0.532 | 0.522 | 0.516 | 0.510 |
| 0.30M | 0.511 | 0.520 | 0.500 | 0.490 | 0.480 |

$\alpha_{CO_2}$ at 38°C in Ringer's soln., 0.537; serum, 0.510.

The effects of individual ions are additive, at least in solutions below 0.5M, and Van Slyke et al. give the following figures for the **decrease** in $\alpha_{CO_2}$ at 38°C per unit molar concentration of the ion present in the solution:

| $H^+$ | $Na^+$ | $K^+$ | $Cl^-$ | $H_2PO_4^-$ | Lactate$^-$ | $HC_2O_4^-$ |
|---|---|---|---|---|---|---|
| 0.0 | 0.085 | 0.053 | 0.029 | 0.137 | 0.066 | 0.026 |

$\alpha_{CO_2}$ in $H_2SO_4$ at 25°C: 0.25M-$H_2SO_4$, 0.727; 0.5M-$H_2SO_4$, 0.705; M-$H_2SO_4$, 0.669.

Further figures for $\alpha_{CO_2}$ in solutions of salts, acids, and non-electrolytes, mainly at 25°C and 40°C, are given in JBC **78**, 765 (1928); International Critical Tables, vol. 3, p. 279 (1928); JACS **63**, 449, 1165 (1941); JACS **65**, 2030 (1943).

(2) Oxygen. The solubility of oxygen (and of hydrogen and nitrogen) in salt solutions is markedly less than in water. For example, values of $\alpha_{O_2}$ at 25°C are: in M-$H_2SO_4$, 0.023; in 2M-NaCl, 0.015.

Chappell — BJ **90**, 225 (1964) — describes a method using an oxygen electrode to determine the concentration of oxygen dissolved in any salt solution. He gives the following figures for $O_2$ concentration in **air**-saturated buffer (pH 7.2) containing 80 mM-KCl, 15mM-$P_i$ and 20 mM-triethanolamine:

| Temperature (°C) | 15 | 20 | 25 | 30 | 35 | 40 |
|---|---|---|---|---|---|---|
| Oxygen conc. of air-saturated buffer ($\mu$g. atom/ml) | 0.575 | 0.51 | 0.474 | 0.445 | 0.41 | 0.38 |

# 25 Atomic weights

ATOMIC WEIGHTS, 1981

*Pure & Appl. Chem.* **55**, 1101 (1983).

The atomic weight scale is based on $^{12}C = 12$ as standard.

| Name | Symbol | Atomic number | Atomic weight |
| --- | --- | --- | --- |
| Aluminium | Al | 13 | 26.98154 |
| Antimony | Sb | 51 | 121.75 |
| Argon | Ar | 18 | 39.948 |
| Arsenic | As | 33 | 74.9216 |
| Barium | Ba | 56 | 137.33 |
| Beryllium | Be | 4 | 9.01218 |
| Bismuth | Bi | 83 | 208.9804 |
| Boron | B | 5 | 10.81 |
| Bromine | Br | 35 | 79.904 |
| Cadmium | Cd | 48 | 112.41 |
| Caesium | Cs | 55 | 132.9054 |
| Calcium | Ca | 20 | 40.08 |
| Carbon | C | 6 | 12.011 |
| Cerium | Ce | 58 | 140.12 |
| Chlorine | Cl | 17 | 35.453 |
| Chromium | Cr | 24 | 51.996 |
| Cobalt | Co | 27 | 58.9332 |
| Copper | Cu | 29 | 63.546 |
| Dysprosium | Dy | 66 | 162.50 |
| Erbium | Er | 68 | 167.26 |
| Europium | Eu | 63 | 151.96 |
| Fluorine | F | 9 | 18.998403 |
| Gadolinium | Gd | 64 | 157.25 |
| Gallium | Ga | 31 | 69.72 |
| Germanium | Ge | 32 | 72.59 |
| Gold | Au | 79 | 196.9665 |
| Hafnium | Hf | 72 | 178.49 |
| Helium | He | 2 | 4.00260 |
| Holmium | Ho | 67 | 164.9304 |
| Hydrogen | H | 1 | 1.00794 |
| Indium | In | 49 | 114.82 |
| Iodine | I | 53 | 126.9045 |
| Iridium | Ir | 77 | 192.22 |
| Iron | Fe | 26 | 55.847 |
| Krypton | Kr | 36 | 83.80 |
| Lanthanum | La | 57 | 138.9055 |
| Lead | Pb | 82 | 207.2 |
| Lithium | Li | 3 | 6.941 |
| Lutetium | Lu | 71 | 174.967 |
| Magnesium | Mg | 12 | 24.305 |
| Manganese | Mn | 25 | 54.9380 |
| Mercury | Hg | 80 | 200.59 |
| Molybdenum | Mo | 42 | 95.94 |
| Neodymium | Nd | 60 | 144.24 |
| Neon | Ne | 10 | 20.179 |
| Nickel | Ni | 28 | 58.69 |
| Niobium | Nb | 41 | 92.9064 |
| Nitrogen | N | 7 | 14.0067 |
| Osmium | Os | 76 | 190.2 |
| Oxygen | O | 8 | 15.9994 |
| Palladium | Pd | 46 | 106.42 |

## 25 Atomic weights

| Name | Symbol | Atomic number | Atomic weight |
| --- | --- | --- | --- |
| Phosphorus | P | 15 | 30.97376 |
| Platinum | Pt | 78 | 195.08 |
| Potassium | K | 19 | 39.0983 |
| Praseodymium | Pr | 59 | 140.9077 |
| Rhenium | Re | 75 | 186.207 |
| Rhodium | Rh | 45 | 102.9055 |
| Rubidium | Rb | 37 | 85.4678 |
| Ruthenium | Ru | 44 | 101.07 |
| Samarium | Sm | 62 | 150.36 |
| Scandium | Sc | 21 | 44.9559 |
| Selenium | Se | 34 | 78.96 |
| Silicon | Si | 14 | 28.0855 |
| Silver | Ag | 47 | 107.8682 |
| Sodium | Na | 11 | 22.98977 |
| Strontium | Sr | 38 | 87.62 |
| Sulphur | S | 16 | 32.06 |
| Tantalum | Ta | 73 | 180.9479 |
| Tellerium | Te | 52 | 127.60 |
| Terbium | Tb | 65 | 158.9254 |
| Thallium | Tl | 81 | 204.383 |
| Thorium | Th | 90 | 232.0381 |
| Thulium | Tm | 69 | 168.9342 |
| Tin | Sn | 50 | 118.69 |
| Titanium | Ti | 22 | 47.88 |
| Tungsten | W | 74 | 183.85 |
| Uranium | U | 92 | 238.0289 |
| Vanadium | V | 23 | 50.9415 |
| Xenon | Xe | 54 | 131.29 |
| Ytterbium | Yb | 70 | 173.04 |
| Yttrium | Y | 39 | 88.9059 |
| Zinc | Zn | 30 | 65.38 |
| Zirconium | Zr | 40 | 91.22 |

ATOMIC WEIGHT MULTIPLES

| | Carbon<br>C = 12.011 | Hydrogen<br>H = 1.00794 | Nitrogen<br>N = 14.0067 | Oxygen<br>O = 15.9994 | |
|---|---|---|---|---|---|
| 1 | 12.01 | 1.01 | 14.01 | 16.00 | 1 |
| 2 | 24.02 | 2.02 | 28.01 | 32.00 | 2 |
| 3 | 36.03 | 3.02 | 42.02 | 48.00 | 3 |
| 4 | 48.04 | 4.03 | 56.03 | 64.00 | 4 |
| 5 | 60.06 | 5.04 | 70.03 | 80.00 | 5 |
| 6 | 72.07 | 6.05 | 84.04 | 96.00 | 6 |
| 7 | 84.08 | 7.06 | 98.05 | 112.00 | 7 |
| 8 | 96.09 | 8.06 | 112.05 | 128.00 | 8 |
| 9 | 108.10 | 9.07 | 126.06 | 143.99 | 9 |
| 10 | 120.11 | 10.08 | 140.07 | 159.99 | 10 |
| 11 | 132.12 | 11.09 | 154.07 | 175.99 | 11 |
| 12 | 144.13 | 12.10 | 168.08 | 191.99 | 12 |
| 13 | 156.14 | 13.10 | 182.09 | 207.99 | 13 |
| 14 | 168.15 | 14.11 | 196.09 | 223.99 | 14 |
| 15 | 180.17 | 15.12 | 210.10 | 239.99 | 15 |
| 16 | 192.18 | 16.13 | 224.11 | 255.99 | 16 |
| 17 | 204.19 | 17.13 | 238.11 | 271.99 | 17 |
| 18 | 216.20 | 18.14 | 252.12 | 287.99 | 18 |
| 19 | 228.21 | 19.15 | 266.13 | 303.99 | 19 |
| 20 | 240.22 | 20.16 | 280.13 | 319.99 | 20 |
| 21 | 252.23 | 21.17 | 294.14 | 335.99 | 21 |
| 22 | 264.24 | 22.17 | 308.15 | 351.99 | 22 |
| 23 | 276.25 | 23.18 | 322.15 | 367.99 | 23 |
| 24 | 288.26 | 24.19 | 336.16 | 383.99 | 24 |
| 25 | 300.28 | 25.20 | 350.17 | 399.99 | 25 |
| 26 | 312.29 | 26.21 | 364.17 | 415.98 | 26 |
| 27 | 324.30 | 27.21 | 378.18 | 431.98 | 27 |
| 28 | 336.31 | 28.22 | 392.19 | 447.98 | 28 |
| 29 | 348.32 | 29.23 | 406.19 | 463.98 | 29 |
| 30 | 360.33 | 30.24 | 420.20 | 479.98 | 30 |
| 40 | 480.44 | 40.32 | 560.27 | 639.98 | 40 |
| 50 | 600.55 | 50.40 | 700.34 | 799.97 | 50 |
| 60 | 720.66 | 60.48 | 840.40 | 959.96 | 60 |
| 70 | 840.77 | 70.56 | 980.47 | 1119.96 | 70 |
| 80 | 960.88 | 80.64 | 1120.54 | 1279.95 | 80 |
| 90 | 1080.99 | 90.71 | 1260.60 | 1439.95 | 90 |
| 100 | 1201.10 | 100.79 | 1400.67 | 1599.94 | 100 |

| | Phosphorus<br>P = 30.97376 | Sulphur<br>S = 32.06 | Chlorine<br>Cl = 35.453 | Water<br>$H_2O$ = 18.0153 | |
|---|---|---|---|---|---|
| 1 | 30.97 | 32.06 | 35.45 | 18.02 | 1 |
| 2 | 61.95 | 64.12 | 70.91 | 36.03 | 2 |
| 3 | 92.92 | 96.18 | 106.36 | 54.05 | 3 |
| 4 | 123.90 | 128.24 | 141.81 | 72.06 | 4 |
| 5 | 154.87 | 160.30 | 177.27 | 90.08 | 5 |
| 6 | 185.84 | 192.36 | 212.72 | 108.09 | 6 |
| 7 | 216.82 | 224.42 | 248.17 | 126.11 | 7 |
| 8 | 247.79 | 256.48 | 283.62 | 144.12 | 8 |
| 9 | 278.76 | 288.54 | 319.08 | 162.14 | 9 |
| 10 | 309.74 | 320.60 | 354.53 | 180.15 | 10 |
| 20 | 619.48 | 641.20 | 709.06 | 360.31 | 20 |
| 30 | 929.21 | 961.80 | 1063.59 | 540.46 | 30 |
| 40 | 1238.95 | 1282.40 | 1418.12 | 720.61 | 40 |
| 50 | 1548.69 | 1603.00 | 1772.65 | 900.76 | 50 |
| 100 | 3097.38 | 3206.00 | 3545.30 | 1801.53 | 100 |

# Index

# Index

# Index

# Index

# Index

# Index

# Index